Health Care Delivery and Clinical Science:

Concepts, Methodologies, Tools, and Applications

Information Resources Management Association
USA

Volume III

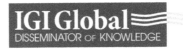

Published in the United States of America by
    IGI Global
    Medical Information Science Reference (an imprint of IGI Global)
    701 E. Chocolate Avenue
    Hershey PA, USA 17033
    Tel: 717-533-8845
    Fax: 717-533-8661
    E-mail: cust@igi-global.com
    Web site: http://www.igi-global.com

Library of Congress Cataloging-in-Publication Data

Names: Information Resources Management Association, editor.
Title: Health care delivery and clinical science : concepts, methodologies,
   tools, and applications / Information Resources Management Association,
   editor.
Description: Hershey PA : Medical Information Science Reference, [2018] |
   Includes bibliographical references.
Identifiers: LCCN 2017025957| ISBN 9781522539261 (hardcover) | ISBN
   9781522539278 (eISBN)
Subjects: | MESH: Medical Informatics | Education, Professional--methods |
   Health Literacy | Patient Participation | Patient-Centered Care
Classification: LCC R858.A2 | NLM W 26.5 | DDC 362.10285--dc23 LC record available at https://lccn.loc.
gov/2017025957

British Cataloguing in Publication Data
A Cataloguing in Publication record for this book is available from the British Library.

All work contributed to this book is new, previously-unpublished material. The views expressed in this book are those of the authors, but not necessarily of the publisher.

For electronic access to this publication, please contact: eresources@igi-global.com.

List of Contributors

Table of Contents

Section 2
Development and Design Methodologies

Section 3
Tools and Technologies

Volume II

Section 4
Utilization and Applications

Volume III

Section 5
Organizational and Social Implications

Section 6
Critical Issues and Challenges

Preface

The constantly changing landscape of Health Care Delivery and Clinical Science makes it challenging for experts and practitioners to stay informed of the field's most up-to-date research. That is why Medical Information Science Reference is pleased to offer this three-volume reference collection that will empower students, researchers, and academicians with a strong understanding of critical issues within Health Care Delivery and Clinical Science by providing both broad and detailed perspectives on cutting-edge theories and developments. This reference is designed to act as a single reference source on conceptual, methodological, technical, and managerial issues, as well as to provide insight into emerging trends and future opportunities within the discipline.

Health Care Delivery and Clinical Science: Concepts, Methodologies, Tools, and Applications is organized into six distinct sections that provide comprehensive coverage of important topics. The sections are:

1.   Fundamental Concepts and Theories;
2.   Development and Design Methodologies;
3.   Tools and Technologies;
4.   Utilization and Applications;
5.   Organizational and Social Implications; and,
6.   Critical Issues and Challenges.

The following paragraphs provide a summary of what to expect from this invaluable reference tool.

Section 1, "Fundamental Concepts and Theories," serves as a foundation for this extensive reference tool by addressing crucial theories essential to the understanding of Health Care Delivery and Clinical Science. Introducing the book is "A Relational Perspective on Patient Engagement: Suggestions From Couple-Based Research and Intervention" by Silvia Donato, a great foundation laying the groundwork for the basic concepts and theories that will be discussed throughout the rest of the book. Section 1 concludes and leads into the following portion of the book with a nice segue chapter, "Application of SMAC Technology" by Manu Venugopal.

Section 2, "Development and Design Methodologies," presents in-depth coverage of the conceptual design and architecture of Health Care Delivery and Clinical Science. Opening the section is "Managing Knowledge Towards Enabling Healthcare Service Delivery" by Tiko Iyamu and Sharol Sibongile Mkhomazi. Through case studies, this section lays excellent groundwork for later sections that will get into present and future applications for Health Care Delivery and Clinical Science. The section concludes with an excellent work by Ignace Djitog, Hamzat Olanrewaju Aliyu, and Mamadou Kaba Traoré, "Multi-Perspective Modeling of Healthcare Systems."

Section 3, "Tools and Technologies," presents extensive coverage of the various tools and technologies used in the implementation of Health Care Delivery and Clinical Science. The first chapter, "Hospital Social Media Strategies: Patient or Organization Centric?" by Fay Cobb Payton and Natasha Pinto, lays a framework for the types of works that can be found in this section. The section concludes with "RFID in Health Care: Building Smart Hospitals for Quality Healthcare" by Amir Manzoor. Where Section 3 described specific tools and technologies at the disposal of practitioners, Section 4 describes the use and applications of the tools and frameworks discussed in previous sections.

Section 4, "Utilization and Applications," describes how the broad range of Health Care Delivery and Clinical Science efforts has been utilized and offers insight on and important lessons for their applications and impact. The first chapter in the section is "Utilisation of Health Information Systems for Service Delivery in the Namibian Environment" written by Ronald Karon. This section includes the widest range of topics because it describes case studies, research, methodologies, frameworks, architectures, theory, analysis, and guides for implementation. The breadth of topics covered in the section is also reflected in the diversity of its authors, from countries all over the globe. The section concludes with "The Power of Words: Deliberation Dialogue as a Model to Favor Patient Engagement in Chronic Care" by Sarah Bigi and Giulia Lamiani, a great transition chapter into the next section.

Section 5, "Organizational and Social Implications," includes chapters discussing the organizational and social impact of Health Care Delivery and Clinical Science. The section opens with "Management of Tacit Knowledge and the Issue of Empowerment of Patients and Stakeholders in the Health Care Sector" by Marc Jacquinet, Henrique Curado, Ângela Lacerda Nobre, Maria José Sousa, Marco Arraya, Rui Pimenta, and António Eduardo Martins. This section focuses exclusively on how these technologies affect human lives, either through the way they interact with each other or through how they affect behavioral/workplace situations. The section concludes with "Patient Privacy and Security in E-Health" by Güney Gürsel.

Section 6, "Critical Issues and Challenges," presents coverage of academic and research perspectives on Health Care Delivery and Clinical Science tools and applications. The section begins with "The Administrative Policy Quandary in Canada's Health Service Organizations" by Grace I. Paterson, Jacqueline M. MacDonald, and Naomi Nonnekes Mensink. Chapters in this section will look into theoretical approaches and offer alternatives to crucial questions on the subject of Health Care Delivery and Clinical Science. The section concludes with "Smart Medication Management, Current Technologies, and Future Directions" by Seyed Ali Rokni, Hassan Ghasemzadeh, and Niloofar Hezarjaribi.

Although the primary organization of the contents in this multi-volume work is based on its six sections, offering a progression of coverage of the important concepts, methodologies, technologies, applications, social issues, and emerging trends, the reader can also identify specific contents by utilizing the extensive indexing system listed at the end of each volume. As a comprehensive collection of research on the latest findings related to using technology to providing various services, *Health Care Delivery and Clinical Science: Concepts, Methodologies, Tools, and Applications* provides researchers, administrators, and all audiences with a complete understanding of the development of applications and concepts in Health Care Delivery and Clinical Science. Given the vast number of issues concerning usage, failure, success, policies, strategies, and applications of Health Care Delivery and Clinical Science in countries around the world, *Health Care Delivery and Clinical Science: Concepts, Methodologies, Tools, and Applications* addresses the demand for a resource that encompasses the most pertinent research in technologies being employed to globally bolster the knowledge and applications of Health Care Delivery and Clinical Science.

Chapter 53
A Reconfigurable Supporting Connected Health Environment for People With Chronic Diseases

Abbes Amira
University of the West of Scotland, UK & Qatar University, Qatar

Naeem Ramzan
University of the West of Scotland, UK

Christos Grecos
University of the West of Scotland, UK

Qi Wang
University of the West of Scotland, UK

Pablo Casaseca-de-la-Higuera
University of the West of Scotland, UK

Zeeshan Pervez
University of the West of Scotland, UK

Xinheng Wang
University of the West of Scotland, UK

Chunbo Luo
University of the West of Scotland, UK

ABSTRACT

Digital healthcare is becoming increasingly important as the ageing population and the number of people diagnosed with chronic diseases is increasing. The face of healthcare delivery has changed radically and at its core is a digital and customer revolution. Connected health is the convergence of medical devices, security devices, and communication technologies. It enables patients to be monitored and treated re

DOI: 10.4018/978-1-5225-3926-1.ch053

motely from their home or primary care facility rather than attend outpatient clinics or be admitted to hospital. This chapter discusses the recent advances in connected health technologies and applications. The authors investigate a reconfigurable supporting connected health solution for people with chronic diseases using reconfigurable hardware and intelligent data interpretation and analysis. In addition, a thorough review of the existing information and communications technologies and challenges in the area of connected health including embedded medical devices, sensors, social networking, knowledge management, data fusion, and cloud computing is presented in this chapter. Finally, future directions and ongoing research in the area of connected health are presented.

INTRODUCTION

The number of elderly is increasing over the world. It is estimated that by the year 2020 the proportion of people aged 60 and over will be 25% worldwide. The ageing process in Europe is even at a higher level. By the year 2020, forecasts say that the percentage of people aged 60 and over will be about 50% in Europe (World, 2003), (UN, 2013).

The ageing of the society comes along with several specific problems. The increased frailty of the elderly, the increasing prevalence of diseases and the increasing resources used per patient have a major impact on the health systems. The ageing of the society comes along with several specific problems. The increased frailty of the elderly, the increasing prevalence of diseases and the increasing resources used per patient have a major impact on the healthcare systems. The awareness of the impact of the growing numbers of elderly has increased. The ageing society has been one of the key actions of the research programs worldwide and in Europe, UK in particular. Within those programs, much attention is paid to effective and efficient delivery of health and social care services to older people diagnosed with chronic diseases (CD) such as Dementia (incl. Alzheimer's disease) and Parkinson disease.

Monitoring different vital signs of patients with CD such as ECG (heart rate), SpO2, blood pressure for example – provides an important source of information to the doctor for defining treatment and planning and for the patients to manage their diseases. It is also an aid for prevention and early diagnosis. Recent advances in information technologies offer the possibility of a new generation of lightweight monitoring systems that a patient diagnosed with CD for example can wear while going about his/her daily business, or which can be carried around easily and used regularly. Such new systems and tools can now provide much more reliable data on multiple parameters, and transmit them to remote locations, so that medical professionals can make better decisions on treatment without having to meet the patients face-to-face. Visual information and remote monitoring of patient's behaviour can also be combined with different vital signs monitored using wireless medical devices for early diagnosis and thus limit the development of the symptoms of CD.

Furthermore, social networks have become a powerful tool for healthcare and helps patients to find remedies and seek advice from other patients with similar conditions or medical experts. For some individuals limited access to healthcare and information on the disease could lead to more severe consequences such as paralysis. Patients often look to the internet to find other people with similar illnesses to aid and advise them where their medical condition is concerned. Patients like these rely on online social media such as Facebook, Twitter, TuDiabetes and PatientsLikeMe Patientslikeme (2013) to find social support. The social networking sites are a powerful and cost effective communication tools.

In addition, modern ICT is increasingly used in healthcare aiming to improve and enhance medical services and reduce costs. In this context, cloud computing has become very appealing when managing the computation and storage resources. E-health clouds offer new possibilities, such as easy and ubiquitous access to medical data, and real-time transmission of heterogeneous data. However, they also bear new risks with respect to security and privacy aspects.

This book chapter discusses an integrated solution for reliable, secure and real-time e-health service delivery at homes and remote locations. It will cover state of the art technologies which can be deployed in a connected health environment such as embedded systems, social networking, data fusion and pattern recognition, cloud computing, security and knowledge management.

We aim to address the following issues required for the development of a complete connected healthcare system:

- Evaluate different embedded medical devices which can be used to acquire and process different vital signs such as ECG, temperature, blood pressure and acceleration signals;
- Analyse the extracted information from health social networking sites and its impact of CD management, treatment and prevention;
- Evaluate existing methods and present real-time solutions for remote heterogeneous data acquisition, fusion and processing and the deployment of secure cloud computing for big data processing, transmission and retrieval; and
- Evaluate knowledge management techniques used for intelligent data analysis and manipulation will be also addressed.

The authors present and discuss different software and hardware related issues to the design and implementation of a heterogeneous reconfigurable computing platform for connected health applications. The proposed solutions cover state of the art technologies which can be deployed in a connected health environment such as intelligent embedded systems, social networking and knowledge management, advanced signal, image and video processing, data fusion and pattern recognition, cloud computing, data security and privacy.

The structure of the remaining of this book chapter is as follows. Next section will present different challenges and an overview about the existing connected healthcare solutions in place. In the future research directions, we will highlight the main features of our proposed solutions. Finally concluding remarks will be included at the end of this chapter.

STATE OF THE ART

In this section, a thorough and comprehensive review will be carried out on the following main pillars in the context of connected health environments:

- Embedded computing systems;
- Social networking and knowledge management;
- Data fusion and pattern recognition; and
- Cloud computing and security

Embedded Computing Systems

The impact of world population ageing in healthcare costs has motivated an increasing effort in the development of Wearable Health-Monitoring Systems (WHMS) by both the research community and industry. Real-time monitoring of patient's health condition can significantly decrease these costs by providing feedback information to either physicians or users so that alerting events and alarms can be triggered for health threatening awareness.

WHMS usually consist of a number of sensors able to measure significant physiological parameters and signals such as blood pressure (BP), oxygen saturation (SaO$_2$), respiration, photoplethysmography (PPG) or electrocardiogram (ECG). Activity patterns obtained from 2D/3D accelerometers and other parameters conveying information on the patient's way of life can also be incorporated to provide context-based information. A central node is linked to these sensors providing connectivity to visualisation displays or transmission nodes for management at point-of-care. This latter connectivity shall be wirelessly provided [different alternatives do exist: Zigbee, bluetooth, 802.11g, etc., Pantelopoulos and Bourbakis (2010)] so that the user's daily activity is not interfered. On the other hand, links between sensors and the main node links can be wired depending on the specific application.

Pantelopoulos and Bourbakis (2010) presented a comprehensive survey on WHMS ranging from research prototypes to commercially available systems. An evaluation of the maturity state of the most relevant systems was also provided. It merely consists of an aggregate scoring of the different system capabilities such as wearability, real applicability, real-time properties, scalability or presence of decision support mechanisms. Each capability was weighted by a pooled "importance" coefficient obtained from different perspectives, namely, patient's, physician's and manufacturer's. The final maturity index consisted on 5 different levels (1=low, 2=medium-low, 3=medium, 4=high, 5=maximum). All the evaluated systems ranged in the 2-4 interval.

Considering research prototypes, those based on microcontroller boards or custom based platforms were evaluated in (Pantelopoulos and Bourbakis, 2010) as being in a medium-low stage of maturity. An example is the AMON (Advanced care and alert portable telemedical monitoring, Hao and Foster, 2008), developed within an EU IST FP5 funded project. The final prototype consists of a wrist-worn device which measures BP, Temperature, SaO$_2$, one-lead ECG and 2D acceleration and provides a GSM link to the telemedicine centre for signal analysis. This allowed the identification of health risk levels according to the world health organization thresholds (WHO). The LiveNet (Sung et al., 2005) mobile platform for long-term health monitoring provides real-time signal processing features and context classification from ECG, Electromyogram (EMG), 3D accelerations, and galvanic skin conductance (GSC). The foreseen applications included Parkinson long-term behavioural modelling, and epilepsy seizure detection.

The effort devoted to the development of smart textiles has leaded to final prototypes whose maturity level according to (Pantelopoulos and Bourbakis, 2010) ranges between medium (3) (Paradiso et al., 2005, Scilingo et al., 2005) and high (4) (Luprano et al., 2006, Di Rienzo et al., 2005, Pandian et al., 2008). Among them, different applications are targeted, from health monitoring in general (Pandian et al., 2008) and specific cases (elderly, chronic diseases) (Paradiso et al., 2005, Scilingo et al., 2005), to more ambitious applications such as prevention and early diagnosis of cardiovascular diseases (Luprano et al., 2006, Di Rienzo et al., 2005). Different signals are measured depending on the application (ECG, respiratory signal, BP, PPG, etc.). Moreover, signal processing and pattern recognition for feature extraction is also performed at different levels in some projects: The MyHeart project (Luprano et al., 2006) incorporated on-body signal processing algorithms to classify activity patterns into resting, walking, running, and going up/downstairs. ECG enhancement techniques were also implemented at body level. The WEALTHY project (Scilingo et al., 2005) and Smart Vest (Pandian et al., 2008) incorporated hardware removal of baseline noise and motion artifacts in the acquired signals.

In order to achieve multi-purpose reconfigurable WHMS, mote-based Body Area Networks (BAN) (Hao and Foster, 2008) are probably the best option. These so-called motes are wireless nodes responsible of collecting one or more types of physiological data and transmitting them to a central node. The wearable wireless BAN prototype described by Milenković et al. (2006) incorporates custom sensor platforms allowing measuring and preprocessing of different signals such as ECG, EMG, and acceleration. These sensors are further integrated on a commercially available platform. The system presented by Chung et al. (2008) integrated ECG and BP measurements with basic signal processing (simple feature extraction and if-then-rules) to extract suspicious patterns for diagnosis support. In they work, Milenković et al. (2006), discuss the lack of standardization in terms of platforms, transmission and wireless communications. Additionally, the authors propose to perform on-board signal processing to reduce the wireless transmission duty cycle and the power consumption. However, dealing with limited computing resources, real-time requirements, and memory space constitutes a challenging task (Pantelopoulos and Bourbakis, 2010).

Mote-based BANs such as (Shimmer, 2013) have attracted the research community interest in the recent years for the development of prototypes. These platforms can be configured to measure different signals and parameters such as 4-lead ECG, EMG, 3D acceleration, and angular velocity in multiple setups. They also provide different drivers and interfaces to signal processing platforms (Labview, Matlab) and smart mobile devices. Actually, incorporating daily-use devices to WHMS will decrease the final cost of the systems and increase their usability. Some specific platforms have also been developed. Microsoft HealthGear (Oliver and Flores-Mangas, 2006), provides SaO_2 and heart rate (HR) measurements and sends them to a cell phone to perform detection of sleep apnea episodes in both time and frequency domain. HealthToGo (Jin et al., 2009) is a cell-phone based platform that performs real-time analysis of the ECG waveform in order to identify abnormal patterns. (Fensli et al, 2005) presented a proposal aimed at the detection of arrhythmias in a similar way. All of these prototypes use mobile devices to perform the signal processing tasks for feature extraction. The recent advances in smart phones and watches technology would additionally allow employing the embedded sensors for signal acquisition.

A final group of devices that is worth mentioning is composed of those which are commercially available for monitoring purposes. Specific health monitoring systems such as Lifeshirt® by Vivometrics (Heilman and Forges, 2007) and Bioharness™ (Zephyr Inc., 2013) provide remote access to ECG, respiration and activity data. These systems do not incorporate sophisticated feature extraction or decision support as is expected from the existing gap between commercially established products and research prototypes. Heart rate chest-belt sensors and wrist displays such as those from Polar (2013) have succeeded in sports applications with proprietary connectivity to fitness equipment (treadmills, bicycles, etc.). Latest releases provide connectivity with mobile devices so that the acquired data can be monitored and processed using Android or iOS applications. Activity monitors such as (Actigraph, 2013) have extensively been used for research purposes. First releases included wired raw data access for prospective analysis and specific software providing sleep reports. Latest ones do also incorporate wireless Bluetooth connectivity.

The preceding paragraphs provide a brief insight into some relevant so far proposed WHMS. The specificity of the customized design approaches can explain the lack of maturity (according to the evaluation by (Pantelopoulos and Bourbakis, 2010)) of these developments. Systems based on smart textiles present desirable wearability properties but are more limited in terms of flexibility and scalability. Mote-based BANs do overcome these problems, providing higher processing capability at the same time. If some of the measurement tasks were performed using smart phone or watch built-in sensors, BAN limited resources would be significantly released. Additionally, adopting daily use devices for health condition monitoring would pave the way for a higher impact of these systems. Nonetheless, the current research challenges in ubiquitous personalized healthcare demand context information to be included in complex signal models to derive physiological parameters of interest (Viswanathan et al., 2012). To this end, computing and storage capabilities beyond those of sensor motes and mobile devices are required. In this context, cloud computing systems and dynamic resource management will play an important role.

SOCIAL NETWORKING

Social networking sites have become very prevalent over the past decade and have stretched at a rapid percentage on the internet. More than one billion active users are using only Facebook. It entices consideration through the competence of the user to create their own personalized profiles, to search long lost friends, to join special interest groups and also to converse with peers all over the world. Most of such types of social networking websites have become an efficient tool that fetches people with similar interests together to interact and discuss the same problems, feelings, thoughts and in some cases seek medical advice from one another (Sheth, 2010). Websites like Facebook, Twitter and Wikipedia can be used in a more health-specific manner to target health professionals and the public, is creating new, cost effective ways to embed a powerful tool into a healthcare system (Khorakhu et al. 2013). In addition, it is very useful tool for healthcare and helps patients to find remedies and seek advice from other patients with similar conditions or medical experts. The research conducted by (Scanfeld, 2010) exhibited that people start to share their health-related information or problems online. This result in a growing number of social networking sites directed towards health and well-being. Recently a number of social applications allowing users to update their health status and health goals via online support groups have been proposed.

Personal devices such as laptops, smartphones and iPads can be used by people to monitor their own health-related behaviour wirelessly (Silva et al. 2011). The work by Afzal et al. (2012) integrated different social media websites such as Facebook, Youtube, Twitter as an input for decision support in healthcare information systems. Furthermore, the investigation in (Norval et al.,2011) proposed the use of social network like Facebook as a framework for telecare. (Griffin et al. 2009) presented the integration of paradigms in social networks into healthcare, i.e. information sharing, monitoring and message alerts. However, only the espousal of the architecture adapted with social networking technologies was proposed, rather than a social media platform. (Detmar et al. 2000) proposed a social network model for health monitoring. Compared to other work, the process has less automation, and did not exploit mobile devices, but did allow patients to control the access to their data. Based on a similar concept, (Ding et al 2012) and (Ayubi et al 2012) employed a monitoring unit, a smartphone and the Facebook platform for monitoring of physical activities. Based on the recent advances in technologies ranging from affordable smart devices to the accessibility of the Internet, along with the popularity of existing social networks, the usage of social media as an input to healthcare platform is already in progress.

Figure 1. Triple synergy of physical, cyber and social paradigm in eHealth framework

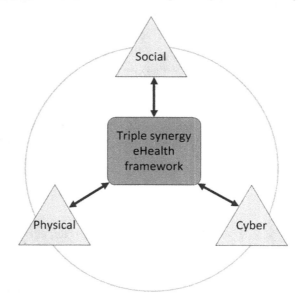

Triple Synergy of eHealth Framework

Triple synergy of physical, cyber and social media is the new and innovative concept to increase the reliability and robustness of the eHealth framework. The cyber-physical system constitutes on the computational and communication components closely interact with physical components. It enables better cyber-mediated observation and interaction with physical components.

Physical-Cyber Platform

We've witnessed significant progress in technology that enhances human-computer interactions. Now we're experiencing increasingly intelligent interfaces which have demonstrated contextual use of knowledge to develop intelligent human–mobile-device interfaces (Sheth et al., 2013). We're also observing progress in how machines especially sensors and device, surroundings, and humans interact, enabled by advances in sensing the body, the mind, and place. Such recent research supports the ability to comprehend human actions, including human gestures and languages in increasingly diverse forms. The extending ability to provide any physical object an identity in the cyber world, will let machines leverage extensive knowledge about the object to complement what humans process. Some of the examples where health applications and tools that monitor a person physically and connect them to care provider is given below.

MedApps

MedApps (MedApps 2013) provides a health information management platform that effectively connects patients to their healthcare providers and electronics medical records to enhance patient cars and drive down the related cost. The example of MedApps system is shown in Figure 2, where the patient

Figure 2. MedApps health monitoring framework (MedApps 2013)

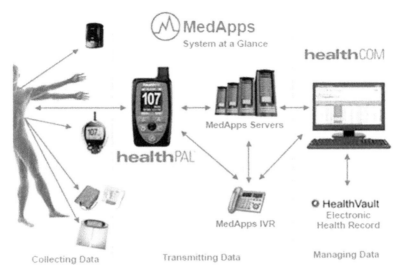

data is collected by remote portable devices and sends it to MedApps server and compare with existing electronic medical record and generate alerts through emails or phone calls if needed.

Cardionet

CardioNet (CardioNet, 2013) provides the next-generation ambulatory cardiac monitoring service with beat-to-beat, real time analysis, automatic arrhythmia detection and wireless ECG transmission. CardioNet prides a comprehensive suite of post-symptom, looping, auto-trigger event monitors as part of its turn-key cardiac event monitoring services.

LifeWatch

LifeWatch, (2013) provides ACT (Ambulatory Cardiac Telemetry), an automatically activated system that requires no patient intervention to either capture or transmit an arrhythmia when it occurs. Upon arrhythmia detection, the system automatically utilizes the integrated cellular phone to transmit the ECG waveform to LifeWatch monitoring sytem, where the ECG is analyzed. The patient's physician is notified of the arrhythmia based on pre-determined notification criteria prescribed by the patient's physician. Patients can be monitored for up to 30 days and all the data is available at the request of the physician during the service period and for 7 days following the end of service.

Intelsense

Intelesens, (2013) offers a flexible Wireless Vital Signs Platform that can be customised to provide a range of monitoring products for in-hospital use and deployment at-home or on-the-move. It can be used as a short range or long range (cellular phone) monitor and specified with a variety of vital sign inputs and wireless systems. Highly miniaturized, light weight and with an extremely long battery life, the monitoring devices are small, unobtrusive and easily worn under clothes allowing patients freedom during monitoring.

Cyber-Social Platform

In cyber-social world, people share their activities, knowledge, experience, opinions, and perceptions. The well-known social websites such as YouTube, Flickr, and Facebook. In such environments, the audio-video content is usually accompanied with metadata, tags, ratings, comments, information about the uploader and their social networks. Analysis of these "social media" shows a great potential in improving the performance of traditional multimedia information analysis/retrieval approaches by bridging the semantic gap between the "objective" multimedia content analysis and "subjective" users' needs and impressions. The integration of these aspects, however, is non-trivial and has created a vibrant, interdisciplinary field of research. There are only few social networks relating to health monitoring like:

Patientslikeme

It is a free patient network where people can connect with others who have the same disease or condition and track and share their own experiences. When people share information on Patientslikeme, (2013), they generate data about the real-world nature of disease that helps researchers, pharmaceutical companies, regulators, providers and non-profits to develop more effective products, services and care.

23andMe

This social networking platform manages risk assessment and provides informed decisions based on gene sequencing (23andMe, 2013). It enables therapeutic developers to evaluate individualized responses to treatment at large scale, while providing research participants with a truly patient-centric study experience.

MedHelp

It is one of the largest online health communities. It provides support for more than 300 different conditions, forums that connect consumers to doctors. (MedHelp, 2013) delivers unparalleled access to trusted information and advice tailored to consumers' personal health needs.

Physical-Cyber-Social Platform

It is an emerging paradigm where physical, cyber, and social information interact with each other as shown in Figure 1. The remote sensors collect observation from the physical world. Data collected from physiological sensors analysed in the social context of similar people (Sheth 2013). The integration and interactions between physical, cyber, and social components need significant human involvement in the interpretation of physiological observations using their knowledge domain and social experiences.

Huge amount of information can be extracted from the social networks and medical sensors; hence there is a real need for knowledge management (KM) techniques which can improve the delivery of healthcare services (Nilakanta et al., 2009). A review on knowledge management in the healthcare industry was presented in (Nicolini et al., 2008, Sheffield, 2008) and has shown different challenges and techniques in this field. (Sheffield, 2008) states that KM is systemically more complex in healthcare because the three domain of knowledge creation, knowledge normalization and knowledge application. (Nicolini et al., 2008) has noted that KM research in healthcare over the years has focused on three overarching themes: "the nature of knowledge in the healthcare sector, the type of KM tools and initiatives that are suitable for the healthcare sector, and the barriers and enablers to adoption of KM practices". Classification and annotation techniques can be also used in KM based healthcare systems for automatic medical data classification and annotation which can help for treatment, diagnosis and disease management.

Data Fusion and Pattern Recognition

With the advancement in ICT and circuit fabrication technologies sensory devices are becoming ubiquitous and smaller in size. ICT technologies have leverages these devices to transmit data over long distances and persist them for offline processing at the point of care. Fabrication technologies have significantly reduced their size and enabled them to add multiple sensors in a single device – today smartphones are equipped with accelerometer, gyroscope, proximity sensor (Scully et al, 2012), and further more sensors (*heart rate sensor, ECG sensors, and glucometer etc.*) can be connected through the Bluetooth protocol. Miniaturization of sensory devices has profound effect on healthcare industry, as it is becoming convenient for patient to use them without any hassle, most importantly a single device equipped with multiple sensors can be used for data acquisition considering multiple physiological and contextual parameters.

Fusing data from diverse sources (*clinical repositories, sensory devices*) is very important both for the patients and healthcare service providers. It can provide an insight view of patient's medical condition and can significantly elevate the efficacy of healthcare services (Craig et al., 2005). Clinical data accumulated at independent healthcare service providers can be fused for advance statistical analysis to develop a deeper clinical understanding of a particular disease. Medical data fusion for telemedicine is a distributed framework for processing clinical images and to facilitate knowledge sharing among physicians and researchers (Megalooikonomou et al., 2007). The proposed framework processes multiple clinical image repositories independently; whereas, distributed processing components synchronize their intermediate results. By utilizing dynamic recursive partitioning (DRP) the framework is able to identify region of interest in medical images (*tumor, lesions etc.*) that are discriminative among groups of subjects. The application of the proposed framework included identifying discriminative brain activation patterns in Alzheimer patients, and studying sexual morphological differentiation of the brain corpus callosum.

Clinical data analysis along with daily clinical observations can be used for medical risk analysis. Kyriacou et al. proposed an integrated system for assessing stroke risk (Kyriacou et al., 2007). The authors collected data from stroke patients by using non-invasive techniques. The collected data is then processed by using automated data analysis techniques and information rich features are extracted. Equipped with extracted information, patients are monitored for a period of 6 to 84 weeks. Statistical correlation techniques are applied to identify patients belonging to a high-risk category. Augmentation of clinical observations with processed clinical data assisted in early identification of critical parameters, thus assisting healthcare service provider to customize clinical services accordingly.

(Brzostowski et al., 2013) demonstrated the practicality of data driver models for e-Health applications. In their proposed model they utilized signals for heart rate, running speed and fatigue; combining expert knowledge with the sensory data – whereas conventional approaches of statistical analysis made use of data only. The authors propose a three tier application model. First tier transmits the data collected by wearable sensory devices, through body area network. Second tier is responsible for modelling and collective processing of transmitted data from all the sensory devices. The third tier works as a presentation layer for results, charts, and reports. The authors demonstrate the efficacy of their data driver model through endurance training for a runner. They utilise a mathematical model of cardiovascular system and fatigue during exercise, in order to evaluate optimized speed of a runner to achieve a particular goal, considering heart rate and level of fatigue.

Yan et al. propose a wireless sensor network based e-Health system to track elderly patients in smart-home environment (Yan et al., 2010). The proposed system integrates information from multiple sensory devices to find location of an elderly along with other contextual information gathered from pressure, fire and pulse sensor node to generate necessary alarm in case of an emergency. Moulton et al. highlight an important issue of data reliability in sensory data fusion for Personal Electronic Health Records (Bruce et al, 2009). They develop a prototype system to understand how the type, quality, installation, maintenance and calibration of the sensors can affect level of confidence practitioners have over the sensory data. Data from sensory devices having level of confidence is fused to make clinical decision. In sensory data processing for clinical purposes considering aforementioned parameters is very important. This is because usually not much consideration is given to these parameters in-home or ambulatory monitoring systems.

In the context of e-Health application situational aware plays an important role in making accurate recommendation and clinical decision. Advancements in sensing technology lead to context-aware devices (Buchmayr et al., 2011), which can assist in realization of effectual e-Health services and applications. (Wolf et al.,2008) proposed SOPRANO, an ambient assistive living platform, which utilizes environmental sensory data obtained from multiple sensors to process the contextual information and generate suitable recommendations / warnings. (Skubic et al., 2009) propose TigerPlace, an active retirement community project, designed specifically for smart-homes equipped with multiple sensory devices i.e., utilizes passive physiological sensor (*motion and bed sensors*) and event-driven video-sensor network. It fuses the output of sensory devices for behavioural activity analysis and to generate appropriate alerts and recommendations. Alarm Net (Wood et al. 2008) is an assistive living and residential monitoring environment for patients with diverse needs. It utilizes Body Area Network to record vital signs and activity information, and emplaced sensors to enable location tracking. Its back-end component provides analysis of the sensed data, whereas user-interface component is utilized by doctors, nurses and residents to query information.

The entire purpose of data fusion is to process data within the correct context e.g., activity information of a patient can be used to decide whether data from blood pressure sensor should be considered or not etc. Another important source of contextual information is social network. Social network analysis can play an important role in learning sentiments of a patient combined with daily routine to make correct and timely clinical recommendations. Fatima et al. proposed SmartCDSS: an integration of Social Media and Interaction Engine (SMIE) in healthcare for chronic disease patients (Fatima et al., 2013). In their proposed system the authors combined tweets, trajectory and email interaction analysis into vMR (*virtual medical record*). Augmented with ontological information (SNOMED CT), vMR assist health practitioners to understand the behaviour and lifestyle of patients for better decision making about their personalized treatment and clinical recommendation.

We are living through a transition phase of healthcare industry, where clinical services are being transformed into wellness services. The proliferation of Smartphone and wearable sensory devices are evidence to this transition phase. However, with the increasing number of sensory devices a normal person or patient can carry, the complexity of data fusion is also increasing. Data fusion methodologies must also take into account any contradiction which may arise among certain sub-group of sensory devices e.g., sensory devices dedicated to activity recognition may state that patient is doing exercise, on the contrary heart rate sensor shows normal heart rate activity. Another important challenge which is faced by data fusion methodologies is that sensory devices transmit data at different rate. For making clinical recommendation or decision it is very crucial that healthcare service provider has a synchronized and accurately correlated data from sensory devices. Even with these open challenges, sensory data fusion will continue to provide a single view of patient's medical condition assisting healthcare service provider to increase efficacy of treatment.

Cloud Computing and Security

Modern ICT is increasingly utilised in healthcare aiming to improve and enhance medical services whilst reducing costs. In this context, cloud computing has become increasingly appealing in light of the vast and cost-effective computation and storage resources available in the cloud. E-health clouds offer new possibilities, such as ubiquitous access to medical data, and real-time transmission of multimedia data. However, they also bear new risks with respect to security and privacy aspects, which must be addressed for wide adoption of cloud-assisted/based e-health services.

Ubiquitous Cloud Healthcare Services

Cloud-based ubiquitous healthcare services exploit the on-demand, location-independent and inexpensive computing and storage resources made available by the widely available Internet clouds. In such systems, the cloud platform is utilised to store the huge volume of data including user information, physiological data, Personal Health Records (PHRs), graphic data to processing and so on, in various databases such as those based on NoSQL (Sakr et al. 2011). The physiological data especially vital signs are collected in real time from the patents' body area networks via wireless biosensors (Benharref 2013) and other monitoring equipment, which can be implantable, wearable, or not (Yang et al. 2012). Computation-intensive tasks such as the visualisation of the monitoring results and massive multimedia data processing are offloaded to the cloud as well. Moreover, the service-oriented nature of clouds well suits the e-health services, which typically require high scalability and flexibility. To facilitate pervasive access to the services, mobile communication technologies including diverse wireless networks (3G/4G, WiFi, Bluetooth, ZigBee etc.) and user devices (smartphones, tablets etc.) are usually utilised. It is essential that all the involved subsystems are integrated carefully to provide a smooth, timely and pervasive service to the users, as shown in Figure 3.

For instance, (He, Fan & Li, 2013) described a city-wide health-monitoring system based on a private cloud platform. A six-layer deployment architecture was proposed, including Service interaction to provide a user interface, Service presentation for high concurrency capability and service interface, Session cache to store/cache user sessions, Cloud engine to coordinate the cloud components based on a message queue method, Medical data mining, and Cloud storage. In this system, users can view the graphical results via TVs as well as web browsers. Pilot testing results demonstrated that the proposed document-oriented system was advantageous compared with non-document-oriented alternative systems such as Amazon's Simple Storage Service or S3 (Amazon, 2013).

Figure 3. Ubiquitous Cloud healthcare services

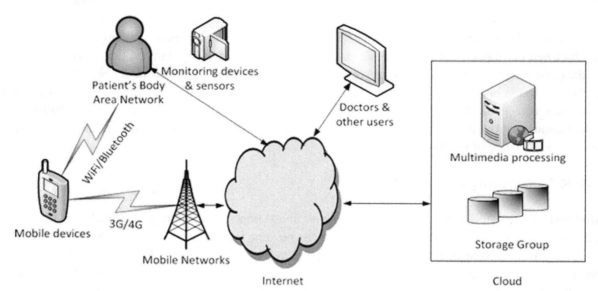

Multimedia Cloud Healthcare Services

Gaining increasing popularity, cloud-based multimedia e-health applications exploit the computation and storage capabilities in clouds whilst benefiting from the advances in multimedia processing technologies. In particular, medical video transmission has been boosted by recent video compression standards such as H.264 Advanced Video Coding (AVC) (ITU-T & ISO/IEC 2010) and H.265 High Efficiency Video Coding (HEVC) (ITU 2013). Reference software implementations of both AVC and HEVC standards are freely available and are widely used in the research community. Currently, H.264/AVC is the predominant video compression standard, and a number of implementations are existing. For instance, real-time, cross-platform AVC video streaming can be realised through VideoLAN's VLC player (VideoLAN, 2013). AVC is also employed by popular cloud-based streaming platforms such as Adobe Media Server (AMS) (Adobe, 2013) and Wowza (Wowza, 2013). For the future, it is expected that the H.265/HEVC standard will replace H.264 as the next-generation video coding standard, providing doubled compression efficiency for the same visual quality. However, real-time HEVC encoding is very challenging owning to the significantly increase computational complexity compared with H.264. Cloud-assisted HEVC processing is therefore a promising approach that should be explored. It is noted that HEVC is featured with built-in parallelisation facilities including the Tiles (rectangular regions of a picture), Wavefront Parallel Processing (WPP) and Dependent Slice Segments tools (Sullivan et al., 2012). These new facilities, in contrast to H.264, allow a more efficient integration of HEVC and clouds, with the latter support parallelisation inherently.

The advantages of HEVC over AVC for developing wireless ultrasound video telemedicine systems were investigated by (Panayides et al., 2012). The authors compared the compression efficiency of AVC and HEVC, and demonstrated the superiority of HEVC in terms of 37% reduction in bitrate requirement for equivalent clinical quality. The wireless transmission of AVC-encoded ultrasound video over a WiMAX network was also evaluated, and simulation results confirmed the feasibility of such a deployment. Due to the clinical nature of medical data, error resilience is essential in medical multimedia delivery, especially when wireless networks are involved (Panayides et al., 2011). The video streaming of HEVC content over loss-prone IP networks was reported in (James et al., 2012), and the system was empirically evaluated on a testbed.

Furthermore, (Wang et al., in press) discuss various mobile video cloud networks that can be further explored by cloud-assisted e-health video services over mobile networks. Moreover, SparkMed (Constantinescu, Kim & Feng, 2012) is a data integration framework that can dynamically integrate various e-health software and databases into a cloud-like peer-to-peer multimedia data store. A web-based transcoding facility was introduced to allow a seamless operation of hospital imaging software at any Internet-enabled devices such as smartphones. Image data are transcoded to lossless JPEG format with metadata provided in XML. For smooth navigation in the web browser-based display environment, SparkMed implemented local preliminary image processing at the end user's devices, and lossy FLV-based streaming of entire image stacks if required. For acceptably interactive performance, the system demands a "near-real-time" updating of the end user's device's data and visualisation content as it was manipulated at the cloud. Through empirical testing, it was found that users considered the system to be responsive when at least 5 frames/s frame rate was achieved for image streaming with a propagation time under 0.5 s.

Security and Privacy in Cloud Healthcare Services

It is imperative that the shift of computational complexity (and potentially operation costs) in an e-health system to the cloud does not compromise the security of the system and the privacy of the clients. Security and privacy protection in cloud-based health systems is inherently tricky due to the combination of the semi-trusted cloud environment and the ever-existing malicious attacks to illegally acquire confidential medical and personal records. Highlighted here are a couple of top concerns including handling a range of potential attacks and risks originated from both outsiders and insiders, and allowing secure yet efficient access to the health data stored in the cloud at the same time.

The insider attacks are typically considered more difficult to be tackled and it was reported that insider attacks had cost the victimised institutions much more than what outsider counterparts had cost (Shaw, Ruby & Post 1998). Whilst outsider attacks could be handled in a rather trivial way such as through cryptographic mechanisms, insider attacks are typically significantly more difficult to deal with. To address insider attacks, a cloud-assisted mobile-Health monitoring system (CAM) was designed by Lin et al. (2013). CAM attempted to achieve a trade-off between privacy constrains and the operability of the system. The added difficulty of cloud environment for both data input and output was taken into account. An identity-based encryption scheme was designed in medical diagnostic branching programs to protect clients' privacy, and the decryption complexity was offloaded to the cloud. In addition, by applying a key private proxy re-encryption mechanism, computational load was shifted to the cloud from resource-constrained small companies for them to enter this market.

PHRs should be stored securely yet be accessed conveniently by the patients and authorised parties. MyPHRMachines (Van Gorp & Comuzzi 2012) is a cloud-based lifelong PHR system that aimed to achieve security and portability of health records. In this system, patients can upload their PHRs, remotely access their records via virtual machines (VMs), and share their remote VM sessions with selected trusted stakeholders, all in a secure manner as the design goals with various security techniques being investigated for different levels in the system. Two case uses including radiology image and sharing and personalised medicine were studied in a prototype. Furthermore, for fine-grained and scalable data access control to PHRs resident in a cloud, (Li et al., 2013) proposed a patient-centric framework and a set of mechanisms. Attribute-based encryption techniques were employed to encrypt the patients PHRs for secure sharing and to handle efficient and on-demand user revocation, and multiple security domains were introduced to reduce security key management complexity, among other considerations. The system's security, scalability, and efficiency were evaluated through analytical and experimental results.

Moreover, in practice, cloud-assisted e-Health systems also need to be compliant with relevant standards, regulations and laws in healthcare. For example, the USA Health Insurance Portability and Accountability Act (HIPAA) should apply to US e-healthcare providers who employ cloud computing technologies. It is reported that Amazon Web Services (AWS), ClearData Networks and other cloud e-health providers have developed HIPAA-compliant services. In addition, to facilitate secure interoperation of different, often heterogeneous cloud-based e-health systems, standardisation work should be intensified. It is expected that more cloud healthcare specific standards, together with national and international regulations and recommendations, will emerge in the near future.

FUTURE RESEARCH DIRECTIONS

The review of existing technologies and systems in connected health applications reveals that most of the approaches can be further improved by looking at new intelligent embedded devices which can handle and interpret the huge amount of medical data coming from different medical sensors and other sources. Our future research directions, which are also aligned with the current trends and research challenges in the area, focus on the development and implementation of a reconfigurable supporting connected health environment for people with CD using reconfigurable hardware in the form of field programmable gate arrays (FPGAs). The research aims at developing a real-time embedded healthcare system for remote management and treatment of people with CD. The proposed environment is innovative and consists of new advanced technologies at both the system and component levels. Appropriate embedded processing platforms and interactive- internet services will be developed where robust intelligent data fusion algorithms can be deployed for data analysis. The main component of the system is an auto-adaptive self-calibrating platform deployed for remote heterogeneous data acquisition and processing. It is a reconfigurable platform which adapts itself depending on the environment changes and parameters. It has advanced on-board processing and communication capabilities which facilitate the wireless communication with different sensors.

Accurate measurement will be carried out at both the sensor and embedded monitoring platform. Advanced filtering, visualisation, processing and analysis techniques and algorithms will be prototyped and embedded in the wireless medical biosensors and the real-time monitoring platform. The system will process heterogeneous data acquired from different medical biosensors, ambient and vision sensors. The system will be used for real-time multi-parametric monitoring of people with CD and will deploy cloud computing for secure data transmission and retrieval. We aim to build wireless medical devices where clinical knowledge can be combined with intelligent algorithms used for data analysis which will provide more accurate decisions that help for early detection and prevention.

Our solution can focuses on remote management and treatment of patients at home but can be also deployed in mobile environments such mobile hospitals and ambulances. The current and future status of the patient will be assessed based on the acquisition of heterogeneous data, videos for behavioural analysis, and robust accurate methods for modelling and prediction.

We will also look at the power of consumption of the devices used and we aim to use advanced low power wearable medical devices for the acquisition of different vital signs. Human-computer interfaces, interactive web and internet services including social networks will be deployed in the system to visualise and analysis heterogeneous data. Intelligent systems, knowledge management techniques and advanced data mining techniques will be investigated for efficient storage of data, modelling and prediction of the current and future patient' status. The system will process and interpret different vital signs for accurate alerting and signalling of risks and for supporting healthcare professionals in their decision making. Novel and robust pattern recognition algorithms to analyse the correlation between the multi-parametric data will be investigated. New modelling and prediction algorithms will be deployed for diagnosing worsening of conditions and prompting early intervention. New advanced encryption and security algorithms and architectures will be developed and implemented for clinical data and other patient's related data transmission and storage in a cloud environment.

CONCLUSION

The number of elderly and people diagnosed specifically with chronic diseases is increasing dramatically in all regions in the world. This has a huge impact on the cost, quality and delivery of healthcare services which are changing from the traditional approach to the connected model. We have discussed in this chapter the recent advances in connected health technologies and applications. We have proposed a reconfigurable supporting connected health framework for people diagnosed with chronic diseases using a reconfigurable hardware and intelligent data interpretation and analysis. In addition, a thorough review on the existing information and communications technologies and challenges in the area of connected health including embedded medical devices, sensors, social networking, knowledge management, data fusion and cloud computing is presented in this book chapter. Finally, future directions and ongoing research in the area of connected health are presented. Our current and future research priorities and problem were discussed and an integrated complete solution which deploys embedded intelligent computing, data fusion, knowledge management, social networking and cloud computing is presented. We anticipate that the proposed solution would have an impact on the medical and scientific communities as it would provide automatically and in real-time a full objective assessment on the current and future status of the patient, something that is difficult to achieve.

ACKNOWLEDGMENT

The authors would like to thank the anonymous reviewers and the editor for their insightful comments and suggestions.

REFERENCES

23andMe. (2013). Retrieved from https://www.23andme.com/

Actigraph. (2013). Available from http://www.actigraphcorp.com

Adobe. (2013). *Adobe media server family.* Available at http://www.adobe.com/uk/products/adobe-media-server-family.html

Afzal, M. Hussain M. Khan W. Lee S. and Ahmad H. (2012). Social media canonicalization in healthcare: Smart cdss as an exemplary application. *IEEE 14th Intl. Conf. on e-Health Networking, Applications and Services (HealthCom),* Oct 2012, pp. 419–422.

Amazon Simple Storage Service (S3) Documentation. (2013). Available at http://aws.amazon.com/documentation/s3/

Ayubi, S., & Parmanto, B., & Person, A. (2012). Persuasive social network for physical Activity. In *Proceedings of IEEE Int. Conf. on Engineering in Medicine and Biology Society (EMBC)* (pp. 2153–2157). IEEE.

Benharref, A. (2013). *Novel Cloud and SOA Based Framework for E-health Monitoring Using Wireless Biosensors. IEEE Journal of Biomedical and Health Informatics.*

Bruce, M., Chaczko, Z., & Karatovic, M. (2009). Data Fusion and Aggregation Methods for Pre-Processing Ambulatory Monitoring and Remote Sensor Data for Upload to Personal Electronic Health Records. *International Journal of Digital Content Technology and its Applications, 3*(4), 120-127.

Brzostowski, K., Drapala, J., & Swiatek, J. (2013). Data-Driven Models for eHealth Applications. *International Journal of Computer Science and Artificial Intelligence, 3*(1), 1–9. doi:10.5963/IJCSAI0301001

Buchmayr, M., & Kurschl, W. (2011). A survey on situation-aware ambient intelligence systems. *Journal of Ambient Intelligence and Humanized Computing, 2*(3), 175–183. doi:10.1007/s12652-011-0055-1

CardioNet. (2013). Retrieved from https://www.cardionet.com/

Chung, W.-Y., Lee, S.-C., & Toh, S.-H. (2008). WSN based mobile u-healthcare system with ecg, blood pressure measurement function. In *Proceedings of IEEE-EMBS 2008. 30th Annual International Conference of the Engineering in Medicine and Biology Society,* (pp. 1533–1536). IEEE.

Constantinescu, L., Kim, J., & Feng, D. D. (2012). SparkMed: A framework for dynamic integration of multimedia medical data into distributed m-Health systems. *IEEE Transactions on Information Technology in Biomedicine, 16*(1), 40–52. doi:10.1109/TITB.2011.2174064 PMID:22049371

Craig, J., & Patterson, V. (2005). Introduction to the practice of telemedicine. *Journal of Telemedicine and Telecare, 11*(1), 3–9. doi:10.1258/1357633053430494 PMID:15829036

Detmar, S., Aaronson, N., Wever, L., Muller, M., & Schornagel, J. (2000). How are you feeling? Who wants to know? Patients and oncologists preferences for discussing health-related quality-of-life issues. *Journal of Clinical Oncology, 18*(18), 3295–3301. PMID:10986063

Di Rienzo, M., Rizzo, F., Parati, G., Brambilla, G., Ferratini, M., & Castiglioni, P. (2005). Magic system: A new textile-based wearable device for biological signal monitoring. applicability in daily life and clinical setting. In *Proceedings of IEEE-EMBS 2005: 27th Annual International Conference of the Engineering in Medicine and Biology Society,* (pp. 7167–7169). IEEE.

Ding, D., Ayubi, S., Hiremath, S., & Parmanto, B. (2012). Physical activity monitoring and sharing platform for manual wheelchair users. In Proceedings of IEEE Intl. Conf. Engineering in Medicine and Biology Society (EMBC) (pp. 5833–5836). IEEE.

Fatima, I., Halder, S., Saleem, M. A., Batool, R., Fahim, M., Lee, Y., & Lee, S. (2013). Smart CDSS: integration of Social Media and Interaction Engine (SMIE) in healthcare for chronic disease patients. *Multimedia Tools and Applications*, 1–21.

Fensli, R., Gunnarson, E., & Gundersen, T. (2005). A wearable ECG-recording system for continuous arrhythmia monitoring in a wireless tele-home-care situation. In *Proceedings of 18ᵗʰ IEEE Symposium on Computer-Based Medical Systems,* (pp. 407–412). IEEE.

Griffin, L., & de Leastar, E. (2009). Social networking healthcare. In *Proceedings of 6th Intl. Workshop on Wearable Micro and Nano Technologies for Personalized Health* (pHealth), (pp. 75–78). pHealth.

Hao, Y., & Foster, R. (2008). Wireless body sensor networks for health-monitoring applications. *Physiological Measurement*, 29(11), R27–R56. doi:10.1088/0967-3334/29/11/R01 PMID:18843167

He, C., Fan, X., & Li, Y. (2013). Toward ubiquitous healthcare services with a novel efficient cloud platform. *IEEE Transactions on Bio-Medical Engineering*, 60(1), 230–234. doi:10.1109/TBME.2012.2222404 PMID:23060318

Heilman, K. J., & Porges, S. W. (2007). Accuracy of the lifeshirt® (vivometrics) in the detection of cardiac rhythms. *Biological Psychology*, 75(3), 300–305. doi:10.1016/j.biopsycho.2007.04.001 PMID:17540493

Intelsense. (2013). Retrieved from http://intellisense.io/

ITU. (2013, April). *High efficiency video coding.* ITU-T H.265.

ITU-T, & ISO/IEC. (2010). *Advanced video coding.* ITU-T Rec. H.264 and ISO/IEC 14496-10.

Jin, Z., Oresko, J., Huang, S., & Cheng, A. (2009). Hearttogo: A personalized medicine technology for cardiovascular disease prevention and detection. In *Proceedings of Life Science Systems and Applications Workshop,* (pp. 80–83). IEEE.

Khorakhu, C., & Bhatti, S. (2013). Remote Health Monitoring Using Online Social Media Systems. In *Proceedings of 6ᵗʰ Joint Wireless and Mobile Networking Conference.* Dubai, UAE: IEEE.

Kshetri, N. (2010, October). Cloud Computing in Developing Economies. *IEEE Computer,* 47–55.

Kyriacou, E. C., Pattichis, C. S., Karaolis, M. A., Loizou, C. P., Christodoulou, C. I., & Pattichis, M. S. et al. (2007). An integrated system for assessing stroke risk. *IEEE Engineering in Medicine and Biology Magazine*, 26(5), 43–50. doi:10.1109/EMB.2007.901794 PMID:17941322

Li, M., Yu, S., Zheng, Y., Ren, K., & Lou, W. (2013). Scalable and Secure Sharing of Personal Health Records in Cloud Computing Using Attribute-Based Encryption. *IEEE Transactions on Parallel and Distributed Systems*, 24(1), 131–143. doi:10.1109/TPDS.2012.97

LifeWatch. (2013). Retrieved from http://www.lifewatch.com/

Lin, H., Shao, J., Zhang, C., & Fang, Y. (2013). CAM: Cloud-Assisted Privacy Preserving Mobile Health Monitoring. *IEEE Transactions on Information Forensics and Security, 8*(6), 985–997. doi:10.1109/TIFS.2013.2255593

Luprano, J., Sola, J., Dasen, S., Koller, J.-M., & Chetelat, O. (2006). Combination of body sensor networks and on-body signal processing algorithms: the practical case of myheart project. In *Proceedings of International Workshop on Wearable and Implantable Body Sensor Networks,* (pp. 76–79). BSN.

Martín-Martínez, D., Casaseca-de-la Higuera, P., Alberola-López, S., Andrés-de Llano, J., López-Villalobos, J. A., Ardura-Fernández, J., & Alberola-López, C. (2012). Nonlinear analysis of actigraphic signals for the assessment of the attention-deficit/hyperactivity disorder (adhd). *Medical Engineering & Physics, 34*(9), 1317–1329. doi:10.1016/j.medengphy.2011.12.023 PMID:22297088

MedApp. (2013). Retrieved from https://healthcom.medapps.net/Login.aspx

MedHelp. (2013). Retrieved from http://www.medhelp.org/

Megalooikonomou, V., & Kontos, D. (2007). Medical Data Fusion for Telemedicine. *IEEE Engineering in Medicine and Biology Magazine, 26*(5), 36-42.

Milenković, A., Otto, C., & Jovanov, E. (2006). Wireless sensor networks for personal health monitoring: Issues and an implementation. *Computer Communications, 29*(13–14), 2521–2533. doi:10.1016/j.comcom.2006.02.011

Mirota, D. J., Wang, H., Taylor, R. H., Ishii, M., Gallia, G. L., & Hager, G. D. (2012). A system for video-based navigation for endoscopic endonasal skull base surgery. *IEEE Transactions on Medical Imaging, 31*(4), 963–976. doi:10.1109/TMI.2011.2176500 PMID:22113772

Nicolini, D., Powell, J., Conville, P., & Martinez-Solano, L. (2008). Managing knowledge in the healthcare sector. A review. *International Journal of Management Reviews, 10,* 245–263. doi:10.1111/j.1468-2370.2007.00219.x

Nightingale, J., Wang, Q., & Grecos, C. (2012). HEVStream: a framework for streaming and evaluation of high efficiency video coding (HEVC) content in loss-prone networks. *IEEE Transactions on Consumer Electronics, 58*(2), 404–412. doi:10.1109/TCE.2012.6227440

Nilakanta, S., Miller, L., Peer, A., & Bojja, V. M. (2009). Contribution of Knowledge and Knowledge Management Capability on Business Processes among Healthcare Organizations. In *Proceedings of System Sciences.* IEEE.

Norval, C., Arnott, J., Hine, N., & Hanson, V. (2011). Purposeful social media as support platform: Communication frameworks for older adults requiring care. In *Proceedings of 5th International Conference on Pervasive Computing Technologies for Healthcare (PervasiveHealth),* (pp. 492–494). Academic Press.

Oliver, N., & Flores-Mangas, F. (2006). Healthgear: A real-time wearable system for monitoring and analyzing physiological signals. In *Proceedings of International Workshop on Wearable and Implantable Body Sensor Networks,* (pp. 1-4). BSN.

Panayides, A., Pattichis, M. S., Pattichis, C. S., & Pitsillides, A. (2011). A tutorial for emerging wireless medical video transmission systems. *IEEE Antennas and Propagation Magazine, 53*(2), 202–213. doi:10.1109/MAP.2011.5949369

Pandian, P., Mohanavelu, K., Safeer, K., Kotresh, T., Shakunthala, D., Gopal, P., & Padaki, V. (2008). Smart vest: Wearable multi-parameter remote physiological monitoring system. *Medical Engineering & Physics, 30*(4), 466–477. doi:10.1016/j.medengphy.2007.05.014 PMID:17869159

Pantelopoulos, A., & Bourbakis, N. (2010). A survey on wearable sensor-based systems for health monitoring and prognosis. *IEEE Transactions on Systems, Man and Cybernetics. Part C, Applications and Reviews, 40*(1), 1–12. doi:10.1109/TSMCC.2009.2032660

Paradiso, R., Loriga, G., & Taccini, N. (2005). A wearable healthcare system based on knitted integrated sensors. *IEEE Transactions on Information Technology in Biomedicine, 9*(3), 337–344. doi:10.1109/TITB.2005.854512 PMID:16167687

Patientlikeme. (2013). Retrieved from http://www.patientslikeme.com/

Polar UK. (2013). Available http://www.polar.com/uk-en

Sakr, S., Liu, A., Batista, D. M., & Alomari, M. (2011). A Survey of Large Scale Data Management Approaches in Cloud Environments. *IEEE Communications Surveys & Tutorials, 13*(3), 311–336. doi:10.1109/SURV.2011.032211.00087

Scanfeld, D., Scanfeld, V., & Larson, E. (2010). Dissemination of health information through social networks: Twitter and antibiotics. *American Journal of Infection Control, 38*(3), 182–188. doi:10.1016/j.ajic.2009.11.004 PMID:20347636

Scilingo, E., Gemignani, A., Paradiso, R., Taccini, N., Ghelarducci, B., & De Rossi, D. (2005). Performance evaluation of sensing fabrics for monitoring physiological and biomechanical variables. *IEEE Transactions on Information Technology in Biomedicine, 9*(3), 345–352. doi:10.1109/TITB.2005.854506 PMID:16167688

Scully, C. G., Lee, J., Meyer, J., Gorbach, A. M., Granquist-Fraser, D., Mendelson, Y., & Chon, K. H. (2012). Physiological parameter monitoring from optical recordings with a mobile phone. *IEEE Transactions on* Biomedical Engineering, *59*(2), 303–306.

Shaw, E., Ruby, K., and Post, J. (1998). The insider threat to information systems: the psychology of the dangerous insider. *Security Awareness Bulletin, 2*(98), 1–10.

Sheffield, J. (2008). Inquiry in health knowledge management. *Journal of Knowledge Management, 12,* 160–172. doi:10.1108/13673270810884327

Sheth, A. (2010). Computing for Human Experience: Semantics-Empowered Sensors, Services, and Social Computing on the Ubiquitous Web. *IEEE Internet Computing, 14*(1), 88–91. doi:10.1109/MIC.2010.4

Sheth, A., Anantharam, P., & Henson, C. (2013). Physical-Cyber-Social Computing: An Early 21st Century Approach. IEEE Intelligent Systems, 78-82.

Shimmer. (2013). Available: http://www.shimmersensing.com/

Silva, B. B., Lopes, I., Rodrigues, J., & Ray, P. (2011). SapoFitness: A mobile health application for dietary evaluation. In *Proceedings of 13th IEEE Intl. Conf. on e-Health Networking Applications and Services (HealthCom)*, (pp. 375–380). IEEE.

Skubic, M., Alexander, G., Popescu, M., Rantz, M., & Keller, J. (2009). A smart home application to eldercare: Current status and lessons learned. *Technology and Healthcare, 17*(3), 183–201. PMID:19641257

Sullivan, G. J., Ohm, J., Han, W.-J., & Wiegand, T. (2012). Overview of the high efficiency video coding (HEVC) standard. *IEEE Transactions on Circuits and Systems for Video Technology, 22*(12), 1649–1668. doi:10.1109/TCSVT.2012.2221191

Sung, M., Marci, C., & Pentland, A. (2005). Wearable feedback systems for rehabilitation. *Journal of Neuroengineering and Rehabilitation, 2*, 17. doi:10.1186/1743-0003-2-17 PMID:15987514

UN. (2013). *Department of Economic and Social Affairs: Population Division: Population database*. UN.

Van Gorp, P., & Comuzzi, M. (2013). *Lifelong Personal Health Data and Application Software via Virtual Machines in the Cloud. IEEE Journal of Biomedical and Health Informatics*.

Video LAN. (2013). *VLC media player*. Available at http://www.videolan.org/vlc/index.html

Viswanathan, H., Chen, B., & Pompili, D. (2012). Research challenges in computation, communication, and context awareness for ubiquitous healthcare. *IEEE Communications Magazine, 50*(5), 92–99. doi:10.1109/MCOM.2012.6194388

Wang, Q., Nightingale, J., Wang, R., Ramzan, N., Grecos, C., & Wang, X. et al. (in press). Mobile Video Cloud Networks. In J. Rodrigues, K. Lin, & J. Lloret (Eds.), *Mobile Computing over Cloud: Technologies, Services, and Applications*. IGI Global. doi:10.4018/978-1-4666-4781-7.ch009

Wolf, P., Schmidt, A., & Klein, M. (2008). *SOPRANO-An extensible, open AAL platform for elderly people based on semantical contracts*. Paper presented at the 3rd Workshop on Artificial Intelligence Techniques for Ambient Intelligence (AITAmI'08), 18th European Conference on Artificial Intelligence (ECAI 08). Patras, Greece.

Wood, A., Stankovic, J., Virone, G., Selavo, L., He, Z., & Cao, Q. et al. (2008). Context-aware wireless sensor networks for assisted living and residential monitoring. *IEEE Network, 22*(4), 26–33. doi:10.1109/MNET.2008.4579768

World, W. P. P. (2003). The 2002 Revision, Highlights (Report No.: ESA/P/WP. 180). New York: United Nations Population Division.

Wowza. (2013). Available at http://www.wowza.com/

Yan, H., Huo, H., Xu, Y., & Gidlund, M. (2010). Wireless sensor network based E-health system implementation and experimental results. *IEEE Transactions on* Consumer Electronics, *56*(4), 2288–2295.

Yang, C., Tsai, C., Member, S., Cheng, K., & Chen, S. (2012). Low-Invasive Implantable Devices of Low-Power Consumption Using High-Efficiency Antennas for Cloud Healthcare. *IEEE Journal on Emerging and Selected Topics in Circuits and Systems, 2*(1), 14–23. doi:10.1109/JETCAS.2012.2187469

Zephyr Inc. (2013). Available: http://www.zephyranywhere.com/

KEY TERMS AND DEFINITIONS

Cloud Security: Cloud security issues such as data protection, privacy, trust/identity management, authentication/authorisation/accounting in a cloud and inter-clouds.

Cloud-Based Video Applications: Video applications that utilise the resources provided by a cloud.

Connected Health: The convergence of medical, security and communication devices. Systems which can be used for remote monitoring.

Data Fusion: The process of integration of multiple data acquired from different medical sensors, social networks and other information sources.

Knowledge Management: Comprises a range of strategies and practices used in the organisation, representation, and distribution, of medical data.

Mobile Cloud Computing: Cloud computing for mobile users.

Reconfigurable Hardware: Type of hardware which can be customised once or as much as needed, usually in the form of field programmable gate arrays.

Social Networking: Platforms to build social networks or social relations among people who, in our case, share experiences, interests, activities, or backgrounds, in healthcare.

This research was previously published in Healthcare Informatics and Analytics edited by Madjid Tavana, Amir Hossein Gha-panchi, and Amir Talaei-Khoei, pages 332-352, copyright year 2015 by Medical Information Science Reference (an imprint of IGI Global).

Chapter 54

Intelligent Risk Detection in Healthcare Contexts of Hip and Knee Athroplasty and Paediatric Congenital Heart Disease

Hoda Moghimi
RMIT University, Australia

Nilmini Wickramasinghe
Deakin University, Australia & Epworth HealthCare, Australia

Jonathan L. Schaffer
Cleveland Clinic, USA

ABSTRACT

Rapid increase of service demands in healthcare contexts today requires a robust framework enabled by IT (information technology) solutions as well as real-time service handling in order to ensure superior decision making and successful healthcare outcomes. Contemporaneous with the challenges facing healthcare, we are witnessing the development of very sophisticated intelligent tools and technologies such as Business Analytics techniques. Therefore, it would appear to be prudent to investigate the possibility of applying such tools and technologies into various healthcare contexts to facilitate better risk detection and support superior decision making. The following serves to do this in the context of Total Hip and Knee Arthroplasty and Congenital Heart Disease.

INTRODUCTION

For some diseases, surgery is not always a final cure and it result in a considerably high rate of disabilities, as well as the possibility of co-morbidities (Goossens, Apers, Gewillig, Budts, & Moons, 2013; Tabbutt et al., 2012); for example, types of cancer and even the development of bowel diseases. Naturally, this also has a direct adverse impact on patients and their families (Landolt, Buechel, & Latal, 2011). Hence,

DOI: 10.4018/978-1-5225-3926-1.ch054

decision-making regarding major surgery is multi-faceted and complex (Noyes, Masakowski, & Cook, 2012; Sox, Higgins, & Owens, 2013).

To facilitate the surgical decision making process, we suggest the application of real time intelligent risk detection decision support would be beneficial. We proffer a suitable solution which combines the application of data mining tools followed by Knowledge Discovery (KD) techniques to score key surgery risk levels, assess surgery risks and thereby help medical professionals to make appropriate decisions.

The aim of this chapter is to outline how it might be possible to improve the outcomes and benefits of surgical interventions and support a healthcare value proposition of excellence for patients, their families, providers, healthcare organizations and society by developing an intelligent risk detection framework to improve surgery decision making processes. While such strategies have been used in other industries (i.e. banking and finance) (Bhambri, 2011; Pulakkazhy & Balan, 2013), it appears that this is one of the first studies focused on healthcare contexts. We focus on the contexts of Total Hip and Knee Arthroplasty and Congenital Heart Disease (CHD) in children to illustrate the potential of this approach.

BACKGROUND

Clinical Decision Support Systems (CDSS) are computer driven technology solutions, developed to provide support to physicians, nurses and patients using medical knowledge and patient-specific information (De Backere, De Turck, Colpaert, & Decruyenaere, 2012). Decision Support systems can be found in widely divergent functional areas. However, in e-health contexts, key features such as intelligent timing, multidimensional views of data and calculation-intensive capabilities become important features given the need for real time outcomes and the multi-spectral nature of care teams (Wickramasinghe, Chalasani, & Koritala, 2012). Hence, systems for healthcare must give advice and support rather than decision making replacing that of clinical staff.

Studies have already proved that CDSS enhance quality, safety and effectiveness of medical decisions through providing higher performance of the medical staff and patient care as well as more effective clinical services. A variety of CDSS programs designed to assist clinical staff with drug dosing, health maintenance, diagnosis, and other clinically relevant healthcare decisions have been developed for the medical workplace (Haug, Gardner, Evans, Rocha, & Rocha, 2007). On the other hand, patients' demand for participation in medical decisions has been increasing (Kuhn, Wurst, Bott, & Giuse, 2006). Therefore, to be respectful of patients and parents/guardians participation and decisions, shared decision-making (SDM) between health care professionals, patients, parents and guardians is widely recommended today (Lai, 2012). SDM is defined as the active participation of both clinicians and families in treatment decisions, the exchange of information, discussion of preferences, and a joint determination of the treatment plan (Barry & Edgman-Levitan, 2012; Charles, Gafni, & Whelan, 1997; Légaré et al., 2011; Makoul & Clayman, 2006).

Although SDM is supported in many disease management domains, some concerns and issues still remain regarding the adoption of SDM solutions such as a perception among some practitioners that the ultimate responsibility for treatment should remain under their authority (Edwards & Elwyn, 2009; Schauer, Everett, del Vecchio, & Anderson, 2007). Moreover, client capacity to participate in decisions (O'Brien, Crickard, Rapp, Holmes, & McDonald, 2011), identifying the SDM components (Sheridan, Harris, & Woolf, 2004; T. van der Weijden et al., 2011) as well as SDM user acceptance (Scholl et al., 2011)are main issues to promote this type of CDCS in the healthcare contexts. However, SDM also has some limitations; for example, SDM is appropriate for situations in which two or more medically reasonable choices exist (O'connor et al., 2009), regardless of whether the degree of risk is high or low (Whitney, McGuire, & McCullough, 2003). Therefore, SDM is not appropriate in these cases while still patients or their families would like to have participation in the care process. Hence, more studies are needed to deepen the understanding of interactions between patient decision aid use and the patterns of patient-practitioner communication as well as format issues such as web-based delivery of patient decision aids. (Cousin, Schmid Mast, Roter, & Hall, 2012; Flight, Wilson, Zajac, Hart, & McGillivray, 2012; O'connor et al., 2009; Parsons et al., 2012).

Research on shared decision making is under way (Barry & Edgman-Levitan, 2012; Deegan & Drake, 2006), but much more is needed in this area. Moreover, it is critical to address the importance of asking right questions in shared decision making process before looking for a right answer, as asking the wrong questions in clinical cases can generate seemingly right answers, but these answers may not be enough to reflect or predict real-life scenarios (Horwitz, Abell, Christian, & Wivel, 2014).

Medical decisions always have to be made in a trade-off between benefit and risk. Unfortunately, many decisions are based upon an incorrect knowledge of risk (Trudy van der Weijden et al., 2011). In addition, different viewpoints concerning risks can result in different optimal choices because of different perspectives (Hsu, Tseng, Chiang, & Chen, 2012). Therefore, the following suggest that an Intelligent Risk Detection (IRD) model which attempts to facilitate and provide decision support for clinicians and patients regarding the treatment risk factors might be beneficial.

To understand the current state and potential for intelligent risk detection, as a first step, more than 500 relevant publications in the period 2003 to 2013 were reviewed. These focused on surgical decision efficiency and/or detecting surgical risk factors. Almost 350 of these publications focused on Information Systems and Health Informatics. From this literature review, the following issues and challenges were identified:

- Lack of communication facilitators to share decisions between clinicians, and between clinicians and patients or their families, in order to support clinical decisions by understanding the treatment risk factors and anticipated outcomes (Bates et al., 2003).
- Lack of some specific Socio-technical components of people, process, technology and environment in healthcare to make a successful implementation of a new technology to address data importance and accuracy issues (Gosain & Kumar, 2009; Kuhn et al., 2006)
- Lack of a dynamic risk assessment system, in the healthcare context (Fortinsky et al., 2004; Gambrill & Shlonsky, 2000; Greenland, 2012; Pancorbo-Hidalgo, Garcia-Fernandez, Lopez-Medina, & Alvarez-Nieto, 2006; Ryan et al., 2012; Twetman, Fontana, & Featherstone, 2013)
- Lack of a multidimensional risk detection model/algorithm (Anderson, Brodie, Vincent, & Hanna, 2012; Aylin, Bottle, & Majeed, 2007; Gran, Fredriksen, & Thunem, 2004; Staal, Hermanns, Schrijvers, & van Stel, 2013; Trucco & Cavallin, 2006).

This in turn makes a real time intelligent risk detection framework the preferred choice. Thus, our study proposes an intelligent application for high-level surgery risk detection and outcome prediction to support surgical decisions. The model is designed based on two steps of the decision making process (surgical and personal) and, includes a decision support system which is suitable for high concentration prediction. Continual model updates inherent in the proposed system results in adaptive and more accurate risk detection and outcome prediction capabilities as compared to a fixed model.

THE CURRENT STUDY

Through this study, it is noted that while data mining is being utilized in various healthcare contexts including applications of text mining and secondary uses for data (Safran et al., 2007), infection control (Iakovidis, Tsevas, Savelonas, & Papamichalis, 2012), physician order entry and electronic health records (Harshberger et al., 2011) and even in the identification of high risk patients (Marschollek et al., 2012) the application of data mining and BI for risk detection is at a nascent state. However, the lack of interaction between healthcare industry practitioners and academic researchers makes it hard to discover surgical risks, and limits opportunities for the application of Business Intelligence and Business Analytics (BI/BA) techniques, and hence weakens the value that knowledge discovery and data mining methods may bring to healthcare risk detection.

In the context of surgical risk detection many dimensions and perspectives (Haga, Ikejiri, Takeuchi, Ikenaga, & Wada, 2012) are of importance and these mainly focus on pathological process, physiological variables, some general health perceptions, social paradigm and also quality of life (Rizzo & Kintner, 2013). Naturally, detecting the risk factors in all of these dimensions is not easy or trivial but based on two approaches to assess the risks, with contribution of clinical experts; this research aims to cover these main dimensions.

Research Design and Methodology

Throughout this research a mixed method approach is conducted incorporating well established qualitative and quantitative data collection techniques. Qualitative and quantitative data are collected by two distinct method; namely, individual semi-structured interviews and questionnaires.

SOLUTIONS AND RECOMMENDATIONS

To capture the inherent complexities of surgery interventions, the conceptual model has been developed. Integral to this model are the two steps of decision making defined over the three key phases of the decision making process for the surgery (Figure 1). The first type of decision making is called "surgical decision making" and is primarily associated with the surgeons while the second type is called "personal decision making" as it is primarily associated with the patients or their family.

Risk Assessment and Detection

Detecting risk factors based on a risk assessment process using BI tools is a useful way to assess improvements in surgery (Larrazabal et al., 2007). Therefore, after first identifying important risk factors in the literature, we will seek expert input at two distinct stages to address this subject. The specific stages involved in the risk assessment process include the following: In the first stage, the specialists in an expert group of clinicians and surgeons are presented with risk factors identified from the literature. The experts will then nominate (or introduce) some main risk categories or dimensions as well as risk factors to be used in the surgical decision making process. In the next stage, the expert group is asked to assess

Figure 1. The conceptual model
Source: adapted from (Moghimi, Seif Zadeh, Cheung, & Wickramasinghe, 2011)

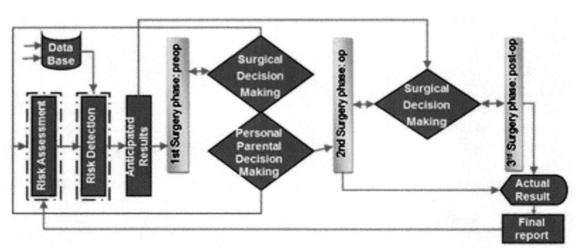

the risk factors and also evaluate the effects of these factors in surgery outcomes. It is also important to document the surgeons' and specialists' recommendations and advice in order to improve the Model.

To incorporate an intelligent technology into the proposed risk assessment process, data mining tasks followed by knowledge discovery will be trained. In the research case, the data types have a significant impact on the data mining tasks. Hence, after completing the data collection phase, techniques such as neural networks and association rules will be used. After the risk assessment process, applying the necessary data mining techniques, and the development and implementation of the model, a database of the patients' data will be used in order to detect risk factors.

Applying Anticipated and Actual Results

To evaluate a risk detection process in the proposed conceptual model, the actual results will be compared with the anticipated results. This provides feedback to assess the accuracy of the process and also provide appropriate modification as new factors are identified. Lastly, the BI reporting tools will be used to create a final report to show important items, and finally apply them to the risk assessment process, for subsequent iterations of evaluations.

CASE STUDIES

To illustrate the benefits of our proposed IRD Model, we look at two specific healthcare contexts: case one, Orthopaedic interventions and case two, Congenital Heart Disease. The following serves to examine the technical and conceptual layers of the IRD Model and also defines some of the associated knowledge driven healthcare services which are supported by the IRD model in order to facilitate superior healthcare delivery.

Case 1: Incorporating IRD Model to Total Hip and Knee Arthroplasty (THA/TKA)

In general, Total Hip and Knee Arthroplasty are successful solutions for people experiencing pain associated with degenerative joints (Malviya et al., 2011). In fracture care for broken hips however, there are other risk factors involved which impact on both the choice of treatment and on patient outcomes (Malviya et al., 2011). This makes the decision process connected with this surgery of significant importance. In addition hip and knee replacements continue to undergo innovation with improvement in technology and it needs to be monitored (Moghimi, Zadeh, Schaffer, & Wickramasinghe, 2012). Taken together, this serves to underscore that performance management in this context is clearly complex, dependent on multi spectral data and information and has far reaching consequences. Therefore, our IRD Model should be an effective and efficient solution in such a context.

Thus, to illustrate the role for our IRD Model, we have categorized the hip and knee arthroplasty, particularly for hip and knee replacement, into four key components as follows in an attempt to systematically capture four key risk factors (Moghimi & Wickramasinghe, 2012):

- **Prosthetic Issues:** Specific to implant that may impact on the outcome of surgery.
- **Financial Issues:** Regarding the costs of these devices in relationship to outcome and type of surgery
- **Physiological and Co-Morbidities:** Patient specific issues that may impact on the outcome of surgery
- **Clinical Issues:** To medical/provider intervention that may impact on the outcome of the surgery.

Table 1 then, serves to illustrate how the key BA techniques can then be transformed and translated into a specific context; in this instance the context of the hip and knee arthroplasty specifically focussing on hip and knee arthroplasty. Implicit in this conceptualisation is that the proposed IRD Model is sufficiently flexible to cover all process from pre-operative, operative and post-operative. In so doing it will then provide most benefit to all key stakeholders.

Case 2: Incorporating IRD Model to the Congenital Heart Disease (CHD)

Congenital Heart Disease (CHD), as a common health problem affecting many children around the world (Marino et al., 2012), is involved a multi-faceted set of considerations including the immediate

Table 1. The role of IRD components to improve performance management in hip and knee arthroplasty

IRD Components	Improvements Subjects	Description (How)
Balanced scorecard	• To improve financial issues • To improve clinical issues	By developing relevant measurements and KPIs
Service line analysis and reporting	• To improve financial issues • To improve clinical issues • To improve physiological issues • To improve prosthetic issues	By making analytical and multidimensional reports
Health and wellness service line management	• To improve biomedical issues • To improve physiological issues	By real-time monitoring and controlling patients' clinical conditions
On-Line Analytical Processing (OLAP)	To improve biomedical issues	By making ad-hoc and real-time analytical reports

medical result, the ongoing increased risk of sudden death, exercise intolerance, neuro developmental and psychological problems as well as long-term impacts on the family unit (Long, Galea, Eldridge, & Harris, 2012). This multi-faceted consideration is important because of the far reaching consequences that can result post-surgery or even mortality or morbidity.

The decision making process in the context of CHD surgery can be divided into three broad phases. In the first phase, or pre-operative phase, the surgeon, having received information about the patient and his/her medical condition, needs to make a decision relating to whether surgery is the best medical option. Once this decision is made but before surgery, the parents must then decide whether to accept or reject the surgeon's decision in consideration of the predicted outcomes. Typically, parents have met many medical staff before they meet the cardiac surgeon. Thus, already at stage one, two key decisions must be made. Once parents and surgeons have agreed to proceed, in phase two, critical decisions pertaining to the unique situations that may arise during the surgery must be addressed. For example, in CHD cases sometimes due to the clinical conditions, surgeons have to change the shunt size during the surgery and regarding this ad-hoc decision, they have to choose the best suitable shunt size with fewer risks, in a very short time. Finally, in the post-operative phase, or phase three, decision making is primarily done at two levels; a) strategies to ensure a sustained successful result for the patient during aftercare and beyond, and b) a record of lessons learnt for use by clinicians in future similar cases.

To clarify the function of the decision making framework across CHD surgery for this study, we summarize current surgery steps and the associated decision making process in one of the common CHD classifications; Hypoplastic Left Heart Syndrome (HLHS) in Figure 2. HLHS patients, usually have three types of surgery during their childhood treatment period, called Norwood, BCPC and Fontan (Hoffman & Kaplan, 2002). These are most recent surgeries suggested to patients in different age and conditions. However, the Norwood surgery is still much more complex and risky with a high rate of mortality and morbidity (Hoffman & Kaplan, 2002). Many factors are likely to be responsible for the improvement in operative survival following the Norwood procedure. These factors include improved surgical techniques, improved peri-operative management, and improved anaesthetic techniques. Despite the improving outcome, early survival for these children is still significantly lower than for other forms of heart disease, which require neonatal surgical intervention (Tabbutt et al., 2012).

In the case of HLHS, it would be diagnosed, either in pre or neonatal and the newborn should be operated, as soon as possible. Hence, as demonstrated at Figure 2, in pre-operative step, the first surgery should be organized by cardiologists and surgeons through making a complex decision regarding the best time and techniques to carry out the surgery. Also, during the surgery surgeons have to make some semi-structured as well as ad hoc decisions such as choosing the best shunt size. In post-operative step, considering the patient conditions, surgeons should make a decision for another surgery or any other clinical treatment. In addition, they should plan a periodic assessment to assess the patient conditions. Thus, our proposed IRD Model will be a valuable Model to apply in the highlighted steps in all three surgery phases and surgery types to predict the operation results by detecting risk factors to assist parents as well as surgeons to make superior decisions.

FUTURE RESEARCH DIRECTIONS

This research cannot attempt to determine all actual risk versus actual benefit. This is because long term risks and rare occurrences are not currently possible to identify using randomized controlled trials, these

Figure 2. Flow diagram of key steps with CHD surgery (Highlighted boxes in the current procedure represent proposed situations to use the IRD Model)
(Adapted from (Moghimi, Schaffer, & Wickramasinghe, 2014))

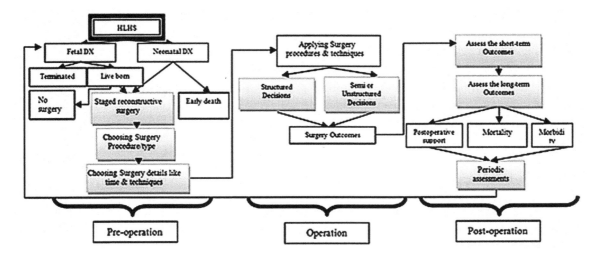

risks and occurrences can only be identified by using methods that were specifically developed for large, observational and longitudinal data sets. This study therefore can only explore the main components of a surgical intelligent risk detection framework to improve clinical decision efficiency.

Although this study supports the benefits of such an intelligent application for healthcare contexts, many issues regarding its implementation into specific healthcare contexts such as Congenital Heart Disease (CHD) and Hip and Knee Arthroplasty remain to be examined. Therefore, the next phase for this research is prototyping and simulation of the solution to trial the model in a selected clinical environment.

DISCUSSION AND CONCLUSION

This study has outlined an exploratory research study aimed at trying to examine the potential benefits of combining a real time intelligent risk detection solution with decision support in a healthcare context. The outcomes from this exploratory research include, early identification of risk factors, providing superior decision support, developing key performance indicators to detect the surgery risk factors, predicting surgical results to identify patients at risk during surgery, standardizing clinical risk assessment and management processes to facilitate superior health outcomes, developing a risk profile for patients, improving risk information sharing, developing a true picture of risk categories and factors, creating a "Risk Aware" alarm to control the risk factors and monitoring the risk factors by using dashboards.

Emphasizing the importance of knowledge sharing between clinicians as well as between clinicians and patients; clinicians' involvement during systems development; acceptability and capability of the system and high demand of outcome predictions to improve decision efficiency are the major contribution to practice.

Providing analytical report to clinicians and patients in three phases of preoperative, operative and post-operative, through different and secure access level, is the other advantages of the IRD model.

In addition, using KPIs as a set of metrics not only is a novel idea to control the risk factors, finding the level and defining their relationships, but it also enables effective monitoring of several key items during surgery.

Another advantage of the proposed IRD model that should be noted is its continuous nature. Most importantly, by comparing anticipated results and actual outcomes and also performing risk auditing, risk factors will be amended to improve future predictions.

A further and final important feature of the proposed IRD model is the integration of the three IT solutions to solve a clinical issue in the definition and assessment of "outcomes" in patients with CHD, combined by some assessment measures. Thus, we believe it will also be one of the valuable contributions to both theory and practice of this research.

REFERENCES

Anderson, O., Brodie, A., Vincent, C. A., & Hanna, G. B. (2012). A systematic proactive risk assessment of hazards in surgical wards: A quantitative study. *Annals of Surgery, 255*(6), 1086–1092. doi:10.1097/SLA.0b013e31824f5f36 PMID:22504280

Aylin, P., Bottle, A., & Majeed, A. (2007). Use of administrative data or clinical databases as predictors of risk of death in hospital: Comparison of models. *BMJ: British Medical Journal, 334*(7602), 1044. doi:10.1136/bmj.39168.496366.55 PMID:17452389

Barry, M. J., & Edgman-Levitan, S. (2012). Shared Decision Making—The Pinnacle of Patient-Centered Care. *The New England Journal of Medicine, 366*(9), 780–781. doi:10.1056/NEJMp1109283 PMID:22375967

Bates, D. W., Kuperman, G. J., Wang, S., Gandhi, T., Kittler, A., Volk, L., & Middleton, B. et al. (2003). Ten commandments for effective clinical decision support: Making the practice of evidence-based medicine a reality. *Journal of the American Medical Informatics Association, 10*(6), 523–530. doi:10.1197/jamia.M1370 PMID:12925543

Bhambri, V. (2011). Application of data mining in banking sector. *International Journal of Clothing Science and Technology, 2*(2).

Charles, C., Gafni, A., & Whelan, T. (1997). Shared decision-making in the medical encounter: What does it mean?(or it takes at least two to tango). *Social Science & Medicine. Social Science & Medicine, 44*(5), 681–692. doi:10.1016/S0277-9536(96)00221-3

Cousin, G., Schmid Mast, M., Roter, D. L., & Hall, J. A. (2012). Concordance between physician communication style and patient attitudes predicts patient satisfaction. *Patient Education and Counseling, 87*(2), 193–197. doi:10.1016/j.pec.2011.08.004 PMID:21907529

De Backere, F., De Turck, F., Colpaert, K., & Decruyenaere, J. (2012). *Advanced pervasive clinical decision support for the intensive care unit.* Academic Press.

Deegan, P., & Drake, R. (2006). Shared decision making and medication management in the recovery process. *Psychiatric Services (Washington, D.C.), 57*(11), 1636–1639. doi:10.1176/ps.2006.57.11.1636 PMID:17085613

Edwards, A., & Elwyn, G. (2009). *Shared decision-making in health care: Achieving evidence-based patient choice*. Oxford University Press.

Flight, I. H., Wilson, C. J., Zajac, I. T., Hart, E., & McGillivray, J. A. (2012). Decision support and the effectiveness of web-based delivery and information tailoring for bowel cancer screening: an exploratory study. *JMIR Research Protocols, 1*(2), e12.

Fortinsky, R. H., Iannuzzi-Sucich, M., Baker, D. I., Gottschalk, M., King, M. B., Brown, C. J., & Tinetti, M. E. (2004). Fall-Risk Assessment and Management in Clinical Practice: Views from Healthcare Providers. *Journal of the American Geriatrics Society, 52*(9), 1522–1526. doi:10.1111/j.1532-5415.2004.52416.x PMID:15341555

Gambrill, E., & Shlonsky, A. (2000). Risk assessment in context. *Children and Youth Services Review, 22*(11), 813–837. doi:10.1016/S0190-7409(00)00123-7

Goossens, E., Apers, S., Gewillig, M., Budts, W., & Moons, P. (2013). *Evaluating quality of life after correction of a cardiac defect*. Academic Press.

Gosain, A., & Kumar, A. (2009). *Analysis of health care data using different data mining techniques*. Paper presented at the Intelligent Agent & Multi-Agent Systems, 2009. IAMA 2009. International Conference on. doi:10.1109/IAMA.2009.5228051

Gran, B. A., Fredriksen, R., & Thunem, A. P.-J. (2004). *An approach for model-based risk assessment. In Computer Safety, Reliability, and Security* (pp. 311–324). Springer. doi:10.1007/978-3-540-30138-7_26

Greenland, P. (2012). Should the resting electrocardiogram be ordered as a routine risk assessment test in healthy asymptomatic adults? *Journal of the American Medical Association, 307*(14), 1530–1531. doi:10.1001/jama.2012.441 PMID:22496268

Haga, Y., Ikejiri, K., Takeuchi, H., Ikenaga, M., & Wada, Y. (2012). Value of general surgical risk models for predicting postoperative liver failure and mortality following liver surgery. *Journal of Surgical Oncology, 106*(7), 898–904. doi:10.1002/jso.23160 PMID:22605669

Harshberger, C. A., Harper, A. J., Carro, G. W., Spath, W. E., Hui, W. C., Lawton, J. M., & Brockstein, B. E. (2011). Outcomes of computerized physician order entry in an electronic health record after implementation in an outpatient oncology setting. *Journal of Oncology Practice, 7*(4), 233–237. doi:10.1200/JOP.2011.000261 PMID:22043187

Haug, P. J., Gardner, R. M., Evans, R. S., Rocha, B. H., & Rocha, R. A. (2007). Clinical decision support at Intermountain Healthcare. *Clinical Decision Support Systems*, 159-189.

Hoffman, J. I., & Kaplan, S. (2002). The incidence of congenital heart disease. *Journal of the American College of Cardiology, 39*(12), 1890–1900. doi:10.1016/S0735-1097(02)01886-7 PMID:12084585

Horwitz, R. I., Abell, J. E., Christian, J. B., & Wivel, A. E. (2014). Right answers, wrong questions in clinical research. *Science Translational Medicine, 6*(221), 221fs225-221fs225.

Hsu, W.-K., Tseng, C.-P., Chiang, W.-L., & Chen, C.-W. (2012). Risk and uncertainty analysis in the planning stages of a risk decision-making process. *Natural Hazards, 61*(3), 1355–1365. doi:10.1007/s11069-011-0032-1

Iakovidis, D. K., Tsevas, S., Savelonas, M. A., & Papamichalis, G. (2012). Image analysis framework for infection monitoring. *Biomedical Engineering. IEEE Transactions on, 59*(4), 1135–1144.

Kuhn, K., Wurst, S., Bott, O., & Giuse, D. (2006). Expanding the scope of health information systems. *IMIA Yearbook of Medical Informatics,* 43-52.

Lai, P. (2012). Shared decision making. *Surgical Practice, 16*(4), 127–127. doi:10.1111/j.1744-1633.2012.00623.x

Landolt, M. A., Buechel, E. V., & Latal, B. (2011). Predictors of parental quality of life after child open heart surgery: A 6-month prospective study. *The Journal of Pediatrics, 158*(1), 37–43. doi:10.1016/j.jpeds.2010.06.037 PMID:20688338

Larrazabal, L. A., Jenkins, K. J., Gauvreau, K., Vida, V. L., Benavidez, O. J., Gaitán, G. A., . . . Castañeda, A. R. (2007). Improvement in Congenital Heart Surgery in a Developing Country: The Guatemalan Experience. *Circulation is published by the American Heart Association, 116,* 1872-1877.

Légaré, F., Stacey, D., Pouliot, S., Gauvin, F. P., Desroches, S., Kryworuchko, J., & Gagnon, M. P. et al. (2011). Interprofessionalism and shared decision-making in primary care: A stepwise approach towards a new model. *Journal of Interprofessional Care, 25*(1), 18–25. doi:10.3109/13561820.2010.490502 PMID:20795835

Long, S. H., Galea, M. P., Eldridge, B. J., & Harris, S. R. (2012). Performance of 2-year-old children after early surgery for congenital heart disease on the Bayley Scales of Infant and Toddler Development. *Early Human Development, 88*(8), 603–607. doi:10.1016/j.earlhumdev.2012.01.007 PMID:22336496

Makoul, G., & Clayman, M. L. (2006). An integrative model of shared decision making in medical encounters. *Patient Education and Counseling, 60*(3), 301–312. doi:10.1016/j.pec.2005.06.010 PMID:16051459

Malviya, A., Martin, K., Harper, I., Muller, S. D., Emmerson, K. P., Partington, P. F., & Reed, M. R. (2011). Enhanced recovery program for hip and knee replacement reduces death rate: A study of 4,500 consecutive primary hip and knee replacements. *Acta Orthopaedica, 82*(5), 577–581. doi:10.3109/17453674.2011.618911 PMID:21895500

Marino, B. S., Lipkin, P. H., Newburger, J. W., Peacock, G., Gerdes, M., Gaynor, J. W., & Johnson, W. H. et al. (2012). Neurodevelopmental Outcomes in Children With Congenital Heart Disease: Evaluation and Management A Scientific Statement From the American Heart Association. *Circulation, 126*(9), 1143–1172. doi:10.1161/CIR.0b013e318265ee8a PMID:22851541

Marschollek, M., Gövercin, M., Rust, S., Gietzelt, M., Schulze, M., Wolf, K.-H., & Steinhagen-Thiessen, E. (2012). Mining geriatric assessment data for in-patient fall prediction models and high-risk subgroups. *BMC Medical Informatics and Decision Making, 12*(1), 19. doi:10.1186/1472-6947-12-19 PMID:22417403

Moghimi, H., Schaffer, J., & Wickramasinghe, N. (2014). *Exploring The Possibilities For Intelligent Risk Detection In Healthcare Contexts* Paper presented at the ECIS Workshop, Tel Aviv.

Moghimi, H., Seif Zadeh, H., Cheung, M., & Wickramasinghe, N. (2011). *An intelligent risk detection framework using business intelligence tools to improve decision efficiency in healthcare contexts.* Paper presented at the Seventeenth Americas Conference on Information Systems (AMCIS).

Moghimi, H., & Wickramasinghe, N. (2012). *Improving e-performance management in healthcare using intelligent IT solutions. In Critical Issues for the Development of Sustainable E-health Solutions* (pp. 3–15). Springer. doi:10.1007/978-1-4614-1536-7_1

Moghimi, H., Zadeh, H., Schaffer, J., & Wickramasinghe, N. (2012). Incorporing intelligent risk detection to enable superior decision support: The example of orthopaedic surgeries. *Health Technology*, *2*(1), 33–41. doi:10.1007/s12553-011-0014-z

Noyes, J., Masakowski, Y., & Cook, M. (2012). *Decision making in complex environments.* Ashgate Publishing, Ltd.

O'Brien, M. S., Crickard, E. L., Rapp, C., Holmes, C., & McDonald, T. (2011). Critical issues for psychiatric medication shared decision making with youth and families. *Families in Society*, *93*(3), 310–316. doi:10.1606/1044-3894.4135

O'connor, A., Bennett, C., Stacey, D., Barry, M., Col, N., Eden, K., . . . Khangura, S. (2009). Decision aids for people facing health treatment or screening decisions (Review). *The Cochrane Collaboration published in the Cochrane Library, 3.*

Pancorbo-Hidalgo, P. L., Garcia-Fernandez, F. P., Lopez-Medina, I. M., & Alvarez-Nieto, C. (2006). Risk assessment scales for pressure ulcer prevention: A systematic review. *Journal of Advanced Nursing*, *54*(1), 94–110. doi:10.1111/j.1365-2648.2006.03794.x PMID:16553695

Parsons, S., Harding, G., Breen, A., Foster, N., Pincus, T., Vogel, S., & Underwood, M. (2012). Will shared decision making between patients with chronic musculoskeletal pain and physiotherapists, osteopaths and chiropractors improve patient care? *Family Practice*, *29*(2), 203–212. doi:10.1093/fampra/cmr083 PMID:21982810

Pulakkazhy, S., & Balan, R. (2013). Data mining in banking and its applications-a review. *Journal of Computer Science*, *9*(10), 1252–1259. doi:10.3844/jcssp.2013.1252.1259

Rizzo, V. M., & Kintner, E. (2013). The utility of the behavioral risk factor surveillance system (BRFSS) in testing quality of life theory: An evaluation using structural equation modeling. *Quality of Life Research: An International Journal of Quality of Life Aspects of Treatment, Care and Rehabilitation*, *22*(5), 987–995. doi:10.1007/s11136-012-0228-1 PMID:22797867

Ryan, P. B., Madigan, D., Stang, P. E., Marc Overhage, J., Racoosin, J. A., & Hartzema, A. G. (2012). Empirical assessment of methods for risk identification in healthcare data: Results from the experiments of the Observational Medical Outcomes Partnership. *Statistics in Medicine*, *31*(30), 4401–4415. PMID:23015364

Safran, C., Bloomrosen, M., Hammond, W. E., Labkoff, S., Markel-Fox, S., Tang, P. C., & Detmer, D. E. (2007). Toward a national framework for the secondary use of health data: An American Medical Informatics Association White Paper. *Journal of the American Medical Informatics Association*, *14*(1), 1–9. doi:10.1197/jamia.M2273 PMID:17077452

Schauer, C., Everett, A., del Vecchio, P., & Anderson, L. (2007). Promoting the value and practice of shared decision-making in mental health care. *Psychiatric Rehabilitation Journal, 31*(1), 54–61. doi:10.2975/31.1.2007.54.61 PMID:17694716

Scholl, I., Loon, M. K., Sepucha, K., Elwyn, G., Légaré, F., Härter, M., & Dirmaier, J. (2011). Measurement of shared decision making–a review of instruments. *Zeitschrift für Evidenz. Fortbildung und Qualität im Gesundheitswesen, 105*(4), 313–324. doi:10.1016/j.zefq.2011.04.012

Sheridan, S. L., Harris, R. P., & Woolf, S. H. (2004). Shared decision making about screening and chemoprevention. *American Journal of Preventive Medicine, 26*(1), 56–66. doi:10.1016/j.amepre.2003.09.011 PMID:14700714

Sox, H. C., Higgins, M. C., & Owens, D. K. (2013). *Medical decision making.* John Wiley & Sons. doi:10.1002/9781118341544

Staal, I. I., Hermanns, J., Schrijvers, A. J., & van Stel, H. F. (2013). Risk assessment of parents' concerns at 18 months in preventive child health care predicted child abuse and neglect. *Child Abuse & Neglect, 37*(7), 475–484. doi:10.1016/j.chiabu.2012.12.002 PMID:23352082

Tabbutt, S., Ghanayem, N., Ravishankar, C., Sleeper, L. A., Cooper, D. S., Frank, D. U., & Goldberg, C. S. et al. (2012). Risk factors for hospital morbidity and mortality after the Norwood procedure: A report from the Pediatric Heart Network Single Ventricle Reconstruction trial. *The Journal of Thoracic and Cardiovascular Surgery, 144*(4), 882–895. doi:10.1016/j.jtcvs.2012.05.019 PMID:22704284

Trucco, P., & Cavallin, M. (2006). A quantitative approach to clinical risk assessment: The CREA method. *Safety Science, 44*(6), 491–513. doi:10.1016/j.ssci.2006.01.003

Twetman, S., Fontana, M., & Featherstone, J. D. (2013). Risk assessment–can we achieve consensus? *Community Dentistry and Oral Epidemiology, 41*(1), e64–e70. doi:10.1111/cdoe.12026 PMID:24916679

van der Weijden, T., van Veenendaal, H., Drenthen, T., Versluijs, M., Stalmeier, P., Loon, M. K., & Timmermans, D. (2011). Shared decision making in the Netherlands, is the time ripe for nationwide, structural implementation? *Zeitschrift für Evidenz. Fortbildung und Qualität im Gesundheitswesen, 105*(4), 283–288. doi:10.1016/j.zefq.2011.04.005

van der Weijden, T., van Veenendaal, H., Drenthen, T., Versluijs, M., Stalmeier, P., Loon, M. K.-, & Timmermans, D. et al. (2011). Shared decision making in the Netherlands, is the time ripe for nationwide, structural implementation? *Zeitschrift für Evidenz. Fortbildung und Qualität im Gesundheitswesen, 105*(4), 283–288. doi:10.1016/j.zefq.2011.04.005

Whitney, S. N., McGuire, A. L., & McCullough, L. B. (2003). A typology of shared decision making, informed consent, and simple consent. *Annals of Internal Medicine, 140*(1), 54–59. doi:10.7326/0003-4819-140-1-200401060-00012 PMID:14706973

Wickramasinghe, N., Chalasani, S., & Koritala, S. (2012). *The role of healthcare system of systems and collaborative technologies in providing superior healthcare delivery to native american patients.* Paper presented at the System Science (HICSS), 2012 45th Hawaii International Conference. doi:10.1109/HICSS.2012.582

KEY TERMS AND DEFINITIONS

Business Analytics: Developing new insights and understanding of business performance based on data and statistical methods.

Clinical Decision Support Systems: Clinical decision support system (CDSS) is an expert system software to assist health professionals in decision making process to improve decision efficiency.

Congenital Heart Disease (CHD): Is a defect in the structure of the heart and great vessels that is present at birth.

Hip and Knee Arthoplasty: A primary hip and knee arthoplasty occurs when the native joint surface(s) are replaced with artificial implants.

Predictive Analytic: Predictive analytics is defined as a variety of statistical techniques to analyse current and historical facts to make predictions about future.

Risk Detection: The ability to capture clinical risks at the earliest time.

This research was previously published in Maximizing Healthcare Delivery and Management through Technology Integration edited by Tiko Iyamu and Arthur Tatnall, pages 1-14, copyright year 2016 by Medical Information Science Reference (an imprint of IGI Global).

Chapter 55
The Power of Words:
Deliberation Dialogue as a Model to Favor Patient Engagement in Chronic Care

Sarah Bigi
Catholic University of the Sacred Heart, Italy

Giulia Lamiani
University of Milan, Italy

ABSTRACT

The concept of patient engagement is attracting growing attention from scholars working on doctor-patient interactions. It refers to the condition in which patients are fully aware of their medical condition and willing to be active both in the relationship with their caregivers and towards the health care institutions. However, the operative steps necessary to achieve patient engagement have not yet been fully described. This chapter focuses on the communicative dimension of engagement. Communication is shown to be a pivotal means to improve patient self-efficacy and commitment, both fundamental components of engagement. In particular, the authors take a closer look at the process of decision making in chronic care settings, and propose a normative model to analyze and evaluate the quality of decision making in consultations. It is argued that the model can also be used as a blueprint to create training materials for clinicians.

INTRODUCTION

Chronic illnesses such as diabetes, hypertension, and asthma - just to name a few - are nowadays common occurrences in the lives of many individuals. Modern Western lifestyle and the aging population will lead, in the next decades, to an increase in the number of people suffering from chronic diseases (Visser, 2000). Chronicity imposes new challenges to the clinician-patient relationship. As chronic diseases are by nature treatable but not curable, it becomes essential for healthcare providers to engage patients in their care and promote patients' self-management and compliance to treatment in order to maintain a good health (Assal, 1999; Coleman, Austin, Brach, & Wagner, 2009; Nuño, Coleman, Bengoa, & Sauto, 2012).

DOI: 10.4018/978-1-5225-3926-1.ch055

Recently, the literature on chronic care has focused on the concept of patient engagement. Patient engagement has been generally described as a result of the relationship between patients and health care providers as they work together to "support active patient and public involvement in health and healthcare and to strengthen their influence on healthcare decisions, at both the individual and collective levels" (Coulter, 2011, p. 10). Engagement has also been described as a complex process of exchanges that occur between the patient and the health care system (Graffigna, Barello, Riva, & Bosio, 2014, p. 87), capable of producing positive psychosocial changes in patients and better quality of life (Barello & Graffigna, 2014). A recent model developed by Graffigna et al. (2014) defined patient engagement as a dynamic process, in which patients experience four phases (blackout, arousal, adhesion and eudaimonic project), each encompassing emotional, cognitive and behavioral dimensions. According to this model, engagement is the final outcome of a series of emotional, cognitive and behavioral reframing of the patient's health condition (Barello & Graffigna, 2014). Specifically, fully engaged patients are able to integrate the disease into their identity and life, manage their own care and mobilize healthcare services proactively if needed. As characterized by the literature, patient engagement can be described as an emotional, cognitive and behavioral change. Patient engagement therefore implies a greater ability and motivation to solve health-related problems, the exchange of relevant information with clinicians, shared decision-making, the capacity to cope with complications and follow through with treatment (Barello & Graffigna, 2014).

In the literature, engagement has been mainly described at an individual level in terms of patient's experience and patient's behaviors. However, engagement is promoted and sustained in the verbal day-by-day interactions between the patient and the healthcare providers (Thompson, 2007). More specifically, as a process supporting a proactive role of patients regarding their own health, patient engagement is promoted in the relationships between patients and clinicians within the consultations (Charles, Gafni, & Whelan, 1997, 1999; Epstein & Street, 2011; Street, Elwyn, & Epstein, 2012).

The process of patient engagement, as proposed in the literature, seems to include at least three dimensions that can only be dealt with through communicative processes: motivation, the exchange of relevant information with clinicians, and shared decision-making (Barello & Graffigna, 2014). Several strategies have been identified for clinicians to help patients move along the process of engagement, such as offering clear information on their condition, strengthening motivation to adopt healthy lifestyles, promoting self-efficacy, reinforcing healthy behaviors, and valuing patients' responsibility towards their own health (Graffigna et al., 2014). However, little is known about what specific clinician-patient communicative behaviors could sustain engagement in clinical consultations. In this contribution, we propose the model of the deliberation dialogue (Walton & Krabbe, 1995; Walton, 2006; Walton, Toniolo, & Norman, 2014) as a tool for the analysis of clinician-patient verbal interactions that can help distinguish and assess the components of engagement-oriented dialogues within chronic care consultations.

Previous studies have taken into account different aspects of the challenge of supporting patients' engagement. The present contribution will focus on the aspects of this challenge pertaining to the dimension of verbal communication, particularly to the process of deliberation. Specifically, in this chapter we will first offer a theoretical background on the studies that have addressed the issue of communication and behavior change in chronic care. Then we will describe the model of the deliberation dialogue as a tool to deepen and specify the analysis of medical consultations, which may lead to a better understanding of the communicative processes that are relevant to achieve patient engagement and behavior change. Finally we will offer examples of the application of this model within the setting of chronic care encounters.

BACKGROUND

In this section we provide a brief overview of studies addressing the complex issue of achieving behavior change by highlighting in particular the factors that have been found to have a significant impact on commitment and task performance.

Among the vast literature on behavior change, our intention is to point out a few significant studies that are helpful to understand which are the factors at play in the complex process of eliciting and sustaining behavior change. More specifically, we will focus on those factors that are communicative in nature (e.g., information sharing) or are realized at least in part through communicative exchanges (e.g., self-efficacy). We address first the literature referring to communication and behavior change in the medical encounter and, following, a few studies that have focused on the connection between goals and commitment.

Communication and Behavior Change

The literature addressing the issue of behavior change in the medical encounter is quite concordant in stressing the pivotal role of participatory communication, collaborative goal setting and shared decision-making.

Proactive, participatory patient-provider communication styles have been acknowledged in the literature as pivotal for the improvement of patient outcomes (Lafata et al., 2013). Studies across several chronic settings - such as diabetes, hypertension, cancer and lupus - suggest that patients who are more communicatively involved in their consultations, who express their concerns and who interact with more patient-centered and informative clinicians experience better outcomes (Street et al., 1993).

Studies also suggest that the most relevant moments in constructing effective patient-provider collaboration are collaborative definition of problems, goal setting and planning (Heisler, Bouknight, Hayward, Smith, & Kerr, 2002). Heisler et al. (2003) show that patients who shared in treatment decision-making and discussed the relevant content areas with their physicians were more likely to display agreement with the physicians. Such agreement is positively correlated with health outcomes. However, it is not clear which are the factors that favor or impede patient-provider agreement on treatment goals and strategies. Moreover, it also looks like collaborative goal setting is not equally beneficial under certain conditions: if, for example, the communication exchanges do not facilitate a positive patient-clinician rapport or patients' confidence to achieve goals set during the exchange (Lafata et al., 2013).

Scholars have also highlighted the importance of involving patients in their health management through the concept of shared decision-making (Epstein & Street, 2011; Elwyn et al., 2012). Addressing more specifically the components of decision-making, Epstein and Gramling (2013) highlight the crucial role of exploring patients' preferences, which in the clinical practice are often contextual, conditional and provisional. Empirical evidence has also shown that patients involved in shared decision-making consultations, where clinicians and patients negotiated a treatment regimen that accommodated patient goals and preferences, reported better adherence and clinical outcomes than patients involved in clinician decision-making consultations (Wilson et al., 2010).

In summary, it seems that more active involvement of all participants in the consultation may achieve better results, both at the clinical level and at the level of participants' satisfaction. However, it is not clear whether this is true under all circumstances, nor how to achieve practically more participatory interaction styles. In order to answer these questions, it is probably useful to take a short detour and take into consideration a few studies from the literature on decision-making and behavior change developed since the late 1950s'.

From Goals to Commitment

Ever since the late 1950s' a growing body of studies developed, which addressed the issue of decision-making and behavior change, trying to explain the processes and factors at play in the formation of goals and in the passage from goals to intentions to actual behavior. Many of these studies suggest that behavior change can be cultivated and sustained. The question is therefore what allows to cultivate and sustain behavior change.

According to the theory of planned behavior (Ajzen, 1988, 1991, 2002; Glanz, Rimer, & Viswanath, 2008), human behavior is guided by three kinds of considerations: positive or negative attitudes towards a certain behavior, which are determined by beliefs about the likely consequences or other attributes of the behavior (behavioral beliefs); perceived social pressure, or subjective norm, which is determined by beliefs about the normative expectations of other people (normative beliefs); and perceived behavioral control, which is caused by beliefs about the presence of factors that may further or hinder performance of the behavior (control beliefs). These three elements in combination give rise to behavioral intention, which is considered to be the immediate antecedent to behavior.

In this description, intention is a concept similar to the idea of commitment, i.e. the decision to allocate resources for the achievement of a goal. However, both intention and commitment need to be triggered and supported through time, especially if the aim is to move from a temporary behavior change to consistent new behaviors (such as is the goal of chronic care, when it comes to the issue of patients' lifestyles) (Becker, 1960; Prochaska, Di Clemente, & Norcross, 1992).

Among the relevant dimensions to take into consideration in order to understand the strength of commitment is the system of values in which individuals form their decisions (Becker, 1960), which is the underlying system that sustains the formation of preferences (Boyd et al., 2012, pp. 32-33). It can sometimes happen that individuals express preferences that deviate from their value system. This happens especially in cases of uncertainty and lack of correct or complete information (Epstein & Gramling, 2013, p. 102S).

Other studies discuss how much the process of goal-setting can impact on task performance. Specifically, studies found that the quality of goal-setting can impact on performance, meaning that goal specificity makes a difference in how a task is carried out (Baca-Motes, Brown, Gneezy, Keenan, & Nelson, 2013). Also the degree of self-efficacy was found to have an impact on goal-setting, so that when the goals are self-set, people with higher self-efficacy will set higher goals, will be more committed to the set goal, find and use better strategies to reach them, and will respond better to negative feedback than people with lower self-efficacy (Locke & Latham, 2002).

Finally, participatory goal-setting does not seem to impact directly on the performance of tasks, but rather via self-efficacy. In other words, the fact that people are given the possibility to self-set their goals has an impact more at a cognitive level than at the motivational one, because it stimulates the exchange of information. Exchanging information appears to be an important element in the quality of performance, because in a number of experiments people who could *self-set* their goals performed much better than people who had been *assigned* goals *only* in the cases in which the latter had received no explanations regarding the goals, i.e. when there had been no exchange of relevant information regarding the goals.

This leads to believe that one relevant component of self-efficacy is having relevant information and training regarding the problem and possible solutions to it (Locke & Latham, 2002).

Summing up and considering only the factors that are relevant on the communicative level: goal specificity; self-setting goals or having goals assigned together with explanations about them; and, information exchanges seem to be pivotal elements around which decision-making develops and, with it, commitment and behavior change. These factors indicate a procedural hierarchy in the steps that lead from the formation of a goal to consistent behavior. First, a value system seems to be the context within which goals are defined according to evaluations of situations or hypothesized outcomes of an action (Becker, 1960). For example, I might decide to stop smoking because I consider good health to be a high value; on the contrary, my friend might refuse to do the same, because she values more highly the pleasure that smoking can give her. Second, self-efficacy seems to play a significant role for the process of goal-setting, for the degree of commitment once the goal has been set or assigned, and for the quality of the effort a person will put into achieving it. One relevant component of self-efficacy seems to be the possession of adequate information to understand the issue at hand, the goal and the resources needed to achieve it. This should also be relevant for the definition of attitudes and perceived behavioral control (Ajzen, 2002). Finally, the possibility to set one's own goals – as opposed to having goals assigned – seems to be more effective only if there is a high degree of self-efficacy.

Open Problems and Possible Pathways to Solutions

The discussion conducted in the previous sections has helped us define more clearly the problem we are addressing: two elements at the core of patient engagement are information sharing and shared decision-making between clinicians and patients. Indeed, literature indicates that better health outcomes are obtained when values and information are shared and specific goals are assigned, or set. These are goals that can be reached through verbal communication, but it is necessary to be able to characterize the dialogical dimension of information sharing and decision-making in order to plan interventions. Therefore it is crucial to proceed from an adequate theoretical model, able to explain the dialogical complexity of chronic care consultations.

In what follows, we will refer to dialogue and not to communication in general because we are addressing, first of all, the dimension of *verbal communication*, and secondly, the structure of the interaction intended as a communicative action, performed with the aim to reach a precise goal and following specific steps to achieve the goal (Grice, 1975; van Eemeren & Grootendorst, 2004). Moreover, the focus of this chapter on the dialogue structure is motivated by the need to address the higher level components first, and then move into the specificities of communication strategies and techniques.

In the following sections, we will first introduce the theoretical approach to the analysis of dialogues we adopted; we will then focus on the deliberation dialogue as a specific type of dialogue, useful to better understand the dialogical process that leads to patient engagement.

DIALOGUE TYPES AND DIALOGUE PROFILES

When we talk about dialogues, we refer to communicative intentions, or aims, like information giving, or deliberation, that have the same value of the aims we have when we want to obtain something, like for example, to build a house. In both cases, we will have to initiate a chain of actions that will lead us to the achievement of the final goal. Depending on the aims that people have when they interact in different contexts, there are different dialogue types. The main dialogue types are: information-seeking, persuasion, deliberation, inquiry, negotiation, and eristics (Table 1) (Walton & Krabbe, 1995).

The single 'acts' to be performed in order to reach one of these goals are the dialogue moves within a dialogue type and they can be represented as 'profiles of dialogue': "a profile of dialogue is a connected sequence of moves and countermoves in a conversational exchange of a type that is goal-directed and can be represented in a normative model of dialogue" (Walton, 1999, p. 53). The profiles of dialogue map out the moves that are dialogically relevant in order to achieve a specific dialogical aim. The notion of *relevance* refers here to the possibilities that each move opens up for the interlocutor and that are most appropriate to reach the dialogical goal. If we look at Figure 1, the profile of an information-seeking dialogue, we notice that the first question by A opens up to B the possibility for only two alternative relevant moves: 'yes' or 'no'. Technically, no other moves (answers) are possible, unless B decided to not reply by either changing the topic ('I surely have a nice doggie') or by a meta-dialogical refusal of the question ('I don't want to talk about this now'). Reading the development of the profile in Figure 1, we could imagine a police officer interrogating a suspect for abusive behavior. The first question and the options it opens up for B are relevant in this context because the final aim of the dialogue is to gain information that will lead to the identification of the culprit. It wouldn't make much sense here to use dialogical moves that could lead, for example, to the suspect talking about his opinions on the advantages of having a spouse.

Table 1. Types of dialogue and their characteristics

Type	Initial Situation	Main Goal	Participants' Aims	Side Benefits
Persuasion Dialogue	Conflicting points of view	Resolution of such conflicts by verbal means	Persuade the other(s)	Develop and reveal positions Build up confidence Influence onlookers, Add to prestige
Negotiation	Conflict of interests & need for cooperation	Making a deal	Get the best out of it for oneself	Agreement, Build up confidence Reveal position Influence onlookers Add to prestige
Inquiry	General ignorance	Growth of knowledge & agreement	Find a "proof" or destroy one	Add to prestige Gain experience Raise funds
Deliberation	Need for action	Reach a decision	Influence outcome	Agreement Develop & reveal positions Add to prestige, Vent emotions
Information-seeking	Personal Ignorance	Spreading knowledge and revealing positions	Gain, pass on, show, or hide personal knowledge	Agreement Develop & reveal positions Add to prestige, Vent emotions
Eristics	Conflict & antagonism	Reaching a (provisional) accommodation in a relationship	Strike the other party & win in the eyes of onlookers	Agreement Develop & reveal positions Gain experience, Amusement Add to prestige, Vent emotions

(Walton & Krabbe, 1995)

Figure 1. Information seeking dialogue

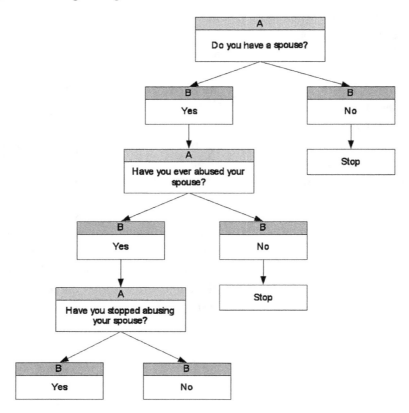

THE DELIBERATION DIALOGUE

As shown in Table 1, deliberation dialogues are abstract patterns that outline the most effective dialogical moves aimed at finding an acceptable course of action to achieve a certain goal (Walton, Atkinson, Bench-Capon, Wyner, & Cartwright, 2010; Walton, 2010). Deliberation dialogues usually take place when there is not a compelling objective way of coping with a problem and parties discuss their reasons for proposing a certain solution.

This is the first relevant feature of this dialogue type that, we think, makes it an adequate model for the analysis of decision-making in chronic care encounters (Bigi, 2014). Indeed, in these consultations the discussions that arise are not about conflicts of opinion *stricto sensu*. In other words, it is seldom the case that clinicians and patients discuss about conflicting opinions in the same way as it could happen during, for example, a dinner, when ideas, interpretations of facts, evaluations are exchanged, which do not have an objective foundation and are different, often non-exclusive, ways of interpreting phenomena.

What happens in chronic care consultations is more often that clinicians and patients may find themselves having one basic kind of discussion about what to do next, given the general health situation of the patient. While trying to answer this question, other kinds of discussions may arise, regarding: wrong or partial information patients have regarding their condition and how to cope with it; different interpretations of symptoms; criteria for preferring one course of action or another.

Secondly, the premise of deliberation dialogues is that parties are out to reach a collective goal, which can be contrary to or different from the individuals' personal goals. In the medical encounter, the patient's health can be construed as a collective goal because it is the only reason for physician and patient to come together in the interaction field of the hospital or outpatient clinic. The discussion is 'task oriented', because the final aim of the relationship between clinicians and patients is to achieve a better health for the latter. In this respect, opinions need to be evaluated against the goal of improved health. In this sense, these discussions are not the same as discussions regarding opinions in a general sense. Chronic patients accumulate lived knowledge on their disease and construct their opinions drawing from their experience and context. As patients' opinions influence their health behavior and lifestyles, it becomes important for clinicians to explore them in order to address possible reasons that support non-healthy behaviors and formulate feasible therapeutic goals. At the same time, it is important that clinicians, who have medical knowledge and more appropriate criteria for evaluation, lead the consultations and, often, the discussions arising within them.

Finally, the dialogical aim of the deliberation dialogue is particularly relevant in the care of chronic patients, where the principle of patient autonomy has partially given back to patients the decisional power regarding their own health and treatment decisions. As mentioned above, clinicians and patients often discuss health goals and treatment options taking into consideration not only clinical evidence but also patients' preferences and values that are usually co-constructed and discovered in the interaction (Truog et al., 2015).

The Structure of Deliberation Dialogues

The structure and development of deliberation dialogues are reported in Figure 2. Deliberation dialogues usually develop in three stages: the opening stage, the argumentation stage and the closing stage. In the

Figure 2. Stages of deliberation dialogue
(Walton et al., 2014)

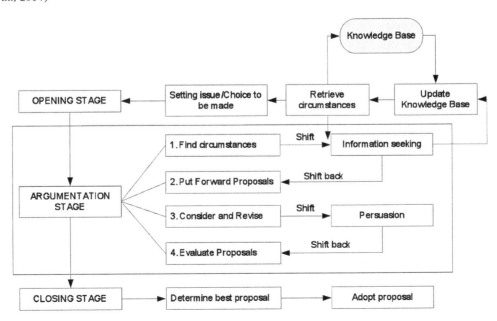

case of the medical consultation, we could consider these stages as the "communicative bricks" of the shared decision-making process. It is important to notice that the stages' names do not necessarily refer to the timeline of the consultation but rather to the communicative content discussed.

Probably the most interesting characteristic of this model, and the one that makes it particularly appropriate for our discussion, is that the deliberation dialogue is represented as a 'hybrid' dialogue, which develops through the intersection with an information seeking and a persuasion dialogue.

Opening Stage and the Role of Information Sharing

In the opening stage the parties become aware that there is a problem and a choice needs to be made (for example, that it is necessary for the patient to lose weight). A process begins in which the parties need to figure out what are the available options for action. In order to do this, they must engage in an information seeking type of dialogue, in which the final aim is to share information regarding the issue. Therefore the pattern of the information seeking dialogue comes into play almost immediately in the deliberation process.

This moment is particularly relevant for the whole deliberation process, for various reasons. When it is conducted effectively, i.e. when the dialogical moves are relevant, it allows the parties to share important information regarding the abilities of the parties to carry out an intended course of action, the values or beliefs behind choices, and any new event that might have changed the configuration of previously shared knowledge between the two. The set of information that is shared during this phase adds to the previously shared knowledge and provides the foundation for the core part of deliberation, in which the parties will put forward actual proposals for action.

The relevance of this process of information is greater than what might be imagined at first. An ongoing study on a corpus of real life interactions between clinicians and patients in an Italian diabetes care setting is revealing that when the information seeking phase is more thorough, the outcome of the deliberation process – i.e. the indication for action – becomes much more specific than in other cases (Bigi, Macagno, & Mayweg-Paus, submitted). This observation can be explained by the fact that, once the relevant information regarding options, ability and criteria for action has been shared, it is much easier for both clinicians and patients to become more specific about the behavior to follow. This finding is interesting because it is coherent with the studies on commitment and goal setting mentioned above, in which goal specificity seemed to be a moderator for commitment (Baca-Motes et al., 2013).

Another reason to stress the importance of the process of information sharing realized through the pattern of the information seeking dialogue is the impact it can have on self-efficacy. As mentioned above, self-efficacy can be bolstered by providing the interlocutor with appropriate information regarding the problem at issue (the disease) and the ways to cope with it (self-management training) (Locke & Latham, 2002). It is worthwhile to work on the strengthening of self-efficacy because it has been shown that, when the difficulty of a goal is controlled, the fact of self-setting the goal or having it assigned does not impact on the quality of performance if the level of self-efficacy is high in both cases (Locke & Latham, 2002). This is a very interesting observation for those patients who need or prefer a more paternalistic and directive relationship, i.e. those who would prefer to have goals assigned to them, rather than self-setting their own goals (Barello & Graffigna, 2014). In these cases, it looks like a well conducted information sharing phase would have the potential to make up – in terms of degree of commitment – for the less participatory style of interaction.

Argumentation Stage and Relevant Persuasion as the Key to Stronger Commitment

Once the problem is clear and relevant information has been shared, the argumentation stage begins, in which the parties actually put forward alternative proposals for the solution of the problem. In chronic care consultations, it means that the clinician and the patient start a discussion about the changes that the patient could adopt in order to achieve a health improvement.

At this point, the most important effect of having shared the information is that both parties are aware of all the circumstances that can have an impact on the proposals they make. Therefore, it will be easier to avoid proposing impossible behaviors or behaviors that the patient will refuse.

The act of proposing is the most relevant move at this stage of the deliberation and the one that calls into play the pattern of the persuasion dialogue. 'Persuasion' is intended here in a neutral sense and it refers to the act of putting forward arguments for or against a certain proposal for action with the aim of finding an agreement on the one that both satisfies the parties and reaches the aim of solving the problem identified at the beginning of the deliberation (on the acceptability of persuasion dialogue within the medical consultation, see Rubinelli, 2013).

Persuasion dialogues are made up of proposals and the arguments to support them, or counter-arguments to oppose a proposal that the interlocutor has put forward. The typical argument scheme (Walton, Reed, & Macagno, 2008) used in deliberations is the one from consequences, because the criteria for deciding on one course of action instead of another are fundamentally the positive effects (consequences) that should ensue from it. The argument from consequences, however, can be off the mark and very weak if the interlocutors do not share the same criteria for considering an outcome as positive or negative. Here, again, we notice how relevant a good information sharing at the beginning of a deliberation can be. We also find a connection with the studies mentioned previously that stress the relevance of the value system within which decisions are made in order to understand commitment (Becker, 1960).

In the argumentation stage of deliberation, clinicians may want to leave room for patients to self-set their goals if possible or desirable. As argued elsewhere (Bigi et al., 2015), asking patients to self-set their goals can even be used as a training strategy by clinicians, to exercise and develop patients' interpretive abilities and skills for self-management. In all cases, this is the stage of deliberation in which the previously shared information is translated into practical indications for action and in which patients' preferences and therapeutic goals are attuned and aligned. This is possible precisely through the combination of the information seeking and persuasion dialogues as components of the deliberation process.

Closing Stage and Patient Commitment

The closing stage, precisely because it comes last, plays a fundamental role for the effectiveness of the whole deliberation. It is at this point that the parties converge on a proposal that best fits the aims of the interaction, regardless of individual goals and desires. A patient may not desire to go on a diet, but may agree to it because during the argumentation stage the positive consequences of losing weight have effectively emerged. At the same time, a physician may want a patient to start treatment with interferon, but may agree to postpone it if the patient during the argumentation phase refused to start the treatment at that moment because of family reasons. However, as mere agreement is not enough, deliberation is effective when patients make an explicit commitment to the agreed course of action (see on this topic, Amrhein, Miller, Yahne, Palmer, & Fulcher, 2003).

APPLICATION OF DELIBERATION DIALOGUE TO CHRONIC CARE ENCOUNTERS

Given its aim, the model of deliberation dialogues can be fruitfully applied to actual clinician-patient conversations where there is a health related problem that calls for action and where there is a decision to be made. As deliberation dialogue is a theoretical model of "best practice", in actual clinical conversations it may happen that only some stages are present. For example, it may happen that the opening stage and the definition of the problem remain implicit, or that the argumentation is missing or is carried out only by one party. It can also happen that there is no closing stage, nor patient commitment. The analysis of the consultations according to the deliberation dialogue model is particularly interesting as it allows the identification of sub-optimal realizations of deliberation and therefore shared decisions within the consultations. The lack of some stages may influence the effectiveness of communication and may hinder patient engagement and adherence. The model can be used to make hypotheses regarding the dialogical components of deliberation dialogues that are more likely to have an impact on patients' commitment, thus also allowing a tentative definition of the pathways that lead from the communication styles used within the consultation to the dimensions of patient engagement and adherence.

To describe the potential of the model, in this section we discuss examples of the application of the deliberation dialogue in the field of hemophilia. Hemophilia is an inherited bleeding disorder, treated by replacing a missing protein responsible for correct coagulation by intravenous injections. The excerpts reported are taken from a set of video-recorded physician-patient consultations collected as a part of a larger multicenter study on patient adherence (Lamiani et al., 2015). The excerpts are extracted from longer check-up visits between different physicians (Md) and patients (Pt). The examples reported in the following sections show two deliberation dialogues where some stages are missing, and one complete deliberation dialogue. The phases of deliberation dialogues are indicated in the left column. The dialogues, which are reported in the right column, are sequential, unless specified.

Incomplete Argumentation and Closing Stage

In excerpt 1 (Table 2), we can observe an incomplete argumentative stage (performed only by the physician) and closing stage.

In this dialogue, we can observe an opening stage where the problem of the patient's suboptimal adherence to treatment is brought up by the physician, but the patient does not seem to be aware of its severity ("Why?"). The physician puts forward a proposal ("3.000 units twice a week") and tries to reach an early closure. As the patient's agreement ("Yes, yes") seems not an actual commitment, a new argumentative stage begins a little later, where the physician argues in favor of a behavior change without asking information regarding the reasons for the patient's non adherence. The dialogue ends without a proper closing stage in which we can find an explicit commitment from the patient. A possible reason for not achieving an effective deliberation, and therefore a closure, could be the lack of information regarding the patient's behavior (information seeking dialogue), and the lack of patient engagement in the argumentation stage.

Lack of Closing Stage

In the second excerpt (Table 3), we can observe a deliberation dialogue where the closing stage is missing.

Table 2. Incomplete argumentation and closing stage

Opening Stage	Md: What have you been doing? Pt: Why? Md: 4000 units once a week, no…stop it!
Argumentation Stage	Pt: Eh, little by little now we'll start again… Md: No, no we should do 3.000 units twice a week, always Pt: Ok
Closing Stage	Md: Do you promise me? Pt: Yes, yes, as I did before Md: Do I have to make you swear? Pt: Eh..by your head?!
Argumentation Stage	Md: No, no by *your* head… It has been proved that once a week is not enough to protect you and you risk that… Pt: …something happens… Md: Moreover, it has been proved that whoever has had such an hemorrhage is more likely to have another one, so no fooling around and no wild experiments Pt: No ok, but it has only been this time. Up until two months ago, we have always being doing the treatment Md: Now you be good, because all the rest is fine. Why should you go looking for trouble? Moreover, also your joints will benefit from it.
	Md: Now we'll let you go….did you stop by the reception for the new appointment? Pt: Yes

Table 3. Lack of a closing stage

Opening Stage	Md: Do you smoke? Pt: Something now and then Md: How much? Pt: Three cigarettes a day Md: Well, this is not "now and then"…it is regularly Pt: Well, compared to people who smoke a packet a day, for me it is now and then …. Yeah, well, you are right though…
Argumentation Stage	Md: You know, I am almost more sympathetic with people who smoke 20 cigarettes a day because it is really an addiction and it's difficult to quit… three cigarettes, you can do without them Pt: No because it is a pleasure! Md: Yes, but you can do without them Pt: Yes, yes, I mean, if I do without them I don't die…I agree…but it's a pleasure!
	Md: Did you take the pill for your pressure today? [Taking the blood pressure]

In this dialogue a problem regarding smoking is raised in the opening stage and both the physician and the patient enter the argumentation stage. In this stage it is interesting to notice that the physician and the patient share a different hierarchy of values. At the top of the physician's priorities is the patient's health and everything else is subordinated to achieving this goal; on the other hand, the patient minimizes the risks of smoking due to the pleasure of it, thus almost implying that this pleasure is more important to him than his own health. The proposals for action they put forward in the argumentation stage ("You can do without it"; "No because it is a pleasure") are based on these different hierarchies. In spite of this, the physician does not explore the reasons behind the patient's apparent disregard for his own health and the patient is not given the opportunity to self-set his goal. As the argumentation stage develops more into a dispute than a deliberation, the closing stage is avoided and the physician moves forward on an easier ground with another medical exam.

Complete Deliberation Dialogue

Excerpt 3 (Table 4) offers a good example of a complete deliberation dialogue where the physician and the patient reach a shared goal regarding the therapeutic regimen that is different from the individual goals.

In this excerpt, all the stages of the deliberation dialogue are present in the communication flow. In the opening stage, the problem regarding treatment adherence is explicitly expressed by the patient ("I am not doing the prophylaxis anymore"). Instead of immediately entering the argumentation stage, the physician explores the reasons of the patient's sub-optimal adherence engaging the patient in an information seeking dialogue ("Why? is the prophylaxis not going well?"). In the argumentative stage, the physician and the patient put forward some proposals to solve the problem and find a compromise. The physician can argue in favor of not giving up prophylaxis based on the knowledge of the patient's lifestyle. The patient is enabled to self-set his therapeutic goal, which is agreed upon by the physician. As the deliberation stage has been conducted effectively, in the closing stage we can observe the patient's commitment ("Ok, we can do like that, 3000 units twice a week").

SOLUTIONS AND RECOMMENDATIONS

As shown in the examples above, applying the model of the deliberation dialogue to chronic care consultations may help analyze the dialogical structure of the decision-making phases, identifying suboptimal realizations and indicating pathways for interventions.

One of the advantages of this model is that it seems possible to integrate it with one of the most known and used methods of analysis for medical consultations, such as the Roter Interaction Analysis System (RIAS). The RIAS takes as the minimal unit of analysis the utterance (Roter & Larson, 2002). By coding each utterance according to categories that describe the 'verbal action' performed by each speaker, the researcher is able to obtain a 'measure' of the degree of patient-centerdness of a consultation[1]. This method however does not allow to reconstruct larger inferential patterns of meaning. On the other hand,

Table 4. Complete deliberation dialogue

Opening Stage	Md: The medicine intake is good? Do you have any problems? Pt: Yes, it is good but...Doc, I am not doing the prophylaxis anymore… Md: Why? is the prophylaxis not going well? Pt: The problem is that I have few venous accesses left, so I try to preserve those I've left for when I really need them. When I see I have some bruises then I understand that that is the time for treatment Md: So let's say that you are doing a "customized" prophylaxis Pt: You got it...
Argumentation Stage	Md: Yes, I understand that you are adjusting your prophylaxis. However, you have to keep in mind that as you are not protected by the drug, then you'll end up moving less and less and you'll give up doing things. You won't feel confident to be doing anything more than what you feel sure about… So I am not saying you must do the prophylaxis three times a week, because now we know that every patient reaches his optimal regimen… however, this does not mean that the patient gives up doing the prophylaxis alltogether. Pt: So, Doc, instead of doing 3000 units three times a week, we could do 3000 units twice a week. Md: I think this is the bare minimum for a person like you who still has an active lifestyle.
Closing stage	Pt: Yes, absolutely, I need to go to work. So, ok we can do like that: 3000 units twice a week (They talk about other issues) Md: Ok, then. Shall we try to do the prophylaxis twice a week? Pt: I'll try it, Doc

an analysis of consultations performed by using the components of the deliberation dialogue allows a description of the macro-structure of the interaction (Bigi & Macagno, submitted). At this point, the two levels of analysis could be combined to gain useful insights into what kind of utterances can more successfully achieve the goal of effective deliberation. An assessment of the effectiveness of the deliberation would be supported by the patient-centerdness evaluation of the consultation obtained through the RIAS coding. This kind of integration between the analysis of the utterance level through the RIAS system and the analysis of the dialogue level through an operationalization of the model of deliberation dialogue is being developed through a joint effort between researchers at the Dept. of Linguistic Sciences of the Catholic University of Milano and colleagues at the Dept. of Health Sciences at the University of Milano, San Paolo Hospital.

From a practical point of view, the results of an analysis conducted by using the model of the deliberation dialogue could enhance the understanding and effectiveness of approaches for behavior change already used in the clinical practice.

For example, the motivational interview suggests a number of techniques to encourage active patient participation and strengthening of commitment (Burke, Arkowitz, & Menchola, 2003; Miller & Rollnick, 2002). These techniques however are not set within a description of the dialogical structure of the consultation and the appropriateness of their use is not related to specific dialogical moves nor to the larger dialogical patterns that typically occur during consultations. We believe that the value of these techniques would not be obliterated if they were observed and reconsidered within a description of the consultation obtained through the analysis conducted at the dialogical level. On the contrary, they could be more easily combined with dialogical goals and stages and become even more focused and effective.

In this sense, the structure of the deliberation dialogue could actually become the blueprint for a 'communication protocol' to conduct more effective decision-making phases and thus be used for clinicians' training. This hypothesis is currently being tested in the framework of an ongoing research project based at Milano's Catholic University (www.unicatt.it/healthyreasoning-eng).

At a more general level, the pattern of the deliberation dialogue constitutes a response to the perplexity that is sometimes expressed by clinicians, that communication skills cannot be taught because they cannot be 'standardized', given the fact that patients are all different one from the other (Bigi & Rossi, 2015). We believe this model shows very well the possibility for a 'standardized' approach able at the same time to incorporate the individual characteristics of every patient. Clinical conversations will vary depending on the information collected in the information sharing stage and the argumentation stage will focus on different arguments based on the patient's individuality.

Finally, the approach to shared decision-making based on the deliberation dialogue is compatible with the most recent formulations of patient-centered care, which values patient autonomy that is expressed in the interaction with clinicians and is not an end to itself (Duggan, Geller, Cooper, & Beach, 2006). Indeed, the ethical preoccupations of respecting patients' individuality and decisional autonomy are matched in this analytical approach with the practical preoccupation of conducting an effective consultation that will have a positive effect on patients. The patient-centered model defines the dialogical objectives of the consultation, but not the dialogical structures that can realize them. The model of the deliberation dialogue outlines the dialogical steps the parties can and should take in order to reach consensus on a behavior by foreseeing 'room' for the expression of both parties' views and reasons.

In conclusion, clinicians' training based on the structure of the deliberation dialogue could improve clinicians' effectiveness in promoting patient engagement and adherence.

FUTURE RESEARCH DIRECTIONS

Elwyn and Miron-Shatz (2009) have convincingly discussed the unsoundness of establishing correlations between the quality of decision-making practices and clinical outcomes. Instead, they argue that decision-making should be assessed based on the quality of deliberation, which ultimately means favoring the definition of the problem and the outline of the different options for its solution. Therefore, their proposal is to link the assessment of the quality of decision-making to the patient's perception about and recall of the deliberation steps. If the model of the deliberation dialogue were used as a blueprint for conducting decision-making phases within consultations, the approach proposed by Elwyn and Miron-Shatz (2009) could be used to test for better recall of and perceptions about the deliberation steps in the consultation.

Further, deliberation dialogue only offers the structural components within which an effective deliberation can occur. It does not explicitly suggest specific communication skills that can be used to achieve the single stages of deliberation dialogues. It should be paired with existing approaches based on specific communication skills in order to create comprehensive and usable training materials for clinicians.

Finally, we know from the literature that, beyond communication skills, relational qualities, such as curiosity, respect, emotional availability and partnership, are essential for a good clinician-patient relationship (Lamiani, Barello, Browning, Vegni, & Meyer, 2012), especially in the field of chronic care where clinicians build long-term relationship with their patients. These qualities are often conveyed by clinicians through the tone of voice, intonation, and non-verbal communication, more than specific words. For this reason, future research could explore the emotional tone of deliberation dialogues in chronic care by assessing whether or not the global degree of affect of the clinician leading the conversation (e.g. dominance, friendliness, respectfulness, interest, anger etc.) impacts on effective deliberation and patient outcomes.

CONCLUSION

The chapter has taken into consideration the concept of patient engagement from the point of view of its dialogical component. Patient engagement refers to a status in which individuals are willing to behave in active and responsible ways with regard to the management of their health conditions. Such status can be fostered, improved and maintained in particular by conscious efforts on the part of clinicians within the boundaries of the medical consultations. It is, however, a complex condition that is achieved by attuning the cognitive, emotional and behavioral levels. Studies on patient engagement are at an early stage and we do not have yet a full-fledged description of the components that contribute to supporting and improving patient engagement. Especially at a practical level, there is still lack of specific and evidence based indications to guide interventions and training for clinicians.

One factor that has been described as fundamental for the achievement of patient engagement is effective communication between clinicians and patients. Moreover, the condition of being fully engaged requires that patients change their attitudes and behaviors with regard to the management of their health, and this is particularly true for chronic conditions. The relevance of the communicative dimension in relation to behavior change calls into play interdisciplinary competences, which are necessary to analyze in particular the dialogical structure and dynamics within the consultation.

In this chapter, we have focused on shared decision-making in chronic care consultations, considered as a pivotal moment for the achievement of patient engagement. We have proposed to consider the dialogical structure of decision-making by the adoption of a normative model – the model of the deliberation dialogue – which was developed within the research field of Argumentation Theory and has already been applied in the domain of AI. This model formalizes the dialogical intention of deliberation through the dialogical moves that are considered the most effective to reach consensus on a solution to a problem. This kind of dialogue seems to be particularly frequent in chronic care setting, where consultations often have the aim to support motivation for behavior change or to find agreement on a therapeutic prescription. In the chapter, the model has been presented on the backdrop of its theoretical setting and explained in its fundamental features. Three examples have been provided to show the analytical potential of this model to guide the scholar to identify suboptimal realizations of decision-making phases in the consultation. It has also been argued that the results of such analyses could be well integrated with results from more traditional analyses of consultations, such as the RIAS coding. Moreover, the same results could be used to improve our understanding and use of techniques such as the ones proposed within the framework of the motivational interview.

We believe that this model is an effective tool for the analysis of real life cases and to provide evidence that could support the design and implementation of interventions to improve clinicians' decision-making skills.

REFERENCES

Ajzen, I. (1988). *Attitudes, personality, and behavior*. Chicago, IL: Dorsey.

Ajzen, I. (1991, December). (1991). The theory of planned behavior. *Organizational Behavior and Human Decision Processes*, *50*(2), 179–211. doi:10.1016/0749-5978(91)90020-T

Ajzen, I. (2002). Perceived Behavioral Control, Self-Efficacy, Locus of Control, and the Theory of Planned Behavior. *Journal of Applied Social Psychology*, *32*(4), 665–683. doi:10.1111/j.1559-1816.2002.tb00236.x

Amrhein, P. C., Miller, W. R., Yahne, C. E., Palmer, M., & Fulcher, L. (2003). Client Commitment Language During Motivational Interviewing Predicts Drug Use Outcomes. *Journal of Consulting and Clinical Psychology*, *71*(5), 862–878. doi:10.1037/0022-006X.71.5.862 PMID:14516235

Assal, J. P. (1999). Revisiting the approach to treatment of long-term illness: From the acute to the chronic state. A need for educational and managerial skills for long-term follow-up. *Patient Education and Counseling*, *37*(2), 99–111. doi:10.1016/S0738-3991(98)00109-8 PMID:14528538

Baca-Motes, K., Brown, A., Gneezy, A., Keenan, E. A., & Nelson, L. D. (2013). Commitment and Behavior Change: Evidence from the Field. *The Journal of Consumer Research*, *39*(5), 1070–1084. doi:10.1086/667226

Barello, S., & Graffigna, G. (2014). Engaging patients to recover life projectuality: an Italian cross-disease framework. *Quality of Life Research,* 24(5), 1087-1096. doi:10.1007/s11136-014-0846-x

Becker, H. S. (1960). Notes on the Concept of Commitment. *American Journal of Sociology*, *66*(1), 32–40. doi:10.1086/222820

Bigi, S. (2014). Key components of effective collaborative goal setting in the chronic care encounter. *Communication & Medicine*, *11*(2), 103–115. doi:10.1558/cam.v11i2.21600 PMID:26596119

Bigi, S., & Macagno, F. (Manuscript submitted for publication). From types of dialogue to dialogue moves - The case of doctor-patient interaction as a communicative practice. *Discourse Processes*.

Bigi, S., Macagno, F., & Mayweg-Paus, L. (Manuscript submitted for publication). Medical consultation as a type of dialogical practice. *Patient Education and Counseling*.

Bigi, S., & Rossi, M. G. (2015). Comunicare (nel)la cronicità [Communicating (within) chronic care]. *MeDIA. Aggiornamento e Formazione in Diabetologia e Malattie Metaboliche, 15*(3).

Bigi, S., Rossi, M. G., Barello, S., Graffigna, G., Mulas, M. F., & Musacchio, N. (2015). *Speaking wisely: pratiche dialogiche appropriate in diabetologia* [Speaking wisely: appropriate dialogical practices in diabetes care]. Paper presented at XX Congresso Nazionale AMD, L'Evoluzione della Diabetologia alla luce del Piano Nazionale Diabete, Genova, Italy.

Boyd, C. M., Singh, S., Varadhan, R., Weiss, C. O., Sharma, R., Bass, E. B., & Puhan, M. A. (2012). *Methods for Benefit and Harm Assessment in Systematic Reviews. Methods Research Report. (Prepared by the Johns Hopkins University Evidence-based Practice Center under contract No. 290-2007-10061-I). AHRQ Publication No. 12(13)-EHC150-EF*. Rockville, MD: Agency for Healthcare Research and Quality.

Burke, B. L., Arkowitz, H., & Menchola, M. (2003). The efficacy of motivational interviewing: A meta-analysis of controlled clinical trials. *Journal of Consulting and Clinical Psychology, 71*(5), 843–861. doi:10.1037/0022-006X.71.5.843 PMID:14516234

Charles, C., Gafni, A., & Whelan, T. (1997). Shared decision-making in the medical encounter: What does it mean? (or it takes at least two to tango). *Social Science & Medicine, 44*(5), 681–692. doi:10.1016/S0277-9536(96)00221-3 PMID:9032835

Charles, C., Gafni, A., & Whelan, T. (1999). Decision-making in the physician-patient encounter: Revisiting the shared treatment decision-making model. *Social Science & Medicine, 49*(5), 651–661. doi:10.1016/S0277-9536(99)00145-8 PMID:10452420

Coleman, K., Austin, B. T., Brach, C., & Wagner, E. H. (2009). Evidence On The Chronic Care Model In The New Millennium. *Health Affairs, 28*(1), 75–85. doi:10.1377/hlthaff.28.1.75 PMID:19124857

Coulter, A. (2011). *Engaging patients in healthcare*. New York: McGraw-Hill Education.

Duggan, P. S., Geller, G., Cooper, L. A., & Beach, M. C. (2006). The moral nature of patient-centeredness: Is it "just the right thing to do"? *Patient Education and Counseling, 62*(2), 271–276. doi:10.1016/j.pec.2005.08.001 PMID:16356677

Elwyn, G., Frosch, D., Thomson, R., Joseph-Williams, N., Lloyd, A., Kinnersley, P., & Barry, M. et al. (2012). Shared Decision-making: A Model for Clinical Practice. *Journal of General Internal Medicine, 27*(10), 1361–1367. doi:10.1007/s11606-012-2077-6 PMID:22618581

Elwyn, G., & Miron-Shatz, T. (2009). Deliberation before determination: The definition and evaluation of good decision-making. *Health Expectations, 13*(2), 139–147. doi:10.1111/j.1369-7625.2009.00572.x PMID:19740089

Epstein, R., & Street, R. L. (2011). Shared Mind: Communication, Decision-making, and Autonomy in Serious Illness. *Annals of Family Medicine, 9*(5), 454–461. doi:10.1370/afm.1301 PMID:21911765

Epstein, R. M., & Gramling, R. E. (2013). What is shared in shared decision-making? Complex decisions when the evidence is unclear. *Medical Care Research and Review. Supplement to, 70*(1), 94S–112S.

Glanz, K., Rimer, B. K., & Viswanath, K. (2008). *Health Behavior and Health Education: Theory, Research, and Practice* (4th ed.). San Francisco: Jossey-Bass.

Graffigna, G., Barello, S., Riva, G., & Bosio, A. C. (2014). Patient engagement: The key to redesign the exchange between the demand and supply for healthcare in the era of active ageing. In G. Riva, P. Ajmone Marsan, & C. Grassi. (Eds.), Active Ageing and Healthy Living (pp. 85-95). Amsterdam: IOS Press.

Grice, H. P. (1975). Logic and conversation. In P. Cole & J. L. Morgan (Eds.), Syntax and Semantics (Vol. 3, pp. 41-58). New York: Academic Press.

Heisler, M., Bouknight, R. R., Hayward, R. A., Smith, D. M., & Kerr, E. A. (2002). The relative importance of physician communication, participatory decision-making, and patient understanding in diabetes self-management. *Journal of General Internal Medicine, 17*(4), 243–252. doi:10.1046/j.1525-1497.2002.10905.x PMID:11972720

Heisler, M., Vijan, S., Anderson, R. M., Ubel, P. A., Bernstein, S. J., & Hofer, T. P. (2003). When do patients and their physicians agree on diabetes treatment goals and strategies, and what difference does it make? *Journal of General Internal Medicine, 18*(11), 893–902. doi:10.1046/j.1525-1497.2003.21132.x PMID:14687274

Lafata, J. E., Morris, H. L., Dobie, E., Heisler, M., Werner, R. M., & Dumenci, L. (2013). Patient-reported use of collaborative goal setting and glycemic control among patients with diabetes. *Patient Education and Counseling, 92*(1), 94–99. doi:10.1016/j.pec.2013.01.016 PMID:23433777

Lamiani, G., Barello, S., Browning, D. M., Vegni, E., & Meyer, E. C. (2012). Uncovering and validating clinicians' experiential knowledge when facing difficult conversations: A cross-cultural perspective. *Patient Education and Counseling, 87*(3), 307–312. doi:10.1016/j.pec.2011.11.012 PMID:22196987

Lamiani, G., Strada, I., Mancuso, M. E., Coppola, A., Vegni, E., & Moja, E. A. (2015). Factors influencing illness representations and perceived adherence in haemophilic patients: A pilot study. *Haemophilia, 21*(5), 598–604. doi:10.1111/hae.12654 PMID:25684356

Locke, E. A., & Latham, G. P. (2002). Building a practically useful theory of goal setting and task motivation. *The American Psychologist, 57*(9), 705–717. doi:10.1037/0003-066X.57.9.705 PMID:12237980

Miller, W., & Rollinck, S. (2002). *Motivational interviewing: preparing people to change*. New York: Guilford Press.

Nuño, R., Coleman, K., Bengoa, R., & Sauto, R. (2012). Integrated care for chronic conditions: The contribution of the ICCC Framework. *Health Policy (Amsterdam), 105*(1), 55–64. doi:10.1016/j.healthpol.2011.10.006 PMID:22071454

Ong, L. M. L., Visser, M. R. M., Kruyver, I. P. M., Bensing, J. M., Van Den Brink-Muinen, A., Stouthard, J. M. L., & De Haes, J. C. J. M. et al. (1998). The Roter Interaction Analysis System (RIAS) in oncological consultations: Psychometric properties. *Psycho-Oncology, 7*(5), 387–401. doi:10.1002/(SICI)1099-1611(1998090)7:5<387::AID-PON316>3.0.CO;2-G PMID:9809330

Prochaska, J. O., Di Clemente, C. C., & Norcross, J. C. (1992). In search of how people change. Applications to addictive behaviors. *The American Psychologist, 47*(9), 1102–1114. doi:10.1037/0003-066X.47.9.1102 PMID:1329589

Roter, D. L. (2002). *The Roter Method for Interaction Process Analysis*. RIAS Manual.

Roter, D. L., & Larson, S. (2002). The Roter interaction analysis system (RIAS): Utility and flexibility for analysis of medical interactions. *Patient Education and Counseling, 46*(4), 243–251. doi:10.1016/S0738-3991(02)00012-5 PMID:11932123

Rubinelli, S. (2013). Rational versus unreasonable persuasion in doctor-patient communication: A normative account. *Patient Education and Counseling, 92*(3), 296–301. doi:10.1016/j.pec.2013.06.005 PMID:23830240

Street, R. L. Jr. (2013). How clinician-patient communication contributes to health improvement: Modeling pathways from talk to outcome. *Patient Education and Counseling, 92*(3), 286–291. doi:10.1016/j.pec.2013.05.004 PMID:23746769

Street, R. L., Elwyn, G., & Epstein, R. (2012). Patient preferences and health care outcomes: An ecological perspective. *Expert Review of Pharmacoeconomics & Outcomes Research, 12*(2), 167–180. doi:10.1586/erp.12.3 PMID:22458618

Street, R. L., Piziak, V. K., Carpentier, W. S., Herzog, J., Hejl, J., Skinner, G., & McLellan, L. (1993). Provider-patient communication and metabolic control. *Diabetes Care, 16*(5), 714–721. doi:10.2337/diacare.16.5.714 PMID:8495610

Thompson, A. G. H. (2007). The meaning of patient involvement and participation in health care consultations: A taxonomy. *Social Science & Medicine, 64*(6), 1297–1310. doi:10.1016/j.socscimed.2006.11.002 PMID:17174016

Truog, R. D., Brown, S. D., Browning, D., Hundert, E. M., Rider, E. A., Bell, S. K., & Meyer, E. C. (2015). Microethics: The ethics of everyday clinical practice. *The Hastings Center Report, 45*(1), 11–17. doi:10.1002/hast.413 PMID:25600383

van Eemeren, F. H., & Grootendorst, R. (2004). *A systematic theory of argumentation*. Cambridge, MA: Cambridge University Press.

Visser, A. (2000). Chronic diseases, aging, and dementia: Implications for patient education and counseling. *Patient Education and Counseling, 39*(2-3), 293–309. doi:10.1016/S0738-3991(99)00002-6

Walton, D. (1999). Profiles of Dialogue for Evaluating Arguments from Ignorance. *Argumentation, 13*(1), 53–71. doi:10.1023/A:1007738812877

Walton, D. (2006). How to make and defend a proposal in a deliberation dialogue. *Artificial Intelligence and Law, 14*(3), 177–239. doi:10.1007/s10506-006-9025-x

Walton, D. (2010). Types of dialogues and burdens of proof. In P. Baroni, F. Cerutti, M. Giacomin, & G. R. Simari (Eds.). *Computational Models of Argument: Proceedings of COMMA 2010* (13-24). Amsterdam: IOS Press.

Walton, D., Atkinson, K., Bench-Capon, T., Wyner, A., & Cartwright, D. (2010). Argumentation in the framework of deliberation dialogue. In C. Bjola, & M. Kornprobst (Eds.), *Arguing Global Governance* (pp. 201-230). London: Routledge.

Walton, D., & Krabbe, E. (1995). *Commitment in Dialogue: Basic Concepts of Interpersonal Reasoning.* Albany, NY: State University of New York Press.

Walton, D., Reed, C., & Macagno, F. (2008). *Argumentation Schemes.* Cambridge, MA: Cambridge University Press. doi:10.1017/CBO9780511802034

Walton, D., Toniolo, A., & Norman, T. (2014). Missing phases of deliberation dialogue for real applications. *Proceedings of the 11th International Workshop on Argumentation in Multi-Agent Systems,* 1-20.

Wilson, S. R., Strub, P., Buist, A. S., Knowles, S. B., Lavori, P. W., Lapidus, J., & Vollmer, W. M. (2010). Shared treatment decision making improves adherence and outcomes in poorly controlled asthma. *American Journal of Respiratory and Critical Care Medicine*, *181*(6), 566–577. doi:10.1164/rccm.200906-0907OC PMID:20019345

KEY TERMS AND DEFINITIONS

Adherence: Extent to which the patient's behavior (e.g. taking medicines, following healthy lifestyles, attending the check-ups) coincides with the recommendations shared with clinicians.

Chronic Care: Care of patients who suffer from chronic diseases. Chronic diseases are treatable, but not curable. They usually have a slow onset, a progressive development and require a complex treatment. When not managed correctly, they can cause acute episodes. On the other hand, badly treated acute conditions may develop into chronic ones.

Deliberation Dialogue: Type of dialogue pattern that takes place when there is a situation that calls for action and the parties aim to reach an optimal collective decision. It is characterized by the combination between the information seeking and the persuasion dialogues.

Dialogical Move: Any of the minimal meaningful units of a dialogue, which contribute to the achievement of the dialogue's aim.

Goal Setting: The specific phase during decision-making in which, after collecting information on the patient's health, it is necessary to decide on the best therapy and behaviors the patient should follow until the next visit.

Patient Engagement: It refers to the condition in which patients have integrated their disease into their identity and are active participants both in the relationship with their caregivers and towards the health care institutions.

Patient-Centered Care: Model of care that takes into account both the patient's disease and the illness experience (e.g. feelings, expectations, interpretations and context). The patient-centered clinical method indicates the communicative aims useful to achieve a patient-centered care.

Persuasion: Used here as a general term to refer to the process of presenting arguments in favor of or against a certain standpoint, also referred to as 'argumentation'. There can be different kinds of persuasion; what usually takes place within medical consultations is not a truth-oriented kind of persuasion process, but rather a pragmatic one, aimed at grounding the acceptability of an opinion on the benefits that can be derived from it.

Shared Decision-Making: Within the healthcare setting, it indicates the process to follow in order to come to a shared decision on therapies and lifestyles. In its early definitions, shared decision-making implied a physician providing medical information and a patient sorting out that information and making choices based on his/her values and preferences. More recent approaches consider it as a process in which both the criteria for choice and decisions are co-constructed in the consultation via a sharing of information and preferences. These recent approaches do not consider physicians as neutral individuals, with no preferences nor biases. Because of this, shared decision-making phases should first of all favor the discussion and sharing of values and preferences before decisions are outlined and assessed.

ENDNOTES

[1]   The RIAS assigns each utterance to a predefined category. Physician communication is classified according to 34 categories, while patient communication to 28. Examples of categories are: Gives information – medical condition; Empathy statements; Asks for opinion (physician only) (Roter, 2002; Ong et al., 1998).

This research was previously published in Transformative Healthcare Practice through Patient Engagement edited by Guendalina Graffigna, pages 66-92, copyright year 2017 by Medical Information Science Reference (an imprint of IGI Global).

Section 5
Organizational and Social Implications

Chapter 56

Management of Tacit Knowledge and the Issue of Empowerment of Patients and Stakeholders in the Health Care Sector

Marc Jacquinet
Universidade Aberta, Portugal

Henrique Curado
Politécnico do Porto, Portugal & Universidade do Minho, Portugal

Ângela Lacerda Nobre
Instituto Politécnico de Setúbal, Portugal

Maria José Sousa
Algarve University, Portugal

Marco Arraya
Universidade Aberta, Portugal

Rui Pimenta
Politécnico do Porto, Portugal

António Eduardo Martins
Universidade Aberta, Portugal

ABSTRACT

There is a growing literature on health and health care dedicated to empowerment of patients; but there is still a gap in the literature to conceptualize knowledge, to extend the discussion of the empowerment of the patients to the stakeholders. The discussion is at the level of managerial processes of empowerment and knowledge management related to health care. The present chapter starts with a review on empowerment, especially focused on the health sector. The following sections will develop a critical analysis

DOI: 10.4018/978-1-5225-3926-1.ch056

of empowerment, mainly around the concept of tacit knowledge (Polanyi) and knowledge management. One key variable is the proximity of the actors involved in the empowerment process. This key variable is very much related to the tacitness issue of knowledge production and flows. The chapter extends the discussion of the empowerment of the patients to that of the stakeholders and the general debate about health literacy. A model is briefly described for the purpose of illustrating the learning process in a knowledge management implemented in health care.

INTRODUCTION

The recent transformations in the economy and society are often referred to as the knowledge economy, the information society or even the knowledge society (Amin & Cohendet, 2004; Amin & Roberts, 2008; Antonelli, Foray, Hall, & Steinmueller, 2006; Carayannis, Pirzadeh, & Popescu, 2011; De la Mothe & Foray, 2001; Foray, 2010; Kahin & Foray, 2006; Lam, 2000). These transformations impact most sectors; and health care is no exception. It is a major provider of knowledge-intensive services that are going through a rather swift adoption of new information systems and knowledge management processes that parallel the concomitant emergence of new management models (J. Birkinshaw, 2010; Julian Birkinshaw, Hamel, & Mol, 2008; Julian Birkinshaw, Nobel, & Ridderstråle, 2002; Raisch & Birkinshaw, 2008). Related to these issues –in public policies, social action and management– the notion of empowerment has spread widely. Now, as discussed here, it is affecting health care models, institutions, businesses and management as much as the structuration and the organization of the whole sector.

Concepts, Context, and Issues

There is a growing literature on health and health care dedicated to empowerment of patients. There is, however, no explicit research on the tacit dimension of the knowledge management of the empowerment process of patients, health care organizations and institutions. There is also a need to clarify the principles for good knowledge management applied in the health care sector; and this is especially true if it goes beyond the implementation of information systems solutions that are only part of the response necessary to tackle the problems of today. Our objective here is to tackle that gap in the literature and to extend the discussion of the empowerment of the patients to the stakeholders more or less concerned or involved with health care. The discussion is at the level of managerial processes of empowerment and the knowledge management aspects of health care provided and organized by professionals for the wellbeing of patients. The authors in this chapter relate empowerment to the issue of health literacy.

The issue of empowerment relates obviously to the notion of health promotion, used by the World Health Organization (WHO) (1986) of the United Nations and is implemented as a guiding principle for many countries around the world (Catford, 2011; Potvin & Jones, 2011). This is an important issue not just for knowledge management specialists and scholars but also for public health and policy makers (Baba, Kearns, McIntosh, Tannahill, & Lewsey, 2016; Banerjee & Duflo, 2008; Bowen & Lawler III, 1992; Brandstetter et al., 2015; Brandstetter, McCool, Wise, & Loss, 2014; Crawford Shearer, 2009; McLaughlin, 2003, 2016; Rappaport, 1985; Wiggins, 2012; Williams, 2016; Marc A. Zimmerman, 2000; Marc A Zimmerman & Rappaport, 1988).

Empowerment can be seen as a way of managing knowledge in specific groups, organizations or sectors, such as the health sector – e.g., the national or regional health systems. Empowerment, broadly construed, is an ancient concept, not just in management but in community development, military organizations, public administration, public policies, and not to mention the associations and religious orders and congregations (McLaughlin, 2016; Rappaport, 1985; Marc A. Zimmerman, 2000; Marc A Zimmerman & Rappaport, 1988). It is, however, of a more recent facture in its modern sense. Although the concept is not new, its *emergence* and *widespread use,* in its modern form, is relatively recent, dating from the 1960s and the 1990s respectively (Carlisle, 2000; McLaughlin, 2016; Nutbeam, 2000, 2008).

There is, nevertheless, still a great lack of studies on knowledge management in health care, and, even more obviously, about empowerment in relation to health issues (Baba et al., 2016; Berkman, Kawachi, & Glymour, 2014; Crondahl & Eklund Karlsson, 2016; Downey, Curado, & Jacquinet, 2016; Karamitri, Talias, & Bellali, 2015; Lam, 2000; MacDonald, 2003; McLaughlin, 2016; Tengland, 2008).

Most studies on the health sector envision a more technological view and functional emphasis of knowledge management that ignore the specificities of the health sector and the broader management issues concerned with information and decision making. In other words, it has to do with management processes, including corporate planning and public policies, strategies and decisions made both at the macro and the micro-levels of the system.

A Preliminary Discussion of the Issue of Knowledge in Health Care

Our discussion of empowerment, in healthcare, is related to health information, health literacy and the logic of knowledge management, i. e., both the vision and the practice. In other words, it goes through the whole spectrum from functional health literacy to critical health literacy (Nutbeam 2000). It is important to mention here that in the specialized literature there is a parallelism or strong association between health literacy and health empowerment (Crondahl & Eklund Karlsson, 2016; Kostenius & Hertting, 2016; Mårtensson & Hensing, 2012; Nutbeam, 2008; Porr, Drummond, & Rishter, 2006).

There are some aspects of knowledge management, namely its imprecision, contradiction and often flawed conceptions of what knowledge is (all about) that are necessary to investigate further. We will study it in greater details in sections two through six below. But before that, it is convenient to tackle a certain number of issues related to knowledge conception, knowledge management and health and health care.

First of all, the notion of knowledge is problematic, not just in the philosophical literature but also in the management literature, not to mention the knowledge management specialization. The problematic nature of knowledge is not new and is even a common feature across all disciplinary borders (Frodeman, 2010; Legendre, 1983, 1996, 2001; Rosenthal & Gutas, 1970).

It is here convenient to make a criticism of traditional or mainstream knowledge management literature, namely Nonaka's model (Ijukiro Nonaka, 1988; Ikujiro Nonaka, 1991, 1994; I Nonaka & H Takeuchi, 1995; Ikujiro Nonaka & Hirotaka Takeuchi, 1995; Ikujiro Nonaka, Toyama, & Konno, 2000; Spender, 1996; Von Krogh, Nonaka, & Ichijo, 2000), that considers knowledge and knowledge processes in management practice or in the implementation of public policies as being too poor or flawed, and lacking evidence (Stephen Gourlay, 2006; S Gourlay & Nurse, 2005). This is in stark contrast with the literature on health and social psychology (Bandura, 1986a, 1986b) that stress the "complex relationships between knowledge, beliefs, and perceived social norms, and provide practical guidance on the content of educational programs to promote behavioural change…" (Nutbeam, 2000: 260).

This is why, in section five, the model based on the tools and concepts from Nonaka and collaborators is adapted to the peculiarities of the health sector. It has to be considered as a heuristic model to help shape practice locally and develop communities of practice in a trial and error fashion and not a descriptive functional model. In this sense it is just a first step to be improved as stakeholders and actors gain experience in the making of knowing, knowledge sharing and interactions.

Too much related to a certain kind of management culture, it used flawed concepts (Dreiling & Becker, 2007; Montuori, 2003; Alexander Styhre, 2003; A. Styhre, 2003; Tsoukas, 2016) and could be indeed clarified and sometimes simplified (Alvesson, 2001; Alvesson & Kärreman, 2001; Alvesson & Sveningsson, 2015), and this is a partial aim of this chapter focused on health literacy and empowerment.

Accordingly, the present chapter will tackle the issue of empowerment and health literacy from a knowledge management focus, leaving aside important issues such as power, power relations, public policies – either social or health, and identity (Alexander, Schallert, & Hare, 1991; Haugaard, 2012). For all these issues we refer to the vast literature already published (Alexander et al., 1991; Haugaard, 2012).

The present chapter will start with a review of the literature on empowerment, especially focused on the health sector and the health providers of health care. The following sections will develop a critical analysis of empowerment, mainly around the concept of tacit knowledge (Polanyi, 1958, 1962, 1966) and knowledge management. One key variable is the proximity of the actors involved in the empowerment process. This key variable is very much related to the tacitness issue of knowledge production and flows.

After considering some limited conceptual issues (section 1), some limitations of empowerment theory (section 2), and the tacit dimension in health care (section 3) we will extend the notion of empowerment to a broader set of stakeholders, and not just patients as object of empowerment policy (section 4).

The chapter extends the discussion of the empowerment of the patients to that of the stakeholders and the general debate about health literacy. In the last two parts of the chapter we will discuss a model for knowledge management in health care (section 5) and discuss the prospects for the future (section 6). Some conclusions and trends to consider in the near future and suggestions for further research and policy action will be presented at the end of the chapter.

EMPOWERMENT THEORY AND APPLICATTIONS TO HEALTH SECTOR

The notion of empowerment in health is very much related to health literacy, health information, and, more recently, to electronic health record (HER) or online portals and databases, and other aspects of the relationship between the patient and the doctor, surgeon or nurse, in brief, the professionals, and this has been casted in terms of the institutionalized knowledge management.

We will not discuss deeply the nature of the relationships between patients and doctors or surgeons for the sake of the present chapter objectives. It is however important to highlight just one aspect that is central to empowerment: the asymmetrical position between the patient and the doctor with respect to knowledge and not just information. It is indeed one of incomplete information, ignorance and uncertainty (Loasby, 1976, 1999).

But here, it is not just the doctor that knows more about the patient health, at least he or she can better interpret the raw data of information, exams, and output from devices than the patient. On the other hand, the patient is or could be more knowledgeable than the doctor, especially about his past and what he did or did not do. Both can know more than they could or would like to tell. But both can also transmit tacit knowledge more than he or she might be aware of.

It is also tantamount to note that patients today not only knows more than those in the past but also are more connected to information and online portals. They are more knowledgeable of current problems, new treatments, debates and secondary or undesired effects of interventions and news coverage. And health professionals are sensitive to these issues, above all when online interactions and social network can amplify certain pieces of information, trends or concerns.

We will come back to some of the tacit dimensions of the relation between the patient and the doctor but also across the whole spectrum of the relationships between patients, health professionals, managers, policy-makers, and the stakeholders (see section 3 and 6). Before that it is important to clarify health promotion on two counts: health literacy and the Ottawa Charter.

Health Promotion and Health Literacy

The three levels of health literacy (Nutbeam, 2000, 2008) can be extended to the notion of empowerment, because both are conceived as proximate concepts and practices (Baba et al., 2016; Banerjee & Duflo, 2008; Brandstetter et al., 2015; Crondahl & Eklund Karlsson, 2016; Cyril, Smith, & Renzaho, 2015; Kostenius & Hertting, 2016; McMillan & Worth, 2015; Rappaport, 1985; Rodwell, 1996; Tengland, 2008; Marc A. Zimmerman, 2000).

The first level of empowerment is the functional health literacy or the most basic component with a focus on factual information. It is typically represented by flyers, folders and information given to the patient on a variety of subjects related to health care, from access, and post intervention recovery, to precautionary behavior (Nutbeam, 2000). It is not limited to information sharing, however; yet, this is its main component. This is related to the more basic concept of literacy focusing on knowledge and information transmission but not much emphasizing on action and management.

The second level of empowerment is called the interactive health literacy that promotes self help as well as the seizing of opportunities to develop individual skills. The focus here is the individual, her or his attitude and behavior. It is also more time oriented, meaning to help change individual perceptions, attitudes and knowledge (Adam, 2004).

Finally, the third level, the critical health literacy, is characterized by a focus on groups and context, with the provision of information on social, economic and group determinants of health and how this can lead to change, both at the individual, group and community levels (Mårtensson & Hensing, 2012; Nutbeam, 2000; WHO, 1998). This third level is the most comprehensive one, going beyond the individual as a learner and getting into matters of management, collective choice, decision and public policies.

It must be stressed that every previous level is integrated in the following one. So in the critical health literacy, we find the content of functional health literacy (such as factual information) and the interactive health literacy that tries to develop skills and characterizes the direct supportive environment. In other words, the focus is getting broader and more and more related to the different factors that have a bearing on health, and moving from the individual to the group and the collective action and policy targets.

In section 3, we will discuss the implications of that model when we take into account the relevance of tacit knowledge.

Ottawa Charter and Health Promotion

We have now to discuss some principles that orient health policies worldwide. To do this, the guidelines defined by the World Health Organization, namely and above all here, the Ottawa Charter (WHO, 1986) are the most relevant. There are other more recent agreements like the Jakarta Declaration of 2013; however they are not changing the essential of the content and objectives, they are getting more in the details. The overall goals are maintained throughout, though, often more precise and more qualified.

The principles and guidelines sketched in the Ottawa Charter connect health policy to health promotion and health literacy and, now, can be related to the empowerment in health care. Other documents are relevant too, but we will not discuss them here and the debates continue, as recently at the world conference on Health promotion organized in June 2016 in Brazil or in China later in the same year convened by the WHO or previous declarations (WHO, 1999) and studies (Catford, 2011). It is important to note that these principles are almost three decades old (Potvin & Jones, 2011). There is room for improvement, namely in terms of integration of policies, instruments and knowledge management initiatives.

The Ottawa Charter, signed in 1986, identified five main areas of action for health promotion: (1) Building healthy public policy; (2) Creating supportive environments; (3) Strengthening community action; (4) Developing personal skills; and (5) Re-orienting health care services toward prevention of illness and promotion of health (WHO 1986). These have implications for knowledge management, namely for going beyond the implementation of information systems, as the concept of informatics is well-known in the health management literature. At this point, knowledge management in health care has to be combined with public policy (see areas 1, 2, 3, and 5) at different levels, namely local or regional (see area 2 and 3). It forces knowledge management to integrate communities and environment where people live and work. This is of far reaching consequences, beyond what traditional or functional knowledge management is designed for.

Furthermore, the rather recent evidence-based approach to health promotion has been introduced to tackle several issues raised by the Ottawa Charter and the implementation of its five areas of health promotion (Juneau, Jones, McQueen, & Potvin, 2011; McQueen & Jones, 2007). The evidence-based approach is a central ingredient in the change process of health policies and the knowledge management systems and processes. This element is part and parcel of the adapted model of knowledge management in section five.

Further complication can be deducted from the fundamental conditions of health promotion: i) peace, ii) shelter, iii) education, iv) food, v) income, vi) a stable eco-system, vii) sustainable resources, viii) social justice, and equity as stated in the Ottawa Charter. We must take into account that even if the conditions are for all countries in the world, yet some of the conditions are barely met in many instances. Even in OECD countries, education, income, food and social justice and equity can be frequent problems and it turns out to be highly correlated. Those lacking food, usually lack income, education, and live in an unstable economic system. This is the problem of intersectionality (Collins, 2015; Crenshaw, 1989; Davis, Collins, & Crenshaw, 2003; Hill-Collins & Bilge, 2016). Issues of sustainable resources and pollution are of increasing concerns as well as social justice and equity, which is one of the concerns of public health and social epidemiology (Berkman et al., 2014).

Finally, the strategies of the World Health Organization in the Ottawa Charter advances three paths of action for health promotion: (1) advocate (advocacy for health) to take defense for the good health, (2) enable (for achieving greater equity), and (3) mediate (relating to the people involved in the processes). The second point – to enable – has to be related to the notion of empowerment. To empower, is it not to enable?

The Human Dimension of Empowerment and Knowledge Management

Finally, it can be very interesting, and even enlightening, at this point, to highlight the relationships of the patient with the health professionals with a citation from a philosopher of science and medicine, Georges Canguilhem and make a few comments to highlight the complexity of the matter and to reinforce our conception of knowledge management for health and health promotion:

Understood as an event in the doctor-patient relationship, healing is at first sight what the patient expects from the doctor, but not what he always obtains from him. There is thus a discrepancy between the patient's hope regarding the power that he attributes to the doctor on the grounds of the latter's knowledge and the doctor's recognition of the limits of his own efficacy. There, without doubt, lies the main reason why, of all the objects specific to medical thought, healing is the one that doctors have considered the least. Yet this is also due to the fact that the doctor perceives in healing an element of subjectivity, a reference to the beneficiary's evaluation of the process, when from his objective point of view, healing is the target of a treatment that can be validated only by a statistical survey of its results. (Georges Canguilhem, 2012: 53)

First of all, the original text, published in 1978, a classic in its own right, from which the current extract comes from, is titled "Is a Pedagogy of Healing Possible?" (G. Canguilhem, 2002) and aims at reflecting on the difficulty of healing and the learning process of the patient.

This is just the idea behind the notion of health promotion, health literacy (we can see a connection between pedagogy, learning and literacy) and empowerment. Accordingly, the second point to highlight is the difficulty of empowering the patient in the process of healing. Health and healing are here defined as capabilities (Horton, 1995; The Lancet, 2009). Indeed, as stated in a recent issue of *The Lancet*, health, following explicitly the steps of Canguilhem, is defined as "the ability to adapt" (The Lancet, 2009: 781).

Another theme is the knowledge asymmetry and the limit of knowledge. There are still other aspects of the problem of health and healing to note. In the following extract it is important to highlight the issue of responsibility, the expectations and vision of the doctor and the patient and their divergent paths at some point in time:

And without making a disparaging comparison to those laughable doctors who would make their patients bear responsibility for therapeutic failure, it has to be acknowledged that the absence of healing in one patient or another does not suffice to induce doubt in the doctor's mind concerning the virtue that he attributes to any prescription. Conversely, whoever claims to speak pertinently about an individual being healed should be able to demonstrate that healing, understood as the satisfaction of the patient's expectation, is really the effect of a prescribed and scrupulously applied therapy. However, it is more difficult to carry out such a demonstration today [...] (Georges Canguilhem, 2012: 53-54)

From this previous extract, we can note one more theme, the difficulty of demonstration of healing and the role played by the doctor – or the health professional – that goes beyond the outcome or the expected outcome. This difference is well highlighted in the next paragraph:

In short, we can say that for the sick man, healing is what medicine owes him, while for most doctors, even today, what medicine owes the patient is the best-studied, best-tested, and most-used treatment currently available. Hence the difference between a doctor and a healer. A doctor who does not succeed in healing anyone would not de jure cease to be a doctor—he continues to be licensed by a diploma that sanctions a conventionally accepted knowledge for the purpose of treating patients whose diseases are outlined in medical treatises in terms of symptomatology, etiology, pathogenesis, and therapy. A healer can be one only de facto, for he is judged on the basis not of his "knowledge," but of his successes. (Georges Canguilhem, 2012: 54)

Finally, the author finished his essay by declaring that for the patient, to heal, it is not the same as coming back to a previous state of health, but a new situation, a change in his or her reality and life: "The lucid consciousness of the fact that healing is not a return helps the patient in his search for the state of the least possible renunciation by liberating him from his fixation upon his previous state" (Canguilhem 2012: 66).

From all these considerations, we would like to stress the complexity of the processes at hand and the importance of the knowledge of the professionals and the patients involved in these very processes. This is relevant to consider for dealing with the promotion of health and the empowerment of agents. What is promotion of health if not enabling people to adapt to new circumstances and changing meanings of live and living. This is here the modernity of Canguilhem at the meeting point with innovation and knowledge management conceived in a complex and evolutionary way (Richard R. Nelson & Winter, 1982; Richard R Nelson & Winter, 2002).

SOME LIMITATIONS OF EMPOWERMENT THEORY

There are a number of limitations to the theory of empowerment and its implementation in management practices and in public policies in the health sector. We will discuss the most important and relevant ones for the health care sector and to orient policies and management decisions that implement knowledge management measures.

One primary limitation, as already hinted at above, is the traditional asymmetry of information between health professionals and patients. The asymmetry can run both ways. This is well covered in the health economics literature (Blaug, 1998; Donaldson, Mugford, & Vale, 2002; Hodgson, 2008; McPake, Kumaranayake, & Normand, 2002; Scott, Maynard, & Elliott, 2003; Wolfe, 2008). It is important to note that it is not just the doctor or health professional that typically knows more about health problems, ailments and diseases as well as factors related to them. On the other hand, the patient knows more about his past history than the professional. The difficulties for knowledge management and for empowering people's health do not stop here. The patient can be less knowledgeable of scientific theories and evidence-based assertions. However, some patients still ignore, before some diagnosis, what their health problem, if any at all, is. The recent literature on downstream and upstream health reveal even professionals may not see the whole picture and proffer misdiagnoses (Ewles & Simnett, 2003; WHO, 1999; Wilkinson & Pickett, 2010).

The second aspect has to do with the tacit dimension of health knowledge and interactions. The concept of knowledge management continues to treat tacit knowledge, despite late criticism of the conception of Nonaka and colleagues (Adler, 1995; Buono, Poulfelt, & København, 2005), as a residual category. Tacitness is not a secondary feature of knowledge but one of its defining aspects (Adler, 1995; Buono et al., 2005; Dreiling & Becker, 2007; Duguid, 2005; Stephen Gourlay, 2006; S Gourlay & Nurse, 2005;

Polanyi, 1958, 1962, 1966; Polanyi & Prosch, 1975; Alexander Styhre, 2003; A. Styhre, 2003). Knowledge has a complex and embedded character that turns its management a difficult and challenging task.

Third, there is a neglect of local and community interactions and knowledge base in the design and implementation of public policies for health promotion and health care. Local knowledge (or indigenous knowledge (Sillitoe, 1998, 2007) as it is called in the anthropology literature) could bridge the gap, at least partially, between science-based knowledge and personal knowledge (as defined by Polanyi). This third limitation is also very relevant for the adoption of new technologies and alternative treatments (Laverack & Wallerstein, 2001; Wallerstein & Bernstein, 1988).

The fourth limitation of the empowerment theory has to do with the limited view of interested parties or stakeholders, most often than not the doctor or surgeon and the patient, neglecting other health, administrative professionals, citizens and associations of public interest or local scope (see the forthcoming section on stakeholders for further considerations). The proposition in this chapter is to involve more key players or stakeholders, from the design of public policies, the measures used and the implementation process, including the management of information and knowledge in an efficient and meaningful way.

The last limitation of the empowerment theory, discussed here, is the lack of an active pedagogy, especially for the patient, and especially the less prepared individuals, namely those that do not have the adequate literacy and skills to fully be aware of what is going on and what can be useful (Laverack & Wallerstein, 2001; Wallerstein & Bernstein, 1988).

TACIT DIMENSION IN HEALTH CARE AND EMPOWERMENT PROCESS

We will discuss here the tacit dimension of health care and the empowerment process as well as health literacy. The tacit dimension here has to be conceived in broad terms, closer to management processes and real life of patients and health professionals. This means that the tacit dimension is not a residual category, as conceived by Nonaka and his group of researchers, but an essential part of knowledge management and social interaction.

The tacit dimension of knowledge as conceived by Michael Polanyi is related to a context of knowing, learning and acting in a scientific community and beyond, including the process of indwelling that focus on the non explicit traits of knowledge creation and transmission (Polanyi, 1958, 1961, 1962, 1966, 1981; Polanyi & Prosch, 1975; Prosch, 1986). His conception received much attention in science and technology studies as well as economics of innovation, technological change, management and philosophy (Jha, 2002).

Our understanding of the tacit here is to be approximated to the knowing how or the "how to" knowledge (contrasted but complementary to the knowing what) as defined by Gilbert Ryle (Ryle, 2009). It is associated to the process view of social action and organization; with philosophical roots in William James, Whitehead and Bergson, *inter alia* (Connolly, 2005, 2011, 2013; Jha, 2002). Without entering in philosophical considerations, tacitness here is construed as a central dimension of knowing. It is not a residual category that can be eliminated through codification, i.e., knowledge management would be essentially a process of transcription, translating tacit knowledge or skills in explicit or codified knowledge. While codification is important and it must be carried out with care in order to avoid loss of knowledge, namely alternatives in any situation where decisions can be made in order to keep the different paths open to social actors or workers or managers in a given organization composed of interdependent subsystems.

There are some aspects of knowledge management, namely, its imprecision, its contradiction and often its flawed conception of what knowledge is (all about). We have studied it in greater details in sections 2 and 3 above, and some more will be tackled in the forthcoming sections. On the other hand, it is convenient to tackle a certain number of issues related to knowledge conception, knowledge management and health and health care.

First of all, the notion of knowledge is problematic, not just in the philosophical literature but also in the management literature, not to mention the knowledge management specialization. The problematic nature of knowledge is not new and is even a common feature across all disciplinary borders (Frodeman, 2010; Legendre, 1983, 1996, 2001; Rosenthal & Gutas, 1970).

Second, we will make a criticism of traditional or mainstream knowledge management literature, namely Nonaka's model (Ikujiro Nonaka, 1994; I Nonaka & H Takeuchi, 1995; Ikujiro Nonaka et al., 2008; Ikujiro Nonaka et al., 2000), that consider knowledge and knowledge processes in management practice or in the implementation of public policies as being too poor or flawed, and lacking evidence (Gourlay 2006, Gourlay & Nurse 2005).

Third, there exists a stark contrast with the literature on health and social psychology (Bandura, 1986a, 1986b) that stresses the "complex relationships between knowledge, beliefs and perceived social norms, and provide practical guidance on the content of educational programs to promote behavioural change …" (Nutbeam 2000: 260).

Too much related to a certain kind of management culture, it used flawed concepts (Dreiling & Becker, 2007; Montuori, 2003; Alexander Styhre, 2003; A. Styhre, 2003; Tsoukas, 2016) and could be indeed clarified and sometimes simplified (Alvesson 2001; Alvesson & Karreman 2001), and this is a partial aim of this chapter focused on health literacy and empowerment.

Finally, the first step is to distinguish and work the difference between beliefs and knowledge. And this step can be taken when dealing with stakeholders and people involved in the processes with different worldviews.

EXTENSION TO VARIOUS STAKEHOLDERS

A final point is our treatment of health literacy as a tool of knowledge management that has to tackle the issue of the widening of the ambit of the actors involved from the specific organization to the whole national or regional health system, beyond just the patient and doctor and integrating institutions, citizens, regulatory agencies, higher education institutions and associations, *inter alia* (Crawford Shearer, 2009).

In a certain sense, we integrate here the conclusions of the previous sections, mainly section 2 and 3, to incorporate them in a model of knowledge organization and management processes that take into account the various stakeholders based on a willingness to learn and improve both the outcomes and the processes at hand.

The first stakeholder in health literacy, health empowerment and health promotion is the state. This is a particularity of the health sector that the state is the most influential decision maker, the promoter, the regulator and the provider (at least of part) the "supply" of health care. Its action goes beyond the regulation of, and provision of, health care. It crosses boundaries, namely in terms of education of health professionals and innovation and research policies.

In the health care sector, the state is the policy maker, defining guidelines, objectives, wielding strong influence on the management of hospitals and professional bodies. It is also the guarantor of patients' rights. It is also defining how and by whom the sector will be regulated. It is often seen as the provider of last resort for health care and the guarantor of some minimum principles for equal access to the health services.

This is also a commitment of the European states to contribute to the empowerment in health, due to the constitutional texts, reflecting the idea of welfare state, not in the role of caregiver, but to foster the development of health education of the people and healthy lifestyle practices (Bambra, Fox, & Scott-Samuel, 2005; Gøsta Esping-Andersen, 1990; Gosta Esping-Andersen, 1999, 2002), as exposed by Esping-Anderson: "The explicit acknowledgement of the political nature of health will lead to more effective health promotion strategy and policy, and to more realistic and evidence-based public health and health promotion practice" (Bambra et al., 2005: 187).

Most literature on empowerment process rightly focuses on patient and on the most extreme cases, those that are marginalized. This is important, but generally the method used and the vision adopted has several drawbacks. It conceives poverty out of the relevant context (much can be done through evidence-based policy) and the diversity of actors and professionals that adopt different vantage points and some of these prevail more than others.

This justifies a more comprehensive approach, taking into account the complexity of the issues and the relevant factors that cannot be neglected. Some of these aspects are related to creativity, innovation and the institutional setting for empowerment (Shalley, Hitt, & Zhou, 2015; Supiot, 2007, 2010, 2015a, 2015b; Todorov, 2001, 2005; Todorov, 2009, 2010, 2013; Vankova, Kerekovska, Kostadinova, & Todorova, 2016).

A MODEL OF KNOWLEDGE TRANSFER AND EMPOWERMENT

In this section, the focus is on a model for knowledge transfer and the development empowerment of medical personnel (and other professionals) through practice. The model presented is based on the model developed by Nonaka and collaborators (see below the combinations of four modes of knowledge transfer – Socialization, Externalization Combination and Internalization, i.e. the SECI Model).

Tacit knowledge is a fundamental knowledge type for organizations and it is disseminated by the employees' networks. The concept was created and defined by Polanyi (1966) in order to identify a type of knowledge that is not possible to be codified or easily explained. It is embodied trough practice with a process named indwelling.

According to this concept we can say that critical skills and knowledge of medical staff are also tacit and emerges from practice. This experiential knowledge can be identified in project context or in communities-of-practice (Wenger, 2000; Yanow, 1999, 2000), and in the healthcare organizations. The success of the medical activities and the organization itself depends on the integration and sharing of this type of knowledge; this is a mean of empowerment and a way of increasing their responsibilities.

Several researchers (Szulanski, 1996, 2000; Szulanski, Cappetta, & Jensen, 2004) refer that knowledge transfer is a process through which knowledge moves between the source and the recipient, with the goal to be applied and used in practical situations. Following this idea, knowledge is an asset that can be transferred among individuals that belong to different departments and hierarchical levels. It is possible to say that knowledge is one of the most important assets to empower employees potentiating their competencies and contributing for their growth within the organization.

SECI Knowledge Transfer Model Applied to Healthcare Sector

There is a heuristic model that can be used in the healthcare sector and by organizations active in providing health care – this model was first introduced by Nonaka (1994) and Nonaka and Takeuchi (1995) and is named the SECI Model. This model explains the knowledge transfer process which is based on the knowledge conversion model and it can assume four forms: socialization, externalization combination and internalization (SECI).

According to Nonaka and Takeuchi (1995: 57), "socialization refers to an organizational process through which tacit knowledge held by some individuals is transferred in tacit form to others with whom they interact. Externalization refers to the transformation of some tacit knowledge into explicit knowledge, via theories, concepts, models, analogies, metaphors and so on. Combination refers to the conversion of codified knowledge into new forms of codified knowledge. Internalization is a process of conversion of explicit knowledge into a tacit form."

The SECI model has to go through some adaptation for the health care sector and to respond do some of the criticisms analyzed in the previous sections. A first modification result from the integration of what Fahey and Prusak (1998) have called the eleven sins of knowledge management in their paper in the California Management Review. The adaptation is also necessary for dealing with organizations active in health care, namely hospitals and specific services providers that are embedded in a very special context with orientations coming from public health policies.

The application of the SECI model to the healthcare sector is as follow. It is possible to analyze the healthcare activities using the Socialization, Externalization, Combination and Internalization dimensions:

Socialization

There are several layers for the socialization process in which health professional are embedded. The socialization process through the practice and the interaction among doctors can help to reduce the doctors' mistakes and to improve the medical practice. This is also true for nurses and other health professionals like therapists, analysts and technicians of diagnosis machines and tools. This process is important at the beginning and at critical points of implementing Information Technology (IT) solutions to manage knowledge flows, inputs and outputs. This process is adequate to discuss beliefs system and clarify the knowledge processes and needs in the implementation of information systems in the test phase or design of its objectives and architecture.

Externalization

The externalization occurs when medical staff explicit the medical routines into new technologies which will raise the quality of services. This is at this level that electronic health record (HER) can be introduced in the model and be integrated with other activities. This process occurs at a further step than socialization when IT solutions are implemented. Here, explicit instruction and procedures are implemented. This dimension of externalization is similar to the concept of codification of knowledge (both explicit and implicit or tacit) to transmit it across organizations or groups in order to promote efficacy and efficiency in production (Cowan, 2001; Cowan & David, 1997; Cowan, David, & Foray, 2000). It is important when writing procedures or codifying knowledge to pay heed to the role and importance of tacit knowledge, as advocated by Fahey and Prusak (1998).

Combination

The combination process occurs when the organization ensures that safety procedures are applied to patients directly by the medical staff and new and better procedures emerges from the practice. In the SECI model it proceeds from explicit knowledge to explicit transformation. It means systematizing procedures and knowledge. It can be the implementation of evidence-based medicine, applying explicit knowledge from scientific research to practical knowledge and procedures in use such as treatments or safety rules.

Internalization

The internalization can emerge when the medical personnel is directly responsible for the quality of services and the treatment process, involving their active participation and using their knowledge in problem solving situations. Sometimes, it means restructuring medical practices that are used on a daily basis. It goes from the explicit knowledge base to tacit transformation. It covers much of what learning means in organizations and health practices. The focus is on improving action and practices.

Having explicitly discussed the SECI model for health, it is important to place it into perspective, namely through its role as improving health care and promoting health, as stated in the Ottawa Charter (Juneau et al., 2011).

It is convenient to combine the different approaches and to foster learning and to improve knowledge in use and practices. In this sense, information science, through such elements as queries, health information seeking, representation, indexing retrieving and evaluation, can be of great help (C. Lopes, 2008; C. T. Lopes & Ribeiro, 2015).

The SECI model is also considered in its effects through a spiral that implies through time improvements in the knowledge base and practices. The engine of the spiral is the learning process that combines the four modes and other modalities of orienting learning in health care organizations and services.

Finally, it must be stressed that the model has to integrate various components and learning processes and this implies complexity, both as a method or way to proceed and as an object of practice or a wicked problem, i.e., issues that are difficult to tackle for the sheer number of elements and nonlinear relationships between them.

Complexity has two different meanings that are of interest for research and must be distinguished: one is complexity as reality or object of study, and this is the most widespread meaning. The other is complexity as a method of inquiry; it is sometimes referred to the science or sciences of complexity (Jacquinet & Caetano, 2010).

FUTURE TRENDS AND META-LEARNING

Several authors address the momentum for social change at a global level, from a knowledge management perspective (e.g., Laszlo & Laszlo, 2002; McMichael, 2016; Pieterse, 2015). The relationship between knowledge processes and organizational learning, represents a radical shift in management thinking (Nobre, 2007). Michael Polanyi, in particular, is highly influential, namely as argued by Sandbrook (2011), through the idea of "re-embedding of economy in society", through community-based alternatives arising from 'reciprocity'.

The social change dynamics is particularly present in the health care sector. Consequently, three critical dimensions may be understood to reflect the reality of the health care system, on one hand, and the evolution of contemporary societies, on the other hand. The present chapter has argued above that tacit knowledge is a core dimension of any knowledge management process, that empowerment strategies potentiate critical health literacy and that stakeholders have to be involved, including communities and the environments in which people live in, when designing effective public health policies. This is a broader perspective on stakeholders and stakeholder theory.

When considering the evolution of societies and the pressure from emergent trends across different disciplinary areas, there is an irrefutable demand for global change, at all levels, socio-political and environmental, which includes precisely the referred above phenomenon. That is, a simplistic and reductive perspective on knowledge imposes a myopic view of the power of science, in particular of social and human sciences. The power of science is substantiated in the quality of life of the populations who are the benefactors of scientific-based public policy design.

Effective decision making, in health care or in any other area, at macro or micro level, implies considering complexity as a social interaction event, ready to be addressed by concepts such as tacit knowledge, empowerment and the role of stakeholders and of communities in helping to design, implement and manage powerful public policies, which indeed have an impact in real lives.

The meta-learning that emerges from the health promotion strategies refers to the prevalence and strength of global change movements. Civic movements represent the hidden, invisible, informal and implicit pressures, which suddenly become operationalized and are systematized into coherent and solid public discourses that, in turn, affect political decision-making as well as the groups and individuals decision-making. Such global processes are present in human's rights movements and they represent a clear cut message to management design functions: to address, again and again, the issues related to the social embeddedness and embodiedness of knowledge, as considered in the concept of tacit knowledge, as a mandatory step towards building more productive, healthy and balanced societies.

CONCLUSION

A number of conclusions can be drawn from our analysis and discussion. First of all, the health care sector is a rather specific arena, diverging on several counts from the mainstream model of business and competition, and this includes most of the knowledge management literature, to heterodox perspectives and alternative frameworks.

Second, there is no easy solution to the problems of the health sector, as it can be construed as a wicked problem (this is equivalent to the notion of complexity as a problem or reality in social science and the philosophy of science).

Third, the implementation and the improvement of knowledge management in healthcare are not easy tasks, not just because of the peculiarities of the sector but because the visions and paradigms in knowledge management are not sufficiently critical and based on evidence. Heuristic models, like the SECI model discusses and adapted in the present chapter, are a possible wedge into the complex problem of health care and better public policies and efficiency of the management of people and resources.

The advocacy of a piecemeal approach is better adapted to the sector needs and to the long-run effectiveness of policies, changes and consolidation of good practices. Learning is central to the success of managing knowledge, health literacy and promoting effectively empowerment of actors.

The empowerment should go beyond the strict action of the patient and include the stakeholders relevant to the issues at hand. And the problem is not just to manage knowledge but to work also at the level of perceptions and beliefs of the significant actors involved in one way or another.

The knowledge approach, that tackles tacitness explicitly, has to integrate learning, with the integration of the different actors' valuations, inertia and attitude.

REFERENCES

Adam, B. (2004). *Time*. Cambridge, UK: Polity.

Adler, P. S. (1995). The Dynamic Relationship Between Tacit and Codified Knowledge: Comments on Ikujiro Nonaka's "Managing Innovation as an Organizational Knowledge Creation Process". In J. Allouche & G. Pogorel (Eds.), *Technology management and corporate strategies: a tricontinental perspective* (pp. 110–124). Amsterdam: Elsevier - North-Holland.

Alexander, P. A., Schallert, D. L., & Hare, V. C. (1991). Coming to Terms: How Researchers in Learning and Literacy Talk About Knowledge. *Review of Educational Research, 61*(3), 315–343. doi:10.3102/00346543061003315

Alvesson, M. (2001). Knowledge Work: Ambiguity, Image and Identity. *Human Relations, 54*(7), 863–886. doi:10.1177/0018726701547004

Alvesson, M., & Kärreman, D. (2001). Odd Couple: Making Sense of the Curious Concept of Knowledge Management. *Journal of Management Studies, 38*(7), 995–1018. doi:10.1111/1467-6486.00269

Alvesson, M., & Sveningsson, S. (2015). *Changing organizational culture: Cultural change work in progress*. Routledge.

Amin, A., & Cohendet, P. (2004). *Architectures of knowledge: Firms, capabilities, and communities*. Oxford, UK: Oxford University Press. doi:10.1093/acprof:oso/9780199253326.001.0001

Amin, A., & Roberts, J. (2008). *Community, economic creativity, and organization*. Oxford, UK: Oxford University Press. doi:10.1093/acprof:oso/9780199545490.001.0001

Antonelli, C., Foray, D., Hall, B. H., & Steinmueller, W. E. (2006). *New Frontiers in the Economics of Innovation and New Technology: Essays in Honour of Paul A. David*. Edward Elgar Publishing, Incorporated. doi:10.4337/9781845427924

Baba, C., Kearns, A., McIntosh, E., Tannahill, C., & Lewsey, J. (2016). Is empowerment a route to improving mental health and wellbeing in an urban regeneration (UR) context? *Urban Studies (Edinburgh, Scotland)*. doi:10.1177/0042098016632435

Bambra, C., Fox, D., & Scott-Samuel, A. (2005). Towards a politics of health. *Health Promotion International, 20*(2), 187–193. doi:10.1093/heapro/dah608 PMID:15722364

Bandura, A. (1986a). The Explanatory and Predictive Scope of Self-Efficacy Theory. *Journal of Social and Clinical Psychology, 4*(3), 359–373. doi:10.1521/jscp.1986.4.3.359

Bandura, A. (1986b). *Social foundations of thought and action: A social cognitive theory*. Prentice-Hall, Inc.

Banerjee, A. V., & Duflo, E. (2008). Mandated Empowerment: Handing Antipoverty Policy Back to the Poor. *Annals of the New York Academy of Sciences*, *1136*(1), 333–341. doi:10.1196/annals.1425.019 PMID:18579890

Berkman, L. F., Kawachi, I., & Glymour, M. M. (2014). *Social epidemiology*. Oxford University Press. doi:10.1093/med/9780195377903.001.0001

Birkinshaw, J. (2010). *Reinventing Management: Smarter Choices for Getting Work Done*. Wiley.

Birkinshaw, J., Hamel, G., & Mol, M. J. (2008). Management innovation. *Academy of Management Review*, *33*(4), 825–845. doi:10.5465/AMR.2008.34421969

Birkinshaw, J., Nobel, R., & Ridderstråle, J. (2002). Knowledge as a Contingency Variable: Do the Characteristics of Knowledge Predict Organization Structure? *Organization Science*, *13*(3), 274–289. doi:10.1287/orsc.13.3.274.2778

Blaug, M. (1998). Where are we now in British health economics? *Journal of Health Economics*, *7*(1), 63–78. doi:10.1002/hec.4730070906 PMID:9744717

Bowen, D. E., & Lawler, E. E., III. (1992). The Empowerment of Service Workers: What, Why, How, and When. In J. S. Ott (Ed.), Classic readings in organizational behavior (Vol. 26, pp. 291-303). Belmont: Wadsworth Pub. Co.

Brandstetter, S., Curbach, J., Lindacher, V., Rueter, J., Warrelmann, B., & Loss, J. (2015). Empowerment for healthy nutrition in German communities: A study framework. *Health Promotion International*, dav092. doi:10.1093/heapro/dav092 PMID:26447192

Brandstetter, S., McCool, M., Wise, M., & Loss, J. (2014). Australian health promotion practitioners perceptions on evaluation of empowerment and participation. *Health Promotion International*, *29*(1), 70–80. doi:10.1093/heapro/das046 PMID:22987842

Buono, A. F., Poulfelt, F., & København, H. i. (2005). *Challenges and Issues in Knowledge Management*. Information Age Pub.

Canguilhem, G. (2002). *Écrits sur la médecine*. Éditions du Seuil.

Canguilhem, G. (2012). *Writings on Medicine*. New York: Fordham University Press.

Carayannis, E. G., Pirzadeh, A., & Popescu, D. (2011). *Institutional learning and knowledge transfer across epistemic communities: new tools of global governance* (Vol. 13). Springer Science & Business Media.

Carlisle, S. (2000). Health promotion, advocacy and health inequalities: A conceptual framework. *Health Promotion International*, *15*(4), 369–376. doi:10.1093/heapro/15.4.369

Catford, J. (2011). Ottawa 1986: Back to the future. *Health Promotion International*, *26*(suppl 2), ii163–ii167. doi:10.1093/heapro/dar081 PMID:22080068

Collins, P. H. (2015). Intersectionalitys Definitional Dilemmas. *Annual Review of Sociology, 41*(1), 1–20. doi:10.1146/annurev-soc-073014-112142

Connolly, W. E. (2005). *Pluralism*. Duke University Press. doi:10.1215/9780822387084

Connolly, W. E. (2011). *A World of Becoming*. Duke University Press.

Connolly, W. E. (2013). *The Fragility of Things: Self-Organizing Processes, Neoliberal Fantasies, and Democratic Activism*. Duke University Press. doi:10.1215/9780822377160

Cowan, R. (2001). Expert systems: Aspects of and limitations to the codifiability of knowledge. *Research Policy, 30*(9), 1355–1372. doi:10.1016/S0048-7333(01)00156-1

Cowan, R., & David, P. A. (1997). The economics of codification and the diffusion of knowledge. *Industrial and Corporate Change, 6*(3), 592–622. doi:10.1093/icc/6.3.595

Cowan, R., David, P. A., & Foray, D. (2000). The Explicit Economics of Knowledge Codification and Tacitness. *Industrial and Corporate Change, 9*(2), 211–253. doi:10.1093/icc/9.2.211

Crawford Shearer, N. B. (2009). Health Empowerment Theory as a Guide for Practice. *Geriatric Nursing, 30*(2), 4–10. doi:10.1016/j.gerinurse.2009.02.003 PMID:19345857

Crenshaw, K. (1989). Demarginalizing the Intersection of Race and Sex: A Black Feminist Critique of Antidiscrimination Doctrine, Feminist Theory and Antiracist Politics. *University of Chicago Legal Forum, 140*, 139–167.

Crondahl, K., & Eklund Karlsson, L. (2016). The Nexus Between Health Literacy and Empowerment. *A Scoping Review, 6*(2). doi: 10.1177/2158244016646410

Cyril, S., Smith, B. J., & Renzaho, A. M. N. (2015). Systematic review of empowerment measures in health promotion. *Health Promotion International*, dav059. doi:10.1093/heapro/dav059 PMID:26137970

Davis, A., Collins, P. H., & Crenshaw, K. W. (2003). An Examination of Racialized Assumptions in Antirape Discourse. *Studies in Practical Philosophy: A Journal of Ethical and Political Philosophy, 3*.

De la Mothe, J., & Foray, D. (2001). *Knowledge management in the innovation process* (Vol. 24). Berlin: Springer Science & Business Media. doi:10.1007/978-1-4615-1535-7

Donaldson, C., Mugford, M., & Vale, L. (2002). *Evidence-Based Health Economics: From effectiveness to efficiency in systematic review*. London: BMJ Books.

Downey, C., Curado, H., & Jacquinet, M. (2016). The Emergence of Biobanks: Between Ethics, Risks, and Governance. In C.-C. Maria Manuela, M. Isabel Maria, M. Ricardo, & R. Rui (Eds.), *Encyclopedia of E-Health and Telemedicine* (pp. 169–178). Hershey, PA: IGI Global. doi:10.4018/978-1-4666-9978-6.ch014

Dreiling, A., & Becker, J. (2007). *Myths, Narratives and the Dilemma of Managerial Support: Organizational learning as an alternative?* Berlin: Deutscher Universitätsverlag.

Duguid, P. (2005). The Art of Knowing: Social and Tacit Dimensions of Knowledge and the Limits of the Community of Practice. *The Information Society, 21*(2), 109–118. doi:10.1080/01972240590925311

Esping-Andersen, G. (1990). *The three worlds of welfare capitalism*. Oxford, UK: Polity Press.

Esping-Andersen, G. (1999). *Social Foundations of Postindustrial Economies*. Oxford University Press. doi:10.1093/0198742002.001.0001

Esping-Andersen, G. (2002). *Why We Need a New Welfare State*. Oxford University Press. doi:10.1093/0199256438.001.0001

Ewles, L., & Simnett, I. (2003). *Promoting health: a practical guide*. Edinburgh, UK: Elsevier Health Sciences.

Foray, D. (2010). *L'économie de la connaissance*. Paris: La découverte.

Frodeman, R. (2010). *The Oxford Handbook of Interdisciplinarity*. OUP Oxford.

Gourlay, S. (2006). Conceptualizing Knowledge Creation: A Critique of Nonakas Theory*. *Journal of Management Studies*, *43*(7), 1415–1436. doi:10.1111/j.1467-6486.2006.00637.x

Gourlay, S., & Nurse, A. (2005). *Flaws in the 'engine' of knowledge creation. In Challenges and Issues in Knowledge Management* (pp. 293–315). Greenwich: Information Age Publishing.

Haugaard, M. (2012). Rethinking the four dimensions of power: Domination and empowerment. *Journal of Political Power*, *5*(1), 33–54. doi:10.1080/2158379X.2012.660810

Hill-Collins, P., & Bilge, S. (2016). *Intersectionality*. New York: John Wiley & Sons.

Hodgson, G. M. (2008). An institutional and evolutionary perspective on health economics. *Cambridge Journal of Economics*, *32*(2), 235–256. doi:10.1093/cje/bem033

Horton, R. (1995). Georges Canguilhem. *Lancet*, *346*(8982), 1094. doi:10.1016/S0140-6736(95)91765-9 PMID:7629760

ISO. (2005). *Health Information and Management Systems Society. EHR: electronic health record*. Retrieved from http://www.himss.org/ASP/topics_ehr.asp

Jacquinet, M., & Caetano, J. C. R. (2010). Complexité. In A.-J. Arnaud (Ed.), Dictionnaire de la globalisation (pp. 72-76). Paris: Librairie Générale de Droit et de Jurisprudence (LGDJ)/Lextenso.

Jacquinet, M., & Curado, H. (2016). Opportunities and Challenges for Electronic Health Record: Concepts, Costs, Benefits, and Regulation. In C.-C. Maria Manuela, M. Isabel Maria, M. Ricardo, & R. Rui (Eds.), *Encyclopedia of E-Health and Telemedicine* (pp. 969–975). Hershey, PA: IGI Global. doi:10.4018/978-1-4666-9978-6.ch075

Jha, S. R. (2002). *Reconsidering Michael Polanyi's Philosophy*. Pittsburgh, PA: University of Pittsburgh Press.

Juneau, C.-E., Jones, C. M., McQueen, D. V., & Potvin, L. (2011). Evidence-based health promotion: An emerging field. *Global Health Promotion and Education*, *18*(1), 79–89. doi:10.1177/1757975910394035 PMID:21721308

Kahin, B., & Foray, D. (2006). *Advancing knowledge and the knowledge economy*. Cambridge, MA: MIT Press.

Karamitri, I., Talias, M. A., & Bellali, T. (2015). Knowledge management practices in healthcare settings: a systematic review. *The International Journal of Health Planning and Management*. doi: 10.1002/hpm.2303

Kostenius, C., & Hertting, K. (2016). Health promoting interactive technology: Finnish, Norwegian, Russian and Swedish students reflections. *Health Promotion International, 31*(3), 505–514. doi:10.1093/heapro/dav021 PMID:25809652

Lam, A. (2000). Tacit Knowledge, Organizational Learning and Societal Institutions: An Integrated Framework. *Organization Studies, 21*(3), 487–513. doi:10.1177/0170840600213001

Laszlo, K. C., & Laszlo, A. (2002). Evolving knowledge for development: The role of knowledge management in a changing world. *Journal of Knowledge Management, 6*(4), 400–412. doi:10.1108/13673270210440893

Laverack, G., & Wallerstein, N. (2001). Measuring community empowerment: A fresh look at organizational domains. *Health Promotion International, 16*(2), 179–185. doi:10.1093/heapro/16.2.179 PMID:11356756

Legendre, P. (1983). Les maîtres de la Loi: Etude sur la fonction dogmatique en régime industriel. *Annales, 38*(3), 507–535. doi:10.3406/ahess.1983.410942

Legendre, P. (1996). *La fabrique de l'homme occidental*. Paris: Mille et une nuits.

Legendre, P. (2001). *Leçons II-L'empire de la vérité. Introductions aux espaces dogmatiques industriels*. Paris: Fayard.

Loasby, B. (1976). *Choice, Complexity and Ignorance: An Inquiry into Economic Theory and The Practice of Decision-making*. Cambridge, UK: Cambridge University Press.

Loasby, B. (1999). *Knowledge, Institutions and Evolution in Economics*. London: Routledge. doi:10.4324/9780203459096

Lopes, C. (2008). *Health Information Retrieval: State of the art report*. Faculdade de Engenharia da Universidade do Porto, Porto. Retrieved from http://www.carlalopes.com/pubs/Lopes_SOA_2008.pdf

Lopes, C. T., & Ribeiro, C. (2015). *Effects of Terminology on Health Queries: An Analysis by User's Health Literacy and Topic Familiarity*. Current Issues in Libraries, Information Science and Related Fields.

MacDonald, M. (2003). Knowledge Management in Healthcare: What Does it Involve? How is it Measured? *Healthcare Management Forum, 16*(3), 7–11. doi:10.1016/S0840-4704(10)60225-6 PMID:14618826

Mårtensson, L., & Hensing, G. (2012). Health literacy – a heterogeneous phenomenon: A literature review. *Scandinavian Journal of Caring Sciences, 26*(1), 151–160. doi:10.1111/j.1471-6712.2011.00900.x PMID:21627673

McLaughlin, K. (2003). Agency, resilience and empowerment: The dangers posed by a therapeutic culture. *Practice, 15*(2), 45–58. doi:10.1080/09503150308416918

McLaughlin, K. (2016). *Empowerment: A Critique*. London: Routledge - Taylor & Francis.

McMichael, P. (2016). *Development and Social Change: A Global Perspective*. SAGE Publications.

McMillan, K. E., & Worth, H. (2015). Problematics of empowerment: Sex worker HIV prevention in the Pacific. *Health Promotion International*, dav069. doi:10.1093/heapro/dav069 PMID:26135585

McPake, B., Kumaranayake, L., & Normand, C. (2002). *Health Economics: An International Perspective*. London: Routledge. doi:10.4324/9780203935040

McQueen, D. V., & Jones, C. M. (2007). *Global perspectives on health promotion effectiveness*. New York: Springer. doi:10.1007/978-0-387-70974-1_1

Montuori, A. (2003). The Complexity of Improvisation and the Improvisation of Complexity: Social Science, Art and Creativity. *Human Relations*, *56*(2), 237–255. doi:10.1177/0018726703056002893

Nelson, R. R., & Winter, S. G. (1982). *An Evolutionary Theory of Economic Change*. Cambridge, MA: Belknap.

Nelson, R. R., & Winter, S. G. (2002). Evolutionary theorizing in economics. *The Journal of Economic Perspectives*, *16*(2), 23–46. doi:10.1257/0895330027247

Nobre, A. L. (2007). Knowledge Processes and Organizational Learning. In C. R. McInerney & R. E. Day (Eds.), *Rethinking Knowledge Management: From Knowledge Objects to Knowledge Processes* (pp. 275–299). Berlin: Springer. doi:10.1007/3-540-71011-6_12

Nonaka, I. (1988). Creating Organizational Order Out of Chaos: Self-Renewal in Japanese Firms. *California Management Review*, *30*(3), 57–73. doi:10.2307/41166514

Nonaka, I. (1991). The knowledge-creating company. *Harvard Business Review*, *69*(November-December), 96–104.

Nonaka, I. (1994). A dynamic theory of organizational knowledge creation. *Organization Science*, *5*(1), 14–37. doi:10.1287/orsc.5.1.14

Nonaka, I., & Takeuchi, H. (1995). *The Knowledge-Creating Company: How Japanese Companies Create the Dynamics of Innovation*. Oxford University Press.

Nonaka, I., & Takeuchi, H. (1995). *The Knowledge Creating Company*. New York: Oxford University Press.

Nonaka, I., Toyama, R., Hirata, T., Bigelow, S. J., Hirose, A., & Kohlbacher, F. (2008). *Introduction: Why We Need a New Theory of the Knowledge-Based Firm. In Managing Flow: A Process Theory of the Knowledge-Based Firm* (pp. 1–5). London: Palgrave Macmillan UK.

Nonaka, I., Toyama, R., & Konno, N. (2000). SECI, Ba and Leadership: A Unified Model of Dynamic Knowledge Creation. *Long Range Planning*, *33*(1), 5–34. doi:10.1016/S0024-6301(99)00115-6

Nutbeam, D. (2000). Health literacy as a public health goal: A challenge for contemporary health education and communication strategies into the 21st century. *Health Promotion International*, *15*. doi:10.1093/heapro/15.3.259

Nutbeam, D. (2008). The evolving concept of health literacy. *Social Science & Medicine*, *67*(12), 2072–2078. doi:10.1016/j.socscimed.2008.09.050 PMID:18952344

Pieterse, J. N. (2015). *Globalization and Culture: Global Mélange*. Rowman & Littlefield Publishers.

Polanyi, M. (1958). *Personal Knowledge: Towards a Post-Critical Philosophy*. Chicago: University of Chicago Press.

Polanyi, M. (1961). Knowing and Being. *Mind*, *70*(280), 458–470. doi:10.1093/mind/LXX.280.458

Polanyi, M. (1962). Tacit Knowing: Its Bearing on Some Problems of Philosophy. *Reviews of Modern Physics*, *34*(4), 601–616. doi:10.1103/RevModPhys.34.601

Polanyi, M. (1966). *The Tacit Dimension*. London: Routledge & Kegan.

Polanyi, M. (1981). The Creative Imagination. In D. Dutton & M. Krausz (Eds.), *The Concept of Creativity in Science and Art* (pp. 91–108). Dordrecht: Springer Netherlands.

Polanyi, M., & Prosch, H. (1975). *Meaning*. Chicago: University of Chicago Press.

Porfírio, J., Jacquinet, M., & Carrilho, T. (2013). *The Impact of ICT and Online Social Networks on Health and Social Services. In Handbook of Research on ICTs and Management Systems for Improving Efficiency in Healthcare and Social Care* (pp. 1224–1243). IGI Global.

Porr, C., Drummond, L., & Rishter, S. (2006). Health literacy as an empowerment tool for low income mothers. *Family & Community Health*, *29*(4), 328–335. doi:10.1097/00003727-200610000-00011 PMID:16980808

Potvin, L., & Jones, C. M. (2011). *Twenty-five Years After the Ottawa Charter: The Critical Role of Health Promotion for Public Health*. doi: 10.17269/cjph.102.2725

Prosch, H. (1986). *Michael Polanyi: A Critical Exposition*. State University of New York Press.

Raisch, S., & Birkinshaw, J. (2008). Organizational ambidexterity: Antecedents, outcomes, and moderators. *Journal of Management*, *34*(3), 375–409. doi:10.1177/0149206308316058

Rappaport, J. (1985). The power of empowerment language. *Social Policy*, *16*(2), 15–21.

Rodwell, C. (1996). An analysis of the concept of empowerment. *Journal of Advanced Nursing*, *23*(2), 305–313. doi:10.1111/j.1365-2648.1996.tb02672.x PMID:8708244

Rosenthal, F., & Gutas, D. (1970). *Knowledge Triumphant: The Concept of Knowledge in Medieval Islam*. London: Brill.

Ryle, G. (2009). *The concept of mind*. Routledge.

Sandbrook, R. (2011). Polanyi and Post-neoliberalism in the Global South: Dilemmas of Re-embedding the Economy. *New Political Economy*, *16*(4), 415–443. doi:10.1080/13563467.2010.504300

Scott, A., Maynard, A., & Elliott, R. (2003). *Advances in Health Economics*. New York: Wiley.

Shalley, C. E., Hitt, M. A., & Zhou, J. (2015). *The Oxford Handbook of Creativity, Innovation, and Entrepreneurship*. Oxford University Press. doi:10.1093/oxfordhb/9780199927678.001.0001

Sillitoe, P. (1998). The Development of Indigenous Knowledge: A New Applied Anthropology. *Current Anthropology*, *39*(2), 223–252. doi:10.1086/204722

Sillitoe, P. (2007). Anthropologists only need apply: Challenges of applied anthropology. *Journal of the Royal Anthropological Institute, 13*(1), 147–165. doi:10.1111/j.1467-9655.2007.00418.x

Spender, J. C. (1996). Making knowledge the basis of a dynamic theory of the firm. *Strategic Management Journal, 17*(S2), 45–62. doi:10.1002/smj.4250171106

Styhre, A. (2003). Knowledge management beyond codification: Knowing as practice/concept. *Journal of Knowledge Management, 7*(5), 32–40. doi:10.1108/13673270310505368

Styhre, A. (2003). *Understanding knowledge management: critical and postmodern perspectives.* Liber.

Supiot, A. (2007). *Homo juridicus: on the anthropological function of the law.* New Left Books.

Supiot, A. (2010). *L'esprit de Philadelphie.* Seuil.

Supiot, A. (2015a). *La Gouvernance par les nombres.* Paris: Fayard.

Supiot, A. (2015b). *La solidarité: enquête sur un principe juridique.* Odile Jacob.

Szulanski, G. (1996). Exploring internal stickiness: Impediments to the transfer of best practice within the firm. *Strategic Management Journal, 17*(S2), 27–43. doi:10.1002/smj.4250171105

Szulanski, G. (2000). The Process of Knowledge Transfer: A Diachronic Analysis of Stickiness. *Organizational Behavior and Human Decision Processes, 82*(1), 9–27. doi:10.1006/obhd.2000.2884

Szulanski, G., Cappetta, R., & Jensen, R. J. (2004). When and How Trustworthiness Matters: Knowledge Transfer and the Moderating Effect of Causal Ambiguity. *Organization Science, 15*(5), 600–613. doi:10.1287/orsc.1040.0096

Tengland, P.-A. (2008). Empowerment: A Conceptual Discussion. *Health Care Analysis, 16*(2), 77–96. doi:10.1007/s10728-007-0067-3 PMID:17985247

The Lancet. (2009). What is health? The ability to adapt. *The Lancet, 373*(9666), 781. doi:10.1016/S0140-6736(09)60456-6

Todorov, T. (2001). *Life in Common: An Essay in General Anthropology.* University of Nebraska Press.

Todorov, T. (2005). *The New World Disorder: Reflections of a European.* Wiley.

Todorov, T. (2009). *Imperfect garden: the legacy of humanism.* Princeton University Press. doi:10.1515/9781400824908

Todorov, T. (2010). *The Fear of Barbarians: Beyond the Clash of Civilizations.* Chicago: University Of Chicago Press. doi:10.7208/chicago/9780226805788.001.0001

Todorov, T. (2013). *Nous et les autres. La réflexion française sur la diversité humaine.* Seuil.

Tsoukas, H. (2016). Don't Simplify, Complexify: From Disjunctive to Conjunctive Theorizing in Organization and Management Studies. *Journal of Management Studies.* doi: 10.1111/joms.12219

Vankova, D., Kerekovska, A., Kostadinova, T., & Todorova, L. (2016). Researching health-related quality of life at a community level: Results from a population survey conducted in Burgas, Bulgaria. *Health Promotion International, 31*(3), 534–541. doi:10.1093/heapro/dav016 PMID:25784305

Von Krogh, G., Nonaka, I., & Ichijo, K. (2000). *Enabling Knowledge Creation: New Tools for Unlocking the Mysteries of Tacit Understanding.* Oxford University Press. doi:10.1007/978-1-349-62753-0

Wallerstein, N., & Bernstein, E. (1988). Empowerment Education: Freires Ideas Adapted to Health Education. *Health Education & Behavior, 15*(4), 379–394. doi:10.1177/109019818801500402 PMID:3230016

Wenger, E. (2000). Communities of Practice and Social Learning Systems. *Organization, 7*(2), 225–246. doi:10.1177/135050840072002

WHO. (1986). *Ottawa charter for health promotion. Genebre.* World Health Organization.

WHO. (1998). *Health Promotion Glossary.* Geneva: Department of Health Promotion (DoHP) Health Promotion Glossary, World Health Organization (WHO). Accessed on September 2016 from http://www.who.int/healthpromotion/about/HPG/en/

WHO. (1999). *Health 21 - Health for all in the 21st Century.* Copenhagen: WHO Europe.

Wiggins, N. (2012). Popular education for health promotion and community empowerment: A review of the literature. *Health Promotion International, 27*(3), 356–371. doi:10.1093/heapro/dar046 PMID:21835843

Wilkinson, R., & Pickett, K. (2010). *The spirit level: why equality is better for everyone.* London: Penguin UK.

Williams, L. (2016). Empowerment and the ecological determinants of health: Three critical capacities for practitioners. *Health Promotion International.* doi:10.1093/heapro/daw011 PMID:26989012

Wolfe, B. (2008). Health economics. In S. N. Durlauf & L. E. Blume (Eds.), *The New Palgrave Dictionary of Economics* (2nd ed.). Retrieved from http://www.dictionaryofeconomics.com/article?id/=pde2008_H000031

Yanow, D. (1999). *The languages of 'organizational learning': A palimpsest of terms.* Paper presented at the Third International Conference on Organizational Learning.

Yanow, D. (2000). Seeing Organizational Learning: A Cultural View. *Organization, 7*(2), 247–268. doi:10.1177/135050840072003

Zimmerman, M. A. (2000). Empowerment Theory. In J. Rappaport & E. Seidman (Eds.), *Handbook of Community Psychology* (pp. 43–63). Boston, MA: Springer US. doi:10.1007/978-1-4615-4193-6_2

Zimmerman, M. A., & Rappaport, J. (1988). Citizen participation, perceived control, and psychological empowerment. *American Journal of Community Psychology, 16*(5), 725–750. doi:10.1007/BF00930023 PMID:3218639

KEY TERMS AND DEFINITIONS

Complexity: Complexity has two different meanings that are of interest for research and must be distinguished: one is complexity as reality or object of study, and the other complexity as method or way of approaching issues. In the first conception, reality is complex because it is composed of distinct and interwoven and intermingled elements that create a whole superior to its parts and structured through different levels of reality. In the second sense, complexity as method, it is a way of understanding and study reality in its multiple dimensions and reciprocal interdependencies. In this second acceptance, complexity is also synonymous of interdisciplinarity or transdisciplinarity. It is also sometimes referred to the science or sciences of complexity.

Critical Health Literacy: (See also interactive health literacy and functional health literacy, in this glossary) Critical health literacy is characterized by a focus on groups and context, with the provision of information on social, economic and group determinants of health and how to lead to change, both at the individual, group and community levels (Mårtensson & Hensing, 2012; Nutbeam, 2000; WHO, 1998). It is the third level of health literacy and the most comprehensive one, going beyond the individual as a learner and getting into matters of management, collective choice, decision and public policies.

EHEALTH, eHealth, or E-Health: A concept comprising all applications used at the level of information technology, including the Internet, to enable more efficient patient care, thereby improving access and the quality of management of clinical processes. The Electronic Health Record (EHR) is part of this set of tools. E-health can be considered as a current avenue for implementing policies that aim at empowering patients and actors in the health care sector (Jacquinet & Curado, 2016; Porfírio, Jacquinet, & Carrilho, 2013).

Electronic Health Record: (EHR and also Electronic Health Registry): See also electronic patient registry, medical electronic record. This is the creation of digital information, its storing, management, transmission, access, modification and use across a health care unit, several units or even a whole system of health care. In its basic generic form, the definition of EHR, according to the document ISO/TR 20514:2005 of the ISO – International Standards Organization, can be stated as followed: "repository of information regarding the health status of a subject of care, in computer processable form" (ISO, 2005).

Empowerment: Empowerment in its modern sense (from the late 1950s to today) must be distinguished from its ancient forms, in which the concept was not considered as a general and adequate character for a wide and not much constrained use like today. Authoritarian regimes and old civilizations retained much its scope. (This theme is central to Polanyi´s philosophical endeavor that we do not discuss here; for a hint, see Jah (2002: 1-47). According to the Cornell empowerment Group: "Empowerment is an intentional, ongoing process centered in the local community, involving mutual respect, critical reflection, caring, and group participation, through which people lacking an equal share of valued resources gain greater access to and control over those resources" (Zimmerman 2000: 43). It is important to stress that empowerment is generally construed at the organizational and the community levels (Zimmerman 2000: 44).

Functional Health Literacy: (See also interactive health literacy and critical health literacy, in this glossary) Functional health literacy is the first level of empowerment, its most basic component with a focus on factual information related to health. It is typically represented by flyers, charts, and information given to the patient on a variety of subjects related to health care, from access to precautionary behavior (Nutbeam, 2000). It is not limited to information sharing, however, yet, this is its main component. This is related to the more basic concept of literacy focusing on knowledge and information transmission but not much focus on action and management.

Health: Health, according to the World Health Organization, is a state of complete physical, mental and social well-being and not merely the absence of disease or infirmity. The modern definition of health is an ability, or, to use, Amartya Sen perspective, a capability.

Health Information: This concept means all kinds of information (past, present or future) directly or indirectly linked to a person's health, or clinical and family history, whether that person is alive or deceased. It is not limited to the knowledge produced and exchange by health professionals. It includes the patient information, among other types of information.

Health Literacy: Health literacy is defined by the World Health Organization (WHO) as the "cognitive and social skills that determine the motivation and ability of individuals to gain access to, understand and use information in ways that promote and maintain good health (Martenson and Hensing 2012: 151; see also WHO 1998) There are, according to Nutebeam (2000), three levels of health literacy: the basic one, functional health literacy, that is centered on factual information; the intermediate level or interactive health literacy that is centered on the development of individual skills and its direct context; and, finally, the critical health literacy that relate the individual to the community and public policies as well as the behavioral change of a population in its global context, not just the direct or obvious one.

Health Promotion: Health promotion can be defined as the process of "enabling people to increase control over and improve their health (WHO, 1998). Health is seen as a resource for everyday life, not the objective of living. Health promotion is not just the responsibility of the health sector, but goes beyond healthy lifestyles to well being." (http://www.who.int/healthpromotion/conferences/previous/ottawa/en/, accessed on September 30 2016).

Interactive Health Literacy: (See also functional health literacy and critical health literacy, in this glossary) Interactive health literacy is the second level of empowerment and promotes self help, seizing of opportunities to develop individual skills. The focus here is the individual, its attitude and behavior. It is also more time oriented, meaning to help change individual perceptions, attitudes and knowledge.

Knowledge Management: Without entering any controversy, following Jashapara (2011: 16), we define knowledge management as "the effective learning processes associated with exploration, exploitation and sharing of human knowledge (tacit and explicit) that use appropriate technology and cultural environments to enhance an organization's intellectual capital and performance." It must be extended in health empowerment to groups and social interaction.

Routines: Routines are repeated and stabilized in time patterns of behaviors in organizations and groups. Processes in organizations, when stabilized, can also be considered as routines.

Tacit Knowledge: As Michael Polanyi (1967: 4) wrote in The Tacit Dimension, we should start from the fact that 'we can know more than we can tell'. Jashapara (2011) identifies tacit knowledge to knowing how or intelligence, in a tentative to approximate the concepts of knowledge developed by Michael Polanyi and Gilbert Ryle. It is frequent in the literature to find an opposition between tacit and codified knowledge, construing tacitness as a residual category. This is not our stance, given the complexity of the notion of knowledge and its dynamics, both in science and technological, technical and professional settings.

This research was previously published in the Handbook of Research on Tacit Knowledge Management for Organizational Success edited by Dhouha Jaziri-Bouagina and George Leal Jamil, pages 436-460, copyright year 2017 by Information Science Reference (an imprint of IGI Global).

Chapter 57

Healthy Avatars, Healthy People:
Care Engagement Through the Shared Experience of Virtual Worlds

Stefano Triberti
Catholic University of the Sacred Heart, Italy

Alice Chirico
Catholic University of the Sacred Heart, Italy

ABSTRACT

Recent literature shows that new technologies can be used to promote patient engagement. The present contribution focuses on Virtual Worlds (VWs), namely virtual environments that multiple users can experience together thanks to the use of avatars. Indeed, VWs offer interesting opportunities for patient engagement interventions on two levels. On the individual level, customized avatars are known to have relationships with users' inner experience and Self-conception, so that they may constitute a peculiar additional tool for psychological assessment. Moreover, they are able to promote healthy behaviors thanks to a strong vicarious reinforcement (Proteus effect). On the collective level, VWs constitute an ideal platform to support the emergence of collective flow states (Networked Flow) which are related to the patients' creative activity and well-being. The present contribution deepens these phenomena, presenting VWs as an innovative and interesting tool for the patient engagement interventions of the future.

INTRODUCTION

In this chapter we will discuss the role of new technologies for patient engagement, according to the model of patient engagement of Barello, Graffigna, Vegni and Bosio (2014), Graffigna and Barello (2015), Barello and Graffigna (2014). In details, we will focus on a specific virtual reality tool called Virtual Worlds (VWs), in order to show their implications for healthcare, from both an individual and a group perspective.

The model of patient engagement (PHE) (Graffina, Barello & Triberti, 2015) depicts a picture of the process in which a patient is involved during his/her everyday life experience of disease management.

DOI: 10.4018/978-1-5225-3926-1.ch057

This process emerged as multi componential and dynamic because it regards the whole people's life, which is embraced in all its complexity.

In details, it is the conjunction of emotional (ability to cope with stress and negative emotions due to illness), cognitive (looking for adequate information regarding one's own illness and comprehending all its implications) and behavioral dimensions (adopting adaptive behaviors; adhering to treatment and medication) of people's lives that is responsible for their health engagement (Graffigna & Barello, 2015). The synergy among these dimensions influences patients' ability to adapt to the situation and to interpret personal disease as a normal experience of life which can be included in the broader perspective of existence.

Further, the model suggests that the above-mentioned process of patient engagement is composed of four phases whose synergy is necessary for a patient to benefit from all the resources provided by the healthcare system:

1. **Blackout:** It refers to the feeling of emotive, cognitive and behavioral blackout in which a patient is involved after the occurrence of a critical event, usually receiving the diagnosis.
2. **Arousal:** The name of this phase reflects its own main feature. Indeed, patients become more "activated", but as the terms "arousal" suggests, it is a general activation that does not lead to adopting adaptive coping strategies.
3. **Adhesion:** Even though the patients become more competent both regarding their health and the treatment rules they have to follow, they are still passive in complying with medical prescriptions because they don't understand deeply the meaning of the actions suggested by the medical professionals.
4. **Eudaimonic Project:** Patients are perfectly aware of their condition and accept it and all its implications. In other words, and in order to summarize this complex process, patient initially experience a state of complete disengagement, then they move to a phase of activation (i.e., arousal), adhesion, in which they are still passive, to the building of their personal "eudaimonic project" in which the person is able to reframe disease into normal everyday life (Graffigna & Barello, 2015).

But, how can this model be so effective in healthcare contexts? Which is the added value that this model can provide?

First, the application of this model in health contexts allows facing the increased demand for health which concerns this period of time in which, thanks to the new discoveries and treatments in medicine, survival leading has been increased and there are more aged people than in the past (Graffigna, Barello, Wiederhold, Bosio, & Riva, 2013). This means that people are more likely to suffer for chronic diseases, a type of pathological situation which entails substantial costs for healthcare system.

According to this model, a chronic patient would become able to activate and maintain adaptive behaviors devoted to the management of the situation (behavioral component); to look for adequate information and cognitively structure both the management of the disease and the adherence to the therapy (cognitive component); to cope with the illness-related stress and negative emotions, and also to recover the ability to positively project his/her own life in the future (emotional component) (Barello et al., 2014; Graffigna, Barello, Libreri, & Bosio, 2014).

Moreover, engaging people in their healthcare helps them to co-build their own health together with healthcare professionals and to maintain social relationships and an active role inside their original community. In other words, people can become "advocates of good health" from a broader perspective.

Finally, one of the most relevant features of this model is its suitability to different types of chronic diseases, such as diabetes (Graffigna et al., 2014), cancer (Graffigna, Vegni, Barello, Olson, & Bosio, 2011), different types of addiction (Simpson, 2004) and chronic pain (Cracken, 2005).

Patients can be supported across all these phases in several ways. One of the most effective can be found in the use of new technologies to sustain patient's care experience (Graffigna & Barello, 2015; Graffigna, Barello, & Riva, 2013a, 2013b; Triberti & Riva, 2015a).

According to the positive technology paradigm (Botella et al., 2012; Riva, Baños, Botella, Wiederhold, & Gaggioli, 2012; Triberti & Riva, 2015a), new technologies can be used to structure, augment or even replace the features of an experience. Indeed, they are able to support the individuals in their daily routine and personal issues, contributing to a change in the perception of individuals' own life.

In details, new technologies can address this issue from three perspectives: Hedonic (using technologies to enhance or support the emerging of positive experiences); Eudaimonic (technologies are used as tools to sustain individuals' self-actualization); Social/interpersonal (technologies are used to promote connectedness among individuals) (Riva et al., 2012).

An interesting and still understudied example of the above-mentioned new technologies able to support the care experience and their level of engagement are Virtual Worlds.

NEW FRONTIERS FOR THE PROMOTION OF PATIENT ENGAGEMENT: THE NEW WORLD OF VIRTUAL WORLDS

As written above, new technologies constitute an interesting resource to foster and promote patient engagement. Indeed, recent literature shows how new technologies in general can be used in the context of interventions to this goal, for example, it is evidenced how a given technology can be used to promote the patient moving from a phase to another in the context of his/her own engagement development (Graffigna et al., 2013a, 2013b; Graffigna et al., 2014; Graffigna et al., 2013; Triberti & Riva, 2015a). However, studies focused on peculiar types of technological tools are still rare. In order to partially fill this gap, the present contribution focuses on Virtual Worlds (VWs), providing insights and examples of how they can be used in the context of patient engagement interventions.

Virtual Words are considered a sort of "successor" of Virtual Reality, in that they provide users with the possibility to share the experience of an interactive virtual environment through the creation, customization and use of avatars (Morie & Chance, 2011). In this sense, they combine the advantages of VR's three-dimensional immersive environments with the connectivity and peer support offered by social networks. On the other hand, VWs, compared to virtual reality, are characterized by persistence. In other words, these worlds do not stop existing and functioning after a participant has left. This property is specific to VWs and leads to new possibilities of interaction among users. Indeed, they allow shared activities among users through a synchronous communication modality (i.e., real time communication).

Famous examples of these peculiar media are *Second Life*, *Active Worlds* and *the Sims*.

VWs have been extensively used in the context of eLearning. According to the critical review by Loke (2015), VWs allow the users to learn knowledge and abilities at least in four ways. First, the users have the occasion to reflect on the events and the activities depicted in the virtual environment; second, they have the occasion to engage into verbal interactions with others, so they are able to share ideas and information; third, they are likely to perform cognitive processes (problem solving, decision making) if invited to resolve/cope with the virtually-simulated problems; fourth, they benefit of vicarious experiences and vicarious learning, in that they are able to see and imitate other people (or at least the digital representations of them) performing desirable actions and decisions.

In the context of learning studies, VWs showed to be more enjoyable, interesting and engaging than other tools and instruments (Pellas & Kazanidis, 2013; Tokel & İsler, 2013; Warburton, 2009).

Precisely, Pellas and Kazanidis (2013, 2014) analyzed the engagement promoted by VWs in users basing on a model entailing multiple factors, similar to the patient engagement which is of interest here. They noticed that the experience in VWs-for-learning features promising components such as the cognitive (self-regulation, investment in learning, learning goals…), the emotional (interest, identification, belonging, positive attitude…) and the behavioral ones (positive conduct, effort, participation…).

Basing on the first experiences as a resource for learning, VWs use made its way in the field of healthcare too. Precisely, both virtual reality and VWs have been used to train health professionals in their relational and communicational skills (Triberti & Liberati, 2014). For example, Sweigart and colleagues (Sweigart, Burden, Carlton, & Fillwalk, 2014) analyzed the effects of using a virtual clinic constructed inside *Second Life* to support nursing students' interviewing skills. The results showed the VW being a useful tool to recreate the setting for unfolding, multicultural, mutigenerational case studies. Similar conclusions are reported by other researchers (El Tantawi, Kashlan, & Saeed, 2013; Sweigart & Hodson-Carlton, 2013; Tiffany & Hoglund, 2014).

However, this intervention goal falls beyond the scope of the present chapter. Here, the focus will be on the possible uses of VWs as directed to patients, in particular in order to promote their engagement in the process of healthcare.

In the next sections, it will be showed how the experience of VWs may be of interest from two different (yet interdependent) viewpoints.

On the one hand, VWs allow the creation and customization of avatars, that are, digital representations of their users; on the individual level, this peculiar phenomenon presents interesting opportunities for healthcare projects.

On the other hand, VWs feature the possibility to build, maintain and transform relationship with others in the context of the virtual experience; rather than being "simply" a resource for social and relational benefits, this characteristic of VWs can be very interesting for patient engagement interventions in that it allows the promotion of shared experiences of knowledge and strategy/activity building.

The next two sections will deepen the above-mentioned aspects.

THE INDIVIDUAL LEVEL: AVATARS AND HEALTH

The word avatar comes from Sanskrit and originally referred to gods incarnating in humans. The word made its way through the field of New Media since the video game *Ultima Online – Quest of the Avatar* (Origin Systems, 1985), where it referred to a single fictional character. Later, this term was used to indicate any digital form or content that identifies the action and/or the communication by a human subject inside digital environments. In the context of video games and VWs, avatars are nearly always anthropomorphic figures.

While in video games it is possible to receive an avatar that is already designed by the game itself, in VWs avatars are often created and customized by the players.

Avatars are an interesting topic for cyber-psychology for at least two reasons.

First, they may have relationships with the identity and/or Self of their users; second, the research demonstrated that they are able to influence their users' behavior.

A debate exists about avatar constituting a more or less accurate representation of the users' Selves or not. According to the first theories (Gee, 2003; Kolko, 1998), when a VW (or video game) user create an avatar, he/she has to perform a "selection" among properties and features of his/her own Self representation, in order to "transfer" them in the avatar. The user can customize the appearance of the avatar resembling characteristics of his/her own appearance, and also artifacts and signs relating to interests, ideas, emotions and personality traits. In their customized features, user-created avatars showed to be sensitive also to age and gender (Martey et al., 2015; Villani, Gatti, Confalonieri, & Riva, 2012). According to these theories, avatars should be considered representations of identity.

Other researchers highlighted that not always users create avatars to represent themselves. One may create an avatar "just to try" to be a different person or even a different creature (Fox & Ahn, 2013); moreover, research showed that avatar creation may be sensitive to the context the avatar has to enter. For example (Vasalou & Joinson, 2009), users who expected to enter a dating-related VW created more attractive avatars.

Another field of research is the "avatar Self-discrepancy" one (Dunn & Guadagno, 2012; Jin, 2012), which sustains that users may create avatars to express *desired* renditions of the Selves. A perceived avatar-Self discrepancy has been associated with users' dissatisfaction with real life (Trepte & Reinecke, 2010) and users' intention to gain better mastery of the VW (Trepte, Reinecke, & Behr, 2009) .

Triberti and Argenton (2013) proposed an identity-construction model to show what identity and context materials are present for the user who want to create/customize an avatar, and what can guide his/her selection according to precise intentions.

The model crosses the theories of Social Identity (Tajfel & Turner, 2004) and Real/Ideal Self (Higgins, 1987). Figure 1 shows that the extremes of these theories are crossed to create four quarters.

The four quarters show possible avatars that can be created by a single user, depending on the virtual context and on his/her personal intentions.

Quarter 1 (Q1) and quarter 4 (Q4) show avatars created to resemble a personal idea of oneself, the first focusing on what the person thinks to be at the present moment, the second focusing on desired/prefigured renditions of the Self.

Quarter 2 (Q2) and quarter 3 (Q3) contains avatars that are created by a user who plan to enter a VW (or a multiplayer online game) where other people are present. These avatars may feature peculiar differences in order to be recognizable by others, or in order to communicate to them precise emotions, personality traits or ideas.

This model is useful to show how the creation of an avatar may be complex and related to one's own Self in many ways.

As said before, avatars not only have interesting relationship with Self and identity. They are also able to influence behavior.

Basing on the mythological figure able to change his own form, researchers labeled *Proteus effect* (Fox, Bailenson, & Tricase, 2013; Yee, Bailenson, & Ducheneaut, 2009; Yee & Bailenson, 2007) the phenomenon of one's behavior modified by guiding a certain avatar. For example, guiding taller avatars moved users to behave more aggressively during virtual reality based negotiation games; using attractive avatars moved users to be more self-confident during virtual interactions.

In the next section, these phenomena will be deepened in the context of healthcare and patient engagement.

Figure 1. Model for avatar identity construction
(adapted from Triberti & Argenton, 2013)

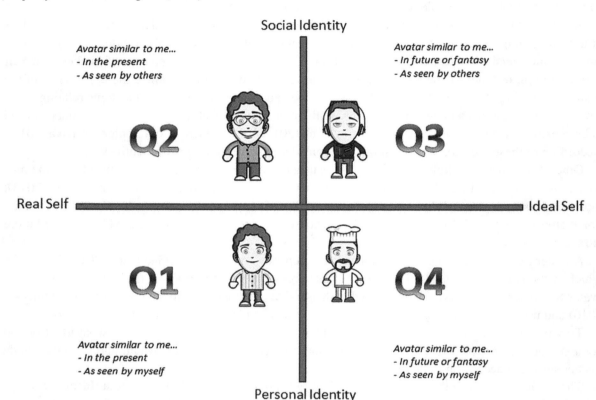

Avatars for Healthcare and Patient Engagement

After the brief introduction about avatars in the last paragraph, the present paragraph will deepen their utility as a resource for healthcare and for patient engagement interventions in particular.

As previously said, avatars maintain some kind of relationship with their users' Selves. Although this relation may be complex and influenced by different factors (e.g., avatars can be representation of the Self; just an identity experimentation; a desired rendition of the Self), it is clear that they can be considered as indicator of the inner experience of people.

Some studies already tested the possibility to use customized avatars as information about the users' characteristics, ranging from personality traits to stages of development (Fong & Mar, 2015; Villani et al., 2012). Other studies explored the virtual representation of life experiences through avatars customization and action inside VWs; for example, Lomanowska and Guitton (2014) analyzed the virtual re-enactment of pregnancy, birth and maternity inside *Second Life*.

Patient engagement, or more precisely, the phase of care engagement a given patient is in, is known to have peculiar influences on his/her own conception of the Self (Barello & Graffigna, 2014). For example, a chronic patient in the blackout phase is living the experience of the establishing of a diagnosis, which means he/she is struggling with the emotional shock deriving from realizing he/she is now a person with a disease: for this reason, the patient perceives him/herself as a "ill body", and is completely absorbed in the illness experience. Differently, the last stages of the patient engagement process allow one to recover his/her own life project despite the presence of the disease and the need to daily adhere to treatment and comply with caregivers and health professionals advices. Again according to Barello and Graffigna (2014), the patient now understands that the "patient self" is only one of the possible Selves, so that he/she is able to recognize his/her internal resources as useful to project satisfactory life trajectories for the future (Barello et al., 2015).

On this basis, if used in conjunction with other assessment tools, the avatar can be considered as a resource to analyze a patient's inner experience, in terms of what he/she thinks to be, or what he/she desires to become/achieve in the future. For example, it is possible to assume that patients in early stages of the engagement process may be driven to represent themselves with a limited number of features, or they may represent themselves highlighting visual features related to the disease or to the emotionally-difficult situation they are living. Differently, patients who start recovering positive conceptions of the Selves projected in the future may customize avatars with a higher number of features identifying passions and interests. In this sense, when imagining a patient engagement intervention which makes use of VWs for patients, the customization of avatars may be a supplemental tool for psychological analysis and assessment, and also a tool to guide patients' interviews deepening their evolving Self-conception.

With regard to the second interesting aspect of avatar, namely their ability in modifying behavior, it has been already used in the context of healthcare interventions.

For example, Murray and colleagues (Murray, Hardy, Spruijt-Metz, Hekler, & Raij, 2013) proposed a classification of avatars' features (physical, behavioral and environmental, that is modification of the environment where the avatar resides) to provide feedback to patients about their progress in disease treatment; for instance, avatar's strength in lifting objects may be an indication of the user's empowered ability due to rehabilitation exercises.

According to Kim and Sundar (2012), participants who created their avatars resembling ideal Selves then obtained positive outcomes (in terms of promotion and prevention-focused Self-regulatory strategies) for health management.

Another experiment (Fox & Bailenson, 2009) showed that participants who saw a digital representation of themselves doing physical exercise then performed more physical exercise comparing with participants who saw a digital representation of another person, due to a stronger effect of vicarious reinforcement. Surveys showed that the effect resisted in a follow-up.

In this sense, both the characteristics and the behavior of an avatar emerged as having an effect on the behaviour of their users. The Proteus effect (Yee & Bailenson, 2007) already demonstrated to be useful in the context of healthcare, so it is possible to prefigure the use of avatars also in order to influence patients in their journey, across the process of activation/engagement in their own care. For example, watching one's own avatar participating in VW-based simulation of medical consultation and gaining positive outcomes from it may positively influence the patient's motivation to recover the consultation also in daily life.

The Social Level: Relationships in Virtual Worlds and Networked Flow

In order to support a patient during all the engagement process, important aspects are personal relationships with care providers, family and also people who are suffering from the same disease.

As above-mentioned, VWs are a powerful tool to support patient engagement also at the level of social relationships.

For example, they are useful tools to share information and experiences regarding healthcare with others. Moreover, they can be used also to gain social support, to find clear guidelines to follow with regard to a specific disease and much more (Suomi, Mäntymäki, & Söderlund, 2014). In other words, they are able to connect people in a new way.

Indeed, considering patients with difficulty in walking or simply in moving, it would be very expensive and almost impossible to help them to keep constantly in contact with other people. On the other hand, the experience of being a part of a group is crucial in order to share emotions, thoughts, coping strategies, receive social support which can have positive health effects (Berkman & Syme, 1979; Bandura, 2001; Buunk, Gibbons, & Buunk, 1997/2013; Cantisano, Rimé, & Muñoz-Sastre, 2013; Cohen & Wills, 1985; Cohen & Syme, 1985). Indeed, first, social support can be both emotional (e.g., emotions sharing) and cognitive (e.g., simple information sharing) (Richmond, Ross, & Egeland, 2007; Buunk et al., 1997/2013; Lin, Dean, & Ensel, 2013) and generally, being part of a group has a great impact on our Self (Suls & Wheeler, 2000).

Therefore, even though the link between the experience in VWs and the real life need to be further analyzed (Beard, Wilson, Morra, & Keelan, 2009), VWs are undoubtedly able (Cohen & Syme, 1985) to create a bridge between these patients and the world outside the hospital, and to give rise to the feeling of being part of a group. VWs allow patients to reframe their Selves as persons and not only as patients.

Therefore the added value provided by VWs is that they allow people with different kinds of disabilities and from a great distance, to become again owners of their lives, moving from a patient-condition to a person-condition (Graffigna & Barello, 2015). This is crucial to engage patients towards their healthcare because it helps them to become active co-builders of their own health, assuming responsibility for it.

In the next paragraph, we will show that being a part of a group can lead not only to all the above mentioned benefits, but also to the emerging of a positive optimal group experience of engagement.

Indeed, recently, according to the model of Networked Flow (Gaggioli, Riva, Milani, & Mazzoni, 2013), it has been found that when a group is entirely focused on a specific activity, it is possible that a positive optimal group experience of engagement emerges, both in a real and in a virtual setting. Sawyer (2003) was the first who investigate this phenomenon which was labeled "group flow". Each time group members are involved in a specific task, it is possible that this experience occurs and it is responsible for optimal group performances and a maximum level of engagement among members.

The potentialities of this optimal group experience to promote patients' active participation towards their healthcare will be discussed in the next paragraph.

A New Way to Engage Patients: From Group Flow to Networked Flow Experience

As said in the previous paragraph, engaging patients in their own healthcare is necessary to help them adapt to the situation and to interpret personal disease as a normal experience of life which can be included in the broader perspective of existence.

However, not all the patients can be easily engaged. Take chronic patients, in particular those who suffer from physical disease (e.g., patients who can't walk). The healthcare system can difficulty bear the costs necessary to engage them.

Therefore, we suggest a new way of supporting patient engagement which can be affordable, amusing and available for all the patients. VWs are the key to address this issue. With this regard, they provide benefits both at an individual level and at a group level. While the first (i.e., individual level) was addressed in the previous paragraphs, the second level will be detailed and discussed in the following.

As we mentioned before, taking part in a group is a fertile field to engage patients in their own care management, showing a double advantage for each member:

1. These group experiences provide social support and sharing of coping strategies, and can support both individual and group well-being through the promotion of connectedness (Ryff & Singer, 2000; Buunk et al., 1997/2013; Cantisano et al., 2013; Cohen & Wills, 1985; Cohen & Syme, 1985).
2. These group experiences can lead people to experience a sense of total absorption in the task so that they feel fully engaged in what they are doing (Gaggioli et al., 2013; Riva et al., 2012; Riva, Milani, & Gaggioli, 2010). Moreover, working together on the same task, patients can be motivated to produce new resources (artifacts, practices, strategies) useful to manage together their own common experience of disease and illness.

While the first aspect has been discussed in the last section of the previous paragraph, the second one deserves to be further explained.

Recently, a new model on group creativity has been developed by Gaggioli and colleagues (Gaggioli et al., 2013), namely, the Networked Flow model. According to this frame, when a group is entirely focused on a specific activity, it is possible that a positive optimal group experience of engagement emerges, both in a real and in a virtual setting.

With the term "optimal group experience", we refer to the phenomenon of *group flow* which was first investigated by Sawyer (2003).

He highlighted that each time group members are involved in a specific task, it is possible that this experience occurs and it is responsible for optimal group performances and a maximum level of engagement among members.

In order to clarify the implications of living this optimal group experience for patient engagement, it is necessary to better introduce this phenomenon, its history and its peculiarities.

First, the domain in which group flow has been first investigated is creativity. In details, the existence of group flow was discovered several years before the development of the Networked Flow model that can be considered as a more general frame in which group flow is included.

As we explained previously, Sawyer (2003, 2006, 2008) was the first to introduce the concept of "group flow" and to investigate it deeply.

Starting from the analysis of improvisational groups engaged in public performances (jazz bands and theaters), he noticed the emergence of a peculiar group optimal experience, closely related to high performances, and highest level of group engagement, which he labeled "group flow". Group flow, far from being the sum of individual optimal experiences of each member (Csikszentmihalyi, 1975; Csikszentmihalyi, 2000), can be considered as an emergent property of group itself, as a sort of "collective state of mind" (p. 43). People feel as a part of a unique body, moving in unison and sharing the same intentions. This phenomenon emerges from the interactions occurring within a group and is able to positively influence overall performance.

He found also several group features able to support the emerging of this experience:

1. The presence of *shared objectives.*
2. The ability to *listen carefully to each other.*

3.   *Deep concentration* on the task.
4.   *Perception of control* on individual actions, autonomy and personal competence.
5.   *Blending egos* so that members feel as if they were a unique body.
6.   *Equal participation* among members.
7.   **Familiarity:** Members should know the performance of colleagues.
8.   *Clear and free communication* among group members.
9.   The ability to *build on other's ideas.*
10. *Possibility of failure* must be clear in members' mind.

Other researches confirmed the relevance of these dimensions to trigger group flow experience (Hart & Di Blasi, 2013; Sawyer, 2008), even though this phenomenon should be explored more deeply in order to discover all its potentialities.

An important integration of this initial perspective towards group engagement is provided by the Networked Flow model which considers group creative collaboration, not only in dynamic terms, but also in structural terms. Therefore, also group structure and artifacts produced need to be considered as a part of the same "creative network".

In other words, the change of perspective occurs from "creative groups" to "creative networks" (Gaggioli et al., 2013) where not only people but also the environment in which creative process takes place and the artifacts produced deserve to be considered.

To better clarify this issue and the implications for patient engagement, the Networked Flow model will be discussed in details.

First, the name of this model itself reminds its main features which are:

1.   The presence of *an optimal group experience among members* (i.e., group flow) closely related to the most creative group performances
2.   The importance of *group structure and social pre-existing environment.*

According to this model, group flow is more than a simple sum of individual interactions (Sawyer, 2003, 2006, 2008), and it can be reached only after the achievement of a "collaborative zone of proximal development" (Gaggioli, Mazzoni, Milani, & Riva, 2015). This condition is characterized by the reach of a balance between individual and group actions which allows the emerging of a sense of Social Presence (i.e., the sensation that we are together in the same place with other Selves in a real or virtual environment) (Biocca & Harms, 2003; Harms & Biocca, 2004; Riva, 2008; Riva et al., 2010).

Simply, when group members feel closely connected to each other and fully absorbed by the group task, even though they are not in the same place, a fertile collaboration field is established and groups are able to achieve their best performance and to create products with a great potential impact on the wider society.

Therefore, this model highlights that this maximum level of group engagement can be reached also in a virtual environment.

The second pilaster of this model refers to the importance that is attributed to group structure, considering also artifacts which emerge from group performance. This feature is due to the "stigmergic" nature of group collaborative processes, namely, each mark left by a member is a trigger for the performance of a next action by the same or by another individual (Elliot, 2006; Grassé, 1959).

Therefore, creativity itself is distributed in the minds, interactions and artifacts of a group. Creativity is not only a matter of people but also concerns artifacts produced by individuals which contribute to create a network, namely a creative network (Gaggioli et al., 2013).

Therefore, in order to engage patients at a group level also artifacts are essential, as it will be detailed.

According to the Networked Flow model, this optimal experience (i.e., networked flow) emerges as a complex phenomenon in which not only the dimension of process but also the structural one is considered. This experience arises concurrently with a process of group creativity which emerges in six stages:

1. **Meeting and Persistence:** From an initial cultural and socio-economical frame, some individuals recognize reciprocal intentions directed towards the present, and something similar to a group begins to emerge.
2. **Reducing the Distance:** People, who recognize to have similar intentions, reduce distance and start to interact more frequently. They start to act as a minority with regard to the original frame.
3. **The Liminality-Parallel Action:** The boundaries of the new subgroup become clearer and definite; therefore the group acts to differentiate itself from the pre-existing frame.
4. **Networked Flow:** This phase is characterized by the emerging of the optimal group experience of Networked Flow in which mainly, individuals' intentions are blended together into group' ones and the new frame becomes explicit.
5. **Creation of the Artifact:** This is the phase in which group's intentions are embedded in one or more artifacts which are, however, used and considered relevant only by the group itself and not by the whole frame. It emerges clearly now the "distributed" nature of optimal creative group process which is not only dependent on individuals but also on artifacts made. Definitely, it is possible to say that group intentions are embedded in the group artifact.
6. **Application of the Artifact:** At this phase, artifacts meet the pre-existing framework. Therefore, "optimal creative group process" does not finish with the creation of the artifact, but with its introduction in the whole pre-existing network.

These phases underline the distributed nature of group creativity which is not only in the mind of group members but also in the produced artifacts (Inghilleri, Riva, & Riva, 2014).

The role of artifacts can now be more clarified.

Indeed, according to the Networked Flow model, during group flow, people are extremely engaged and concentrated on group task which has the delicate function of creating an artifact in which all group's intentions are incorporated. Therefore, also the artifact is part of group collaboration process and represents group identity.

It is now clear how these experiences can affect patients' attitude towards their healthcare by promoting their engagement through group creative tasks: being a part of a group who is involved in the creation of an artifact relevant for all the group members, can lead to a maximum level of group engagement, namely, group flow.

Because this experience (i.e., group flow) can occur both in natural and in virtual environments (Gaggioli et al., 2013; Riva et al., 2012; Riva et al., 2010; Sawyer, 2003, 2006, 2007, 2008), VWs are particularly suitable to promote these experience.

At this point, also the link between the process of patients' engagement, new technologies (in this case VWs) and group flow, emerges clearly.

Given that VWs are democratic tools able to extend the possibility of social interaction also to patients who, differently, could not have been connected with other people; and, according to the frame of Networked Flow, group collaboration can lead to the emergence of a group optimal experience also in mediated environments, and patients can be effectively engaged also through VWs. Indeed, they can be involved in group creative activities and can be motivated to produce new resources (artifacts, practices, strategies) useful to manage together their own common experience of disease. Social interactions through VWs can be another way to gain social support. Moreover, the experience of being able to create useful artifacts is closely related also to people's self-efficacy and self-esteem, which are key components of well-being (Bandura, 1982, 2001; Brown, Hoye, & Nicholson, 2012; Kernis, 2013; Thoits, 2013; Wu et al., 2012). Indeed, our efficacy beliefs are linked to our sense of engagement regarding a task, both at an individual and at a group level (Simbula, Guglielmi, & Schaufeli, 2011; Vera, Le Blanc, Taris, & Salanova, 2014).

Both group flow and Networked Flow are extremely engaging experiences, in which each member of a group is fully concentrated and absorbed by the group task. But, which kind of task can be effective for the emerging of group flow and networked flow? In other words, which task can better sustain patients' engagement with regard to their healthcare? If we analyze the literature regarding VWs and patients' engagement, one of the most used VW platforms is *Second Life* (Beard et al., 2009; Suomi et al., 2014). *Second Life* is an online VW in which it is possible to interact with other people by means of avatars. Despite the high number of health-related interventions on Second Life (informative, supportive, training, or recruiting for researches), Suomi et al. (2014) evidenced that little social interactions occur in this environment. Even though users have many opportunities of interacting with each other also through non verbal communication cues, it seemed that no intervention was really able to support this social interaction feature. For this reason we suggest group creative activities in which users (i.e., patients) can build together one or more artifacts that have an impact also on the real world. Indeed, the high sense of presence and social presence that users can experience during the execution of tasks, even in a VW, are able to support their engagement and sense of self-efficacy. In other words, thanks to the features of Second Life platform, patients can feel as if others were actually present with them in that environment. Patients can actually work in group creating something meaningful for them and also for the entire society. Doing so, in this mediated environment, patients would be able to enter a state of flow which could enable them to feel more engaged in their own care management giving them the opportunity of feeling again owners and active co-builder of their own lives (Csikszentmihalyi, 1997; Riva, Castelnuovo, & Mantovani, 2006).

Consider the example of a chronic patient who is never going to be able to walk, or who can only moves fingers on a keyboard. This person may feel not competent to do something useful for his own condition, experiencing his own dependency by caregivers and care providers every day. A patient engagement plan may be particularly difficult when directed to patients who, due to a peculiar pathological condition, are actually impaired in basic functions. VWs such as Second Life offer the possibility of overcoming these hindrances and make also people who suffer from severe chronic disease able to become again owner of their healthcare and of some aspects of their everyday life. Imagine that chronic patients unable to move, except of their fingers and heads, are asked to think and realize a project for other people who are experiencing their same conditions. They are invited to share their personal backgrounds in order to make something useful and meaningful for other real people, and also for themselves. Therefore, they can participate and contribute to the design of new projects of healthcare. Finally, also a completely different task as managing a virtual place (say: a facility in which new patients' avatars may be welcomed when entering the VW) can foster the emerging of a group flow experience. Creativity is the first step requested to healthcare professionals, but it is not the only one. Care providers have to be sensitive towards the intrinsic patient's needs, giving voice to them in an innovative way, until patients will be able to do it by their own. The combination between patients' actual needs and patients' expectations towards the future will be the bases of the fascinating architecture of patient engagement in VWs. With this regard, VWs can actually become worlds in which everything is possible and with an impact on the real life too (Beard et al., 2009).

An example in this direction can be found in the system of online support groups (Shopler & Galinsky 2014). Patients suffering from cancer benefited of online support groups, reducing symptomatology, distress and promoting wellbeing. The dimension of sharing provided by this typology of intervention is easily reproducible trough VWs, which could also put distant patients in contact and could offer the possibility for a complete anonymity too. Finally, we suggest that some kinds of disease force patient to social isolation (e.g., immunodeficiency), so VWs could help to overcome this hindrance.

A final example in this direction is the research protocol proposed by Gaggioli et al. (2014), who evidenced the possible positive implications of group reminiscence therapy for institutionalized elderly adults in terms of increased self-esteem, life satisfaction, quality of life and decreased depressive symptoms. Among the different possible reminiscence modalities (Haber, 2006) we suggest here the one based on "life review" that seems the most suitable approach to promote the reach of an Eudaimonic project, according to the model of patient engagement. Indeed, this approach allows patient to concentrate on both positive and negative life time memories, in order to help patient to achieve ego integrity again. This could be a powerful tool to reframe disease in to normal everydaylife. Further, the positive implications of reminiscence interventions could be enriched by the social dimension of sharing provided by VWs also for those patients unable to move.

CAVEATS

Despite the relevant and extraordinary possibilities provided by new technologies in healthcare, there is also a "dark side" regarding the use of these tools for patient engagement. In this contribution we have focused on the positive outcomes that could be originated by the use of VWs only. Nevertheless, there are also some negative aspects which should be considered regarding the use of new technologies. Indeed, some possible negative outcomes are related to the patient engagement phase the patient is involved in. For example, according to the PHE model, at the beginning (blackout phase) patients are not prepared to effectively face the disease, and they are not aware of the situation. Therefore, it could be really difficult to use technologies such as VWs in this phase. In this context, the main challenges are (i) to make patients aware of the fact that they are not alone while facing their own illness; (ii) to make them aware of the most important information they should know concerning their illness. Therefore, it could be difficult to persuade them of the add value of new technologies regarding the two above-mentioned aspects. Instead, some patients may prefer traditional procedures, such as talking with their own doctor or directly with their own family.

For what regards the following phases, it is important to guarantee that patients are not considering VWs as a video game or "just fun". Otherwise, it should be made clear that they are using a healthcare tool. Moreover, both medical professionals and patients could not feel enough competent regarding the use of VWs which would be perceived as hindrances instead of facilitators, able to help patients to adequately face their own disease and its implications. Finally, patients suffering from cognitive deficits should be accompanied in the exploration of WVs by medical assistants, since the use of some virtual reality-based technology requires attention and cognitive abilities.

FUTURE RESEARCH DIRECTIONS

In light of the above-mentioned literature and observations made before, a possible future challenge for researchers in this field could be investigating the long-term effects of avatars for users. For example, can avatars be able to (i) change over time offering useful feedback to patients about their own body changes and (ii) to help them better understand their own health situation (for example, aging avatars, or avatars visibly recovering from disease symptoms)? To this purpose, a possible way could be to adopt longitudinal perspective of analysis. Further, almost all features of WVs can be manipulated. Therefore, this aspect opens the possibility of building infinite types of VWs, so that customization emerges as the main feature of these environments. Moreover, it is possible to modify a pre-existing environment provided, for example, by the *Second Life* platform, in order to reach a specific therapeutic goal. On the other hand, this potentiality deserves to be further investigated with regard to the implications of manipulating some features with respect to others. To address this issue, it could be very useful to adopt a multidisciplinary approach towards VWs design, in order to improve all their potentialities and understanding the implications due to some choices regarding designs with respect to others. For example, User-Centered Design, as a design based on a prior research/analysis of users' needs and intentions, has been already associated to the use of new technologies for patient engagement and patient centered medicine (Triberti & Liberati, 2014; Triberti & Riva, 2015b).

Other possible future research directions relate to the current development of virtual reality technologies, which may be adapted to Virtual Worlds too in the future. Total immersion inside computer-generates experiences is today more and more reachable. For example, research on the so-called body-swapping illusion (Petkova & Ehrsson, 2008; Riva, in press; Serino et al., 2015) suggest that it is possible to induce the sensation to own a virtual body, even different from the real one. The relevance of this technology is evident in the field of diseases characterized by alteration of bodily self-consciousness, which can be manipulated according to patient's needs. These new scenarios expand the potentialities of virtual reality-based tools of generating meaningful experiences for their users.

Finally, virtual reality is moving to mobile devices and it is becoming more affordable. New head-mounted displays are available on the market, such as Google Cardboard, able to adapt mobile phones for the fruition of virtual reality-based contents. Therefore, everyone can experience an immersive VR environment with a low economic investment. Since these VR devices are intuitive and easy to use, they constitute a concrete opportunity to expand actual possibilities in the healthcare field.

CONCLUSION

To conclude, the model of patient engagement offers a picture of the process patients go through during their everyday life experience of disease management. The final expected outcome is the reaching of a complete awareness towards their own disease with the assumption of an active role in managing their healthcare.

New technologies are one of the best ways to support patients across all the phases of this complex process. They can be used to structure, augment or even replace the features of an experience. Indeed, they are able to support the individuals in their daily routine and personal issues, contributing to a change in the perception of individuals' own life.

An example of new technologies which emerges as effective tools for patient engagement are Virtual Words.

Their impact can be seen both at an individual level, relating to the utilization of an avatar, and at a group level. Indeed, avatars can be used as an assessment tool in that they have relationships with the users' inner experience and Self-conception. Moreover, the opportunities provided by VWs are mainly two: (i) the democratic nature of this tool which can be used also by people unable to move and living from a great distance; (ii) the economic benefits due to the fact that the majority of VWs platforms are free.

Moreover, at a group level, VWs can be used to foster optimal group experiences responsible for high levels of engagement and group performance. This experience emerges when all group members are involved in a specific task relevant for each of them. There are many examples of task that groups of patients can do in a virtual world. Therefore, all patients can feel engaged towards their healthcare using VWs.

We suggest deepening the analysis of the opportunities for patient engagement provided by these kinds of digital environments, so that the people suffering from different diseases could benefit from their use regarding their own healthcare. VWs can be actually considered "unexplored worlds" for what regards their social dimension; therefore, we hope that future researchers and web developers would be interested in deepening VWs tools as a resource to promote patient engagement and well-being.

REFERENCES

Bandura, A. (1982). Self-efficacy mechanism in human agency. *The American Psychologist, 37*(2), 122–147. doi:10.1037/0003-066X.37.2.122

Bandura, A. (2001). Social cognitive theory: An agentic perspective. *Annual Review of Psychology, 52*(1), 1–26. doi:10.1146/annurev.psych.52.1.1 PMID:11148297

Barello, S., & Graffigna, G. (2014). Engaging patients to recover life projectuality: An Italian cross-disease framework. *Quality of Life Research: An International Journal of Quality of Life Aspects of Treatment, Care and Rehabilitation, 24*(5), 1087–1096. doi:10.1007/s11136-014-0846-x PMID:25373927

Barello, S., Graffigna, G., Vegni, E., & Bosio, A. (2014). The challenges of conceptualizing patient engagement in healthcare: A lexicographic literature review. *Journal of Participatory Medicine, 6*, e9.

Barello, S., Graffigna, G., Vegni, E., Savarese, M., Lombardi, F., & Bosio, A. C. (2015). 'Engage me in taking care of my heart': A grounded theory study on patient–cardiologist relationship in the hospital management of heart failure. *BMJ Open, 5*(3), e005582. doi:10.1136/bmjopen-2014-005582 PMID:25776041

Beard, L., Wilson, K., Morra, D., & Keelan, J. (2009). A survey of health-related activities on second life. *Journal of Medical Internet Research, 11*(2), e17. doi:10.2196/jmir.1192 PMID:19632971

Berkman, L. F., & Syme, S. L. (1979). Social networks, host resistance, and mortality: A nine-year follow-up study of Alameda County residents. *American Journal of Epidemiology, 109*(2), 186–204. doi:10.4236/health.2012.49087 PMID:425958

Biocca, F., & Harms, C. (2003). *Guide to the Networked Minds Social Presence Inventory v. 1.2: Measures of co-presence, social presence, subjective symmetry, and intersubjective symmetry.* Michigan State University. Retrieved from http://cogprints.org/6743/

Botella, C., Riva, G., Gaggioli, A., Wiederhold, B. K., Alcaniz, M., & Banos, R. M. (2012). The present and future of positive technologies. *Cyberpsychology, Behavior, and Social Networking, 15*(2), 78–84. doi:10.1089/cyber.2011.0140 PMID:22149078

Brown, K. M., Hoye, R., & Nicholson, M. (2012). Self-esteem, self-efficacy, and social connectedness as mediators of the relationship between volunteering and well-being. *Journal of Social Service Research, 38*(4), 468–483. doi:10.1080/01488376.2012.687706

Buunk, B. P., Gibbons, F. X., & Buunk, A. (1997/2013). *Health, coping, and well-being: Perspectives from social comparison theory.* Mahwah, NJ: Erlbaum.

Cantisano, N., Rimé, B., & Muñoz-Sastre, M. T. (2013). The social sharing of emotions in HIV/AIDS: A comparative study of HIV/AIDS, diabetic and cancer patients. *Journal of Health Psychology, 18*(10), 1255–1267. doi:10.1177/1359105312462436 PMID:23129833

Cohen, S., & Wills, T. A. (1985). Stress, social support, and the buffering hypothesis. *Psychological Bulletin, 98*(2), 310–357. doi:10.1037/0033-2909.98.2.310 PMID:3901065

Cohen, S. E., & Syme, S. (1985). *Social support and health.* New York: Academic Press.

Csikszentmihalyi, M. (1975). *Beyond boredom and anxiety.* San Francisco, CA: Jossey-Bass.

Csikszentmihalyi, M. (1997). *Finding flow: The psychology of engagement with everyday life.* New York: Basic Books.

Csikszentmihalyi, M. (2000). *Beyond boredom and anxiety.* San Francisco: Jossey-Bass.

Dunn, R. A., & Guadagno, R. E. (2012). My avatar and me–Gender and personality predictors of avatar-self discrepancy. *Computers in Human Behavior, 28*(1), 97–106. doi:10.1016/j.chb.2011.08.015

El Tantawi, M. M., El Kashlan, M. K., & Saeed, Y. M. (2013). Assessment of the Efficacy of Second Life, a Virtual Learning Environment, in Dental Education. *Journal of Dental Education, 77*(12), 1639–1652. PMID:24319136

Elliot, M. (2006). Stigmergic collaboration: The evolution of group work. *journal of media and culture, 9*(2).

Fong, K., & Mar, R. A. (2015). What Does My Avatar Say About Me? Inferring Personality From Avatars. *Personality and Social Psychology Bulletin, 41*(2), 237–249. doi:10.1177/0146167214562761 PMID:25576173

Fox, J., & Ahn, S. J. (2013). Avatars: Portraying, Exploring, and Changing Online and Offline Identities. In R. Luppicini (Ed.), *Handbook of Research on Technoself: Identity in a Technological Society* (Vol. 1, pp. 255–271). Hershey: IGI Global. doi:10.4018/978-1-4666-2211-1.ch014

Fox, J., & Bailenson, J. N. (2009). Virtual self-modeling: The effects of vicarious reinforcement and identification on exercise behaviors. *Media Psychology*, *12*(1), 1–25. doi:10.1080/15213260802669474

Fox, J., Bailenson, J. N., & Tricase, L. (2013). The embodiment of sexualized virtual selves: The Proteus effect and experiences of self-objectification via avatars. *Computers in Human Behavior*, *29*(3), 930–938. doi:10.1016/j.chb.2012.12.027

Gaggioli, A., Mazzoni, E., Milani, L., & Riva, G. (2015). The creative link: Investigating the relationship between social network indices, creative performance and flow in blended teams. *Computers in Human Behavior*, *42*, 157–166. doi:10.1016/j.chb.2013.12.003

Gaggioli, A., Riva, G., Milani, L., & Mazzoni, E. (2013). *Networked Flow: Towards an Understanding of Creative Networks*. Heidelberg: Springer. doi:10.1007/978-94-007-5552-9

Gaggioli, A., Scaratti, C., Morganti, L., Stramba-Badiale, M., Agostoni, M., Spatola, C. A., & Riva, G. et al. (2014). Effectiveness of group reminiscence for improving wellbeing of institutionalized elderly adults: Study protocol for a randomized controlled trial. *Trials*, *15*(1), 408. doi:10.1186/1745-6215-15-408 PMID:25344703

Gee, J. P. (2003). *What videogames have to teach us about learning and literacy* (2nd ed.). New York: Palgrave Macmillan.

Graffigna, G., & Barello, S. (2015). Modelling Patient Engagement in Healthcare: Insight for Research and Practice. In G. Graffigna, S. Barello, & S. Triberti (Eds.), *Patient Engagement: A consumer-centered model to innovate healthcare*. Berlin: DeGruyter Open. doi:10.1515/9783110452440-004

Graffigna, G., Barello, S., Libreri, C., & Bosio, C. A. (2014). How to engage type-2 diabetic patients in their own health management: Implications for clinical practice. *BMC Public Health*, *14*(1), 648. doi:10.1186/1471-2458-14-648 PMID:24966036

Graffigna, G., Barello, S., & Riva, G. (2013a). How to make health information technology effective: The challenge of patient engagement. *Archives of Physical Medicine and Rehabilitation*, *94*(10), 2034–2035. doi:10.1016/j.apmr.2013.04.024 PMID:24075414

Graffigna, G., Barello, S., & Riva, G. (2013b). Technologies for patient engagement. *Health Affairs (Project Hope)*, *32*(6), 1172. doi:10.1377/hlthaff.2013.0279 PMID:23733998

Graffigna, G., Barello, S., & Triberti, S. (2015). *Patient Engagement: A consumer-centered model to innovate healthcare*. Berlin: DeGruyter Open. doi:10.1515/9783110452440

Graffigna, G., Barello, S., Triberti, S., Wiederhold, B. K., Bosio, A. C., & Riva, G. (2014). Enabling eHealth as a pathway for patient engagement: A toolkit for medical practice. *Studies in Health Technology and Informatics*, *199*, 13–21. PMID:24875682

Graffigna, G., Barello, S., Wiederhold, B. K., Bosio, A. C., & Riva, G. (2013). Positive technology as a driver for health engagement. *Studies in Health Technology and Informatics, 191*, 9–17. PMID:23792833

Graffigna, G., Vegni, E., Barello, S., Olson, K., & Bosio, C. A. (2011). Studying the social construction of cancer-related fatigue experience: The heuristic value of Ethnoscience. *Patient Education and Counseling, 82*(3), 402–409. doi:10.1016/j.pec.2010.12.017 PMID:21292426

Grassé, P. P. (1959). La reconstruction du nid et les coordinations interindividuelles chezBellicositermes natalensis et Cubitermes sp. la théorie de la stigmergie: Essai d'interprétation du comportement des termites constructeurs. *Insectes Sociaux, 6*(1), 41–80. doi:10.1007/BF02223791

Haber, D. (2006). Life review: Implementation, theory, research, and therapy. *International Journal of Aging & Human Development, 63*(2), 153–171. doi:10.2190/DA9G-RHK5-N9JP-T6CC PMID:17137032

Harms, C., & Biocca, F. (2004). Internal Consistency and Reliability of the Networked Minds - Measure of Social Presence. *Proceedings of the Seventh Annual International Workshop: Presence*. Valencia, CA: Universidad Politecnica de Valencia press.

Hart, E., & Di Blasi, Z. (2015). Combined flow in musical jam sessions: A pilot qualitative study. *Psychology of Music, 43*(2), 275-290. doi:0305735613502374.

Higgins, E. T. (1987). Self-discrepancy: A theory relating self and affect. *Psychological Review, 94*(3), 319–340. doi:10.1037/0033-295X.94.3.319 PMID:3615707

Inghilleri, P., Riva, G., & Riva, E. (2014). *Enabling Positive Change: Flow and Complexity in Daily Experience*. Berlin: De Gruyter Open.

Jin, S. A. A. (2012). The virtual malleable self and the virtual identity discrepancy model: Investigative frameworks for virtual possible selves and others in avatar-based identity construction and social interaction. *Computers in Human Behavior, 28*(6), 2160–2168. doi:10.1016/j.chb.2012.06.022

Kernis, M. H. (2013). *Self-esteem issues and answers: A sourcebook of current perspectives*. New York: Psychology Press.

Kim, Y., & Sundar, S. S. (2012). Visualizing ideal self vs. actual self through avatars: Impact on preventive health outcomes. *Computers in Human Behavior, 28*(4), 1356–1364. doi:10.1016/j.chb.2012.02.021

Kolko, B. E. (1998). Representing bodies in virtual space: The rhetoric of avatar design. *The Information Society, 15*(3), 177–186. doi:10.1080/019722499128484

Lin, N., Dean, A., & Ensel, W. M. (2013). *Social support, life events, and depression*. New York: Academic Press.

Loke, S.-K. (2015). How do virtual world experiences bring about learning? A critical review of theories. *Australasian Journal of Educational Technology, 31*(1), 112–122.

Lomanowska, A. M., & Guitton, M. J. (2014). My avatar is pregnant! Representation of pregnancy, birth, and maternity in a virtual world. *Computers in Human Behavior, 31*, 322–331. doi:10.1016/j.chb.2013.10.058

Martey, R. M., Stromer-Galley, J., Consalvo, M., Wu, J., Banks, J., & Strzalkowski, T. (2015). Communicating age in Second Life: The contributions of textual and visual factors. *New Media & Society*, *17*(1), 41–61. doi:10.1177/1461444813504270

Morie, J. F., & Chance, E. (2011). Extending the reach of health care for obesity and diabetes using virtual worlds. *Journal of Diabetes Science and Technology*, *5*(2), 272–276. doi:10.1177/193229681100500211 PMID:21527093

Murray, T., Hardy, D., Spruijt-Metz, D., Hekler, E., & Raij, A. (2013). Avatar interfaces for biobehavioral feedback. In A. Marcus (Ed.), *Design, User Experience, and Usability. Health, Learning, Playing, Cultural, and Cross-Cultural User Experience* (pp. 424–434). Heidelberg: Springer. doi:10.1007/978-3-642-39241-2_47

Pellas, N., & Kazanidis, I. (2013). On the value of Second Life for students' engagement in blended and online courses: A comparative study from the Higher Education in Greece. *Education and Information Technologies*.

Pellas, N., & Kazanidis, I. (2014). Engaging students in blended and online collaborative courses at university level through Second Life: Comparative perspectives and instructional affordances. *New Review of Hypermedia and Multimedia*, *20*(2), 123–144. doi:10.1080/13614568.2013.856958

Petkova, V. I., & Ehrsson, H. H. (2008). If I were you: Perceptual illusion of body swapping. *PLoS ONE*, *3*(12), e3832. PMID:19050755

Richmond, C. A., Ross, N. A., & Egeland, G. M. (2007). Social support and thriving health: A new approach to understanding the health of indigenous Canadians. *American Journal of Public Health*, *97*(10), 1827–1833. doi:10.2105/AJPH.2006.096917 PMID:17761564

Riva, G. (2008). *Psicologia dei nuovi media*. Bologna: Il Mulino.

Riva, G. (in press) Embodied Medicine: What Human-Computer Confluence Can Offer to Health Care. In A. Gaggioli, A. Ferscha, G. Riva, S. Dunne, and I. Viaud-Delmon (Eds.), Human Computer Confluence: Transforming Human Experience Through Symbiotic Technologies, Berlin: De Gruyter Open

Riva, G., Banos, R. M., Botella, C., Wiederhold, B. K., & Gaggioli, A. (2012). Positive technology: Using interactive technologies to promote positive functioning. *Cyberpsychology, Behavior, and Social Networking*, *15*(2), 69–77. doi:10.1089/cyber.2011.0139 PMID:22149077

Riva, G., Castelnuovo, G., & Mantovani, F. (2006). Transformation of flow in rehabilitation: The role of advanced communication technologies. *Behavior Research Methods*, *38*(2), 237–244. doi:10.3758/BF03192775 PMID:16956100

Riva, G., Milani, L., & Gaggioli, A. (Eds.). (2010). Networked Flow: comprendere e sviluppare la creatività di rete. Milano, IT: LED.

Ryff, C. D., & Singer, B. (2000). Interpersonal flourishing: A positive health agenda for the new millennium. *Personality and Social Psychology Review*, *4*(1), 30–44. doi:10.1207/S15327957PSPR0401_4

Sawyer, R. K. (2003). *Group creativity: Music, theater, collaboration*. Mahwah, NJ: LEA.

Sawyer, R. K. (2006). Group creativity: Musical performance and collaboration. *Psychology of Music, 34*(2), 148–165. doi:10.1177/0305735606061850

Sawyer, R. K. (2007). *Group genius: The creative power of collaboration*. New York: Basic Books.

Sawyer, R. K. (2008). *Group genius: The creative power of collaboration* (2nd ed.). New York: Basic Books.

Schopler, J., & Galinsky, M. (2014). Expanding our view of support groups as open systems. In M. Galinsky & J. Schopler (Eds.), *Support groups: Current perspectives on theory and practice* (pp. 3–10). New York: The Haworth Press, Inc.

Serino, S., Pedroli, E., Keizer, A., Triberti, S., Dakanalis, A., Pallavicini, F., & Riva, G. et al. (2015). Virtual Reality Body Swapping: A Tool for Modifying the Allocentric Memory of the Body. *Cyberpsychology, Behavior, and Social Networking*. doi:10.1089/cyber.2015.0229 PMID:26506136

Simbula, S., Guglielmi, D., & Schaufeli, W. B. (2011). A three-wave study of job resources, self-efficacy, and work engagement among Italian schoolteachers. *European Journal of Work and Organizational Psychology, 20*(3), 285–304. doi:10.1080/13594320903513916

Simpson, D. D. (2004). A conceptual framework for drug treatment process and outcomes. *Journal of Substance Abuse Treatment, 27*(2), 99–121. doi:10.1016/j.jsat.2004.06.001 PMID:15450644

Suls, J., & Wheeler, L. (Eds.). (2000). *Handbook of social comparison*. New York: Kluwer Academic/Plenum. doi:10.1007/978-1-4615-4237-7

Suomi, R., Mäntymäki, M., & Söderlund, S. (2014). Promoting Health in Virtual Worlds: Lessons From Second Life. *Journal of Medical Internet Research, 16*(10), e229. doi:10.2196/jmir.3177 PMID:25313009

Sweigart, L., Burden, M., Carlton, K. H., & Fillwalk, J. (2014). Virtual simulations across curriculum prepare nursing students for patient interviews. *Clinical Simulation in Nursing, 10*(3), e139–e145. doi:10.1016/j.ecns.2013.10.003

Sweigart, L., & Hodson-Carlton, K. (2013). Improving student interview skills: The virtual avatar as client. *Nurse Educator, 38*(1), 11–15. doi:10.1097/NNE.0b013e318276df2d PMID:23222623

Tajfel, H., & Turner, J. C. (2004). The Social Identity Theory of Intergroup Behavior. In J. T. Jost, & J. Sidanius (Eds.), Political Psychology: Key Readings (pp. 276–293). New York: Psychology Press.

Thoits, P. A. (2013). Self, identity, stress, and mental health. In C. S. Aneshensel, J. C. Phelan, & A. Bierman (Eds.), *Handbook of the sociology of mental health*. New York: Springer. doi:10.1007/978-94-007-4276-5_18

Tiffany, J. M., & Hoglund, B. A. (2014). Facilitating Learning Through Virtual Reality Simulation: Welcome to Nightingale Isle. In Virtual, Augmented Reality and Serious Games for Healthcare 1 (pp. 159-174). Springer Berlin Heidelberg.

Tokel, S. T., & İsler, V. (2013). Acceptance of virtual worlds as learning space. *Innovations in Education and Teaching International*.

Trepte, S., & Reinecke, L. (2010). Avatar creation and video game enjoyment: Effects of life-satisfaction, game competitiveness, and identification with the avatar. *Journal of Media Psychology: Theories, Methods, and Applications*, 22(4), 171–184. doi:10.1027/1864-1105/a000022

Trepte, S., Reinecke, L., & Behr, K.-M. (2009). Creating virtual alter egos or superheroines? Gamers' strategies of avatar creation in terms of gender and sex. *International Journal of Gaming and Computer-Mediated Simulations*, 1(2), 52–76. doi:10.4018/jgcms.2009040104

Triberti, S., & Argenton, L. (2013). *Psicologia dei videogiochi*. Milano: Apogeo.

Triberti, S., & Liberati, E. G. (2014). Patient centered virtual reality: an opportunity to improve the quality of patient's experience. In P. Cipresso & S. Serino (Eds.), *Virtual Reality Technologies, Medical Applications and Challenges* (pp. 1–30). New York: Nova Science.

Triberti, S., & Riva, G. (2015a). Positive Technology for Enhancing the Patient Engagement Experiences. In S. Barello, G. Graffigna, & S. Triberti (Eds.), *Patient Engagement: a comsumer- centered model to innovate healthcare*. Berlin: De Gruyter Open. doi:10.1515/9783110452440-005

Triberti, S., & Riva, G. (2015b). Engaging Users to Design Positive Technologies for Patient Engagement: the Perfect Interaction Model. In S. Barello, G. Graffigna, & S. Triberti (Eds.), *Patient Engagement: a comsumer- centered model to innovate healthcare*. Berlin: De Gruyter Open. doi:10.1515/9783110452440-006

Vasalou, A., & Joinson, A. N. (2009). Me, myself and I: The role of interactional context on self-presentation through avatars. *Computers in Human Behavior*, 25(2), 510–520. doi:10.1016/j.chb.2008.11.007

Vera, M., Le Blanc, P. M., Taris, T. W., & Salanova, M. (2014). Patterns of engagement: The relationship between efficacy beliefs and task engagement at the individual versus collective level. *Journal of Applied Social Psychology*, 44(2), 133–144. doi:10.1111/jasp.12219

Villani, D., Gatti, E., Confalonieri, E., & Riva, G. (2012). Am I my avatar? A tool to investigate virtual body image representation in adolescence. *Cyberpsychology, Behavior, and Social Networking*, 15(8), 435–440. doi:10.1089/cyber.2012.0057 PMID:22823468

Warburton, S. (2009). Second Life in higher education: Assessing the potential for and the barriers to deploying virtual worlds in learning and teaching. *British Journal of Educational Technology*, 40(3), 414–426. doi:10.1111/j.1467-8535.2009.00952.x

Wu, L. M., Austin, J., Hamilton, J. G., Valdimarsdottir, H., Isola, L., Rowley, S., & Rini, C. et al. (2012). Self-efficacy beliefs mediate the relationship between subjective cognitive functioning and physical and mental well-being after hematopoietic stem cell transplant. *Psycho-Oncology*, 21(11), 1175–1184. doi:10.1002/pon.2012 PMID:21739524

Yee, N., & Bailenson, J. (2007). The Proteus effect: The effect of transformed self-representation on behavior. *Human Communication Research*, 33(3), 271–290. doi:10.1111/j.1468-2958.2007.00299.x

Yee, N., Bailenson, J., & Ducheneaut, N. (2009). The proteus effect: Implications of transformed digital self-sepresentation on online and offline behavior. *Communication Research*, 36(2), 285–312. doi:10.1177/0093650208330254

KEY TERMS AND DEFINITIONS

Avatar: Any representation of a human user's action and/or communication inside a digital environment. In VWs and video games, these are typically 3d graphical representations.

Group Flow: An optimal group experience of fully engagement often described as sense of "*collective mind*" by people who experienced it.

Networked Flow Model: An innovative framework to understand networks creativity which is seen as a process culminating in the generation and sharing of an artifact.

Patient Engagement: A process of disease/illness management which culminates in patients' experience of feeling responsible for their own healthcare and able to manage it adequately. At the highest level, patients recover a positive life project despite the presence of a chronic disease.

PHE Model: A theoretical model explaining the evolutionary phases of the patient engagement process.

Positive Technology: A theoretical, research and design paradigm that consider new technologies a resource to improve the quality of people's personal experience by structuring, augmenting or even replacing its features.

Proteus Effect: The phenomenon of avatars modifying the behavior of their own users.

Virtual Words: Internet-based virtual environments where people can interact by means of their avatars.

This research was previously published in Transformative Healthcare Practice through Patient Engagement edited by Guendalina Graffigna, pages 247-275, copyright year 2017 by Medical Information Science Reference (an imprint of IGI Global).

Chapter 58
Patients' Rights and Medical Personnel Duties in the Field of Hospital Care

Bogusław Sygit
University of Łódź, Poland

Damian Wąsik
Nicolaus Copernicus University in Torun, Collegium Medicum in Bydgoszcz, Poland

ABSTRACT

The aim of this chapter is to describe selected universal rights of the patient. The authors specify the seven types of patient rights: the right to appropriate organization of treatment on equal terms, the right to respect patient's dignity and privacy, the right to full and comprehensible information on the state of health, the right of access to medical documentation, the right to self-determination - to agree to provide health care services, the right to respect for private and family life and religion and the right to seek compensation and other benefits in the event of damage to the result of medical malpractice. This classification is the basis to discuss the specifics of each of them with reference to specific examples of their implementation or violations. The chapter specifically addresses the issues such as the obligation to inform the patient of the medical procedure, the legal conditions for the effectiveness of consent to treatment and the principle of access to medical documentation. Presentation of patients' rights is made from the perspective of fulfilling the duties of medical personnel working in hospitals. The authors make extensive use of current case law of the European Court of Human Rights. The undeniable advantage of the publication is to present selected theses of Polish court rulings issued in cases of violation of patient rights.

DOI: 10.4018/978-1-5225-3926-1.ch058

INTRODUCTION

The Concept and the Source of the Patient's Rights

In the literature we can find the statement that patients' rights are an integral part and concretization of wider human rights and are a consequence of the evolution that took place in the twentieth century in the field of these rights. This fundamental rights increase from a common sense of threat subjective rights and the dignity of the human person (G. Iwanowicz-Palus, 2000).

In the 70s there were opinions criticizing the privileged position of the medical community in making most of the decisions affecting the way of organizing health care. It was thought that it is necessary to change the situation by weakening the position of the doctors and strengthening the position of the patient. Then also began to appear the concept of patient rights. Sometimes the transition to patient rights was seen as an attack on the power providers, leading to resistance and protests. With time, however, all interested parties have started to realize that this way of shaping the relationship is the only possible (D. Karkowska, 2012).

As a source of patients' rights generally the Universal Declaration of Human Rights is indicated. It is noted that the patient's rights were at "the inherent dignity" and the "equal and unalienable rights of all members of the human family". World Health Organization indicates that patients' rights vary in different countries and in different jurisdictions, often depending on the prevailing cultural and social norms. Different models of the patient-physician relationship—which can also represent the citizen-state relationship—have been developed, and these have informed the particular rights to which patients are entitled. In North America and Europe, for instance, there are at least four models which depict this relationship: the paternalistic model, the informative model, the interpretive model, and the deliberative model. Each of these suggests different professional obligations of the physician towards the patient. For instance, in the paternalistic model, the best interests of the patient, as judged by the clinical expert, are valued above the provision of comprehensive medical information and decision-making power to the patient. The informative model, by contrast, sees the patient as a consumer who is in the best position to judge what is in their own interest, and thus views the doctor chiefly as a provider of information. There continues to be an enormous debate about how to conceive of this relationship best, but there is also a growing international consensus that all patients have a fundamental right to privacy, to the confidentiality of their medical information, to consent to or to refuse treatment, and to be informed about the relevant risk to them of medical procedures (see http://www.who.int/genomics/public/patientrights/en/).

The literature emphasizes that the modern concept of patient's rights is based on the values that presented in 1994 by WHO in the document called *Declaration on the Promotion of Patients' Rights in Europe* and prepared in 2002 by the organization Active Citizenship Network (European non-governmental civic organizations) document called *the European Charter of Patients' Right*. These acts refer to the laws dedicated to the protection of basic human and civil rights. In the field of international and European law sources of patients' rights are especially the International Covenant on Civil and Political Rights, the European Convention on the Protection of Human Rights and Fundamental Freedoms and the European Social Charter. This thesis is confirmed by extensive case law of the European Court of Human Rights given in cases of human rights violations in terms of treatment. At national level, one of the first European countries that have adopted the regulation of the issue, was France. Currently, the EU Member States that regulate the patient's rights issues in an act include: Finland (1992), The Netherlands (1994), Greece, Hungary, Lithuania, Latvia and Portugal (1997), Denmark (1998), Belgium and

Estonia (2002), Cyprus (2005) and Poland (2006). Such regulations are also formed outside the EU, for example in Israel (1996). However, in some EU countries such as the UK and Germany, the cards are a type of patient's rights guidelines in the healthcare system and do not take the form of legislation (D. Karkowska, 2012).

Catalogue of patients' rights legislation is similar in almost all the countries in which there is such a legal instrument. Frequently includes the right to receive health care benefits on equal terms and in the same quality, the right to maintain the confidentiality of information related to the patient, the right of access to medical records, the right to consent to surgery, or the right to respect for family life. However, when examined in detail and compare the various legal acts, you can find many specific rules which further extend the patient's right or limit them.

Danish Law No. 482 of 1 July 1998 on patients' rights (Lottidende, 1998, Part A, 2 July 1998, No. 99, pp. 2883-2888), in article 14 concerns hunger strike provides that if it is clear that a patient has begun a hunger strike and has been informed of its consequences for his health, the health care provider shall not have the right to terminate it. In addition, there are large Danish law restrictions on the freedom to decide by doctors to treatment with blood. According to article 15 a treatment involving the transfusion of blood or blood products may not be begun or continued without the patient's informed consent. The patient's refusal to receive blood or blood products shall be expressed in connection with the current state of the disease and based on information supplied by the health care provider concerning the health-related consequences of omitting to provide blood or blood products as part of the treatment.

The Lithuanian law, concretely Law on the rights of patients and compensation of the damage to their health (October 3, 1996. No I – 1562) specifies the rules for so-called compensation. medical malpractice and other negligence in treatment.. In implementing individual health care, the health care institutions of the National Health System of Lithuania, accredited for individual health care, must insure their civil responsibility for the damage caused to patients through the lawful actions of physicians or nursing staff members. The State Patients' Fund shall implement the compulsory insurance for civil responsibility for the damage caused to patients, of the individual health care institutions of the National Health Care system of Lithuania, in instituting for this purpose, an independent Individual Health Care Institution Insurance Fund for the damage caused to patients. The Government shall approve the statutes of this fund. The health care institutions of the National Health System of Lithuania, which provide in-patient assistance shall pay 0.2 per cent, while those not providing in-patient assistance shall pay 0.1 per cent from the added on work compensation fund of physicians and nursing staff members. The health care institutions, accredited for individual health care which are independent of the National Health Care System of Lithuania must, in implementing individual health care, insure their civil responsibility for the damage inflicted upon patients, as a result of the legitimate actions by physicians and nursing staff members, through arranging insurance agreements with insurance companies, which have a right to implement general civil responsibility insurance in accordance with the laws of the Republic of Lithuania or by entering into agreements with the State Patients' Fund. If the health care organisations, which do not belong to the National Health System of Lithuania, in implementing individual health care, shall insure their civil responsibility for the damage caused to patients through the lawful actions of physicians and nursing staff members by forming insurance contracts with insurance companies, the terms of insurance, size of insurance payments, procedure of the payment thereof, etc., shall be established in the insurance contracts. If the health care institutions, which do not belong to the National Health System of Lithuania, form contracts with the State Patient's Fund, the same insurance conditions and procedure of contribution payment shall apply to them as to the National Health System of Lithuania health care institutions. Compensation for damage caused to patients shall be paid from the State Patients' Fund monies from the Insurance Fund of the Health Care Institutions Civil Responsibility for Damage Caused to Patients, if damage was caused to the patient at a health care institution which had formed an insurance contract with the State Patients' Fund, in accordance with the requirements of this Law. The compensations shall be paid per decision of the Commission in accordance with the procedure and amounts approved by the Government, but not to exceed the 15 minimal monthly pay amount. The damage shall be compensated in accordance with the minimum monthly pay amount, in effect on the day the request, concerning compensation of the damage incurred, was submitted to the commission on compensation. 2. If the patient sustained damage at a health care institution not under the National Health System and one not having formed an insurance contract with the State Patients' Fund, the insurance compensation shall be paid in accordance with the conditions provided in the contract between the health care institution and an insurance company.

Turkish regulations of 1998 of the Ministry of Health on patients rights (Turkiye Cumhurzjveti Resmi Gazete, 1 August 1998, No. 23420, pp. 67-76) directly relates to the issue of euthanasia, indicating that tt shall be prohibited to take life, by medical methods or in any other manner whatsoever. The taking of a person's life shall not be permitted, either at his request or at the request of another person.

Israeli Patient's Right Act (1996) also limits the patient's right to self-determination of their treatment or withdraw from it. Should the patient be deemed to be in grave danger but reject medical treatment, which in the circumstances must be given soon, the clinician may preform the treatment against the patient's will, if an Ethics Committee has confirmed that all the following conditions obtain: a) the patient has received information as required to make an informed choice, b) the treatment is anticipated to significantly improve the patient's medical condition; c) there are reasonable grounds to suppose that, after receiving treatment, the patient will give his retroactive consent.

TYPES AND CLASSIFICATION OF PATIENTS' RIGHTS

The patient has the right to be informed of their rights. This information should be placed in a public place, in the case of patients who cannot move - in a room where the patient is located.

Taking into consideration the conditions of hospital treatment and the principles for the provision of healthcare services, the universal rights of the patient can be grouped into the following categories:

1.   The right to appropriate organization of treatment on equal terms:
     °   The right to free healthcare services;
     °   The right to equal access to health care services;
     °   The right to obtain healthcare services consistent with the current medical knowledge;
     °   The right to request to consult another doctor or medical council to convene;
2.   The right to respect patient's dignity and privacy:
     °   Presence at providing healthcare services only those that are necessary because of the type of service;
     °   The right to prepare for the test in a separate room, a room or behind a screen in the hospital dormitory room;
     °   The right to request the presence of a person close to the investigation;
     °   The right to a dignified death;

3. The right to full and comprehensible information on the state of health:
   ○ The right to demand a thorough explanation of the specific nature of the proposed treatment, its purpose and benefits of alternatives;
   ○ Right to request information about the disease, for which the patient suffers, methods of treatment, the prognosis for the future;
   ○ The right to decide to whom and what information will be disclosed;
   ○ The right to authorize a close relative or other person to have access to medical records, even after the death of the patient;
4. The right of access to medical documentation;
5. The right to self-determination - to agree to provide health care services;
6. The right to respect for private and family life and religion:
   ○ The right to personal contact, telephone or correspondence with other people;
   ○ The right to additional care on the part of the people designated by the patient;
   ○ The right to pastoral care.
7. The right to seek compensation and other benefits in the event of the damage being the result of medical malpractice.

The Right to Appropriate Organization of Treatment on Equal Terms

The right to appropriate organization of treatment on equal terms is mainly about ensuring equal access to health care services, in particular publicly-funded state. If the national law provides for any restrictions on the ability to provide appropriate services, the patient has the right to a transparent, objective, based on medical criteria procedure for access to these benefits. In addition, anyone who has the right to health care services, receives medical treatment at the same level. An important aspect of this law is also entitled to immediate medical assistance in the state of emergency - if it is risk of health or life of the patient.

Organization of hospital treatment should take into account the patient's autonomy and the need of proper care for it adequate to the nature of the illness or the type of healthcare services provided. In particular, so the patient has the right to free pharmaceuticals and medical supplies during hospitalization, and medical staff cannot ask him to supply in any medical materials while in hospital. The patient has the right to a room and meals adequate to his health. The patient should also guarantee free medical transport (including air transport) to the nearest hospital and back. The patient is entitled to medical transport in particular in the case of immediate need for treatment in a medical facility, in order to maintain continuity of care and in the case of musculoskeletal diseases that prevent the use of public transport. Patient has the right not to agree to donate organs or tissues after their death. Likewise, they have the right to refuse to carry out an autopsy after their death, unless an autopsy require generally applicable laws.

With the patients' right to receive medical care in conditions that meet certain standards of sanitation involves the medical staff obligation to care about maintaining appropriate sanitary requirements to ensure the safety of the patient while providing health care services. To meet these requirements, the attention has to be put to proper maintenance and periodic verification of whether a room or medical devices continue to meet the standards to ensure the safety of patients. These obligations also apply to people who directly provide health services, because they are required the routine inspection of each used in the diagnostic and therapeutic device for any visible and easily detectable faults and defects. The person providing health services should continue to monitor the operation of the equipment used for the purpose of providing health services to react immediately to unexpected failures. They may pose a threat to the health or life of patients (e.g. medical equipment generating the erroneous records research).

The patient has the right to obtain health services by people with appropriate qualifications and experience, i.e. those performing basic medical professions (e.g. doctors, nurses) and people in other medical professions authorized to provide health benefits (e.g. physiotherapists). Members of the medical staff should be in the right state of psycho-physical in the award of healthcare services and respect the scope allowances (e.g. the nurse may provide only certain benefits without doctor's orders).

The method of providing medical and related procedures must comply with current medical knowledge. This means that the physician should discontinue the use of methods of practice widely rejected, that is, those in the view scientific studies have been found to be ineffective, faulty or even dangerous for patients. Moreover, in principle the universally accepted method of procedure should be used, that is, those that are recognized by the relevant medical organizations as appropriate to take in certain cases, medical facilities, and for which there is virtually no doubt as to the validity of their application. It may also be used practices questioned only in a situation when in a particular case there are no methods widely accepted. Challenge by the notion of methods should be understood as a method that in truth are accepted by the medical organizations, but not commonly (it is a subject to criticism). If, in a given situation, there are several equivalent methods commonly accepted, procedure or some equivalent method should be questioned as the patient while using this method of conduct in the specific case is given the most likely the expected positive effect of a diagnostic or therapeutic. It should be remembered that the final choice of the method of procedure depends on the decision (approval) of the patient, which should provide all possible and acceptable in a given situation treatments (T. Filarski, T. Sroka, 2013, p. 16).

In the literature, it is noted that there are situations in which the respect of the standards relating to current medical knowledge will be impossible. For justified restrictions that will permit the use of such methods, which did not correspond to current medical knowledge, but in the circumstances, constitute a medical procedure to ensure the patient the best kind of help that can be obtained, include: 1) a large number of different types of medical procedures, a person performing medical profession may not have the necessary skills to perform certain therapeutic functions; 2) lack of access to specific medical devices or medicinal products; 3) legal barriers, i.e. the patient's refusal to permit the particular method of treatment; 4) economic considerations and the shortage of financial resources for the provision of health services (T. Filarski, T. Sroka, 2013, p. 18).

Patient has the right to request the situation in which a doctor providing health care services has to consult another doctor or the situation of convening of a medical council. The physician may, however, refuse to consult another doctor, if it considers it to be unfounded.

The Right to Respect Patient's Dignity and Privacy

The patient's right to dignity and privacy when receiving health care services means that in the course of providing medical care to the patient only those which are necessary because of the type of health care benefits should be present. The participation of other people, including medical professionals and students of medical colleges should be subject to the consent of the patient and the doctor's approval.

In granting health care services a person close to the patient may be present. The doctor has the right not to accept the presence of a close relative, if there is a possibility of the threat of epidemic or due to health safety of the patient.

The patient has the right to prepare for the examination or treatment in a separated and protected place so that could not be seen or overheard. If they are confined to bed or bed-ridden and are in a hospital dormitory room, they are entitled to expect that the examination or treatment will be carried out with respect for privacy and dignity - behind a screen or curtain. The doctor should not discuss the patient's illness and ask them questions in the intimate presence of other patients.

The element of respect for the dignity of the patient is also the right attitude towards them from the medical staff. A patient has the right to expect that the medical profession will not underestimate them and requests formulated by them. They should ask the patient culturally and kindly, in an appropriate and comprehensible manner, maintaining patience and understanding. Breach of the duty to respect the dignity of a man is such treatment which causes the feeling of fear and humiliation, which could lead to the collapse of the physical and mental health (T. Filarski, T. Sroka, 2013, p. 40).

The patient has the right to data protection and to keep secret about themselves obtained by those medical professionals in relation to the provision of health services. The medical confidentiality includes all information relating to health, diagnosis and course of treatment, as well as private and family life and professional activity. This information must be treated as confidential and not be disclosed to unauthorized persons, even after the death of the patient. Medical practitioners are required to disclose information when medical secrecy can cause danger to life and health of the patient or others (G. Iwanowicz-Palus, 1999).

The right to dignity includes the right to a dignified death. If the patient is in a terminal state, has the right to health care services providing pain relief and minimize the suffering of another type. It should be remembered that the breach of the patient's right to die in peace and dignity may be appropriate with respect to the so-called, aggressive medical treatment. By persistent treatment should be read as the use of medical procedures, technical equipment and pharmaceuticals in order to maintain vital functions terminally ill, which prolongs the dying, bound to the dignity of the patient, especially with excessive suffering; persistent therapy does not include basic treatments, relieve pain and other symptoms, and feeding and watering, if designed well-being of the patient.

The Right to Full and Comprehensible Information on the State of Health

The patient has the right to be informed in different forms. Information can be communicated to them verbally, in writing, but also recorded in any other form, i.e. in any medium that contains information about the patient. This is all more important, if the information is based on evidence of actual events that concern it and regardless of the manner in which it was fixed, especially when that message is the evidence of the law. It is important for individuals facing risks to their health to have access to information enabling them to assess those risks. The states are bound, by virtue of this obligation, to adopt the necessary regulatory measures to ensure that doctors consider the foreseeable consequences of a planned medical procedure on their patients' physical integrity and to inform patients of these consequences beforehand, in such a way that the latter are able to be given the informed consent. In particular, as a corollary to this, if a foreseeable risk of this nature materialises without the patient having been duly informed in advance by doctors, the concerned State may be directly liable under the Article 8 of the European Convention on the Protection of Human Rights and Fundamental Freedoms for this lack of information (see Vo v. France [GC], no. 53924/00, § 89, ECHR 2004-VIII).

The right of access to such information falling within the ambit of the notion of private life can be said to comprise on the other hand, a right to obtain available information on one's condition. The European Court of Human Rights stated that further considers that during the pregnancy the foetus' condition and health constitute an element of, for example, the pregnant woman's health (see Eur. Comm. HR, Brug-geman and Schouten v. Germany, § 59, mutatis mutandis). The effective exercise of this right is often decisive for the possibility of exercising personal autonomy by deciding, on the basis of such informa-tion, on the future course of events relevant for the individual's quality of life (e.g. by refusing consent to medical treatment or by requesting a given form of treatment).

The information about the state of health should be accessible and relevant to diagnosis, proposed and possible methods of diagnosis and treatment, and foreseeable consequences for the health and life of the patient using or discontinuing certain medical procedures. Doctor should explain exactly what conducted treatments and tests consist of and for what purpose the patient is to take the medication. The patient has the right to be informed of the results of the research. The patient also has the right to obtain from a nurse accessible information about the care and treatment.

In the literature, it is rightly pointed out that all information on the health status and methods of treatment should be communicated to the patient using the vocabulary and terminology understandable to the patient because of their age, education, health and mental state. For example, patients generally do not need to be informed that in their case it is necessary to perform hysterectomy. The patient should be given the message while there is the need to make hysterectomies with a precise explanation of its impact on their health condition performed by this procedure, particularly in the view of the possibility of having children. The patient should be given clear information on the current condition of psycho - physical, diagnosed diseases (diseases), carried out in relation to the effectiveness of diagnostic and therapeutic procedures and the outlook for their health for the future. Telling the truth about the results of the diagnosis of the patient should not be synonymous with hope to the patient receiving. It happens sometimes that inexplicable things happen from the perspective of modern medicine. Therefore, it is needed to clearly distinguish between the transmission of the disease to the patient information about the expected date of the determination of its duration. The information about the used medical procedures should indicate the proposed and possible diagnostic and therapeutic methods and foreseeable conse-quences of their use or omission. Responsibility of the person providing health care services is to give the patient all medical procedures (treatment), which, according to the current medical knowledge could be applied due to a specific health condition of the patient. This information should also include at least basic information indicating the way of the implementation of a particular treatment. The information about the foreseeable consequences of the use of a particular method of treatment should include both data on the desired effects of a particular treatment, and of the possible undesirable effects, i.e. the side effects (T. Filarski, T. Sroka, 2013, p. 27; M. Nesterowicz, 2012, pp. 111-221; M. Świderska, 2007; R. Kubiak, 2000).

The person providing health care services is under no obligation to inform the patient about any possible undesirable effects, including those that occur rarely or incidentally. The information about all the possible complications could in fact lead to a deterioration of the patient's health, including its well-being, and sometimes unfounded refusal to agree to provide specific health benefits, due to the received information about possible complications. The person providing health care services should inform the patient only about normal, typical, frequent complications. However, detailed coverage of data transmission should always be such as to allow the patient to take the decision to consent to the treatment with full knowledge of what is accepted and what should be expected (T. Filarski, T. Sroka, 2013, I. Adrych, 2009; W. Borysiak, 2008; M. Świderska, 2003).

Therefore, the scope of information always depends on the purpose and nature of the specific treat-ments and "what a reasonable person who is in the patient's situation, objectively should hear from the doctor to be able to make an informed and wise decision to surrender to the proposed medical treatment." For the transmission of information to the patient of the proper range, it is necessary to determine whether the indications for the use of a particular method of treatment are absolute (implemented due to the health of the patient) or only relative (that should be used due to the patient's health status, but there is no absolute necessity). The less is necessary to indicate the use of a particular method of treatment, the greater the amount of information the patient must be given before agreeing to surgery (T. Filarski, T. Sroka, 2013, p. 28).

The physician may not take or refrain from treatment, unless there is a case of urgency, and the failure to provide medical care for the patient does not pose a danger: loss of life, serious injury, serious health disorder, and another case of an urgent. The withdrawal of treatment cannot be a surprise for the patient. The reason for withdrawal from the follow-up treatment may be, for example, the doctor's opinion of possessing insufficient knowledge and skills to ensure an effective medical treatment or that taking into account the patient's condition all treatment possibilities available to them were used. In this case, however, the patient has the right to notice it early enough, by a doctor of its intention to withdraw from the treatment and indicate to them the real possibility of obtaining health care benefits from another physician or other medical facility. Such information should be communicated to the patient early enough to give them enough time to contact another doctor and the opportunity to continue treatment without interruption. There is a possibility to withdraw from treatment by a doctor, especially in case one uses aggression, obscene and abusive words towards them or notoriously challenges the professional competence and treatment. The annotation of the refusal of health care benefits can be given the form of statement, which is prepared and signed by the physician (justify its refusal in writing), and then presents it to sign the patient or their legal representative (T. Filarski, T. Sroka, 2013, p. 28).

The patient may also decide to whom and what information about their health may be communicated. They have the right to require from the hospital to inform the people close to them or designated institution about threat to their life or their death. The hospital has a duty to fulfill the patient's request promptly and effectively.

The Right of Access to Medical Documentation

The entity providing health care services (e.g. hospital, clinic, private institution) makes the medical records of the patient, or their legal representative or a person authorized by the patient. After the death of the patient, a person who was authorized by a patient has got the access to their medical records. The medical records can be made available for inspection (free of charge, at the registered office of the entity, in which the patient to be treated), through the production of its statements, a copy or copies of the original, or by issuing a confirmation of receipt. The standard should be that the hospital after treatment of the patient receives the information sheet on the diagnosis, test results of the treatment, appointments made during treatments, further indication, time off from work, the annotation of stored drugs and the dates of the planned consultation (U. Drozdowska, 2012; P. Pochopień 2013).

The Right to Self-Determination: To Agree to Provide Health Care Services

The Article 8 of the European Court of Human Rights encompasses the physical integrity of a person, since a person's body is the most intimate aspect of private life, and medical intervention, even if it is of minor importance, constitutes an interference with this right (see Y.F. v. Turkey, no. 24209/94, §

33, ECHR 2003-IX, V.C. v. Slovakia, no. 18968/07, §§ 138-142, ECHR 2011; Solomakhin v. Ukraine, no. 24429/03, § 33, 15 March 2012; and I.G. and Others v. Slovakia, no. 15966/04, §§ 135 - 146, 13 November 2012).

After receiving the doctor's full and comprehensible information about the health, the patient has the right to consent to the examination. It is expressed a separate agreement to stay in the hospital and all other research and medical benefits. Consent may be oral, written or expressed through behavior that is not in doubt as to the decision. Written consent is required for the surgery or the use of methods of treatment or diagnosis of posing an increased risk of having an impact on the health of the patient or his life. It is not allowed to receive a blanket consent from patients, usually on a variety of ready-made forms, and for all medical activities to be undertaken in the future in relation to the patient. It is the responsibility of the person performing the medical profession to immediately before granting consent for health care benefits apply only particular, giving expression method of treatment (T. Filarski, T. Sroka, 2013, p. 31).

As a rule effective are also the *pro futuro* statements or the statements made by the patient in the event of loss of consciousness, in which they express their opposition to the use of specific terms of the method of treatment. Such a declaration is important and should be respected by those providing health care services, if it is made in a clear, unambiguous way and there is no doubt about it. It is necessary to be analyzed by a health care professional whether due to the age and health of the patient they were able to give such a statement fully consciously. In case of any doubt, assume that the statement made by the patient is not binding, and the person performing the medical profession has an obligation to obtain consent a foster or, in certain circumstances, even to provide health care benefits without permission (T. Filarski, T. Sroka, 2013, p. 33).

In certain cases, because of the threat to life or health of the patient, it is possible to provide health care benefits without the consent of the patient (the legal representative, guardian actual), or without the permission of the court. The necessity of this occurs when: 1) the patient requires immediate medical attention, and because of health or age of the patient cannot give consent, and at the same time it is not possible to communicate with their legal representative (guardian actual); 2) the patient requires surgery or the use of increased risk surgery and is not a person capable of informed consent because of their age or state of consciousness, and the delay would risk the danger of loss of life to the patient or to cause grievous bodily harm (T. Filarski, T. Sroka, 2013, p. 33).

It should be remembered that the exception to the above rules is not only regarded as a violation of patient rights, but primarily as a violation of fundamental human rights, which was confirmed in the case law of the European Court of Human Rights. In case of Juhnke v. Turkey (no. 52515/99) the Court decided that in the situation where a female detainee complains of a sexual assault and requests a gynaecological examination and the obligation of the authorities to carry out a thorough and effective investigation into the complaint would include the duty promptly to carry out the examination (see, for example, Aydın v. Turkey, judgment of 25 September 1997, Reports 1997 VI, § 107), a detainee may not be compelled or subjected to pressure to such an examination against her wishes. As noted above, the applicant in the present case made no complaint of sexual assault against those who detained her and did not request a gynaecological examination. No reason has been advanced to suggest that she was likely to do so. The gynaecological examination which was imposed on the applicant without her free and informed consent has not been shown to be "in accordance with the law" or to be "necessary in a democratic society". There has accordingly been a violation of the applicant's rights under the Article 8 of the European Convention on the Protection of Human Rights and Fundamental Freedoms.

In view of this issue it seems problematic to decide by a woman giving birth home and abandonment of hospitalization. This problem has also been the subject of litigation before the European Court of Human Rights. In case of Dubska and Krejzova v. The Czech Republic (no. 28859/11 and 28473/12) the Court notes that the Czech Republic Government focused primarily on the legitimate aim of protecting the best interests of a child, which - depending on their nature and seriousness - may override those of the parent who cannot, in particular, be entitled under the Article 8 to have taken the measures that would harm the child's health and development (see Haase v. Germany, no. 11057/02, § 93, ECHR 2004-III (extracts)). The Court considers that while there is generally no conflict of interest between the mother and her child, certain choices made by the mother as to the place, circumstances or method of delivery may be seen to give rise to increased risk to the health and safety of the newborns whose mortality rate shown in figures for perinatal and neonatal deaths, is not negligible, despite all the advances in medical care. The Court accepted that the situation in question had a serious impact on the freedom of choice of the applicants who were required, if they wished to give birth at home, to do so without the assistance of a midwife and, therefore, with the attendant risks posed to themselves and to the newborns, or to give birth at hospital. The applicants were free to give birth in a hospital of their choice, where in theory their wishes relating to matters concerning the birth would be respected. However, the material before the Court suggests that the conditions in most local hospitals, as far as respecting the choices of mothers, were questionable. In this context the Court notes that the Committee on the Elimination of Discrimination against Women, recommended to the respondent State that it should ensure respect for patients' rights, avoiding unnecessary medical interventions. Accordingly, the mothers' free choice of the hospital in which they give birth to their child did not weaken the applicants' interest in having assisted home births. Meanwhile, on the one hand, that the majority of the research studies presented to it do not suggest that there is an increased risk for home births, when compared to births in a hospital, but only if certain preconditions are fulfilled. First, home births would be acceptable only in case of "low-risk" pregnancies. Second, the home birth has to be attended by a qualified midwife who is able to detect any complications during a delivery and to refer a woman in labour to a hospital if necessary. Third, the transfer of mother and child to the hospital should be secured within a very short period of time. Thus, a situation such as the one in the Czech Republic in which medical professionals are not allowed to assist mothers who wish to give birth at home and where no specialised emergency aid is available, may be said to increase rather than reduce the risk to the life and health of the mother and newborn. On the other hand, the Court, noting the Government's argument that the risk for newborns is higher in respect of home births than in respect of deliveries in fully staffed and equipped maternity hospitals, is aware that, even if a pregnancy seems to be without any particular complications, there can arise unexpected difficulties during the delivery, such as the acute lack of oxygen supply to the foetus or profuse bleedings, or events which require specialised medical intervention, such as a caesarean section or the need to put a newborn on neonatal assistance. Moreover, in the course of a hospital birth, the institution can immediately provide the necessary care or intervention, which is not true of a home birth, even one attended by a midwife. The time spent on getting to a hospital should such complications occur could indeed give rise to increased risks to the life and health of the newborn or of that of the mother. Finally, the Court finds it appropriately to add that the State authorities should keep the relevant provisions under a constant review which reflects medical, scientific and legal developments. The Court ordered the Czech authorities to re-examine the health policy women with low risk pregnancies may choose whether they wish to remain in hospital for a period of 72 hours after delivery, following the recommendation of medical specialists, or to give birth in hospital under the care of a midwife and leave the hospital 24 hours after the birth.

The Right to Respect for Private and Family Life and Religion

Patient has the right to personal contact, telephone or correspondence with others during his stay in hospital. They are also entitled to refuse such contact. The hospital does not in any way hinder the patient contact, and should determine the time and place of meetings and telephone contact or opportunity stationery. Using the patient's right to personal contact, telephone or correspondence may be limited due to the organizational capacity of the entity.

The patient has the right to additional care on the part of individuals indicated by him. Additional home care also involves the care of a patient during pregnancy, childbirth and postpartum period. If the patient exercise this right, the medical staff cannot replace the family in care. The staff still has oversight responsibility proper patient care and concern for them. Stay patient's legal guardian of a minor or a person who has actual care of the patient is restricted in case of emergency epidemic, health safety of patients or because of the organizational capacity of the facility (housing conditions of other people sick in the hospital, no rooms available, visiting hours). The costs associated with the operation of the hospital premises and facilities of the caregiver are the costs of implementing powers of the patient to additional nursing care conducted by a close person. It should be noted that these charges may not be excessive and should not constitute significant material loss for caregiver.

If the patient's condition is getting worse or their life is threatened hospital is obliged to allow them the access to proper religious clerics.

The Right to Seek Compensation and Other Benefits in the Event of Damage to the Result of Medical Malpractice

Therefore decisive responsibility providing medical benefits to prove two conditions: violation of patients' rights above and culpability in this matter the service provider without having to show damage. It does not matter whether it is the claim of a violation due to willful or unintentional. Assessment of the degree fault may be the only meaningful for the amount claimed in the amount of money (M. Safjan, 1999).

The European Court of Human Rights reiterates that in the specific sphere of medical negligence, if the legal system affords victims full access to civil proceedings or to disciplinary proceedings which may lead to liability for medical negligence being established and a corresponding award of compensation, this could in principle be sufficient to discharge the State's positive obligation to provide an effective judicial system (see Calvelli and Ciglio v. Italy [GC], no. 32967/96, §§ 48-51, ECHR 2002-I).

Cases of alleged medical negligence, that the positive obligations under the Article 2 of the European Convention on the Protection of Human Rights and Fundamental Freedoms require States to set up an effective independent judicial system so that the cause of death of patients in the care of the medical profession, whether in the public or the private sector, can be determined and those responsible held accountable (see Erikson v. Italy (dec.), no. 37900/97, 26 October 1999; Powell v. the United Kingdom (dec.), no. 45305/99, ECHR 2000-V; and Byrzykowski v. Poland, no. 11562/05, § 104, 27 June 2006). If the infringement of the right to life or to personal integrity is not caused intentionally, the positive obligation imposed by the Article 2 of the Convention to set up an effective judicial system does not necessarily require the provision of a criminal-law remedy in every case. In the specific sphere of medical negligence the obligation may, for instance, also be satisfied if the legal system affords victims a remedy in the civil courts, either alone or in conjunction with a remedy in the criminal courts, enabling any liability of the doctors concerned to be established and any appropriate civil redress, such as an order for damages and/or for the publication of the decision, to be obtained. The disciplinary measures may also be envisaged (see Šilih v. Slovenia [GC], no. 71463/01, §§ 159, 161-163, 9 April 2009, § 194). In order to satisfy its positive obligation under the Article 2 of the Convention, the State has a duty to ensure, by all means at its disposal, that the legislative and administrative framework set up to protect patients' rights is properly implemented and any breaches of those rights are put right and punished (see Konczelska v. Poland (dec.), no. 27294/08, § 35, 20 September 2011).

PROTECTING THE PATIENTS' RIGHTS IN THE POLISH JURISPRUDENCE

Legal act which regulates patient rights issues in Poland is Patient Rights Act and the Patient Ombudsman (*ustawa o prawach pacjenta i Rzeczniku Praw Pacjenta*). The explanatory memorandum of the bill pointed out that it refers to the protection of individual and collective rights of the patient and is a normative act of ordering the Polish legal system of patients' rights issues. For the first time at the level of a single act of universally binding formulated the most important rights of the patient. So far, this was a potential difficulty for both the patients and the providers of health care services to familiarize themselves with the content of those rights, in consequence of their compliance. Form of the project was therefore logical and reasonable treatment from the point of view of the entities involved in the providing health services. Patient Rights Act and the Patient Ombudsman entered into force in 5th June 2009.

So far, on the basis of Polish law courts have issued a number of decisions relevant to the protection and realization of the rights of the patient. They form the practice of therapeutic activity by medical staff and physicians relationships with patients. The Polish court rulings are fully consolidated from the line of case-law, *inter alia*, ECHR. For this reason also scheduled to present themes from the case may be useful for the implementation of patient rights outside Poland, particularly in the matters concerning the right to self-determination and agreement to providing health care services, the right to respect for private and family life and religion and the right to seek compensation and other benefits in the event of damage to the result of medical malpractice:

1. Manifestation of the autonomy of the individual and the freedom of those choices is the right to decide about himself - including the choice of treatment. Informed choice must be preceded by information about the existing and available alternative methods of treatment or diagnosis. The final decision is up to the patient and the doctor is obliged to respect it, even if in his assessment of the patient's decision it is not correct (Appeal Court in Łódź, 18 IX 2013, I ACa 355/13).
2. The doctor is obliged to provide information about the patient's health status, prognosis and course of treatment. In certain situations (therapeutic privilege) doctor may be repealed of this obligation. Then, in the case of the request, updated medical obligation to provide information to the patients' family. This obligation also arises in the case of loss of consciousness of the patient. (...) However, if it was observed a significant deterioration of general condition occurred shortly before losing consciousness by the patient, the hospital staff could not have a real opportunity to comply with its disclosure obligations (Appeal Court in Lublin, 17 X 2012, I ACa 420/12).

3. The written anesthesia consultation card does not contain an exhaustive explanation of the scope of the information that the claimant received while agreeing to anesthesia and surgery. On the date of the consultation and admission to hospital the claimant was preparing for natural childbirth, cesarean section was included as optional with insensitive proposition. According to the testimony of the doctor the claimant was informed about complications, but not all. Frequently, doctor shall inform headaches and treatment options. The consultation exercise is to encourage, reassure the patient and ensure that doctors will do everything to the patient and the baby to be healthy. (…) Toning information in this field, certainly deprives the patient's choice and decision making on the choice of treatment. The lack of information is the violation of patients' rights. Consent is the right to decide for themselves. The result of consent in relation to the provision of medical risk is to accept and adopt it on themselves by the patient. (…) Consent to a specific medical action is not a legal act. It is a statement in the field of consciousness and will of a unilateral (Appeal Court in Katowice, 15 I 2014, I ACa 922/13).

4. The patient has the right to consent or refuse treatment - after obtaining the relevant information. The condition of the legality of medical action is properly informed consent of the patient. In the doctrine of consent is defined as the conscious, explained. The point, therefore, the consent which must precede appropriate to inform the patient. The doctor has a duty to provide reasonable patient health information, diagnosis, proposed and possible methods of diagnosis, treatment, foreseeable consequences of their use or omission, the results of treatment and prognosis (Appeal Court in Białystok, 20 XI 2013, I ACa 531/13).

5. Information provided by the doctor before the surgery should include data that will allow the patient to take the decision to consent to the treatment with full knowledge of what is accepts and what to expect (The Supreme Court, 29 IX 1999, II CKN 511/98).

6. Undoubtedly, medical facilities are obliged to inform the patient about the planned medical treatment, the expected effects and possible complications. The scope of this obligation does not include the notification of planned medical treatment of people designated by the patient, whom they trust and would like to be present when making their decision to consent to treatment. The law does not provide for the obligation to provide the medical information in writing. The obligation written form only applies to the patient's consent to perform surgery or the use of methods of treatment or diagnosis of causing an increased risk for the patient. In other situations, the patient's consent to conduct research or provide other health benefits can be expressed verbally or even through such behavior, which clearly indicates a willingness to undergo operations proposed by the doctor (Appeal Court in Poznań, 25 III 2014, I ACa 142/14).

7. The medical operation performed without the patient's consent is the act illegal, even if made in accordance with the principles of current medical knowledge (The Supreme Court, 31 III 2006 r., I ACa 973/05).

8. If, for a predictable, even occurring infrequently, the consequences of surgery are complications that are of the particularly dangerous nature of the health or life threatening, the patient should be informed of them. However this does not mean that in each case the doctor is obliged to inform about any possible serious consequences even surgery, regardless of the type of surgery and the probability of their occurrence. The scope of information provided to the patient must be dependent on the type of surgery, in particular whether in this case speak for their performing absolute indications (in terms of life-saving treatment), or to indicate the relative or whether it is merely a cosmetic treatment. This range extends furthest in the case of treatments carried out only for aesthetic purposes.

In a situation where there is an absolute need for surgery, the doctor should explain to the patient only the purpose and type of operations and its usual consequences. It does not need, or even due to the well-being and health of the patient should familiarize them with unusual consequences, not covered by the normal risk of surgery undertaken that in special cases, complications can occur. If surgery is necessary to save the life of the patient the physician does not give the patient information about complications that occur very rarely, because it might adversely affect the psyche of the patient and lead to a deterioration of health, the unfounded refusal to consent to perform surgery, or to increase the risk of the operation (Appeal Court in Białystok, 20 XI 2013, I ACa 531/13).

9.   Referring to the appellate complaint of violating patient's right to pastoral care it should be noted that the hospital acted pastors various faiths and organized hospital chapel. On the bulletin board of each of the branches were included information on how to contact the pastors. There is thus no reason to believe that the hospital staff prevented the patient contact with a priest of the Catholic religion. It is impossible to assume that this obligation had to rely on hospital visits initiated by the patient's pastor. Due to the fact that neither the patient nor the person closest to him is initiated in the said pastor visits could not be a violation of their rights (Appeal Court in Lublin, 17 X 2012, I ACa 420/12).

10.   The claimants' harm is not related to the health upset, injury or repeating surgery, but it results from the violation of their *personal*. The claimants' non-pecuniary damage expressed in the extension of the recognition process of spontaneous diseases and thereby prolong the healing process, and thus the exposure of the patient's health and life. Such an understanding of the harm is the result of violations of the rights guaranteed to medical care (including diagnostics) conforming to the requirements of current medical knowledge, the right to the immediate provision of health care benefits and the right to health services provided with reasonable care. (…) When assessing the conduct of a doctor should always be borne in mind not to rechallenge to aggravate medical condition. The test based on the question of whether the doctor in this case should have been and could do more (better) may be particularly useful. In the present case, the answer to this question is positive decided and prejudge the guilt of involuntary the claimant in an infringement of rights as a patient (Appeal Court in Lodz, 27 XI 2014, I ACa 745/14).

11.   For the jurisdiction it cannot be irrelevant that in another lawsuit compensation it has been included in a much higher level. Each case is subjected to an individual assessment. It is impossible to assess whether the harm suffered by the victim is greater or less than the harm suffered by the another victim for whom in an another case it was ordered to pay a different amount (Appeal Court in Katowice, 5 II 2014, V ACa 683/13).

12.   The criteria defining the amount of compensation are evaluative and only if it is shown a manifest infringement of those criteria, it could be justified to accept a plea over- or understatement of compensation, which should be kept within reasonable limits, corresponding to the current conditions and the average standard of society living (The Supreme Court, 15 II 2006, IV CK 384/05; 27 II 2004, V CK 282/03; 6 VI 2003, IV CKN 213/01).

13.   The compensation for harm caused by the infringement relates to specific patient's rights. It should be borne in mind that the rights of patients matter, because they are different and protect different values, including dignity, privacy and autonomy of the patient, similarly as the right to a proper standard of care which may cause the patient experience negative psychological discomfort, loss of confidence healing, even if there was no medical harm (Appeal Court in Katowice, 28 III 2013, V ACa 604/12).

REFERENCES

Adrych, I. (2009). Informed consent – informed consent of the patient's treatment in US law. *Prawo i Medycyna, 3.*

Borysiak, W. (2008). *No informed consent of the patient and the responsibility for the lack of care and case* (Vol. 49). Studia Iuridica.

Drozdowska, U. (Ed.). (2012). *The medical documentation.* Warszawa: Cegedim.

Filarski, T., & Sroka, T. (2013). *Understand the patient's rights. Basic information about the healthcare system in Poland.* Warszawa: Akademia Narodowego Funduszu Zdrowia.

Iwanowicz-Palus, G. (1999). Observance of medical secrecy as a patient's right. *Zdrowie Publiczne*, 11.

Iwanowicz-Palus, G. (2000). *Patients' rights in Poland.* Prawo i Medycyna.

Karkowska, D. (2012). *Patient Rights and the Patient Ombudsman Act. Commentary.* LEX.

Kubiak, R. (2000). *Cases absence of the required consent as a prerequisite for healing and therapeutic treatments* (Vol. 42). Studia Prawno-Ekonomiczne.

Nesterowicz, M. (2012). *Medical law. Comments and glosses to judgments.* Warszawa: Lexis Nexis.

Pochopień, P. (Ed.). (2012). *The medical documentation.* Warszawa: Wolters Kluwer.

Safjan, M. (1999). *Claims for damages against doctors and patients health care institutions.* Prawo i Medycyna.

Świderska, M. (2003). *Obligation of information and the patient's consent to medical treatment under French law.* KPP.

Świderska, M. (2007). *Consent to medical treatment.* Toruń: TNOiK.

This research was previously published in Organizational Culture and Ethics in Modern Medicine edited by Anna Rosiek and Krzysztof Leksowski, pages 282-297, copyright year 2016 by Medical Information Science Reference (an imprint of IGI Global).

Chapter 59
Missing Link of the Health Information Exchange Loop:
Engaging Patients

Alice Noblin
University of Central Florida, USA

Kendall Cortelyou-Ward
University of Central Florida, USA

ABSTRACT

Since 2004, the services of the Florida Health Information Exchange (HIE) have grown, and in 2011, the state contracted with Harris Corporation to provide some basic services to the Florida health care industry and provide functional improvements to the expanding state-wide HIE. The endeavors of this public-private partnership continue to the present day; however, as HIE services have expanded, challenges continue to be encountered. Ultimately, successful exchange of medical data requires patient engagement and "buy-in." The purpose of this article will consider why patient engagement is important for HIE success, offer recommendations to improve both patient and provider interest, and consider the importance of online patient portals to increase the effectiveness of health record keeping and the sharing of vital patient medical information needed by caregivers and their patients.

INTRODUCTION

Efforts toward building a Health Information Exchange (HIE) in Florida began in 2004. The Agency for Health Care Administration (AHCA) laid the foundation for a statewide HIE by organizing health care stakeholders and providing initial funding to local Regional Health Information Organization (RHIO) projects through its grants program. Florida worked to achieve a secure and sustainable approach to health information technology adoption and exchange resulting in better health care outcomes with lowered total costs. In 2010, the Office of the National Coordinator for Health Information Technology (ONC) provided grant funds to significantly advance Florida's plans to build a statewide health information

DOI: 10.4018/978-1-5225-3926-1.ch059

infrastructure. Since the funding from ONC has now ended, sustainability has been at the forefront for HIEs across the country, including Florida.

To date, key services implemented in the Florida HIE include the following:

- Patient look-up (accessing patient information)
- Secure messaging (transmitting password protected & encrypted data)
- Event notification (sharing healthcare encounter information)-

The purpose of this paper is to describe the current services of Florida HIE, identify future HIE goals including the need to increase patients' access to their own health records, define the obstacles to goals, and offer recommendations to overcome obstacles and reach the desired goals. As networks are established throughout the state, the ability of patients to access health information becomes an added benefit for the citizens of Florida. As has occurred throughout the nation, privacy concerns have been at the forefront of all networking efforts in Florida. In addition to describing the current structure and services available, the ways the Florida HIE can improve communication and engagement with patients will be explored.

BACKGROUND

The initial goal of the Florida Health Information Network (FHIN) was to provide a data set consisting of hospital inpatient and outpatient encounters including laboratory results and diagnoses, as well as medications and demographic information (Rosenfeld, Koss, Caruth & Fuller, 2006). One of the major obstacles encountered in implementing a statewide network was legal and regulatory issues surrounding existing privacy laws (Rosenfeld, et al., 2006).

In March 2010, the Office of the National Coordinator (ONC) announced the State Health Information Exchange Cooperative Agreement Program awardees as part of the Health Information Technology for Economic and Clinical Health (HITECH) Act. Florida received $20,738,582 (HHS, 2012). Following an Invitation to Negotiate, this federal funding resulted in Florida awarding a contract to Harris Healthcare Solutions (hereafter referred to as "Harris" or "Harris Corporation") to create the Florida HIE infrastructure.

Through the Agency for Healthcare Administration (AHCA), a designated state entity, Florida looked to Harris to create a Florida Health Information Exchange Infrastructure under the ONC funding. The infrastructure includes open-source technologies where appropriate and gives the highest priority to privacy, security, and interoperability with existing and future electronic patient medical records. Agreements that establish the obligations and assurances between the FHIN, Harris Corporation and other health care organizations in the network were created for the exchange of health information (AHCA, 2011). Consumers are given the ability to explicitly grant permission for disclosure and use of sensitive data as required by state and federal law through the use of consents and authorizations. In the event of a medical emergency when the patient or his/her legal representative is unable or unavailable to authorize access, the participant user may access the information. Written documentation in the patient's record immediately following the disclosure is required by the requesting participant user.

The structure of the HIE is a network within other health networks without a centralized master patient index. The patient lookup service within the HIE enables participating users to locate and retrieve patient records. An authoritative provider directory facilitates communication between participating providers. Secure messaging to facilitate sharing of clinical summaries (a meaningful use criterion) uses national standards to ensure security. Event notification services (ENS) is the newest service, alerting providers and payers when patients are admitted, discharged or transferred from a participating facility. ENS allow for improved continuity of care and case management.

STUDY DESCRIPTION

The American Recovery and Reinvestment Act (ARRA) provided incentive payments to hospitals and physicians who engaged in the meaningful use of electronic health records (EHR). Meaningful use is a set of standards meant to ensure that EHRs are not only purchased, but utilized for certain key functions. The main goals of the HIE meaningful use standards include to 1) provide health records for the treating physician (from prior episodes of care) 2) improve the quality and coordination of care, and 3) provide patients access to their health information. The administration, planning and implementation of HIE services must take into account the broad scope and complex nature of electronic data exchange and location (e.g., computer network, dedicated servers, cloud servers) of electronic patient records.

In Florida, the HIE is federated, meaning data is housed locally, not in a centralized format (AHCA, 2011). The HIE serves as the location for patient information exchange but the provider maintains the data. This allows providers to query for patient records across various participating networks via the Patient Look-Up.

Patient Look-Up Services

Patient Look-Up enables the search and retrieval of a patient's health information, such as labwork, medication history, and discharge summaries from disparate sources (i.e., a "pull" function). AHCA recognizes that the majority of patient care is delivered locally, and that the goal of local HIE efforts will be connecting providers with local sources of patient data. Public health officials will also use the HIE to prevent disease outbreaks and to investigate reported disease cases of significance to the public (FHIE, 2015).

If the provider has a Master Patient Index (MPI) in place, the Florida HIE provides an Express Lite application option that allows the provider to connect directly to the FHIN. If the provider does not have an MPI in place, another type of Express app is available-that allows the provider to connect to the FHIN or create a HIE (Shim, 2011). Both the Express Lite and Express applications need to connect to the appropriate provider system to create and package information conforming to the required standard profiles to participate in the Florida HIE. These profiles are variations of the base standards such as the Clinical Document Architecture (CDA), Continuity of Care Document (CCD), Continuity of Care Record (CCR), and HITSP C32 that build upon the HL7 CCD component. A Minimum Data Set for Patient Look-Up and Delivery Services has also been established as follows (FHIE, 2015):

- Encounter information for each emergency department visit, primary care or hospital visit (depending on participant type) shall include: patient demographic information, reason for visit, treating health care provider(s), date and place of visit, diagnoses, and procedures.

- Vital signs, discharge summaries, medications, alerts (i.e., allergies), immunizations, patient functional status, laboratory test results, and other diagnostic test results which are available electronically.

DIRECT MESSAGING SERVICE

The Florida HIE provides a Direct Messaging Service (DMS) to all subscribers to support communication between physicians and/or health care organizations for transition of care or patient referral purposes. DMS can also support the provision of clinical documents or information in response to medical information requests. Supported national and best practice security standards enable the transmission of encrypted information directly to trusted recipients via the Internet. The service is hosted at the Florida HIE data center and can be accessed securely by subscribers using a Web-enabled client. In this manner, providers can meet the requirements of meaningful use incentives. The Florida HIE DMS is nationally accredited through Direct Trust. The Direct Trust specifications represent a national standard model meant to streamline transmission of encrypted health information directly to known trusted recipients over the Internet.

EVENT NOTIFICATION SYSTEMS

In 2013, the Florida HIE developed the Event Notification System (ENS) which sends patient admit-discharge-transfer (ADT) notifications to participating health plans and providers when a patient is admitted or discharged from a hospital (system) or when the patient is seen in the emergency department (AHCA, 2013). To participate, subscribers (health plans or providers) provide patient rosters to the Florida HIE, and patient names are matched against hospital ADT events. If a match is detected, the subscriber is notified. The ENS improves coordination of care by lowering readmission rates and diverting non-urgent care to the primary care provider (AHCA, 2015). In addition to real time monitoring of events, the ENS can be used to alert hospitals if a patient is admitted to another facility within 30 days of discharge from the initial facility (AHCA, 2015).

CURRENT CHALLENGES

The Florida HIE has made significant strides in the development of services allowing healthcare organizations to share information. However, in order to "close the loop" and make the Florida Health Information Exchange a valuable link in the healthcare process, patients must have access to this data and be actively engaged in their own care. The Florida HIE does not currently offer this service, but research shows that including patients in the healthcare process increases quality and reduces health care costs (Aberger, Migliozzi, Follick, Malick & Ahern, 2014; Ricciardi, Mostashari, Murphy, Daniel & Siminerio, 2013).

In the current model of health information exchange, providers are the key participants and patients must "opt in" to participate through the use of consents. This means that patients are not given direct access to the HIE, nor are they are included in the DMS services. This can result in patients having numerous specialists with multiple patient portals and no linkage to provide a comprehensive overview of the individual's health. Although patients may want to engage in their own care, this type of disjointed technology does not encourage patient involvement (Landi, 2016).

Why is Patient Engagement Important?

An engaged patient is one who seeks out health information to become an active participant in his or her own care, rather than a compliant patient who simply follows his or her provider's orders. These engaged patients are motivated to search for information and perceive significant value in the information obtained. The HIE can provide information from multiple sources and present a cohesive overview, but the patient must be willing to look at and use the information for it to be of value to continuing care and contribute to engagement.

Empowering patients to be active participants in their own care has been extensively researched and found to have a positive impact on care and cost. The benefits include higher quality care, fewer errors, (Osborn & Squires, 2012) improved medication adherence (Roebuck, Liberman, Gemmill-Toyama & Brennan, 2011), reduced hospitalizations, (Laurance, Henderson, Howitt, Matar, Kuwari Edgman-Levitan, & Darzi, 2014) as well as reduced cost and improved health (Coulter, 2012).

The primary challenges to the management and functioning of health information exchanges for patient engagement include awareness, access, usability, and health literacy. Improving these areas can increase patient engagement and offer the Florida HIE an opportunity to improve patient health outcomes and reduce costs in the state of Florida.

Awareness

Awareness of electronic health records has increased in recent years, but studies show that the majority of patients are not offered access to their health records by providers (Birth, 2016; Patel, Barker & Siminerio, 2015). A 2015 Harris Poll found that 25% of patients have online access to their medical record compared to 17% in 2012, while e-mail access is at 19%, up from 12% in 2012 (Birth, 2016). In addition to their own access, 65% of patients valued the accessibility of their prior medical history by a physician highly, with a "very important" rating. This Poll also found that 44% of patients found it very important to be able to communicate with their doctor outside of an appointment, either by phone or e-mail.

Access

Access to medical information has been shown to provide numerous benefits, such as improved communication with providers, improved understanding of treatment regimens; and ultimately, improved compliance with healthcare plans (Green et al., 2008; Hassol et al., 2004; Winkelman, Leonard, & Rossos, 2005). Ancker, et al. (2014) conducted research involving challenges to providing HIE access to patients in New York. Technical aspects in terms of how the patient would access information (including how patients are enrolled) and what information would be accessed were considered in interviews with product developers, project managers, and outreach staff. The specific information to be released included encounters, allergies, medications and billing, but not laboratory results due to clinician concerns about patient misinterpretation. The challenge of managing patient identity resulted in manually enrolling patients into the HIEs to avoid multiple accounts for one patient (Ancker, et al., 2014).

The Pew Center reports that Internet access has reached full saturation for individuals falling within certain groups including those with high educational attainment, younger age, and more affluent living arrangements (Perrin & Duggan, 2015). This penetration is significant in attempts to engage patients using health information technology. However, some patient groups that traditionally use a lot of health-care services, such as the elderly, are being left behind (Perrin & Duggan, 2015). It should be noted that many individuals access the Internet only through the use of a smart phone or tablet. While these devices are convenient, they have limited capabilities when it comes to high usage activities such as streaming videos, which might be useful for patient education.

Differences in access to the Internet also exist according to socioeconomic categories. Kontos, Blake, Chou and Prestin (2014) found that people making less than $20,000 per year were 46% less likely to use the Internet to help with diet and physical activity than those consumers making $75,000 or more. Conversely, those making less than $20,000 were found to be twice as likely to use social networking sites to investigate health topics as those making $75,000 or more. Additional research in a medical practice revealed that 75% of patients surveyed (majority with less than $20,000 annual income and a high school education) indicated willingness to adopt an online health record if it is made available to them (Noblin, Wan & Fottler, 2012).

Usability

Perceived ease of use has been shown to be important in the behavioral intention to use a new technology (Davis, 1989). Some basic administrative issues can impede the use of health information technology to engage patients. A difficult to use interface can deter the most willing patient to forgo engaging in his or her own care (Irizarry, Devito Dabbs & Curran, 2015). This is particularly true for individuals using a smart phone or tablet to access portals. To best serve this large population and more readily reach consumers, patient portals should be designed to fit mobile screens, and/or have an app that a patient can download to his or her phone.

In the age of increasing identity theft, one major concern of patients wishing to access their health information through a patient portal is that of security of their sensitive and personal medical information. A recent meta-analysis of patient portal research found that 41% of articles mentioned security of health records as an issue inhibiting the growth of the patient portal market (Kruse, Argueta, Lopez & Nair, 2014).

Passwords are also a major cause for concern and one of the issues for physicians looking to implement patient portal technology. To ensure patient privacy, all access to records must be password protected. However, when a patient forgets his or her password or locks him or herself out the system, the password recovery process can be burdensome to the provider and the patient. This can discourage the patient from proceeding with current or future engagement activities.

Health Literacy

Health literacy is defined as the degree to which individuals have the capacity to obtain, process and understand basic health information and services needed to make appropriate health decisions (Dept of

HHS, 2010). While some of the traditional assumptions about who would demonstrate high levels of literacy hold true, research has shown that individuals with chronic diseases or individuals caring for those with a chronic disease, have high levels of health literacy regardless of age and socio-economic status (Zide, Caswell, Peterson, Aberle, Bui & Arnold, 2016).

In their meta-analysis examining the prevalence of limited health literacy, Paasche-Orlow, Parker, Gazmararian, Nielsen-Bohlman, and Rudd (2005) found low education levels and race were significant predictors of low health literacy. People who speak English as a second language are less confident in their ability to obtain needed health information (Moen & Brennan, 2005). In addition, in cities with diverse patient populations, it may not be possible to provide translations for all languages (Ancker, et al., 2014).

RECOMMENDATIONS

Given the challenges to patient engagement in health planning and behavior as relates to the Florida HIE, it is important to consider a variety of strategies to address these issues. Communication has the potential to educate, persuade and motivate patients to engage in healthy behaviors (Schulz & Nakamoto, 2013). Improving competence of patients can allow more autonomy in healthy decision making.

Three primary strategies identified in the literature include engaging patients through 1) inclusion in design and implementation of patient portals 2) involvement in social media, and 3) education about technology and health information exchange.

Patient Portals

Patient portals are the entry point for patients to access their records, and they are generally offered through a physician's office and are typically part of an electronic health record. Currently, portals are specific to a health system and do not allow the patient to share among outside providers which significantly reduces usefulness in seeking a holistic view of one's health.

Having the ability to fill in knowledge gaps with credible information from a variety of sources is a challenge for all health care providers. Allowing patients to download HIE data into a personal health record is one way to collect information and can also allow patients to track who has accessed their information through an audit log (Ancker et al., 2014). Patient portals can be used to push relevant educational information to patients based on specific diagnoses. Tailoring information to the patient is an important consideration and can include unique content based on laboratory test results or medication prescriptions, as well as personalized decision support for treatment option decision making (Prey, et al., 2014). Physicians and other providers (as well as HIE support staff) must play an active role as the change agents for adoption, but ultimately the patient can control his/her destiny through continued active use of the patient portal or other electronic access to health information.

To improve patient engagement, including behavior change, portals must be user friendly like common applications in Apple, Facebook and Google. According to Brian Eastwood, a lead analyst with Chilmark Research, "Portals capture information about episodes of care but they are not built for coordinated care and are inadequate for population health management" (Landi, 2016).

Social Media

The use of social media is pervasive in today's culture, with its use crossing diverse demographic and social boundaries. Engaging patients in their own space can limit user interface concerns and help individuals feel comfortable with the mechanisms to access their information. Providing information and marketing of services using social media can increase participation and thus engagement.

As another factor, often chronic diseases provide a common thread for patients to interact with online sources for information about their conditions (e.g., Medline, WebMD). These patients can be highly literate, having researched extensively about their condition. Kalichman et al. (2003) reported that a group of people living with HIV/AIDS who use the Internet for health information searches are better informed about the disease and also use the Internet for social support. Improving Internet usage among this population is felt to be important for both education and coping strategies.

Chung (2014) confirmed that the strongest motivation for online support group participation is information seeking. This includes learning about one's own health condition, treatment options, and seeking advice from others who have the same condition and have tried various treatment options. Patients are also motivated to provide support to others who are coping with the same issue(s) (Chung, 2014). While this type of sharing is not ideal for an HIE environment, the ability of patients to collect their data and discuss it with others they trust outside of the healthcare team has been shown to improve engagement in medical care (Fox, 2014).

Education

Education on the importance of engagement and ways that patients can take control over their own health is essential to the success of any patient engagement program. In the case of patient portals, technical aspects of the system, security and the importance of engagement must be stressed in all educational materials.

Health literacy is also a key attribute of the educational recommendations. Without at least a foundational level of health literacy, patients could at best be confused by information contained in their record and at worst follow incorrect medical advice. Health literacy could be improved by simple outreach programs by either physicians or Florida Department of Health personnel.

For example, to offset literacy challenges, Baorto and Cimino (2000) reported on the development of an "infobutton" for use by women to access Pap smear results online. This is part of the Patient Clinical Information System (PatCIS) provided by New York Presbyterian Hospital. Definitions for frequently encountered diagnostic terms are made available to aid patients in reading and understanding their reports. Providing patients with such a tool is an important step in allowing patients to take ownership of their healthcare outcomes.

CONCLUSION

As healthcare costs continue to rise, individual patients do have an option to directly impact their outcomes through self-management and communication with providers (Windham, Bennett, & Gottlieb, 2003).

A survey found that 79% of adult Americans believe that maintaining a personal health record would provide major benefits in healthcare management (Connecting for Health, 2008). A distinct advantage of health information access is the ability it affords the patient to be an active member of the medical team and not just a passive consumer of healthcare services. An active team member will seek the ability to understand the content of the health record, including diseases and medications. Giving the patient the ability to refer (back) to treatment plans can result in improved care and, more importantly, prevent an untoward event (The Joint Commission, 2007).

The current state of health information exchange in Florida does not include patient input or engagement. Until patients are included, and encouraged to access their own medical information, the complete mission of the HIE cannot be accomplished. The Florida HIE should consider challenges including a digital divide among age groups and socioeconomic status when engaging patients using HIT. Also, improving the health literacy of vulnerable populations is a necessary step to engaging patients.

REFERENCES

Aberger, E. W., Migliozzi, D., Follick, M. J., Malick, T., & Ahern, D. K. (2014). Enhancing patient engagement and blood pressure management for renal transplant recipients via home electronic monitoring and web-enabled collaborative care. *Telemedicine Journal and e-Health*, *20*(9), 850–854. doi:10.1089/tmj.2013.0317 PMID:25046403

AHCA. (2011). State health information exchange cooperative agreement program strategic and operational plans. State Health Information Exchange Cooperative Agreement Program. Retrieved February 10, 2017 from http://www.nashp.org/wp-content/uploads/sites/default/files/Florida%20Strategic%20Plan.pdf

AHCA. (2013). Event notification service overview for the Florida HIE. Retrieved February 10, 2017, from https://www.florida-hie.net/Files/DSM/ENSGenOverviewFAQ.pdf

AHCA. (2015). Health information exchange coordinating committee meeting minutes, November 20, 2015. Retrieved February 10, 2017 from http://www.fhin.net/committeesAndCouncils/docs/hiecc/Nov2015/HIECCminutesNov2015.pdf

Ancker, J. S., Miller, M. C., Patel, V., & Kaushal, R. (2014). Sociotechnical challenges to developing technologies for patient access to health information exchange data. *Journal of the American Medical Informatics Association*, *21*(4), 664–670. doi:10.1136/amiajnl-2013-002073 PMID:24064443

Baorto, D., & Cimino, J. (2000). An "infobutton" for enabling patients to interpret on-line Pap smear reports. *Proceedings of the AMIA 2000 Symposium* (p. 47).

Birth, A. (2016). Satisfaction with doctor visits on the rise, January 20, 2016. Retrieved January 30, 2017 from http://www.theharrispoll.com/health-and-life/Doctor-Visit-Satisfaction.html

Chung, J. E. (2014). Social networking in online support groups for health: How online social networking benefits patients. *Journal of Health Communication*, *19*(6), 639–659. doi:10.1080/10810730.2012.757396 PMID:23557148

Connecting for Health. (2008). *Americans overwhelmingly believe electronic personal health records could improve their health.* Markle Foundation. Retrieved February 10, 2017 from https://www.markle.org/sites/default/files/ResearchBrief-200806.pdf

Coulter, A. (2012). Patient engagement—what works? *The Journal of Ambulatory Care Management,* *35*(2), 80–89. doi:10.1097/JAC.0b013e318249e0fd PMID:22415281

Davis, F. (1989). Perceived usefulness, perceived ease of use, and user acceptance of information technology. *Management Information Systems Quarterly,* *13*(3), 319–340. doi:10.2307/249008

Fox, S. (2014, January 15). The social life of health information. Pew Research Center. Retrieved January 30, 2017 from: http://www.pewresearch.org/fact-tank/2014/01/15/the-social-life-of-health-information/

Green, B., Cook, A., Ralston, J., Fishman, P., Catz, S., Carlson, J., & Thompson, R. et al. (2008). Effectiveness of home blood pressure monitoring, web communication, and pharmacist care on hypertension control: A randomized controlled trial. *Journal of the American Medical Association,* *299*(24), 2857–2867. doi:10.1001/jama.299.24.2857 PMID:18577730

Hassol, A., Walker, J., Kidder, D., Rokita, K., Young, D., Pierdon, S., & Ortiz, E. et al. (2004). Patient experiences and attitudes about access to a patient electronic health care record and linked web messaging. *Journal of the American Medical Informatics Association,* *11*(6), 505–513. doi:10.1197/jamia.M1593 PMID:15299001

Irizarry, T., DeVito Dabbs, A., & Curran, C. R. (2015). Patient Portals and Patient Engagement: A State of the Science Review. *Journal of Medical Internet Research,* *17*(6), e148. doi:10.2196/jmir.4255 PMID:26104044

Kalichman, S. C., Benotsch, E. G., Weinhardt, L., Austin, J., Luke, W., & Cherry, C. (2003). Health-related Internet use, coping, social support, and health indicators in people living with HIV/AIDS: Preliminary results from a community survey. *Health Psychology,* *22*(1), 111–116. doi:10.1037/0278-6133.22.1.111 PMID:12558209

Kontos, E., Blake, K. D., Chou, W. Y. S., & Prestin, A. (2014). Predictors of eHealth usage: Insights on the digital divide from the Health Information National Trends Survey 2012. *Journal of Medical Internet Research,* *16*(7), e172. doi:10.2196/jmir.3117 PMID:25048379

Kruse, C. S., Argueta, D. A., Lopez, L., & Nair, A. (2015). Patient and Provider Attitudes Toward the Use of Patient Portals for the Management of Chronic Disease: A Systematic Review. *Journal of Medical Internet Research,* *17*(2), e40. doi:10.2196/jmir.3703 PMID:25707035

Landi, H. (2016, October 6) Patient engagement technology: Moving beyond patient portals? *Healthcare Informatics.* Retrieved January 30, 2017 from http://www.healthcare-informatics.com/article/patient-engagement/patient-engagement-technology-moving-beyond-patient-portals

Laurance, J., Henderson, S., Howitt, P. J., Matar, M., Al Kuwari, H., Edgman-Levitan, S., & Darzi, A. (2014). Patient engagement: Four case studies that highlight the potential for improved health outcomes and reduced costs. *Health Affairs,* *33*(9), 1627–1634. doi:10.1377/hlthaff.2014.0375 PMID:25201668

Moen, A., & Brennan, P. (2005). Health@home: The work of health information management in the household: Implications for consumer health informatics innovations. *Journal of the American Medical Informatics Association*, *12*(6), 648–656. doi:10.1197/jamia.M1758 PMID:16049230

Noblin, A., Wan, T., & Fottler, M. (2012). The impact of health literacy on a patient's decision to adopt a personal health record. *Perspectives in Health Information Management*, 9, 1-13. PMID:23209454

Osborn, R., & Squires, D. (2012). International perspectives on patient engagement: Results from the 2011 Commonwealth Fund Survey. *The Journal of Ambulatory Care Management*, *35*(2), 118–128. doi:10.1097/JAC.0b013e31824a579b PMID:22415285

Paasche-Orlow, M., Parker, R., Gazmararian, J., Nielsen-Bohlman, L., & Rudd, R. (2005). The prevalence of limited health literacy. *Journal of General Internal Medicine*, *20*(2), 175–184. doi:10.1111/j.1525-1497.2005.40245.x PMID:15836552

Patel, V., Barker, W., & Siminerio, E. (2015). *Trends in Consumer Access and Use of Electronic Health. ONC Data Brief, no.30*. Washington, DC: Office of the National Coordinator for Health Information Technology.

Perrin, A., & Duggan, M. (2015). Americans' Internet Access: 2000-2015. *Pew Research Center*. Retrieved February 10, 2017 from http://www.pewinternet.org/2015/06/26/americans-internet-access-2000-2015/

Prey, J. E., Woollen, J., Wilcox, L., Sackeim, A. D., Hripcsak, G., Bakken, S., & Vawdrey, D. K. et al. (2014). Patient engagement in the inpatient setting: A systematic review. *Journal of the American Medical Informatics Association*, *21*(4), 742–750. doi:10.1136/amiajnl-2013-002141 PMID:24272163

Ricciardi, L., Mostashari, F., Murphy, J., Daniel, J. G., & Siminerio, E. P. (2013). A national action plan to support consumer engagement via e-health. *Health Affairs*, *32*(2), 376–384. doi:10.1377/hlthaff.2012.1216 PMID:23381531

Roebuck, M. C., Liberman, J. N., Gemmill-Toyama, M., & Brennan, T. A. (2011). Medication adherence leads to lower health care use and costs despite increased drug spending. *Health Affairs*, *30*(1), 91–99. doi:10.1377/hlthaff.2009.1087 PMID:21209444

Rosenfeld, S., Koss, S., Caruth, K., & Fuller, G. (2006). Evolution of state health information exchange: A study of vision, strategy, and progress. The Agency for Healthcare Research and Quality. Retrieved February 10, 2017 from https://healthit.ahrq.gov/sites/default/files/docs/medicaid/hie-statebased-finrep-20130731.pdf

Schulz, P. J., & Nakamoto, K. (2013). Health literacy and patient empowerment in health communication: The importance of separating conjoined twins. *Patient Education and Counseling*, *90*(1), 4–11. doi:10.1016/j.pec.2012.09.006 PMID:23063359

Shim, S. (2011). The evolution of health information exchanges. *Paper presented at the meeting of the Florida Health Information Management Association*, Orlando, FL.

Subscription Agreement, F. H. I. E. (2015). Retrieved February 10, 2017 from https://www.florida-hie.net/Files/Resources/PLU_Subscription_Agreement.pdf

The Joint Commission. (2007). *What did the doctor say? Improving health literacy to protect patient safety*. Oakbrook Terrace, IL: Author.

U.S. Department of Health & Human Services. (2012). The office of the national coordinator for health information technology. Retrieved February 10, 2017 from https://www.healthit.gov/policy-researchers-implementers/state-health-information-exchange

US Department of Health and Human Services. (2010). Healthy People cited in National Network of Libraries of Medicine. "Health Literacy." Retrieved from http://nnlm.gov/outreach/consumer/hlthlit.html

Windham, B., Bennett, R., & Gottlieb, S. (2003). Care management interventions for patients with congestive heart failure. *The American Journal of Managed Care*, 9(6), 447–459. PMID:12816174

Winkelman, W., Leonard, K., & Rossos, P. (2005). Patient-perceived usefulness of online electronic medical records: Employing grounded theory in the development of information and communication technologies for use by patients living with chronic illness. *Journal of the American Medical Informatics Association*, 12(3), 306–314. doi:10.1197/jamia.M1712 PMID:15684128

Zide, M., Caswell, K., Peterson, E., Aberle, D. R., Bui, A. A., & Arnold, C. W. (2016). Consumers' Patient Portal Preferences and Health Literacy: A Survey Using Crowdsourcing. *JMIR research protocols, 5*(2).

This research was previously published in the International Journal of User-Driven Healthcare (IJUDH), 6(2); edited by Ashok Kumar Biswas, pages 46-55, copyright year 2016 by IGI Publishing (an imprint of IGI Global).

Chapter 60
Why Do Patients Protest? Collective Action Processes in People With Chronic Illnesses:
A Psychosocial Perspective

Davide Mazzoni
University of Bologna, Italy

Augusta Isabella Alberici
Università Cattolica del Sacro Cuore, Italy

ABSTRACT

Despite the relevance of the topic, an exhaustive psychosocial reflection on the processes that may facilitate patients' protest is still missing. The chapter provides a theoretical and empirical overview of psychosocial pathways for patients' collective action. Five core factors are reviewed: perceived injustice, group efficacy, group identification, moral convictions and social embeddedness. Each of them provides a different explanation of collective action processes and is examined for its potential impact among patients. The chapter closes suggesting some core elements for a theoretical explanation of patients' collective action and its relationship with patient engagement. Practical and theoretical implications of patients' collective action are discussed to identify new directions for future research and interventions.

Quel che ci accomuna è, soprattutto, la scelta di prendere in mano il nostro destino, di essere noi i protagonisti di questo movimento civile ed umano, senza deleghe in bianco a chicchessia.

[What we share is, most of all, the choice to be protagonists of our fate, to be ourselves the protagonists of this civil and human movement without proxies to anyone.]

– Alberto Damilano, From the homepage of the Italian network of people with amyotrophic lateral sclerosis (website: http://www.comitato16novembre.org/).

DOI: 10.4018/978-1-5225-3926-1.ch060

INTRODUCTION

Looking at local and national news in many European countries, it is not surprising to see and read about patients taking part in demonstrations, holding flags and posters to defend their own rights. Just to make some examples, we can refer to the pro-Stamina stem cell treatment demonstration that took place on December 2013 in the center of Rome (Italy). The police attempted to block the march and two protesters were stopped by the police. Few months later (June 2014), a group of workers and patients of the Bellvitge University Hospital (Spain) demonstrated against the healthcare budget cuts and blocked a nearby highway for several minutes. Again, on October 2014, a mass protest of patients was hold in Kiev and in some regions of Ukraine. The protest was titled "Black Tuesday". Patients picketed the Cabinet of Ministers, and demanded from the government to procure medicines for critically ill Ukrainians. They brought hundreds of shoe pairs that symbolized the death of the patients in case the government did not procure the necessary medicines.

As suggested by most patient engagement literature, nowadays, patients appear to be increasingly aware of their rights, and more demanding in the fruition of healthcare services. They are concerned with their own needs and preferences, and have become more critical in expressing judgments about the received health services (e.g., Guyatt, Mulla, Scott, Jackevicius, & You, 2014). On the other side, healthcare organizations do not always recognize and accept patients' active role. This may be a source of strain that, under certain circumstances, can result in a real collective mobilization.

Despite the relevance of the question we ask in the title, for patients and society, an exhaustive psychosocial reflection on the processes that may facilitate patients' protest is still missing. The available analyses focused on single groups or episodes (e.g., Rabeharisoa, 2006), while a broader theorization is actually desirable. This echoes Zoller (2005), when she wrote that we are more likely to heardiscussion of AIDS activism or breast cancer activism than we are tohear 'health activism' or other converging terms.

This chapter contributes to the book "Promoting Patient Engagement and Participation for Effective Healthcare Reform" by enlarging the analysis of patient engagement and participation with a group-based perspective, which is distinctive of the social psychology approach. Among the disciplines that were interested on the topic, our chapter focuses on the psychosocial processes at the basis of patients' collective action, conceived as one of the ways through which patients can produce (or resist to) a change in their health care system. Before we proceed to the social psychological answer as to why patients protest, we devote a few words to describe patients' collective action itself.

BACKGROUND: PATIENTS AS ACTIVISTS

In the psychosocial domain, collective action is often defined as a specific form of participation where individuals undertake actions as group members, with the aim to improve the group's conditions (e.g. Wright, Taylor, & Moghaddam, 1990; see also Van Zomeren & Iyer, 2009). According to Wright et al. (1990), collective action is proposed in contrast to individual action, that is specifically directed at improving one's personal conditions rather than group.

A wide range of behaviors can be classified as collective action, ranging from participation in protest demonstrations and strikes to seemingly individualistic acts such as signing a petition (Van Zomeren & Iyer, 2009) or contributing to a cause through an individual donation. More generally, despite some limitations that are discussed in the next paragraphs, patients' participation can potentially cover the broad spectrum of social and political engagement as classified by Ekman and Amnå (2012), including both legal and illegal forms of participation. In all cases, the aim of improving the patients' group conditions coincides with the aim of improving their health by influencing the healthcare system and the society. This influence can be expressed either toward the production of a social change (e.g., a desirable health care reform), and the resistance to an unwanted social change, (e.g., against money cuts for health services).

Moreover, like many other expressions of dissent, patients' collective actions represent the concerted efforts by committed supporters of the cause. Indeed, activists are usually defined as people who actively work for social or political causes. This group includes not only "protesters", that is patients who, for example, concretely march at the front of a demonstration, but also people who recruit for and mobilize people, and sustain the organizational structures that support them (see also Stuart, Thomas, Donaghue, & Russell, 2013; Simon & Klandermans, 2001).

In this sense, we should note that our discourse on patients' collective action must take into account not only the actions concretely run by patients, but also by the community of individuals that support, and sometimes are the only way to make possible, patients' mobilization. Concretely, supporters may include patients' familiars, friends, medical and paramedical professions also with a wide range of actors: researchers (biologists and clinicians), industry, public authorities, institutions, patient organizations, the local communities, etc.

PATHWAYS TO PATIENTS' PROTEST

Why do people protest? Which psychosocial processes are involved in their engagement in collective actions? These questions, despite rarely referred to patients, have occupied social psychologists for at least three decades, and have received diverging answers over the years (see Klandermans, 1997; Van Zomeren, Postmes, & Spears, 2008; Van Stekelenburg, 2013; Van Stekelenburg & Klandermans, 2013; Klandermans & Van Stekelenburg, 2013, for reviews). As suggested by Van Zomeren (2011), the first decade of the 21st century can be rightly called an 'age of integration' for the collective action literature. Before this period, various perspectives on collective action existed side-by-side (Van Zomeren & Spears, 2009; Van Zomeren et al., 2008).

Building on the existing literature, in this chapter we describe the social-psychological motives for undertaking collective action through three 'classical' core variables, such as perceived injustice, group identification, and group efficacy (Gamson, 1992; Klandermans, 1997; Stürmer & Simon, 2004; Van Zomeren et al., 2008; Van Zomeren, 2011). Considering more recent developments, two more factors will be considered: moral convictions (e.g., Van Zomeren, Postmes, & Spears, 2012) and social embeddedness (e.g., Van Stekelenburg & Klandermans, 2013).

Compared to other populations (e.g., migrants, no-global, environmentalist, etc.), patients have not been object of systematic analysis from a psychosocial perspective. In the following sections, we will review each of these psychosocial motives for collective mobilization and we will examine how they can specifically influence collective action processes among patients. Finally, the chapter closes suggesting some core elements for a theoretical explanation of patients' collective action and discussing some lines for further research.

Perceived Injustice

As suggested by some authors (Marwell & Oliver, 1993; Klandermans, 2004), even in view of significant changes in their environment and lives, most people continue to do what they were doing, namely nothing. A consequence of this observation is that, even in contexts of deprivation and cuts to health services, only a minority of patients decide to engage in some forms of collective action.

This is coherent with the idea that (objective) deprivation is neither necessary nor sufficient to determine collective action. At this regard, the study focus should include the subjective experience involved and its presumed connection to objective deprivation. Stouffer and colleagues (Stouffer, Suchman, DeVinney, Star, & Williams, 1949) introduced the concept of relative deprivation to explain why objective deprivation does not always predict peoples' dissatisfactions with their lost. Similar research led to the development of relative deprivation theory (e.g., Folger, 1986, 1987; Pettigrew, 1967; Runciman, 1966; Walker & Smith, 2002), which focused on the subjective experience of unjust disadvantage. Relative deprivation theory proposes that feelings of deprivation develop on the basis of social comparisons, while theory and research have suggested that social inequality in distributions can be perceived as even fair (e.g., Jost & Major, 2001; Major, 1994).

The notion that the subjective experience of inequality has greater weight than its objective, material origins has been considered also in recent developments in the social-psychological literature on fairness judgments, which focuses on how people respond to distributive and procedural fairness and their emotional consequences (e.g., anger, resentment) (Leventhal, 1980; Lind & Tyler, 1988; Miller, 2001; Tyler, Boeckmann, Smith, & Huo, 1997; Van den Bos & Lind, 2002).

Similar conclusions can be found also in patient engagement literature. For example, in a UK qualitative study involving patients who have experienced rationing associated with morbid obesity or breast cancer care, participants had a choice whether to accept that decision, to contest it, or to opt out of the public healthcare system and pay for private care. Results showed that the perception of decision-making being unjust led some patients to contest decisions (Owen-Smith, Coast, & Donovan, 2009). Moreover, among the most important factors affecting how patients reacted to rationing were their sense of entitlement to National Health Service care, and the attitude of the clinical team providing treatment. The importance of perceived fairness of decision-making suggests that it is important to continue to explore the acceptable bases for rationing alongside the accountability of the process of decision making, which has been the focus of much of the recent priority setting literature (Daniels, 2000; Kapiriri, Norheim, & Martin, 2007). In this sense, the authors conclude that patients need to be provided with sufficient information and support to make an informed decision following the revelation of rationing, and that clinicians need training to assist them in communicating rationing decisions.

(Group) Efficacy

In the 1970s, theories like relative derivation were criticized by scholars arguing that grievances do not provide a sufficient reason to participate in protest. In some way, the key question to address was: why do some aggrieved people become mobilized, while others do not? At this regard, in the last decades, personal and group *efficacy* beliefs have become one of the key explanations of collective action. The idea behind group efficacy is that people engage in collective action if they believe this will make it more likely that relevant goals are achieved by the group (e.g., Van Zomeren et al., 2008). Several studies have shown that feelings of efficacy are highly correlated with participation in protest and this relation was confirmed also meta-analytically (Van Zomeren et al., 2008).

In the analysis by Van Zomeren and Spears (2009), efficacy beliefs were grouped together with cost-benefit calculations (Olson, 1965), as motivations of the 'intuitive economists' metaphor. The assumption here about human motivation is that people are individual-based intuitive economists (Edwards, 1962) who make social judgments and decisions by calculating the costs and benefits of a particular action and its consequences. This motivation for collective action is reflected in early sociological work on collective action (e.g., Olson, 1965), which strongly influenced later approaches to collective action in terms of its individual rationality assumption (e.g., Hardin, 1971; Klandermans, 1984; McCarthy & Zald, 1977; Simon et al., 1998). In this sense, the idea that personal commitment depends on expectations that one's group is able to achieve the social change, can be considered an instrumental path to collective action.

It is plausible that similar efficacy beliefs are relevant for patients' collective action. However, we must recognize that efficacy beliefs among patients may be lower than in other populations. As described by Jennings (1999), the effects of pain and loss may reduce efficacy beliefs: people experiencing pain and loss may be disinclined toward political participation because they feel depressed, overwhelmed, and helpless, especially if they also face stigma by others. Even if, in theory, it would be also possible that sometimes pain and loss can "trigger" emotional and cognitive responses that provide incentives and motivations for political action (Jennings, 1999), this is rarely the case. The results of a nationally representative survey in the United States confirmed that several measures of efficacy that help predict-political activity were found to be significantly lower among people with disabilities than among similar people without disabilities (Schur, Shields, & Schriner, 2003).

At this regard, we note that some patients decide to express their dissent and protest against decisions that are hardly possible to modify. For example, it seems unlikely that protests run by patients with amyotrophic lateral sclerosis in Italy, as expressed in the citation we reported at the beginning of this chapter, are moved by instrumental motives only. Even, if it is quite difficult to fully obtain the desirable change, and the costs of the protest for patients are quite high, some people still decide to engage in some forms of collective action. This suggests that also other factors, some of which will be discussed in the next paragraphs, different from efficacy, could be relevant for patients.

However, also the distinction between the individual and the group level of analysis can be useful. Individual efficacy, that is the belief in the achievement of individual goals through one's own actions is an important predictor of such action. Similarly, group efficacy beliefs are important in motivating people to achieve group goals through collective action. Some authors recently suggested that *participative* efficacy, that is the belief that individual's participations matters – i.e., that the individual's participation is seen as having a potential incremental effect on collective action – could be more relevant than group efficacy (Van Zomeren, Saguy, & Schellhaas, 2013).

Group Identity

In the 1980s it become clear to many researchers that instrumental motivation was not a sufficient reason to engage in collective actions. From that time, the literature devoted greater attention to the key-role played also by group identification processes (Tajfel & Turner, 1986; Turner, Hogg, Oakes, Reicher, & Wetherell, 1987). More specifically, some social-psychological studies report consistently that the more people identify with a group, the more they are inclined to protest (e.g., Reicher, 1984; Simon et al., 1998; Stryker, Owens, & Wite, 2000; Mazzoni, Van Zomeren, & Cicognani, 2015). Indeed, identification with others is accompanied by an awareness of similarity and shared fate with those who belong to the same category. When group members perceive a collective disadvantage, they may decide to act as a group to reduce it (Ellemers, 2002).

According to Simon and Klandermans (2001), group identity politicizes when group members become aware of shared grievances and of an opponent who is to blame; when they share a sense of the possibility and normative requirement to act collectively for social change; and when they become aware that the power struggle has to be fought in the public arena, where third parties need to be involved (Simon & Klandermans, 2001). There is strong evidence that politicized identity is a crucial predictor of collective action as it implies that group members, through their struggle, achieve a sense of themselves as being collectively agentic (Blackwood & Louis, 2012; Van Zomeren, Spears, Fischer, & Leach, 2004). Psychosocial research also highlighted that collective identity facilitates beliefs and emotions that, in turn, predict collective action (Van Zomeren at al., 2008). At the same time, collective identity encapsulates beliefs and emotions relevant to action, and mediates their effect on collective action (Thomas, Mavor, & McGarty, 2012).

More recent developments in this area of research pointed out that "dual identity" is particularly important in the collective action processes (e.g., Simon & Grabow, 2010). Social psychology showed that people can hold many different identities at the same time (e.g., as patient, as patient with AIDS, as citizen, as human being, etc.). In the context of collective action, dual identity involves both identification with the aggrieved ingroup (e.g., a group of patients) and identification with a more inclusive group or community (e.g., the same country of residence) that entitles them to societal support for their claims.

Similar processes can be described for patients, where this identification may become even stronger, since, borrowing the term from Rabinow (2002), they are ''biosocially'' linked to one another. Brown et al. (2004) use the term "collective illness identity" to describe the intersection of social constructions of illness and the personal illness experience of a biological disease process. When patients develop a 'cognitive, moral, and emotional connection' with other illness sufferers, a collective illness identity emerges. Moreover, for a politicized collective illness identity to form, the collective illness identity must be linked to a broader social critique that views structural inequalities and the uneven distribution of social power as responsible for the causes and/or triggers of the disease.

Even in case of patients and disabled people, collective action intentions are enhanced by processes of identification (Scotch, 1988). As described by Brown et al. (2004), when "institutions of science and medicine fail to offer disease accounts that are consistent with individuals' experiences of illness, or when science and medicine offer accounts of disease that individuals are unwilling to accept, people may adopt an identity as an aggrieved illness sufferer, and even progress to collective action" (p. 55).

However, the group identity formation presents also some specific features and obstacles for patients. For example, people normally desire to retain an ordinary healthy identity and its value. For this reason, the identification with a group if patients can be initially hindered by feelings of pain and loss (Allsop, Jones, & Baggott, 2004; Kostova, Caiata-Zufferey, & Schulz, 2014). Together with the process of gradual identification, patient engagement is as a multidimensional psychosocial process resulting from the conjoint cognitive, emotional, and behavioral enactment of individuals. The process starts with the "blackout position" that follows the onset of the disease condition. In the "adhesion position" patients start to see him/herself as patient. Only in the last position of the engagement process (i.e., eudaimonic project), patients have fully accepted their condition and their patients' identity is only one of their possible selves (elaboration) (Graffigna, Barello, Riva, & Bosio, 2014).

In this sense, we suggest that is properly in the last position of the engagement (eudamonic) that patients collective action can potentially take place. Indeed, the "adhesion position" is individually characterized by the recognition of him/herself "as a patient", and this is, of course, a prerequisite to identify with the patients' group. However, only in the eudamonic position patient see him/herself "as a person" who can advocate for the health of his/her community (Graffigna et al., 2014). In psychosocial terms, this can be considered the basis for a politicized identity to develop.

Another key point is that communication among group members contributes to the development of group identity. The interactive model of identity formation (IMIF; Postmes, Haslam, & Swaab, 2005) postulates that in interactive groups two different paths are involved in social identity formation: a deductive path and an inductive path (Postmes, Spears, Lee, & Novak, 2005). In the latter case, group identity is inferred via the individual attempts of group members to shape consensus and it is deduced from commonalities at a superordinate group level. Consensus within the group can be obtained through a process through which group members interact with each other and negotiate a common group definition that is more than the sum of the distinctive individual positions. Consistently, Thomas and colleagues (Thomas, Smith, McGarty, & Postmes, 2010) proposed that, to pursue social change, emerging political forces need to consensualize and share their grievances through group interaction.

In a similar way, research on patients' illness narratives has highlighted how some patients can use stories to develop a coherent self, to make sense of their experiences, and to empower their existence (Charmaz, 1991; Frank, 1997; Kleinman, 1988). Moreover, telling stories about one's illness experience may allow both the speaker and the audience to cope with illness, to exchange information, and to reflect and reconstruct their new identities (Dickerson, Posluszny, & Kennedy, 2000; Hsieh, 2004). In this sense, for some patients storytelling may play an important role in the illness identity construction and can be considered a process through which such patients share a common identity potentially linked to social change.

Moral Convictions

Undoubtedly, in many cases, the motivations explained in the above paragraphs are sufficient to explain many people's collective behavior. However, in the last decade, some authors "rediscovered" the importance of moral convictions (e.g. Goodin, 1992), suggesting a special relationship with politicized identities and collective action. More specifically, moral convictions can be defined as strong and absolute stances on moral issues, they do not tolerate any exceptions to the general 'higher-order' principle (Tetlock, 2002). A violation of a moral conviction therefore motivates individuals to actively change that situation (Skitka, Bauman, & Sargis, 2005; Van Zomeren & Lodewijkx, 2005). According to authors, this mechanism would refer not only to moral absolutism - as a distinctly minority position – but could be a motivating factor for many people taking part in collective actions.

Moreover, moral convictions seem to represent a unifying motivation between 'advantaged' and 'disadvantaged' people. Once moral convictions acquire a moral status, they become subjectively universal and thus transcend group boundaries. For example, when moral convictions of 'advantaged' are against social inequality and they are confronted with a disadvantaged group, this constitutes a violation of their moral conviction, which can motivate them to change the situation (Van Zomeren, Postmes, Spears, & Bettache, 2011). Similar processes can be described also in patients' literature.

Moral conviction may also motivate collective action to support universal human rights. Two recent studies showed that the perceived violation of human rights (conceived as moral principles) can motivate activists through their group identity (Mazzoni et al., 2015). Despite its controversial definitions, the right to health is present in many national and international declarations (e.g., Backman et al., 2008). If a detailed review is out of the scopes of the present chapter, what we want to emphasize here is that the right to the highest attainable standard of physical and mental health may represent a strong moral motivator for both patients and supporters who decide to engage in many forms of collective action to defend it.

At this regard, we can refer to the 9th European Patients' Rights Day took place on May 2015, launched by the Active Citizenship Network. That was also the occasion to discuss the European Charter of Patients' Rights to guarantee a "high level of human health protection" (Article 35 of the Charter of Fundamental Rights of the European Union) and to assure the high quality of services provided by the various national health services in Europe.

However, other examples can be found, in which the moral motivation lies behind the manifest behavior, even if it represents an important and strong motivation. Using the metaphor in the classification by Van Zomeren and Spears (2009), "intuitive theologians" are primarily moved by the defense of "sacred" values (like health) then by instrumental motives.

Social Embeddedness

Some sociologists revised previous models of collective action, emphasizing the idea that the decision to take part in protest is not taken insocial isolation (Van Stekelenburg, 2013). On the contrary, individual grievances and feelings are transformed into group-based grievances and feelings within social networks. Networks provide space for the creation and dissemination of a critical discourse toward authorities, and this represents a way for active opposition to authorities to grow (Paxton, 2002). For this reason, being part of a network increases the chances that one will be targeted with a mobilizing message and that people participate (Klandermans & Oegema, 1987).

The literature on new social movements has shown the importance of face-to-face interactions and conflicts in the shaping of a collective reality (Klawiter, 1999; Mueller, 1994). Psychosocial research demonstrated that when people share their opinions within a group, this constitutes a basis for developing new collective identities strictly linked to collective action (e.g. Gee, Khalaf, & McGarty, 2007; Thomas & McGarty, 2009). The underlying idea is that through communication and consensualization people reach agreement upon a shared sense of "we" and, at the same time, crystallize norms for social action (Postmes, Haslam, & Swaab, 2005a).

However, we suggest here that for patients, even if face-to-face interactions are important, web-interactions have a specific value and allows patients to create the necessary network at the basis of mobilization. This is particularly true for patients who experience more difficulties in face to face interactions because of physical impairments. A similar discourse can be true for (but it is not limited to) rare diseases, where a casual meeting is difficult, and for stigmatizing conditions, in which patients show some resistance in showing their condition (e.g., Frohlich & Zmyslinski-Seelig, in press).

There is consensus around the idea that the web 2.0 is deeply changing the health communication paradigm (Laubie & Elie-Dit-Cosaque, 2012). Until the wide adoption of the Internet, health communication was limited to top-down approaches where health professionals and third parties involved were those communicating information to patients. Together with the development of more recent online 2.0 tools, wide connected and bottom-up spaces are opening: patients connect with others by experiencing the same disease, by sharing information about symptoms and treatments and by exchanging ideas about their decision-making processes when coping with the disease (Orizio, Schulz, Gasparotti, Caimi, &

Gelatti, 2010). Many have argued that the web is facilitating the creation of health-related virtual communities (Radin, 2006). For example, online communication allows patients to maintain a continuous link with the community members, and to quickly receive information which is understandable and that can be tailored on their personal needs (van Uden-Kraan et al., 2008). Health communication research conceptualized these communities as online support groups, and showed that patients often use these groups to seek informational and emotional support, and to help other patients (e.g. Braithwaite, Waldron, & Finn, 1999; Shaw, McTavish, Hawkins, Gustafson, & Pingree, 2000; Sullivan, 2003; Turner, Grube, & Meyers, 2001; Weinberg, Schmale, Uken, & Wessel, 1996; Wright, 2002; Mazzoni & Cicognani, 2014). Moreover, online patient groups are often aimed at calling the attention of the public opinion and at mobilising consensus around health-related topics. In this sense, online groups may become a kind of collective action itself as well as a basis of other online/offline forms of collective mobilization.

Psychosocial research on collective action has recently showed that online interaction stimulates collective action (Brunsting & Postmes, 2002; Shah, Cho, Eveland, & Kwak, 2005). Online communication facilitates place- and time-independent interaction making it easier for members of less powerful groups to exchange uncensored and dissenting opinions. Furthermore, some have shown that communicating online within social movements shapes the effect of the psychosocial predictors of collective action (Alberici & Milesi, 2013). For example, discussing online frequently enhances the predicting effect of collective efficacy on willingness to act collectively, probably because activists become aware and believe in the potential of the web as a tool for mobilising social support; this in turn empowers users and stimulates collective action (Postmes, 2007). Some studies have consistently found that participating in online support groups empowers patients as they have the chance to exchange knowledge and share experiences. Unwanted isolation is one of the most significant psychosocial stressors that patients face when they receive the diagnosis of a chronic illness. It has been shown that online support groups can help to reduce these stressors, and can enhance collective empowerment especially because of the presence of other participants who have been through similar experiences (Høybye et al., 2010; van Ulden- Kraan et al., 2008). A qualitative analysis of messages posted in an online support group for breast cancer sufferers, survivors and supporters showed that information-gathering became one of the main strategies to reduce uncertainty and produced feelings of control and hope (Radin, 2006).

Online interactions have also a positive influence on well-being. For example, consistent with work showing the benefits of public action (e.g., Putnam, 2000; Freund & McGuire, 1999; Foster, 2015), tweeting actively about a common discrimination increases well-being and decreases negative affect among participants (Foster, in press). Similarly, a study involving activists of web-based social movements found that the more users interacted online, the less it was likely that group-based anger was a driver to collective action (Alberici & Milesi, 2013). Indeed, while angry messages may go viral on online discussions, it has been shown their real influence on participants' behaviour may be much less than one might expect (Choi, 2014). Certainly, the peculiar way in which patients' share their emotions online (e.g., without non-verbal cues), and the consequent influence on collective behaviour is an underresearched point that deserves to be systematically investigated by future studies.

On the whole, in psychosocial terms, these results show that online interactions can be considered as a communication context where psychosocial drivers to collective action are affected and transformed. This seems especially true for group identity. Grounded in the social identity theory, the Social Identity model of De-individuation Effects (SIDE; Reicher, Spears, & Postmes, 1995; Spears & Lea, 19 94) postulates that that group identity can become especially salient during computer-mediated communication. Empirical findings support the idea that group norms become group-defining in online contexts thanks to the anonymity of CMC (e.g., Spears, Lea, Corneliussen, Postmes, & Ter Haar, 2002). Following this perspective, it has been found that participating in online political discussions affects the way in which activists gradually build the meaning of their group politicized identity (i.e., "who we are" and "what we do"), and this indirectly makes collective action more likely. For example, interacting online in an encouraging and 'safe' context makes participants feel that many others support the same cause; sharing these empowering beliefs makes participants understand what it means to be a group member and this in turn stimulates collective action (Alberici & Milesi, in press). A study conducted among patients participating in an online breast cancer online community revealed that sharing group norms was a driver to collective action. Patients reported that when browsing on the forum, they realized they shared the same vision with other patients. Although they were surrounded by their family, they said they needed to talk to people, to women sharing the same disease (Laubie & Elie-Dit-Cosaque, 2012). This collective self-definition was a psychological determinant of patients' willingness to mobilize around the disease-related issues. Thus, on the one hand perceiving a homogeneity of experiences and sharing a common point of view may strengthen the patients' sense of collective identity and empowerment when coping with the disease. On the other hand, however, interacting online with like-minded others may shift to extreme and polarized positions during discussions. In psychosocial terms, polarization is a function of social identity salience and it has to be understood as the convergence of group members upon a group prototypical position or norm (Turner, 1982; Turner et al., 1987). Groups use polarization to signal their consensual and distinctive position, hence comparing themselves with one or more out-groups. Some studies have shown that during online interactions, people are more likely to polarize their opinions (Lee, 2007; Postmes et al., 2005b). Although the weak-ties nature of most online networks may provide people with diverse and non-redundant views, some evidence suggests that online communication encourages self-segregation into homogenous groups (e.g., Wojcieszak, 2011). Consistently, the Internet is often perceived to be an ideal medium for radicalized groups (Back, 2002; Douglas, 2007) because the support of like-minded others can lead to heightened expression of in-group extremist views (Douglas & McGarty, 2002). As a consequence, online interactions may in some cases favor patients' support of polarized and inflexible points of view, challenging medical views. For example, it was found that exposure to vaccine-critical Websites increases perceptions of the risks of vaccinations and decreases perceptions of their benefits (Betsch, Renkewitz, Betsch, & Ulshöfer, 2010). Some of these alternative movements may have positive effects in the long run, but others may not (see the polarization of the online vaccination debate). However, some have suggested that social media technologies may provide patients with novel opportunities for advocating for particular treatments: for example, the chance to combine efficacious narrative-based content (e.g., personal experience diaries posted online or via You Tube) with scientific and medical knowledge (e.g., posting historical statistics about the impact of a vaccine) represents a promising communication strategy which future research should investigate (Witteman & Zikmund-Fisher, 2012; Mazanderani, O'Neill, & Powell, 2013).

On the whole, the effects of perceived similarity among patients sharing via the web the experience of a same disease/treatment certainly represents a critical point which deserve to be better investigated by future research. Psychosocial studies highlighted that similarity forms the basis for the development of a collective (and politicized) identity on the one hand, but on the other it was found that the more members of a group feel the pressure to group norms and standards, the greater they may support polarized points of view. Adopting a psychosocial perspective would enrich research on patients' engagement, for example, by focusing on how the peculiarities of online interactions among patients (e.g., anonymity, lack on non verbal cues) shape perceptions of similarity, and how this would indirectly influence the meaning they give to their collective/politicized identity.

Another critical point regards the quality of online discussions and their effects on mobilization. Online deliberation may be both positively and negatively related to political engagement (Halpern & Gibbs, 2013). On the one hand, the written and asynchronous character of online interactions may stimulate more reflexive, rational and argumentative conversations (Stromer-Galley & Wichowski, 2010). On the other hand, computer-mediated communication (CMC) has been historically regarded as an impersonal phenomenon that deindividuates participants, encouraging uncivil political discourse (e.g., flaming). A recent study found that when online discussions are perceived as being constructive (e.g., with a high conversational coherence), a sense of moral responsibility to act stimulates collective action. On the contrary, when online discussions are unproductive, intention to act collectively is discouraged (Alberici & Milesi, 2015). By extending this line of research to health-care online communication contexts, the psychosocial perspective could help to understand why the effectiveness of online support groups on collective behavior may often be limited, especially on the long term. Indeed, it seems that online interactions have mobilizing effects for some patients, but not for others who are more hard to mobilize. We claim that, besides investigating the role that patients' individual differences may play in stimulating vs. discouraging online collective action, future studies could focus on individuating the peculiar online deliberative practices that can sustain an enduring patients' collective engagement with online health-related communities.

Discussion

This chapter presented a theoretical and empirical overview of important factors that can influence patients' potentially strong collective action. Among the disciplines who are interested in studying such process, we based on psychosocial literature to draw five most important pathways toward collective action. They include perceived injustice, efficacy, group identity, moral convictions and social embeddedness. Paraphrasing them in simple terms, they provide different possible answers to the question in the title (why do patients protest?): because of a perceived injustice, because they believe that their efforts matter, because they belong to a group they identify with, because they want to defend a threatened moral principle, and because they are embedded in on-line and off-line social networks.

We separately discussed each of these concepts, but obviously, in practice they are all connected. These factors act jointly to propel collective action among patients. As anticipated in the introduction, the last years are sometimes called "age of integration" for collective action literature and many attempts have been done to integrate different factors in more complex models of collective action.

For example, in the famous meta-analysis by Van Zomeren et al. (2008), identity was the key factorthat bridged the injustice and efficacy explanations of collective action. Subsequent attempts tried to integrate in a similar model also moral convictions: in this case, the moral convictions have a special relationship with politicized identities and collective action because of their potentiallystrong normative fit with the action-oriented content of politicized identities (Van Zomeren et al., 2012).

In other models, shared identity was placed before other factors. For example, the model by Van Stekelenburg and Klandermans (2009) combined grievances, efficacy, identity and emotions. This model, that assigns a central and integrating role to processes of identification, suggests that in order to develop the shared grievances and shared emotions a shared identity is needed (Van Stekelenburg & Klandermans, 2009). More recent developments of such model combine important predictors in a model comprising two routes: an efficacy route steered by social embeddedness and a grievances route (Van Stekelenburg, 2013).

Some limitations of these research approaches must be recognized also in terms of the opportunity of deriving practical implication. Indeed, in the attempt to develop general models, they lose part of the explanatory power of concrete and contextualized situations. Patients represent an heterogeneous population that shares some common concrete experiences and needs. For example, we do not sustain that to make the unfairness go away, all we have to do is to change patients' perception of injustice. Collective action models must be necessarily applied with some cautions and considering the specific context and situation.

At this regard, more research is needed to provide more evidence of the underlying process that may guide patients' collective action. We must recognize, for example, that collective action may assume meanings that are not so relevant for other populations. For example, protests may represent a specific stigma-reduction strategy by diminishing negative attitudes about mental illness (Corrigan & Penn, 1999). On the other side, as we showed in this chapter, it is possible that other factors, like group efficacy, may be less important for patients' motivation.

In this chapter, we focused on factors that can have an impact on patients' collective action. However, this relationship is necessarily more complex, and other outcomes then collective action could be considered. For example, it is possible to sustain that collective action processes may have a more or less direct effect also on patients' health and well-being. For example, identifying with a group can impact (positively) upon group members' health, and this can be explained (in part) through the social relations that a shared identity allows (Khan et al., 2014). To this regard, some authors have recently defined shared social identity in terms of a "social cure" showing that the sense of "we-ness" with other group members results in better health and well-being (Jetten, Haslam, & Haslam, 2012). Moreover, in a study by Brashers and colleagues, activists with HIV or AIDS perceived that their collective behaviors impacted also on the physician-patient communication. Differences between activist and nonactivist individuals showed that activists used more problem-focused coping (and less emotion-focused coping), had a greater knowledge of treatment information sources, and had a greater HIV social network integration (Brashers, Haas, Klingle, & Neidig, 2000). All these positive effects of collective action could serve also as soft incentives (Olson, 1965; Opp, 1986) for patients that, in turn, can sustain their future participation.

FUTURE RESEARCH DIRECTIONS

In our chapter, across the five concepts we discussed, we also suggested some critical points which future research on patients' engagement could investigate. A first point regards the importance to include the examination of subjective experience of injustice and its presumed connection to objective deprivation. For example, future research will clarify how objective deprivation is perceived by patients, and which factors discriminate between mobilization from non-mobilization.

A second point regards the study of patients' perceived efficacy. Here we stressed the opportunity to distinguish the efficacy level of analysis (from the individual to the group). Indeed, patients could be motivated by the perception that their participation can have a potential incremental effect on the group effort, rather than to obtain a real change in the status quo.

As regards patients' collective identity, we argue the focus should be more on the processes and barriers through which patients can build and develop a politicized identity. To do this, it would be interesting to investigate how the other motivations interact with patients' collective identity and their intention to act collectively.

For example, future research will examine the specific role played by moral convictions. Indeed, the defense of an important moral principle could represent a strong motivator, also for other people, to overcome group boundaries and to support patients' collective action.

Moreover, the investigation of the role of patients' collective action could be enriched by the analysis of the ways though which patients consensualize and share their experiences through group interaction, both offline and online. As regards online interactions, we suggested that more research is needed to understand how the peculiarities of online interactions (e.g., anonymity) shape patients' motivations to adhere to collective actions. For example, we stressed the importance to better understand the effects of online perceived homogeneity/similarity on attitudes polarization, as well as the deliberation practices that can sustain or discourage collective mobilization.

CONCLUSION

On the whole, we argue that the study of patients' collective action can strongly enrich the existing research on patient engagement, as it helps to develop practices aimed at making patients/clients co-producers of their health, thus enhancing their collective responsibility in both care and prevention (Graffigna et al., 2014). It is already known that, through their engagement, patients gain a positive approach to health management and recapture an active role in the society. We emphasize here that patients have even more chances to influence their health care system if they are prompted to think and act collectively. A recent and notable result in this direction is the news that in May 2010, the Canadian Agency for Drugs and Technologies in Health (CADTH) added patient group input to its Common Drug Review (CDR) process. This initiative helps ensure that health outcomes and issues important to patients are incorporated into the CDR process in a formal and meaningful way.

Finally, we must also recognize that patients' collective action, as defined the beginning of this chapter (see Wright et al., 1990; Van Zomeren & Iyer, 2009) is not a synonymous and it does not necessarily includes all the features of patient engagement as defined in the literature (see Barello, Graffigna, Vegni, & Bosio, 2014). According to some definitions of patient engagement, it usually requires an alliance, a partnership among patients and health care providers. This alliance is useful to obtain better clinical outcomes as it contributes to foster a collaborative approach to the symptoms' cure and supports the development of effective coping strategies for disease management. On the other hand, collective action often represents an expression of dissent. When patients' collective action take place, from patients' point of view, 'something was not going in the right direction' and a social change is desirable. In this case, health care providers may become close allies for the cause or, alternatively, part of the system to challenge.

In this sense, the value of studying patients' collective action is twofold. From one side, it may represent a good example of patients' empowerment, in which they become able to perceive themselves as patients and citizens, and are consequently able to join together to reach a common goal. For example, as we showed in the paragraph about identification, collective action requires an acceptance of the disease that usually characterized the last positions of the engagement process.

From the other side, collective action may sometimes represent an example in which the alliance between patients and health care system manifests some problems. In this case, collective action is a symptom of a break in patients' trust, that should be carefully considered.

Our suggestion is that further research to better understand processes at the basis of patients' collective action is strongly needed. This could give important insights about how to promote a constructive group-based patients' involvement in the healthcare system. At the same time, it would provide instruments to better understand and prevent radicalization of behaviours, in an even more sustainable exchange between healthcare services and demand.

REFERENCES

Alberici, A. I., & Milesi, P. (2013). The influence of the internet on the psychosocial predictors of collective action. *Journal of Community & Applied Social Psychology, 23*(5), 373–388. doi:10.1002/casp.2131

Alberici, A. I., & Milesi, P. (2015, July 7-10). "The right thing to do": discussing online and the moral pathway to collective mobilization. *Paper presented at The 14th European Congress of Psychology*, Milan (Italy).

Alberici, A. I., & Milesi, P. (in press). Online discussion, politicized identity, and collective action. *Group Processes & Intergroup Relations*. doi:10.1177/1368430215581430

Allsop, J., Jones, K., & Baggott, R. (2004). Health consumer groups in the UK: A new social movement? *Sociology of Health & Illness, 26*(6), 737–756. doi:10.1111/j.0141-9889.2004.00416.x PMID:15383039

Back, L. (2002). Aryans reading Adorno: Cyber-culture and twenty-first century racism. *Ethnic and Racial Studies, 25*(4), 628–651. doi:10.1080/01419870220136664

Backman, G., Hunt, P., Khosla, R., Jaramillo-Strouss, C., Fikre, B. M., & Rumble, C. et al. (2008). Health systems and the right to health: An assessment of 194 countries. *Lancet, 372*(9655), 2047–2085. doi:10.1016/S0140-6736(08)61781-X PMID:19097280

Barello, S., Graffigna, G., Vegni, E., & Bosio, A. C. (2014). The challenges of conceptualizing patient engagement in health care: A lexicographic literature review. *Journal of Participatory Medicine, 6*.

Betsch, C., Renkewitz, F., Betsch, T., & Ulshöfer, C. (2010). The influence of vaccine-critical websites on perceiving vaccination risks. *Journal of Health Psychology, 15*(3), 446–455. doi:10.1177/1359105309353647 PMID:20348365

Blackwood, L. M., & Louis, W. R. (2012). If it matters for the group then it matters to me: Collective action outcomes for seasoned activists. *The British Journal of Social Psychology, 51*(1), 72–92. doi:10.1111/j.2044-8309.2010.02001.x PMID:21294752

Braithwaite, D. O., Waldron, V. R., & Finn, J. (1999). Communication of social support in computer-mediated groups for people with disabilities. *Health Communication, 11*(2), 123–151. doi:10.1207/s15327027hc1102_2 PMID:16370973

Brashers, E., Haas, M., Klingle, S., & Neidig, L. (2000). Collective AIDS activism and individuals' perceived self-advocacy in physician-patient communication. *Human Communication Research*, 26(3), 372–402. doi:10.1111/j.1468-2958.2000.tb00762.x

Brown, P., Zavestoski, S., McCormick, S., Mayer, B., Morello-Frosch, R., & Gasior Altman, R. (2004). Embodied health movements: New approaches tosocial movements in health. *Sociology of Health & Illness*, 26(1), 50–80. doi:10.1111/j.1467-9566.2004.00378.x PMID:15027990

Brunsting, S., & Postmes, T. (2002). Social movement participation in the digital age: Predicting offline and online collective action. *Small Group Research*, 33(5), 525–554. doi:10.1177/104649602237169

Charmaz, K. (1991). *Good days, bad days: The self in chronic illness and time*. New Brunswick, NJ: Rutgers University Press.

Choi, S. (2014). Flow, diversity, form, and influence of political talk in social-media-based public forums. *Human Communication Research*, 40(2), 209–237. doi:10.1111/hcre.12023

Corrigan, P. W., & Penn, D. L. (1999). Lessons from social psychology on discrediting psychiatric stigma. *The American Psychologist*, 54(9), 765–776. doi:10.1037/0003-066X.54.9.765 PMID:10510666

Daniels, N. (2000). Accountability for reasonableness. *BMJ (Clinical Research Ed.)*, 321(7272), 1300–1301. doi:10.1136/bmj.321.7272.1300 PMID:11090498

Dickerson, S. S., Posluszny, M., & Kennedy, M. C. (2000). Help seeking in a support group for recipients of implantable cardioverter defibrillators and their support persons. *Heart & Lung*, 29(2), 87–96. doi:10.1067/mhl.2000.104138 PMID:10739484

Douglas, K. M. (2007). Psychology, discrimination and hate groups online. In A. N. Joinson, K. Y. A. McKenna, T. Postmes, & U. D. Reips (Eds.), *The Oxford handbook of Internet psychology* (pp. 155–163). Oxford: Oxford University Press.

Douglas, K. M., & McGarty, C. (2002). Internet identifiability and beyond: A model of the effects of identifiability on communicative behavior. *Group Dynamics*, 6(1), 17–26. doi:10.1037/1089-2699.6.1.17

Edwards, W. (1962). Dynamic decision theory and probabilistic information processings. *Human Factors: The Journal of the Human Factors and Ergonomics Society*, 4(2), 59–74.

Ekman, J., & Amnå, E. (2012). Political participation and civic engagement: Towards a new typology. *Human Affairs*, 22(3), 283–300. doi:10.2478/s13374-012-0024-1

Ellemers, N. (2002). Social identity and relative deprivation. In I. Walker & H. Smith (Eds.), *Relative deprivation: Specification, development and integration* (pp. 239–264). Cambridge, UK: Cambridge University Press.

Folger, R. (1986). A referent cognitions theory of relative deprivation. In J. M. Olson, C. P. Herman, & M. P. Zanna (Eds.), *Relative deprivationand social comparison: The Ontario symposium* (Vol. 4, pp. 217–242). Hillsdale, NJ: Erlbaum.

Folger, R. (1987). Reformulating the conditions of resentment: A referent cognition model. In J. C. Masters & W. P. Smith (Eds.), *Social comparison, social justice, and relative deprivation* (pp. 183–215). London: Erlbaum.

Foster, M. D. (2015). Tweeting about sexism: The well-being benefits of a social media collective action. *The British Journal of Social Psychology*, *54*(4), 629–647. doi:10.1111/bjso.12101 PMID:25639601

Frank, A. W. (1997). Enacting illness stories: When, what, and why. In H. L. Nelson (Ed.), *Stories and their limits: Narrative approach to bioethics* (pp. 31–49). New York: Routledge.

Freund, P., & McGuire, M. (1999). *Health, illness, andthe social body: A critical sociology*. Upper Saddle River, NJ: Prentice Hall.

Frohlich, D. O., & Zmyslinski-Seelig, A. N. (in press). How Uncover Ostomy challenges ostomy stigma, and encourages others to do the same. *New Media & Society*. doi:1461444814541943

Gamson, W. A. (1992). The social psychology of collective action. In A. D. Morris & C. M. Mueller (Eds.), *Frontiers in social movement theory* (pp. 53–76). New Haven, CT: Yale University Press.

Gee, A., Khalaf, A., & McGarty, C. (2007). Using group-based interaction to change stereotypes about people with mental disorders. *Australian Psychologist*, *42*(2), 98–105. doi:10.1080/00050060701280581

Goodin, R. E. (1992). *Motivating political morality*. Oxford: Wiley–Blackwell.

Graffigna, G., Barello, S., Riva, G., & Bosio, A. C. (2014). Patient Engagement: The key to redesign the exchange between the demand and supply for healthcare in the era of active ageing. In G. Riva, P. Ajmone Marsan, & C. Grassi (Eds.), *Active Ageing and Healthy Living* (pp. 85–95). Amsterdam, The Netherlands: IOS Press; doi:10.3233/978-1-61499-425-1-85

Guyatt, G. H., Mulla, S. M., Scott, I. A., Jackevicius, C. A., & You, J. J. (2014). Patient engagement and shared decision-making. *Journal of General Internal Medicine*, *29*(4), 562. doi:10.1007/s11606-013-2727-3 PMID:24464283

Halpern, D., & Gibbs, J. (2013). Social media as a catalyst for online deliberation? Exploring the affordances of Facebook and YouTube for political expression. *Computers in Human Behavior*, *29*(3), 1159–1168. doi:10.1016/j.chb.2012.10.008

Hardin, R. (1971). Collective action as an agreeable "n"-Prisoners' dilemma. *Behavioral Science*, *16*(5), 472–481. doi:10.1002/bs.3830160507

Høybye, M. T., Dalton, S. O., Deltour, I., Bidstrup, P. E., Frederiksen, K., & Johansen, C. (2010). Effect of Internet peer-support groups on psychosocial adjustment to cancer: A randomised study. *British Journal of Cancer*, *102*(9), 1348–1354. doi:10.1038/sj.bjc.6605646 PMID:20424614

Hsieh, E. (2004). Stories in action and the dialogic management of identities: Storytelling in transplant support group meetings. *Research on Language and Social Interaction*, *37*(1), 39–70. doi:10.1207/s15327973rlsi3701_2

Jennings, M. K. (1999). Political responses to pain and loss. *The American Political Science Review*, *93*(1), 1–15. doi:10.2307/2585757

Jetten, J., Haslam, C., & Haslam, S. A. (2012). *The social cure: Identity, health, and well-being*. London, UK: Psychology Press.

Jost, J. T., & Major, B. (2001). *The psychology of legitimacy: Emerging perspectives on ideology, justice, and inter-group relations*. New York: Cambridge University Press.

Kapiriri, L., Norheim, O. F., & Martin, D. K. (2007). Priority setting at the micro-, mesoandmacro-levels in Canada, Norway and Uganda. *Health Policy (Amsterdam)*, *82*(1), 78–94. doi:10.1016/j.healthpol.2006.09.001 PMID:17034898

Khan, S. S., Hopkins, N., Reicher, S., Tewari, S., Srinivasan, N., & Stevenson, C. (2014). Shared identity predicts enhanced health at a mass gathering. *Group Processes & Intergroup Relations*, *18*(4), 504–522. doi:10.1177/1368430214556703

Klandermans, B. (1984). Mobilization and participation: Social-psychological expansions of resource mobilization theory. *American Sociological Review*, *49*(5), 583–600. doi:10.2307/2095417

Klandermans, B. (1997). *The social psychology of protest*. Oxford: Basic Blackwell.

Klandermans, B. (2004). The demand and supply of participation: Social-psychological correlates of participation in social movements. In D. A. Snow, S. A. Soule, & H. Kriesi (Eds.), *The Blackwell Companion to Social Movements* (pp. 360–379). Blackwell Publishing; doi:10.1002/9780470999103.ch16

Klandermans, B., & Oegema, D. (1987). Potentials, networks, motivations, and barriers: Steps toward participationin social movements. *American Sociological Review*, *52*(4), 519–531. doi:10.2307/2095297

Klandermans, B., & Van Stekelenburg, J. (2013). Social movements and participation in collective Action. In D. O. Sears, L. Huddy, & R. Jervis (Eds.), *Oxford handbook of Political psychology* (pp. 774–812). Oxford: University Press; doi:10.1093/oxfordhb/9780199760107.013.0024

Klawiter, M. (1999). Racing for the cure, walking women, andtoxic touring. Mapping cultures of action within the BayArea terrain of breast cancer: Programs and organizationalprocesses. *Social Problems*, *46*(1), 104–126. doi:10.2307/3097164

Kleinman, A. (1988). *The illness narrative: Suffering, healing, and the human condition*. New York: Basic Books.

Kostova, Z., Caiata-Zufferey, M., & Schulz, P. J. (2014). The process of acceptance among rheumatoid arthritis patients in Switzerland: A qualitative study. *Pain Research & Management*, *19*(2), 61–68. doi:10.1155/2014/168472 PMID:24527466

Laubie, R., & Elie-Dit-Cosaque, C. (2012, December 16-19). Exploring and predicting online collective action on patients' virtual communities: a multi-method investigation in France. *Research Paper presented at ICIS12*, Orlando, Florida, USA.

Lee, E. J. (2007). Deindividuation effects on group polarization in computer-mediated communication: The role of group identification, public-self-awareness, and perceived argument quality. *Journal of Communication*, *57*(2), 385–403. doi:10.1111/j.1460-2466.2007.00348.x

Leventhal, G. S. (1980). What should be done with equity theory? Newapproaches to the study of fairness in social relationships. In K. Gergen, M. Greenberg, & R. Willis (Eds.), *Social exchanges: Advances in theoryand research* (pp. 27–55). New York: Plenum. doi:10.1007/978-1-4613-3087-5_2

Lind, E. A., & Tyler, T. R. (1988). *The social psychology of proceduraljustice*. New York: Plenum.

Major, B. (1994). In M. P. Zanna (Ed.), *From social inequality to personal entitlement: The role of social comparisons, legitimacy appraisals, and group membership* (Vol. 26, pp. 293–355). Advances in experimental social psychology San Diego, CA: Academic Press.

Marwell, G., & Oliver, P. (1993). *The critical mass in collective action: A micro-social theory*. Cambridge: Cambridge University Press. doi:10.1017/CBO9780511663765

Mazanderani, F., O'Neill, B., & Powell, J. (2013). "People power" or "pester power"? YouTube as a forum for the generation of evidence and patient advocacy. *Patient Education and Counseling*, *93*(3), 420–425. doi:10.1016/j.pec.2013.06.006 PMID:23830239

Mazzoni, D., & Cicognani, E. (2014). Sharing experiences and social support requests in an Internet forum for patients with Systemic Lupus Erythematosus (SLE). *Journal of Health Psychology*, *19*(5), 689–696. doi:10.1177/1359105313477674 PMID:23479300

Mazzoni, D., Van Zomeren, M., & Cicognani, E. (2015). The motivating role of perceived right violation and efficacy beliefs in identification with the Italian Water Movement. *The Journal of Positive Psychology*, *36*(3), 315–330. doi:10.1111/pops.12101

McCarthy, J. D., & Zald, M. N. (1977). Resource mobilization and social movements: A partial theory. *American Journal of Sociology*, *82*(6), 1212–1241. doi:10.1086/226464

Miller, D. T. (2001). Disrespect and the experience of injustice. *Annual Review of Psychology*, *52*(1), 527–553. doi:10.1146/annurev.psych.52.1.527 PMID:11148316

Mueller, C. (1994). Conflict networks and the origins of women's liberation. In H. Johnston, E. Larana, & J. R. Gusfield (Eds.), *New Social movements. From ideology toidentity* (pp. 234–263). Philadelphia: Temple University Press.

Olson, M. (1965). *The logic of collective action: public goods and the theory of groups*. Cambridge, MA: Harvard University Press.

Opp, K. D. (1986). Soft incentives and collective action. Participation in the Anti-Nuclear Movement. *British Journal of Political Science*, *16*(01), 87–112. doi:10.1017/S0007123400003811

Orizio, G., Schulz, P., Gasparotti, C., Caimi, L., & Gelatti, U. (2010). The world of e-patients: A content analysis of online social networks focusing on diseases. *Telemedicine Journal and e-Health*, *16*(10), 1060–1066. doi:10.1089/tmj.2010.0085 PMID:21070131

Owen-Smith, A., Coast, J., & Donovan, J. (2009). "I can see where they're coming from, but when you're on the end of it ... you just want to get the money and the drug.": Explaining reactions to explicit health-care rationing. *Social Science & Medicine*, *68*(11), 1935–1942. doi:10.1016/j.socscimed.2009.03.024 PMID:19375210

Paxton, P. (2002). Social capital and democracy: An interdependentrelationship. *American Sociological Review*, *67*(2), 254–277. doi:10.2307/3088895

Pettigrew, T. F. (1967). Social evaluation theory. In D. Levine (Ed.), *Nebraska symposium on motivation* (pp. 241–315). Lincoln: Nebraska University Press.

Postmes, T. (2007). The psychological dimensions of collective action, online. In A. N. Joinson, K. Y. McKenna, T. Postmes, & U. D. Reips (Eds.), *The Oxford handbook of Internet psychology* (pp. 165–184). Oxford: Oxford University Press.

Postmes, T., Haslam, S. A., & Swaab, R. I. (2005). Social identity and social influence in small groups: Communication, consensualization and socially shared cognition. *European Review of Social Psychology*, *16*, 1–42. doi:10.1080/10463280440000062

Postmes, T., Spears, R., Lee, A. T., & Novak, R. J. (2005). Individuality and social influence in groups: Inductive and deductive routes to group identity. *Journal of Personality and Social Psychology*, *89*(5), 747–763. doi:10.1037/0022-3514.89.5.747 PMID:16351366

Putnam, R. (2000). *Bowling Alone: The Collapse and Revival of American Community*. New York: Simon and Schuster. doi:10.1145/358916.361990

Rabeharisoa, V. (2006). From representation to mediation: The shaping of collective mobilization on muscular dystrophy in France. *Social Science & Medicine*, *62*(3), 564–576. doi:10.1016/j.socscimed.2005.06.036 PMID:16051407

Rabinow, P. (2002). Artificiality and enlightnment: From sociobiology to biosociality. In M. Biagioli (Ed.), The Science Studies Reader. New York: Routledge.

Radin, P. (2006). "To me, it's my life": Medical communication, trust, and activism in cyberspace. *Social Science & Medicine*, *62*(3), 591–601. doi:10.1016/j.socscimed.2005.06.022 PMID:16039031

Reicher, S. (1984). The St Paul's riot: An explanation ofthe limits of crowd action in terms of a socialidentity model. *European Journal of Social Psychology*, *14*(1), 1–21. doi:10.1002/ejsp.2420140102

Reicher, S., Spears, R., & Postmes, T. (1995). A social identity model of deindividuation phenomena. *European Review of Social Psychology*, *6*(1), 161–198. doi:10.1080/14792779443000049

Runciman, W. G. (1966). *Relative deprivation and social justice: A study of attitudes to social inequality in twentieth-century England*. Berkeley: University of California Press.

Schur, L., Shields, T., & Schriner, K. (2003). Can I make a difference? Efficacy, employment, and disability. *Political Psychology*, *24*(1), 119–149. doi:10.1111/0162-895X.00319

Scotch, R. K. (1988). Disability as the basis of a social movement: Advocacy and the politics of definition. *The Journal of Social Issues*, *44*(1), 159–172. doi:10.1111/j.1540-4560.1988.tb02055.x

Shah, D. V., Cho, J., Eveland, W. P., & Kwak, N. (2005). Information and expression in a digital age: Modeling Internet effects on civic participation. *Communication Research*, *32*(5), 531–565. doi:10.1177/0093650205279209

Shaw, B. R., McTavish, F., Hawkins, R., Gustafson, D. H., & Pingree, S. (2000). Experienceso f women with breast cancer; Exchanging social support over the CHESS computer network. *Journal of Health Communication, 5*(2), 135–159. doi:10.1080/108107300406866 PMID:11010346

Simon, B., & Grabow, O. (2010). The politicization of migrants: Further evidence that politicized collective identity is a dual identity. *Political Psychology, 31*(5), 717–738. doi:10.1111/j.1467-9221.2010.00782.x

Simon, B., & Klandermans, B. (2001). Politicized collective identity: A social psychological analysis. *The American Psychologist, 56*(4), 319–331. doi:10.1037/0003-066X.56.4.319 PMID:11330229

Simon, B., Loewy, M., Stürmer, S., Weber, U., Freytag, P., & Habig, C. et al. (1998). Collective identification and social movement participation. *Journal of Personality and Social Psychology, 74*(3), 646–658. doi:10.1037/0022-3514.74.3.646

Skitka, L. J., Bauman, C. W., & Sargis, E. G. (2005). Moral conviction: Another contributor to attitude strength or something more? *Journal of Personality and Social Psychology, 88*(6), 895–917. doi:10.1037/0022-3514.88.6.895 PMID:15982112

Spears, R., & Lea, M. (1994). Panacea or panopticon? The hidden power of computer-mediated communication. *Communication Research, 21*(4), 427–459. doi:10.1177/009365094021004001

Spears, R., Lea, M., Corneliussen, R. A., Postmes, T., & Ter Haar, W. (2002). Computer mediated communication as a channel for social resistance - The strategic side of SIDE. *Small Group Research, 33*(5), 555–574. doi:10.1177/104649602237170

Stouffer, S. A., Suchman, E. A., DeVinney, L. C., Star, S. A., & Williams Jr, R. M. (1949). Adjustment during army Me. In *Studies in social psychology in World War II* (Vol. 1, pp. 379-387).

Stromer-Galley, J., & Wichowski, A. (2010). Political discussion online. In R. M. Burnett, M. Consalvo, & C. Ess (Eds.), *The handbook of Internet studies* (pp. 168–187). Chichester, UK: John Wiley & Sons.

Stryker, S., Owens, T. J., & White, R. W. (2000). *Self, identity, and social movements* (Vol. 13). Minneapolis: University of Minnesota Press.

Stuart, A., Thomas, E. F., Donaghue, N., & Russell, A. (2013). "We may be pirates, but we are not protesters": Identity in the Sea Shepherd Conservation Society. *Political Psychology, 34*, 753–777. doi:10.1111/pops.12016

Stürmer, S., & Simon, B. (2004). The role of collective identification in social movement participation: A panel study in the context of the German gay movement. *Personality and Social Psychology Bulletin, 30*(3), 263–277. doi:10.1177/0146167203256690 PMID:15030619

Sullivan, C. F. (2003). Gendered cybersupport: A thematic analysis of two online cancersupport groups. *Journal of Health Psychology, 8*(1), 83–104. doi:10.1177/1359105303008001446 PMID:22113903

Tajfel, H., & Turner, J. (1986). The social identity theory of intergroup behaviour. In S. Worchel & W. G. Austin (Eds.), *Psychology of intergroup relations* (pp. 33–47). Chicago: Nelson.

Tetlock, P. E. (2002). Social functionalist frameworks for judgment and choice: Intuitive politicians, theologians, and prosecutors. *Psychological Review*, *109*(3), 451–471. doi:10.1037/0033-295X.109.3.451 PMID:12088240

Thomas, E. F., Mavor, K. I., & McGarty, C. (2012). Social identities facilitate and encapsulate action-relevant constructs: A test of the social identity model of collective action. *Group Processes & Intergroup Relations*, *15*(1), 75–88. doi:10.1177/1368430211413619

Thomas, E. F., & McGarty, C. (2009). The role of efficacy and moral outrage norms in creating the potential for international development activism through group-based interaction. *The British Journal of Social Psychology*, *48*(1), 115–134. doi:10.1348/014466608X313774 PMID:18534045

Thomas, E. F., Smith, L. G. E., McGarty, C., & Postmes, T. (2010). Nice and nasty: The formation of prosocial and hostile social movements. *Revue Internationale de Psychologie Sociale*, *23*(2), 5–43.

Turner, J. C. (1982). Towards a cognitive redefinition of the social group. In H. Tajfel (Ed.), *Social identity and intergroup relations* (pp. 15–40). Cambridge: Cambridge University Press.

Turner, J. C., Hogg, M. A., Oakes, P. J., Reicher, S. D., & Wetherell, M. S. (1987). *Rediscovering the social group: A self-categorization perspective*. Oxford: Basil Blackwell.

Turner, J. W., Grube, J. A., & Meyers, J. (2001). Developing an optimal match within online communities: An exploration of CMC support community and traditional support. *Journal of Communication*, *51*(2), 231–251. doi:10.1111/j.1460-2466.2001.tb02879.x

Tyler, T. R., Boeckmann, R. J., Smith, H. J., & Huo, Y. J. (1997). *Social justice in a diverse society*. Oxford, England: Westview Press.

Van den Bos, K., & Lind, E. A. (2002). In M. P. Zanna (Ed.), *Uncertainty management by means of fairness judgments* (Vol. 34, pp. 1–60). Advances in experimental social psychology San Diego, CA: Academic Press.

Van Stekelenburg, J. (2013). The political psychology of protest: Sacrificing for a cause. *European Psychologist*, *18*(4), 224–234. doi:10.1027/1016-9040/a000156

Van Stekelenburg, J., & Klandermans, B. (2009). Social movement theory: Past, present and prospect. *Movers and shakers: Social movements in Africa*, *8*, 17.

Van Stekelenburg, J., & Klandermans, B. (2013). The social psychology of protest. *Current Sociology Review*, *61*(5-6), 886–905. doi:10.1177/0011392113479314

van Uden-Kraan, C. F., Drossaert, C. H., Taal, E., Shaw, B. R., Seydel, E. R., & van de Laar, M. A. (2008). Empowering processes and outcomes of participation in online support groups for patients with breast cancer, arthritis, or fibromyalgia. *Qualitative Health Research*, *18*(3), 405–417. doi:10.1177/1049732307313429 PMID:18235163

Van Zomeren, M. (2011). Four core social-psychological motivations to undertake collective action. *Social and Personality Psychology Compass*, *7*(6), 378–388. doi:10.1111/spc3.12031

Van Zomeren, M., & Iyer, A. (2009). Introduction to the social and psychological dynamics of collective action. *The Journal of Social Issues, 65*(4), 645–660. doi:10.1111/j.1540-4560.2009.01618.x

Van Zomeren, M., & Lodewijkx, H. F. M. (2005). Motivated responses to 'senseless' violence: Explaining emotional and behavioural responses through person and position identification. *European Journal of Social Psychology, 35*(6), 755–766. doi:10.1002/ejsp.274

Van Zomeren, M., Postmes, T., & Spears, R. (2008). Toward an integrative social identity model of collective action: A quantitative research synthesis of three socio-psychological perspectives. *Psychological Bulletin, 134*(4), 504–535. doi:10.1037/0033-2909.134.4.504 PMID:18605818

Van Zomeren, M., Postmes, T., & Spears, R. (2012). On conviction's collective consequences: Integrating moral conviction with the socialidentity model of collective action. *The British Journal of Social Psychology, 51*(1), 52–71. doi:10.1111/j.2044-8309.2010.02000.x PMID:22435846

Van Zomeren, M., Postmes, T., Spears, R., & Bettache, K. (2011). Can moral convictions motivate the advantaged to challenge social inequality? Extending the social identity model of collective action. *Group Processes & Intergroup Relations, 14*(5), 735–753. doi:10.1177/1368430210395637

Van Zomeren, M., Saguy, T., & Schellhaas, F. M. H. (2013). Believing in "making a difference" to collective efforts: Participative efficacy beliefs as a unique predictor of collective action. *Group Processes & Intergroup Relations, 16*(5), 618–634. doi:10.1177/1368430212467476

Van Zomeren, M., & Spears, A. (2009). Metaphors of protest: A classification of motivations for collective action. *The Journal of Social Issues, 65*(4), 661–680. doi:10.1111/j.1540-4560.2009.01619.x

Van Zomeren, M., Spears, R., Fischer, A. H., & Leach, C. W. (2004). Put your money where your mouth is!: Explaining collective action tendencies through group-based anger and group efficacy. *Journal of Personality and Social Psychology, 87*(5), 649–664. doi:10.1037/0022-3514.87.5.649 PMID:15535777

Walker, I., & Smith, H. J. (2002). *Relative deprivation: Specification, development, and integration.* Cambridge, England: Cambridge University Press.

Weinberg, N., Schmale, J. D., Uken, J., & Wessel, K. (1996). Online help: Cancer patients participate in a computer mediated support group. *Health & Social Work, 21*, 24–29. doi:10.1093/hsw/21.1.24 PMID:8626154

Witteman, H. O., & Zikmund-Fisher, B. J. (2012). The defining characteristics of Web 2.0 and their potential influence in the online vaccination debate. *Vaccine, 30*(25), 3734–3740. doi:10.1016/j.vaccine.2011.12.039 PMID:22178516

Wojcieszak, M. E. (2011). Computer-mediated false consensus: Radical online groups, social networks and news media. *Mass Communication & Society, 14*(4), 527–546. doi:10.1080/15205436.2010.513795

Wright, K. (2002). Social support within an online cancer community: An assessment of emotional support, perceptions of advantages and disadvantages, and motives for usingthe community from a communication perspective. *Journal of Applied Communication, 30*(3), 195–209. doi:10.1080/00909880216586

Wright, S. C., Taylor, D. M., & Moghaddam, F. M. (1990). Responding to membership in a disadvantaged group: From acceptance to collective protest. *Journal of Personality and Social Psychology*, *58*(6), 994–1003. doi:10.1037/0022-3514.58.6.994

Zoller, H. (2005). Health activism: Communication theory and action for social change. *Communication Theory*, *15*(4), 341–364. doi:10.1111/j.1468-2885.2005.tb00339.x

KEY TERMS AND DEFINITIONS

Active Citizenship Network: An umbrella association of about 100 civic organizations from 30 countries aimed towards developing a European Active citizenship.

Collective Action: A specific form of participation where individuals undertake actions as group members, with the aim to improve the group's conditions. It is proposed in contrast to individual action, that is specifically directed at improving one's personal conditions rather than group.

European Charter of Patients' Rights: Drafted in 2002 by Active Citizenship Network in collaboration with 12 citizens' organizations from different EU countries, it states 14 patients' rights that together aim to guarantee a "high level of human health protection" and to assure the high quality of services provided by the various national health services in Europe.

Moral Convictions: Strong and absolute stances on moral issues, they do not tolerate any exceptions to the general 'higher-order' principle.

Participative Efficacy: The belief that individual's participations matters – i.e., that the individual's participation is seen as having a potential incremental effect on collective action.

Self-Efficacy: Individual's belief in his/her ability to execute behaviors necessary to reach goals and to produce specific performance attainments.

Social Psychology: The scientific field that seeks to understand the nature and causes of individual behavior in social situations.

This research was previously published in Promoting Patient Engagement and Participation for Effective Healthcare Reform edited by Guendalina Graffigna, pages 128-150, copyright year 2016 by Medical Information Science Reference (an imprint of IGI Global).

Chapter 61
Confrontation of Human Rights in Daily Clinical Situations

Anna Konieczna
University of Applied Sciences in Nysa, Poland

Przemysław Słomkowski
Ministry Hospital in Bydgoszcz, Poland

ABSTRACT

The chapter concerns human rights as they are enacted in daily clinical situations. It invokes basic documents describing human rights as well as legislative acts dealing more specifically with the rights of doctors and patients. Basing on the theoretical legislative background, the text presents cases of conflict and misunderstanding between various participants of clinical situations. The authors are mainly concerned with the clash of values and beliefs concerning terminal care treatment of ICU patients and with the issue of patient's autonomy and self-determination. The concepts of informed consent and moral distress are explained and visualized with real life examples.

INTRODUCTION

The issue of human rights has been the topic of numerous social discussions and the subject matter of many documents proclaimed in different spheres of life after the Second World War and later. Some of the most recent documents narrow their focus and discuss the concept of human rights with reference to one particular milieu or a specific profession. Following this trend the chapter specifies its focus and talks about the way human rights are being enacted in clinical situations (that is situations involving patients and medical care providers: physicians, nurses or pharmacy staff). The text invokes selected legislative acts describing the rights of the patient and the rights and duties of the medical staff, and presents sample situations in which these particular rights and duties come into conflict. The discussion here presented draws from earlier research studies as well as from two interviews realized on our own and involving physicians as respondents. (The physicians are referred to as dr Y and dr Z later in the text).

At the very start of the chapter it needs to be admitted that sometimes it is difficult to draw a clearly-cut borderline between what constitutes rights, privileges and duties. Moreover, the different rights are

DOI: 10.4018/978-1-5225-3926-1.ch061

not always certain to be ascribed to just one of the parties: the patients or the medical staff. For example, making the decision to withhold terminal care treatment, which is allowed within some legislative systems, may be considered the patient's right or the health care providers' right, depending on the perspective taken (see the discussion later in the chapter). The point is that patients and medical staff are in constant cooperation and interdependence. What is the right of the patient may for example invade in some way the right of a doctor. The interdependencies may be sometimes quite complicated. The patients' rights may in some cases be the source of doctors' moral dilemmas, or may stay in contradiction to particular doctors' beliefs. The approach adopted in this chapter consists in taking the perspective of a third party, not involved with either of the groups being discussed, and not favouring any particular opinions. Ethical issues are often intricate, that is why it might be more beneficial to discuss the complexity of certain problems rather than argue for particular opinions. In fact, if there is a problem involving human rights, it usually concerns not just patients, but also to various extent the medical personnel. That is why this chapter quotes documents applying to both doctors and patients. What also needs to be emphasized is the fact that for obvious reasons the discussion presented here must be limited. That is why only selected clinical problems are described. The text most directly refers to the situations concerning terminal care and to the issues of patient's autonomy.

HUMAN RIGHTS DOCUMENTS

Numerous international acts describe fundamental human rights. Among these acts there can be enumerated, as the most important ones, the Universal Declaration of Human Rights (1948) and the European Convention for the Protection of Human Rights and Fundamental Freedoms (1950), whose text has been amended several times throughout the years. The Universal Declaration of Human Rights enshrined the concept of human dignity. It also provided the background for the developments of universal standards concerning the treatment of human beings based on our common responsibilities as society members. The values recognized by the Universal Declaration of Human Rights are "the inherent dignity" (art. 1) and the "equal and unalienable rights of all members of the human family" (preamble). Basing on the above cited statements concerning human dignity and equality, the concept of patient rights was developed. As subsequent legislative documents proliferated, declarations concerning more specifically the rights and privileges of a patient appeared. An example here could be the European Convention on Bioethics announced in 1997. This and other similar conventions were intended to stand on the side of ethics and protect the rights and the freedoms of people. An important role within this movement was played by World Health Organization (WHO) and World Medical Association (WMA), organizations which have proclaimed numerous important documents dealing with medical health care and patient rights. Among the many documents announced, the one that deserves special attention is the Declaration on the Promotion of Patient Rights in Europe (1994). The document states that patients should be treated with dignity and respect which is owed to all human beings. That also means that they are entitled to be provided with access to medical care and to be offered safe clinical services, that their autonomy and privacy are to be respected, and that confidentiality of information concerning individual patients should be the norm.

As the document states, the development of the complexity of health care systems as well as greater hazardousness of many of the medical treatments result in the fact that medical practice becomes more impersonal and bureaucratic, but at the same time more dehumanized and mechanical. The document emphasizes the fact that enormous progress in the development of technology and medical science puts new and stronger emphasis on the importance and the need of recognizing the human rights of patients. The very basic rights articulated in the declaration concern patient self-determination, independence, integrity, privacy and moral values. With reference to human rights the Declaration on the Promotion of Patients' Rights in Europe (1994) states that:

- Everyone has the right to respect of his or her person as a human being.
- Everyone has the right to self-determination.
- Everyone has the right to physical and mental integrity and to the security of his or her person.
- Everyone has the right to respect for his or her privacy.
- Everyone has the right to have his or her moral and cultural values and religious and philosophical convictions respected.
- Everyone has the right to such protection of health as is afforded by appropriate measures for disease prevention and health care, and to the opportunity to pursue his or her own highest attainable level of health. (p. 9)

Having the right to self-determination means being entitled to get the information concerning one's health condition and the medical procedures to be taken, but also being informed on the potential risk of those procedures and the expected benefits stemming from them. It also refers to the right to agree or refuse medical treatment. The right to physical and mental integrity refers to patient's consent. It means that unless the patient is unable to express consent and urgent treatment is necessary, the medical staff is not allowed to perform any interventions. Similarly, the patient cannot be subdued to medial experiment without his or her consent. Respecting privacy means that all the medical data concerning patient's health condition, diagnosis, prognosis and treatment as well as all other personal information are confidential and to be protected.

As far as information provided to the patient is concerned, the declaration states, among others, that it is the right of the patients to be fully informed about their health condition and about the recommended medical procedures to be taken. The patient needs to be informed about the potential risks and about the likely benefits of each particular procedure suggested, as well as about the alternative forms of treatment. The patient is also entitled to be offered the information about the possible consequences of non-treatment. He or she is to be informed about the diagnosis, about the health prognosis and the procedures to be taken (point 2.2 of the declaration). The only situation when the information may be withheld from the patients is when their physical and psychical condition indicates that it will have no obvious positive effects on them but will rather harm them seriously (point 2.3). The very important right stated in the declaration is the one concerning informed consent for any medical interventions. This consent, as the document says, is to be treated as a prerequisite for any medical procedures. The patient also has the right to refuse treatment. If the patient refuses treatment, the attending physician is obliged to explain in detail all the possible consequences of not taking the medical procedure recommended. In a situation of emergency, when medical intervention needs to be provided urgently, and the patient is unconscious or not able to state his or her will, the consent for treatment is to be assumed and taken for granted, except the situations when the patient had previously in an explicit way stated otherwise (section 3 in the declaration, points 3.1-3.3). The separate sections of the declaration dealing with confidentiality and privacy state that all information concerning patient's health, diagnosis, prognoses, medical procedures taken and planned as well as whatever personal information the medical staff may have about the patient is to be kept confidential, both during the patient's life or after his or her death. The act also states that the patient's privacy is to be protected. That means that any kind of medical interventions should be performed with appropriate respect for the privacy of the patient. Medical treatment may be provided only in the presence of necessary medical or technical staff unless the patient agrees for other people to be present (points 4.1, 4.7) With reference to care and treatment the document states that patients should be treated with respect to their dignity as human beings, regardless of any aspects, racial, individual or others. They should be treated with respect for what are their cultural values and beliefs. Finally, the document also states that "patients have the right to humane terminal care and to die in dignity" (point 5.11). This is an important statement as, surprisingly, in spite of its alleged simplicity, it evokes numerous ethical dilemmas resulting from its possible different interpretations (the issue will be discussed further in the chapter). Yet, what needs to be emphasized now is the fact that all the statements included in the Declaration on the Promotion of Patients' Rights in Europe can be considered embodiments of the ideas first formally and universally proclaimed in the Declaration of Human Rights.

DOCTORS' RIGHTS

The rights of the doctors are being discussed less often, possibly due to the fact that doctors enjoy higher position in the patient-doctor relationship and this higher position is less vulnerable[1]. There are probably no widely known doctors' bills of rights being proclaimed. Doctors' rights are normally specified by the legislative acts valid for particular countries. Still, doctors' performance is also subject to the rules formulated in a general way in the Hippocratic Oath and to the rules included in the Medical Code of Ethics. The rules define the priorities of physicians' professional practice and present the principles concerning physicians' responsibility and behaviour towards the patients, other physicians and towards the community.

The rules of physicians' ethics and deontology that are valid in Europe and many other countries stem form the laws first written by the Greek doctor Hippocrates in the fifth century B.C. The oath is taken by the graduates of Polish medical universities and of many other medical universities in the world. In its original version written by Hippocrates the doctors swore to treat the patients to the best of their ability, to respect the ill people's privacy, and to teach medicine to younger practitioners. Nowadays in many countries modernized versions of the original oath are used. The modern Hippocratic Oath text (Tyson, 2001) varies across its versions and across languages, with some statements, for example, absent in the Polish text but present in the English one. The English text of the oath seems to appeal more to the values of humanism. It emphasizes the need for humanistic approach towards the treatment of a patient, whatever the procedures to be taken are. Passages selected from the oath state the following:

I will remember that there is art to medicine as well as science, and that warmth, sympathy, and understanding may outweigh the surgeon's knife or the chemist's drug.

I will remember that I do not treat a fever chart, a cancerous growth, but a sick human being, whose illness may affect the person's family and economic stability. My responsibility includes these related problems, if I am to care adequately for the sick. - (Tyson, 2001)

These statements show certain respect that supposedly medicine should have for other values reigning social relationships, not only for its own achievements. The statement talking about not treating "a fever chart, a cancerous growth, but a sick human being" is probably most significant here. It emphasizes the need for humanistic approach to all kinds of medical procedures - an approach in which the patient as a human being stays at the centre of the physician's attention, together with all the related problems and all his or her fears, weaknesses and needs. The physician, as the oath says, cannot ignore the problems but needs to treat a human being as a "whole person" (the notion of a whole person is known in psychology and refers to humanistic approaches in education[2]), dealing with whatever issues might appear important to that person. The English version of the oath also alludes to the notion of the commonwealth of society and the physicians obligations towards it, stating the following: "I will remember that I remain a member of society, with special obligations to all my fellow human beings, those sound of mind and body as well as the infirm" (Tyson, 2001). The commonwealth is emphasized by the statement that a physician is one of the whole structure (of society) and that other members are his or her fellow human beings. Finally, the English version of the Hippocratic Oath includes a statement saying that the physician will be willing to sincerely admit his of her lack of knowledge on a specific issue and ask other professionals for help if needed: "I will not be ashamed to say «I know not», nor will I fail to call in my colleagues when the skills of another are needed for a patient's recovery" (Tyson, 2001). The humanistic approach to the profession of a physician as envisaged in this statement consists in the readiness to accept one's limitations and putting the patient's welfare beyond personal pride.

Medical Code of Ethics (KEL[3]) proclaimed in Poland (whose counterparts also exist in some other countries) defines the priorities of physicians' professional practice and presents the principles concerning physicians responsibility and behaviour towards patients, other physicians and towards the community. Medical Code of Ethics obliges the physician to respect human rights. It states that the highest ethical law is the welfare of the patient, according to the statement "salus aegroti suprema lex esto". Whatever the social, administrative or economical circumstances surrounding the doctor are, he or she is obliged to follow this law (KEL, art. 2).

Other paragraphs concerning the rights of the doctor state for example that unless the case is urgent, the physician has the right not to undertake the treatment of a patient or to withhold his or her treatment for reasons which can be justified with serious arguments. Still, in such situation the duty of the physician is to provide the patient with the information concerning other possibilities of medical treatment (KEL, art. 7). If the patient offends doctor's dignity or does not obey his or her orders, the doctor has the right to refuse or stop treatment. The only exception to this rule is the situation when the patient needs urgent help (KEL, art. 17). In case of refusal the doctor should indicate to the patient another possibility of medical help. Some of the paragraphs of the Medical Code of Ethics mirror the statements formulated in different patients' bills of rights. And so KEL mentions the physician's duty to provide the patient with all the information concerning the details of his or her treatment (this includes the risks and benefits of the procedures suggested, the alternatives for the treatment and the risks of not undergoing the treatment). It also reminds that the information given to the patient needs to be formulated in a way which is comprehensible to that particular person (KEL, art. 13). Medical Code of Ethics also includes the "respecting the rights of patients" section, where the statements cited before with reference to Declaration on the Promotion of Patient Rights in Europe reappear.

With reference to terminal treatment, which will be discussed in greater detail in the following parts of the chapter, KEL states that "the physician is forbidden to use euthanasia or to help the patient commit a suicide" (art. 31). At the same time, it says that in terminal states there is no obligation for the physician to provide resuscitation or futile treatment or to use extraordinary means to prolong the patient's life (art. 32). In Poland it is obligatory to respect the Medical Code of Ethics. Failing to comply with the code means not respecting the standards of professional conduct, which can be sued to the court.

The rights discussed so far, referring to both patients and medical staff, will form the basis for the discussion of the issues presented in the ongoing parts of the chapter. As it appears, many of the ethical dilemmas surrounding clinical situations that are discussed further in the chapter stem from the difficulty of applying the nicely described humanistic theory to everyday reality and practice.

Further Exploration of Rights and Duties: More About Informed Consent

Informed consent should be based on most appropriate information provided to the patient. The information should include the rationale for particular treatment. It should also explain what are the risks and possible side effects, what are the possibilities of alternative procedures and the consequences of refusing treatment. Informed consent is normally the prerequisite for any medical intervention. Many of the judicial cases described by Nesterowicz (2013) deal with the situations of violating the patient right 'to know and decide'.

Polish legislative acts allow the physician to act without the consent of the patient only in two cases. The first situation takes place when the treatment is absolutely necessary but due to patient's condition the consent cannot be obtained. The other situation takes place when getting a consent is possible but could cause a delay dangerous for the patient. One other extraordinary situation allowing the physician to act even if contradicting the earlier expressed wishes of the patient takes place when the patient faces the risk of death. Yet, "except from life threatening cases, the physician has no obligation to act against the consciously expressed will of the patient" (Nesterowicz, 2013, p.166).

As far as the patient's consent is concerned, some situations are quite controversial. Performing tests for diagnosing HIV infection could be an example here. In the USA and many other countries it is forbidden to perform the test without the patient's consent. Patient's autonomy and privacy in this respect are protected by the law. The patient must be informed of the fact that the test is not obligatory and that he or she can submit the consent any time. The patient also needs to be informed about the purposes of doing the test (Nesterowicz, 2013). If hospitals or other health care institutions break these rules, they are often sued to the court as patients demand to be paid punitive damages for the harm caused to their health, for distress and humiliation (Nesterowicz, 2013). In Poland it is legally allowed to perform the HIV test without the patient's consent (Nesterowicz, 2013). These judicial differences enshrine the quite differing conceptions of what constitutes patient's autonomy for a particular country.

Another controversial issue concerns the witnesses of Jehovah, who give their consent for operations but not for blood transfusions. And so for example in England a physician who had given blood transfusion to a Jehovah's Witness in a life-threatening situation was declared guilty, as there was no consent for the procedure (Nesterowicz, 2013). A similar case took place in France where a Jehovah's Witness sued the hospital and demanded to be paid compensation for moral damages that she suffered as a result of blood transfusion done against her will during an operation. The court admitted the patient's rights to integrity but stated at the same time that the physician rescuing patient's life cannot be considered guilty. The court declared saving human life as a value superior to individual patient's wishes and thus set limits to individual freedom and autonomy (Nesterowicz, 2013). In Poland the issue is also controversial. The case described by Nesterowicz (2013) concerns a Jehovah's Witness who had a car accident. The woman had a note stating that she refuses blood transfusion, whatever the circumstances are. The case was taken to the district court who gave consent for blood transfusion for the sake of rescuing the patient's life. Yet, the Supreme Court stated differently and declared that the patient's will, when expressed clearly and without ambiguities, is legally binding. This statement emphasized the priority of patient's autonomy and their right to self-determination (Nesterowicz, 2013). These differing interpretations concerning the same or similar situations present not only the clash of values and beliefs but also the difficulty of finding an ethically acceptable solution to these problems. Nesterowicz (2013) states that Jehovah's Witnesses should be taken to a hospital where alternative methods of treatment are used, without the use of blood. Otherwise the physicians may be faced with the moral dilemma of whether to follow the patient's will and let the person die, or whether to stand on the side of life and against the will of the patient (Nesterowicz, 2013).

Information and Truth

The rule says that the patient has the right to "truth", even though the range of information given to the patient may vary according to his or her level of intelligence, psychic condition and sensitivity (Nesterowicz, 2013). There are situations in which the physician does not need to provide the patient with information. This may happen: a) when the patient is not conscious or for some other reason not able to understand the information, and the treatment is necessary, and b) when providing the information would be medically harmful for the patient (Nesterowicz, 2013). That is why in certain situations, when the prognosis is poor, the physician may decide to limit the information given to a patient (Nesterowicz, 2013). Telling the whole truth about a poor prognosis might not be a good strategy, as the patient may get depressed or even refuse further treatment. Thus physicians are faced with one more dilemma as have to decide how extensive and how explicit the information given to patients should be.

Some clinical cases concern "excessive information" given to the patient. In Germany a physician was declared guilty when he openly informed his patient of a growing brain tumour, stating at the same time that it might be malicious and not operable. The patient reacted with a violent shock whose consequences were heart disease, partial paralysis and speaking difficulties. The court stated that even though the physician had the right to inform the patient about the diagnosis, he still broke the law. According to the court statement, it is the physician's duty to find balance between the patient's right to know and the danger the information might pose to the patient (Nesterowicz, 2013). The right to limit the information (or sometimes an obligation to do it – as could be seen in the last of the examples quoted) is called "the therapeutic privilege" (or "a humanitarian lie", see Zajdel, 2008, p. 367). As this privilege is very controversial, the law of some countries does not allow for its use. It is also forbidden to use the 'privilege' when it is the patient or the proxy who openly demand to be told all the truth. When discussing the issue of informed consent, one should also point to what can be called "informed refusal". This means that even though the patient may refuse treatment, he or she needs to be informed about the consequences of doing so.

Informed Consent of Intensive Care Unit Patients

Jeffery, Lanken, & Taichman (2004) summarize what the elements of informed consent in an intensive care unit are[4]. These elements can be described as: data referring to patient's diagnosis, information concerning the proposed treatment and its alternatives, together with the likely benefits and dangers of those particular procedures and information about the consequences of refusing medical treatment. What is also taken into account is whether the patient is free of coercion.

The requirements of informed consent are quite extensive and in the majority of cases rather impossible to be applied to patients at the moment of admitting them to intensive care units. The patients admitted are most often unconscious or in very poor condition. As the cases are often acute, urgent treatment is needed. And so in such cases the consent for medical intervention is presumed. The rule for such situations is "to err on the side of life" (Jeffery, Lanken, & Taichman, 2004, p. 5) and provide the patient with the necessary treatment as quickly as possible. However, as Jeffery, Lanken, & Taichman (2004) report, in the state Philadelphia the physician is obliged to withdraw the treatment if later the patient or the surrogate decides against it. This means that the patient's autonomy and self-determination, even in those most acute and life-threatening cases, are prioritized and must be respected.

In Poland the requirements for ICU informed consents look quite differently. First of all, there is no institution of a proxy for the patient that would have the right to make medical decisions. If the patient is adult, none of the members of his or her family are entitled to decide about the treatment. Of course the overwhelming majority of the patients admitted to ICU are unconscious and so in their case the consent is assumed and legalized by the court. Yet, even if the patient stays conscious and is able to communicate logically, his or her words cannot be per se considered as valid. They require to be formally validated in the presence of lawyers. The cases reported by Doctor Z that can be quoted here are two quite similar histories of young male patients admitted to ICU as they suffered from the injury of neck backbone and were paralyzed from neck to waist. The patients were fully communicative and psychically able to make decisions but physically unable sign documents. They talked being connected to respirators but their messages were clear to the medical staff. Still, as they could not sign the document stating their will, a notary needed to be called. The formal procedure for such cases includes the notary visiting the hospital with the presence of two other lawyers acting as witnesses. Having talked to the patient, the notary prepares a document stating the patient's will and all three of them confirm what has been stated by the patient by putting their signatures. The whole procedure is quite troublesome and sometimes difficult to arrange. It may exemplify the formality of Polish procedures. The regulations and examples quoted above show very clear differences in what are considered patient's rights to autonomy and self-determination in different legislative systems. These differences concern not only legislative measures but also the social perception of what the rights to autonomy and self-determination imply. The differences in the enactments of these rights may be the source of misunderstandings and discussions. What clearly is the matter of discussion here is the range of individual patient rights and the extent to which those rights can be limited.

TERMINAL CARE ETHICAL DILEMMAS

Intensive care units (ICUs) are the place where human rights are being challenged to the extremes. The challenge consists in the many ethical dilemmas that all the people involved in the life of an ICU are made to confront. First of all, the patients admitted to ICU are defined as critically ill. Most of them are on respirators. Those who are admitted to the unit are typically in the sickest and most acute phases of illnesses. Many of the patients die soon after being admitted to ICU. Of course, due to the advances of medical technology and pharmacologic therapies it is often possible to extend life. The advancement of modern technology makes it possible for more and more patients to survive the critical phase. This does not solve the ethical problems, though. Quite surprisingly, in some situations the use of the newest technology can be considered as a mixed blessing. It prolongs biological existence but at the same time fosters the appearance of even more ethical and moral dilemmas. Thus the health providers become responsible for making more ethical and medical decisions. Kälvemark and colleagues (2004) confirm this statement saying that the newest development in technology, and consequent changes in medicine "have made health care more complex and [thus] ethics has increasingly become a required component of clinical practice" (p.1).

The recurring dilemmas appearing in ICUs concern: a) patients lingering on (futile treatment), b) transferring patients too soon, c) limiting the age of patients undergoing certain surgical operations, and d) shortages of technical resources as well as of professionally trained staff resources (Bunch, 2000). The author calls the atmosphere of an ICU as "hidden drama" (Bunch, 2000, p. 2), and the notion concerns not just the medical state of the patients. The drama, as she states, is also "hidden in a context full of difficult interacting and ethical problems. The actors in this hidden drama [...] face ethical issues surrounding end of life and ambiguous clinical data on which [they base their] decisions on what the ethically right action is in a specific situation" Bunch (2000, p. 40). The drama concerns, first of all the problem of limited resources of both the nursery staff and equipment.

Access to Limited Resources

ICUs are said to be specially equipped and specially staffed departments of hospitals, but of course, resources are never infinite. The development of advanced medical technology has made critical care treatment more effective but also more expensive. Another problem is that technological advancement is accompanied by raising social expectations. Nowadays medicine offers more, but patients also expect more. That is why many of the ICU physicians are made to be the "gate-keepers" responsible for the inflow of patients. Of course, there are regulations dealing with that inflow, but these are not always very clear when applied in practice. Skowronski (2001) quotes the American Thoracic Society statement of fair allocation of resources in ICUs. The statement includes among others the following points:

- Access to ICU care requires that patients have sufficient medical need.
- ICU care should provide the patient a certain degree of potential benefit. On grounds of insufficient benefit to the patient, those who are permanently unconscious or who suffer form severe irreversible lack of cognitive function should generally be excluded from intensive care.
- Whenever feasible, patients should give their informed consent for initiation and continuation on ICU care. (p. 481)

The author admits at the same time that applying these rules to particular patients is not always an easy task. It is sometimes difficult, as he says, to estimate the benefit and it is highly subjective to talk about the quality of life. There appear many ethical questions, too. Looking at the rules regulating ICU admission, Skowronski (2001) asks the question whether patients qualifying to the unit but representing low predicted mortalities should be admitted (as they are more likely to survive and get benefit from the treatment) or refused due to the fact that they possibly could manage in a general care ward. Other, more thorny dilemmas, concern terminal care treatment and situations when the benefits are not very clear.

Medical Futility

The concept of "medical futility" implies not being able to offer effective treatment, not being able to achieve the goals of treatment and a very low likelihood of recovery (Chow, 2014).

The concept was also described as "using considerable resources without a reasonable hope for recovery" (Sibbald et al., cited in Chow, 2014, p. 259). The issue of providing futile treatment is often an ethical dilemma. In 1985 Weinberg asked: "are we carrying out expensive and ceremonial treatments which we know are futile because we lack the courage to make realistic therapeutic decisions?" (p. 141). It seems the question still remains valid. Futile care is often being provided due to the pressure of patient's family or because there is no consensus between those who are responsible for medical decisions (Chow, 2014). The family even realizing the futility of the treatment will often insist to continue with it. An example here could be the situation reported by Chow (2014) in which a husband rejecting the argumentation presented to him insists on futile therapy and declares to be "still hoping for a miracle" (p. 258). It must be admitted that lingering on ICU patients whose clinical prognosis remains unclear pose a problem to both medical staff and their families. As it appears, there is no unique and universally valid solution to the problem of futile treatment, as whatever the arguments are, they can always be discussed and questioned. Skowronski's evaluation of terminal care treatment seems practically minded, but also, if you go into its meaning, possibly cruel. He states that "the limitations for terminal care treatment should not only depend on what is medically possible, but also on what is socially, ethically and economically appropriate" (2001, p. 483).

Dying in Dignity

As has been stated before, the perceptions of what are the limits for medicine have changed over the years. Modern sophisticated medical therapies have made it possible for many critically ill patients to recover, but even the highly advanced technology has its limits. And the use of this sophisticated technology also has its consequences. Thus the question may arise whether the prolonging of life on ICU should not be considered rather as the prolonging of the dying process. If it is the prolonging of the dying process, then those interested (patients and families) may not really consider the therapies as beneficial. It seems then that the development of technology has created new possibilities which in fact can be considered as both: benefit and harm to critically ill patients (Bresnahan, 1990). At the same time "discussions about withholding or withdrawing care in the ICU can be the source of miscommunication, misunderstanding, and even conflict" (Jeffery, Lanken, & Taichman, 2004, p. 2). Quite clear, the participants in medical decision making may be guided by differing beliefs concerning moral values. It may also happen that the same shared values are prioritized differently by the people. And so for example one person may believe in the prolongation of life (biologic existence) as a primary value, and the other may believe that relief in suffering is crucial (Bresnahan, 1990). These two values tend to stay in tension with one another. It is also possible for people to agree on values and their ranking in theory but differ in the practical implication of their beliefs. The opposite situation is also possible, namely that people do not agree theoretically but come to the same practical conclusions (Bresnahan, 1990).

Yet, whatever the opinions are, it should be admitted that the usage of sophisticated life sustaining technology for clearly futile cases can endanger the patients' humanity. Bresnahan visually describes a situation when technology and patient's right to autonomy and self-determination come into play:

We encounter limit situations. Where patient cry out, "too much," we have to pause. Where "medical futility" in some sense becomes evident to one or another decision maker, we must take time to speak together of what we really intend and how we can achieve it. (Bresnahan, 1990, p. 414)

Nurses About Not Allowing to Die

Nurses are caregivers, staying at the bedside and accompanying the patients in their daily existence, and so they often develop a kind of emotional attachment towards patients and their families. That is possibly why they are more likely to notice the human aspects of the clinical situations they experience. One of the nurses interviewed by Kälvemark and colleagues (2004) openly stated the fact that intensive care technology may dehumanize patients, especially the older ones, in situations when it clearly deprives them of their 'right' to die a natural death. Still, on the other hand, it seems that nurses are more likely to 'give everybody a chance'. Nurses interviewed in Bunch's research (2000) said they never gave up hope for patient's recovery. They were unwilling to discuss the withholding of intensive care treatment saying "who am I to determine what quality of life means" (p. 39). This nursing ideology of hope and support permeated the ICU unit described by Bunch (2000), though, as the author suggests, this ideology was not necessarily shared by physicians.

Sample ICU Cases

The following part of the chapter reports sample ICU cases where the values, beliefs and wishes of various parties involved in the treatment came into conflict. These reports may help to visualise the many ethical challenges posed to ICU staff and to patients' families. All the cases will be cited after Bresnahan (1990).

The first case concerns a patient (Mr B), aged 85, suffering from pneumonia and of a fragile overall condition. The patient was transferred to ICU and proposed to be intubated while the treatment with the use of antibiotics continued. The patient was conscious, thus all the details concerning the treatment on ICU and possible dangers were discussed with him. Mr B. was warned of the risk of having to stay under ventilation and not being able to return to independent function. The degree of medical and technological help was agreed with the patient before intubation and the possible consequences were discussed. The patient agreed to undergo the treatment and gave his informed consent but also set limits to the treatment by demanding to put the 'do not resuscitate' (DNR) order on his bed. The order forbids cardiac resuscitation beyond the use of pressors. The procedure discussed with the patient was applied but after the treatment it resulted that Mr B required chronic ventilatory support. The patient was conscious and was informed about the problems. He was transferred from ICU to another unit where the use of ventilator was possible. Yet, after 10 days the patient communicated to the medical staff of the unit that he demanded to be taken out of the ventilator. He also clearly communicated he recognized the fact that this would result in his dying. He wrote "this is too much to bear" (p. 416). Still, when the medical staff brought this message to the long-standing physician of Mr B, the doctor reacted with surprise as such course of action had not been agreed. The doctor refused to comply with this request. And so the patient spent one other month under a ventilator. He kept requiring to be removed from it. The care givers of Mr B again passed the message to the doctor. Both the care givers and the physician realized that the patient was not "abnormally depressed" and he had the right to change the earlier expressed consent. Still, the values to which the doctor adhered quite visibly came into conflict with the patient's rights. Bresnahan (1990) describes the dilemma as follows:

Although the doctor could not deny the reasonableness of this competent patient's request, it appeared that he had great personal difficulty in accepting discontinuing aggressive treatment once begun – although he might, perhaps, have been ready to more readily accept a decision not to begin it. (p. 417)

Finally, Mr B's case is resolved with the help of a committee panel, to whom the patient communicates his will. Mr B is taken off the ventilator and dies 48 hours later. The problem here described visualises the clash of values and beliefs, and the difficulty to accept the arguments of "the other side". In the described case the moral and ethical values of the doctor make him break the rules of "informed consent" (which can be always withdrawn). The doctor is unwilling to take part in what he possibly envisages as "passive euthanasia", meaning that he passively (by not intervening) allows the patient to die. On the other hand, the arguments of the patient also seem reasonable. The patient considers the treatment as excessively burdensome and futile. Bresnahan (1990) suggests that if the doctor's moral conviction come into conflict with what the patient demands, then the physician should resign care to another physician who would be more likely to accept the patient's position. In this particular case doctor X believes that biological existence must be prolonged with the use of all the possible means of modern technology and that the intensive care treatment once begun cannot be stopped. The patient clearly objects to that. The conflict seems unresolvable. It is finally taken to a medical committee panel who confirms the patient's rights - quite controversial ones, as they are the rights to die. Yet, it should be added that the case took place in the USA, where medical decisions like the one described above are protected by the courts from being punished. Such decisions have also been declared as morally acceptable by the American Medical Association (Bresnahan, 1990).

The second case reported by Bresnahan concerns a case of an ICU patient – Mr F – who had not stated himself his will concerning the intubation and ICU treatment. Yet, the family of the patient claimed he had talked about his preferences to them and he had always objected to life sustaining therapies. When the medical staff stated it was impossible for Mr F to awake again to consciousness, and that the patient might continue in that state for about a month if given aggressive support, the family requested that Mr B be extubated. In this particular case the doctor again was not willing to take the step, "although he wished he had not permitted Mr F to be intubated in the first place" (p. 420). After a few days the patient suffered a cardiac arrest and died, so the conflict concerning life-sustaining therapy used for this particular case as if 'got resolved by itself'. Still, the moral and ethical dilemma concerning clinical situations similar to the one described here remained.

The two cases quoted point to an interesting ethical issue, namely to the fact that it seems easier for some physicians not to start intensive care treatment than to withhold the treatment once begun. Once they get involved in the treatment, they are unwilling to interrupt it, even if the case appears futile. In his conclusion summarizing the two cases, Bresnahan (1990) argues for the patient's right to medical treatment, but also for the right to refuse it (as long as there is no clear evidence of suicidal attempts). The author also supports patient's right to decide about the extent of end-of-life medical treatment (Bresnahan, 1990).

More on Patient Autonomy

The respect for the patient's autonomy means that the patient has the right to refuse medical interventions, including life-sustaining interventions (Jeffery, Lanken, & Taichman, 2004). In the jurisdiction of the USA it is accepted that it is the patient's decision to undergo an intervention or a treatment or to refuse it, even if the refusal will result in a certain death. And so a patient may for example refuse to be given blood-transfusion due to the fact that it is not in accordance with his or her religious beliefs and the health providers need to respect this decision (Nesterowicz, 2013). The US courts evoke here various legislative measures, among others the right to privacy, the right to die, the right to control one's body and the right to profess a particular religion. Patients, as Jeffery, Lanken, & Taichman (2004) state, are allowed to act according to their personal values, evaluate the quality of their life during and after the treatment, compare the prognosis to their life expectations and their living standards and finally, refuse treatment even if the refusal may bring about the likely death. Of course, the refusal needs to be expressed clearly in a written or spoken form and cannot be ambiguous. Then the doctor should respect the patient's right to refuse the therapy (Jeffery, Lanken, & Taichman, 2004).

What is fundamental to the concept of patient's autonomy, as Jeffery, Lanken, & Taichman (2004) notice, is the patient's capacity to undertake medical decisions. This decision-making capacity is determined by well-established clinical standards. The standards require that the patient be in a condition that makes it possible to him or her to understand the information concerning the diagnosis, prognosis and treatment alternatives, as well as the consequences of refusing medical intervention. Jeffery, Lanken, & Taichman (2004) pay attention to the fact the patient's decision-making capacity can be crippled by the use of medicines, stress, sleep deprivation, anxiety and so on. As a result the patient may be confused and disorientated and not really in the condition to make decisions. It is the responsibility of the ICU staff to assess the patient's decision-making capacity before they start discussing with him or her important treatment issues. Possibly, intensive care patients will be able to make some decisions but not others, depending on the gravity and complexity of the issues to be discussed. The estimation of patient's decision making capacity should also be based on patient's history, and on the opinion of other care professionals and members of patient's family. If there is still some doubt or ambiguity, a psychiatrist should be called for consultation (Jeffery, Lanken, & Taichman, 2004). According to schemas provided by Jeffery, Lanken, & Taichman (2004), the criteria for adequate decision-making capacity include: "a) ability to comprehend information relevant to the decision, b) ability to compare alternatives of the decision with personal values and goals, and c) ability to communicate in a consistent and meaningful manner" (p. 3). The right to autonomy and self-determination does not apply to cases where suicidal attempts take place and to patients who are mentally incompetent. In situations involving these two groups of people it is the court who makes medical decisions and provides consent for medical treatment (Nesterowicz, 2013).

Compulsory Treatment

Louis Kornprobst, a French expert in medical law, said that no one is obliged to cure if he or she prefers to suffer, die or if he or she does not trust medicine (cited in Nesterowicz, 2013). Yet, in some cases this statement, calling for patient's full autonomy and self-determination, appears not valid. And so for example if due to somebody's illness public health is endangered, the individual patient's rights need to be subdued to the rationale concerning the welfare of the society. Compulsory treatment of particular patients or whole groups of people is meant to protect public health. And so in Poland it applies to drug-addicts, alcoholics, and people diagnosed with *venereal diseases. Protective vaccination against certain diseases is also obligatory.*

When Family or Surrogates Can Decide

Chow writes that in some states of the USA it is enough for two attending physicians to agree that the case is "medically futile" to make decisions concerning the withholding of terminal treatment. In other states, agreement of the family is required, which makes the case much more complicated, and sometimes even frustrating for the medical staff as individual members of the patient's family often "dictate care without any previous health care knowledge" (Chow, 2014, p. 259). Thus, if the burden of making the ending-of-life decision is left to the family the situation becomes even more difficult. Cultural and religious beliefs as well as limited knowledge on critical care very often prompt people to insist on futile care in spite of the contradicting medical advice. Sometimes family members agree to place the "do not resuscitate" order on the bed of the patient. Still, there are a lot of emotional aspects that play a role here. Quite often family members admit they still have the hope for the patient's recovery, even if the situation is critical. That is why they often reject the argumentation presented by physicians. Sometimes the lack of consensus within one family is also a problem. Bresnahan (1990) relates the history of a patient – Mr H - whose family all agreed on the decision to be taken except one person – a son, who had always lived away from house but who had suddenly appeared after the father's death. The son tried to counteract the decisions of other family members and he succeeded in doing so, as due to his objection, no steps concerning the withdrawal of life-sustaining therapy could not be taken. The case was quite complicated due to the conflicts within the family of the patient. It also clearly showed that when the family is legally allowed to make decisions, all problems become even more burdensome as the physicians, willing or not, become involved in what normally would be considered private issues. And of course, waiting for the family's decision, physicians cannot act according to what they consider medically appropriate. Mr H finally died, still being joined to a ventilator. Here again, even though the particular case was 'resolved' with the patient's death, the problem concerning decision-making procedure in similar cases remained. Bresnahan suggests problems of that kind should be consulted with psychologists and ethics.

Most of the patients in intensive care units do not have the capacity to make decisions concerning their treatment. In such situations the American law allows for the surrogates to decide, sustaining in this way the autonomy of the patient. Surrogates can be designated in different ways, though it is best if the patient does it for himself or herself in advance. This can be done in the form of signing a living will, which is a document stating in advance what the person's preferences for medial care are (Jeffery, Lanken, & Taichman, 2004). Of course, intensive care units patients very often do not formally designate a surrogate before losing capacity. Thus many American states have promulgated regulations which establish a legal hierarchy of order for the selection of surrogates. The hierarchy will normally mention the spouse as the first, and further on the list parents, an adult child, and later possibly other more distant family members (Jeffery, Lanken, & Taichman, 2004). In some states of the USA the wishes of surrogates are legally considered as having the same value as the wishes of the patient. Within the legislative act of the British Commonwealth, the problem of surrogate decision making is not explicitly stated, thus the important decisions concerning the ICU patients' medical care are solved in the court, who is supposed to take into account the best interests of the patient. In Poland, as was stated earlier, there is no legislative act allowing for the use of surrogates, thus all the important decisions concerning medical treatment of adult patients whose conditions do not allow them to decide for themselves need to be taken to the court.

DNR ORDER, FUTILE TREATMENT, AND OTHER ICU DILEMMAS IN POLAND

In Poland the patient's right to autonomy seems to be more limited, especially if it concerns end-of-life decisions. As has been stated earlier, the decisions of ICU patients are hardly ever considered to be valid per se and their validation most often requires the presence of lawyers (that is sending the case to the court or calling notaries to the hospital). Obtaining a valid informed consent, as one of the interviewed physicians said, is quite impossible in an ICU due to patients' condition and the characteristics of the place. "We assume that a patient being treated at ICU is not able to make objective medical decisions and has no decision making capacity", states doctor Y. This happens, as he explains, due to the mere fact that staying at ICU is very stressful for the patient. In this unit the lights are always on, something is happening all the time, there is continuous knocking, hissing, there is no silence at night, but continuous movement all the time. The patients stay in the same room, and so even though there are curtains separating particular beds, the patients still may hear and notice what is happening. They can hear and see when somebody dying. Moreover, ICU patients are often under the influence of medicines and that may also influence their decision making capacity. Staying at ICUs is also likely to produce depression. Patients there undergo regular medical interventions. So even if they are conscious, they are normally given sedatives. That is why doctors in Poland seem to believe that ICU patients are rather not likely to able to make medical care decisions. Even if they make decisions, these probably would not be considered valid as ICU patients are mostly under the influence of sedatives. That is why ICU patients are often considered not to have full legal decision-making capacity. This argumentation, confirmed by one of the physician interviewed, shows that patient's autonomy in an ICU is often assumed to be restricted.

Quite unlike the situations described earlier with reference to ICUs in the USA, in Poland there is no possibility for the patient to decide about not being reanimated. The patient has no right to make such a decision. Neither before the treatment nor during the treatment can he or she decide that. Similarly, there is no option allowing the patient to decide about applying only certain resuscitating procedures and not others. The patient has no right to demand that, either. One might say that patient's autonomy becomes endangered here. Yet, by way of response, the interviewed physician says "we are not the ones to decide about life or death. And the patient also is not allowed to decide that". Here the right to live is prioritized over any other rights.

The regulations in Poland say that in case of futile treatment doctors can organize a case conference to decide about the withdrawal of some of the treatment procedures. This decision however needs to be thoroughly explained in appropriate documents. The decision cannot be taken by one physician. "It may happen that we are curing a patient with the best and most expensive antibiotics, but we clearly see the is no improvement, so we do not really help", says the interviewed doctor. "Or if the patient's brain in damaged after SEPSA and she is unconscious for several months, then we can limit the patient's treatment". Yet there are no clear formal criteria as to when these limitations can take place. If the patient's condition is definitely terminate, doctors may call for a case conference and decide to put the DNR order in the patient's documentation. Still, as doctor Y admits, physicians in Poland tend to avoid doing that. He quotes the numbers saying that whereas the percent of DNR orders in Western Europe stays at the level of 85-90% of those who would in fact qualify for it, in Poland the percent is much smaller and amounts to about 59% (Kübler, 2015). That is, as the doctor states, due to the fact that physicians feel emotionally burdened when faced with the decision to place the order. Doctor Y quotes a case which will be reported here as it very clearly shows the dilemma discussed. The case concerns a 14 year old girl with leukemia who suffered from lung infection and sepsis. There were complications, she was diagnosed with disseminated intravascular coagulation which caused brainstem bleeding and the death of the brainstem. After that, following the required medical examinations and procedures for such cases, a team of three physicians declared the girl dead. So since that very moment the patient was legally considered dead.

And so we have the following situation [says doctor Y]: formally the person is dead. But the family can see in the monitor that the heart is beating, the person is warm, there is pulse, she is under a respirator and unconscious but seems to be alive. The family does not agree to quit the room. And now I am supposed to turn the respirator off. In the presence of the family...

The situation is very difficult. The family has the right to stay next to the patient. And so physicians admit they are often made to turn the respirator off when the family is present. That is why, due to the tension of the situation, but also taking into account the emotions of the family and their own emotions, they often decide not to do that. "It's easier not to do it. Other physicians don't do it either. One cannot be so insensitive" (Doctor Y). They do not disconnect the respirator even though the regulations say they should, as a person legally declared as dead should not stay at a hospital bed and be provided with medical treatment. The reasons given by doctors point mainly to the emotions of the family who is more likely to accept the "more traditional" death, when they notice the heart stop beating. Another example quoted by doctor Y concerned a child born with almost no brain. The child remained under respirator for a year. And even though it was clear the child would not survive and its treatment was futile, nobody disconnected the respirator. The cases cited here are worth reflecting over. They display the conduct and the values of the society and of the physicians clearly pointing to the 'more traditional' ways of looking at life and death. The word "traditional" would mean here standing more on the side of life as well as prioritizing life and existence over any other rights.

Appealing for the Right to Die

Medical graduates swear always to serve life and health. Yet very often ethical discussions concern patients' rights to die. The first in the world legislative document concerning natural death was proclaimed in California and was called the Natural Death Act. The act stated that every adult person has the right to decide about the medical treatments being given to him or her. The document also entitles an adult person to decide about not using or withdrawing the use of life-sustaining procedures in a medically critical condition. The legislative acts of California also enshrines the right of an adult person to declare in a written form his or her living will. The document may tell that the particular person does not agree for the use of life sustaining procedures in a terminal condition. In order to be legally valid the document needs to be signed by the patient and by two witnesses who are not relatives of the patient and who are not entitled to inherit from him or her. The patient and the witnesses declare that the patient is sound of mind at the moment of signing the document and that he or she is not under coercion. In the USA the law includes the 'right to life' but also 'right to death with dignity'. The arguments of those who support the right to choose death – not life – state that artificial life-sustaining therapies involving the use of sophisticated technology imply certain 'dehumanization' of life (Nesterowicz, 2013), where the patient seems to be treated more as 'medical object' (on which certain procedures are to be performed) rather than as a human being. Prolonging futile treatment with medical machinery may be perceived as denying the patient's right to die a natural death. It seems a denial of the right to die in peace and dignity.

Those who advocate the right to choose death emphasize the fact that the newest medical technology makes it possible to prolong life beyond its natural length, but in conditions which are not only extremely burdensome for the patient but which can also be considered inhumane. Such unnatural prolongation of human life can in fact be considered as prolongation of the dying process, which might be perceived as humiliating for the patient. What is also believed to be unethical here, is giving the patient no choice as to the way he wants to die, when death is inevitable. That is probably why as early as in 1986 the Californian Court of Appeals stated that in a terminal condition each mentally sane patient has a full right to demand being disconnected from life-sustaining equipment. At the same time the court warned that the diagnosis stating terminal condition needs to be confirmed by two physicians. In California the patient's decision to be disconnected is declared to be valid if it is taken consciously and when it is based on all the necessary information. As the US court stated, a doctor who is not willing to act according to such decision is obliged to resign care to another physician willing to follow what is the patient's right (Nesterowicz, 2013).

Polish legislative acts (KEL, art 32) state that in terminal states there is no obligation for the doctor to continue futile treatment or to use extraordinary life-sustaining techniques. The decision to stop the therapy belongs to the physician and involves the estimation of treatment chances. To make it more valid and to reduce any possible doubt, it is recommended that the decision about disconnecting life-sustaining equipments be taken by a team of doctors (Nesterowicz, 2013). Yet, as one could learn from the interviewed doctors, the practices of Polish ICUs most often aim to sustain life, even if the patient wishes otherwise. Whether a particular patient had previously declared to agree or to refuse terminal treatment is rather not taken into account. And even if the person had earlier expressed his or her will refusing medical intervention, the doctor will still act in favour of saving life, assuming that the will could have been changed, were the patient conscious. In a similar way, in urgent and life-threatening cases the doctors will always provide treatment. As doctor Y says, in majority of the acute cases the physician will assume that the patient wishes to be rescued, even if he or she had earlier explicitly declared otherwise.

Exposure to Death: Nurses

The stress concerning medical situations and accompanying ethical dilemmas has increased during the recent decades. As a result nurses are also ethically challenged and they often suffer from stress evoked by ethical conflicts. They are also the group which is most likely to be influenced by the discrepancies of opinions and emotions emerging in intensive care units. Nurses accompany patients in their daily existence and in their suffering and are the closest caregivers staying at the patient's bedside. They witness the drama of the patient and of the family. They are exposed to death and to ethical dilemmas surrounding life-extending therapies. ICUs nurses are very likely to undergo a burnout in cases thought to be futile. They often admit their feeling of frustration and lack of support. Corley researched the problem and found out that 60% of the nurses interviewed had experienced the situation of having to compromise their values due to the standards and policy of the hospital and physicians' requests or due to limitations of nursing staff and organizational constraints (Kälvemark et al., 2004). The different studies show that the most common sources of moral distress between nurses are concerns related to pain management and the prolongation of life. Nurses also report to feel distressed when they are made to perform unnecessary tests or when they have the desire to tell the truth (Kälvemark et al., 2004). Different studies also show nurses' frustration and sorrow when they feel unable to act according to what are their moral rules (Kälvemark et al., 2004).

MORAL DISTRESS

As a result of all the problems described earlier stress-related disorders have become a common affliction of health care professionals. Moreover, medical staff is often reported to suffer from what is called 'moral distress', which refers more specifically to the circumstances of their work. Moral distress can be described as

...traditional negative stress symptoms, such as feelings of frustration, anger and anxiety, which might lead to depressions, nightmares, headaches and feelings of worthlessness, that occur due to a conviction of what is ethically correct but [impossible due to] institutional and structural constraints [which] prevent the desired course of action. (Kälvemark et al., 2004, p. 1077)

The background for moral distress is the perception of moral and ethical responsibility which cannot be enacted due to the fact that one is restricted by circumstances. The stress appears when "one knows the right thing to do, but institutional or other constraints make it difficult to pursue the desired course of action" (Kälvemark et al., 2004, p. 1076). Raines (cited in Kälvemark et al., 2004) describes two situations which are likely to produce moral distress: a) when the person needs to act against his or her beliefs in order to follow regulations, and b) when one is not acting according to the rules because of his or her moral convictions (so the person is doing what is legally not allowed). The majority of research studies performed on moral distress refer to nurses, even though the problem concerns all categories of health care providers. Basing on the study of Kälvemark and colleagues (2004), the following text reports sample situations when the medical staff breaks legal rules and follows what is believed the right thing to do.

And so for example, the nurses consulted by Kälvemark and colleagues admit that responding to doctors' orders they often place patients in the hospital corridor, which is against the formal regulations. In this situation nurses have no possibility to act legally, as they are expected to follow the doctors' orders. "We then treat patients illegally when we put them in corridors", admits one of the nurses, adding that these rules are being broken almost every day (p. 1080). Of course, it is quite clear that the rules are broken for the patients' benefit, as otherwise some of them would have to leave the hospital. Doctors explain they brake the rules for the patients' sake. And because not doing so would be even worse for their conscience. "You do it for he patient", says one of the nurses. "You do it because it is more ethical [and] humanitarian", admits a doctor" (Kälvemark et al., 2004, p. 1081). So rules are often voluntarily broken when there is a conflict between regulations and the welfare of the patient. Similar situations, being potentially the source of moral distress, are also reported by pharmacy staff. One of the pharmacist talking to Kälvemark and colleagues admits: "yes, we break rules sometimes. One person came in and had an attack of asthma but no prescription. And then you feel "oh, my God!" ...[and] I gave her the medicine" (p. 1080). So again for the patient's welfare the legal rules were broken as the pharmacist reacted according to what she considered appropriate. Situations like that are possibly much more numerous. Sometimes the hierarchy between medical staff may play a role in the extent to which particular individuals are allowed to act according to what they perceive is appropriate. It happens that the person being subordinate – lower in the hierarchy – is made to act against his or her own beliefs in order to respond to orders given by the superior. This may concern the relations within the same institution, for example between a doctor and a nurse, or relations between representatives of different organizations, for example between a doctor and a pharmacist. Sample situation reported by a pharmacist can be quoted here:

Another thing ...is when we feel that the prescription isn't right. You check with the doctor maybe two times whether the dosage should be like this. He says yes, and we... in our experience it isn't a good dosage. We have tried to make him aware. It's the same thing when there are prescriptions from different doctors and you see that it's not good. The total situation for the customer isn't good. But what are you to do? (Kälvemark et al., 2004, p. 1081)

In case of nurses, the problem of moral distress is even more acute. As has been mentioned earlier, most of the studies concerning moral distress refer to this particular medical staff group. Nurses are most likely to suffer from moral distress. That may be because they are often unable to act on their beliefs as they do not take the final decisions concerning patients' care. Nurses were shown to use different strategies for coping with situations involving moral stress. Sometimes they were trying to influence the physician or they called the head nurse. Sometimes they submitted a report to the head of the unit (Kälvemark et al., 2004). Greater overall exposure to situations provoking moral distress may contribute to nurses' professional burnout.

Limited Time and Staff Resources

The situations involving medical dilemmas are often concerned with the lack of resources. This refers to equipment and financial resources as well as human resources. Shortages in medical staff mean that doctors and nurses do not have enough time and are faced with the need to prioritize between equally important tasks. The issue of distribution of the care givers' time between individual patients is at stake here. And so if one patient urgently needs help, the time and effort devoted to this particular person influences what is being offered to other patients. It applies both to nurses and physicians. Quite often the time to be spent on visiting patients is established. These visits are expected and calculated to last a certain, limited amount of time. Thus if for some reasons the physician stays longer with one patient, this is at the cost of the time devoted to others. These restrictions can be the source of various moral dilemmas. Sometimes it is impossible to inform a patient about everything he or she needs to know in the short time scheduled for the consultation. Even the mere recording of the patient's personal and medical data takes some time. Not mentioning the situation when an unexpected serious diagnosis needs to be provided. Then the typically established limits of time are never long enough. In such cases the physician cannot hurry. "What if [the patients] get to know that they have a cancer that is to be treated with cyotoxin and you just move on?", one of the doctors asked (Kälvemark et al., 2004, p. 1081). So again moral dilemmas and distress appear. The doctor can choose between limiting the consultation time (which in serious and acute cases appears to be quite inhumane) or breaking time regulations at the expense of being late for his or her other duties (and possibly suffering some kind of distress because of that too.). The interesting psychological phenomenon, also noticed by medical staff, is that they tend to prioritize what happens 'at present'. "We prioritise the customer who's at the counter right now, but not the customer we know will come in within two hours of time, says one of the pharmacists (Kälvemark et al., 2004). That might be because the needs of the person who stands in front of us are most evident, thus the person is more likely to get more attention at the cost of those who will come later. Doctors admit that some cases require more time than others. They also add that if you inform your patients that some of them need more urgent help than others, they will be willing to respect your decisions.

When we treat a patient, we do it well, I think it's better to do it well with that patient and let someone else wait for a while. And we always pioritise those who are acutely ill, I think. … Even if it isn't good for the one who is less acutely ill to have to wait the patients understand, if they are properly informed that others are worse out. (Doctor, Kälvemark et al., 2004, p. 1079)

Of course meeting patients is just one of the tasks of health care stuff. Much time is also devoted to administrative work. And that is often reported to produce frustration. Administrative work and documentation is very time-consuming and very often the IT technology, as applied in practice, does not make it shorter. As a consequence both doctors and nurses often feel distressed, as they believe that is not what should concern them most. They all agree that their prime task is to take care of the patients, not of papers. Members of the medical staff interviewed in the research performed by Kälvemark and colleagues (2004) also expressed their willingness to have more time for patients, and to be less overwhelmed with administrative work. Being unable to act to what they believe the priority, medical care givers often express frustration, stating they are not able to live up to their own standards.

Bed Allocation and Financial Shortages

The medical and human resources available in a hospital are never infinite. Intensive care units, which are said to be specially staffed and specially equipped, also face limitations. Moreover, as has been mentioned earlier, social expectations concerning medical treatment are now greater, as the up-to-date medical technology offers more. The technology is costly but gives us the possibility to extend and sustain life, sometimes for a long time. In this situation intensive care units are challenged even more, as: a) within the aging society the number of ICU patients grows bigger, b) particular patients may linger on in the unit quite long, c) the costs of ICU therapy are very high, and d) there are always new patients who need to be admitted to the unit. All that results in the fact that the amount of resources is probably never satisfactory and that the ICU medical staff is required to make judgments concerning those who can stay in the unit and those who can be admitted. These judgments may not be easy and may evoke ethical dilemmas, as in fact all the patients staying at ICU and arriving to the unit are very ill. As a consequence intensivists are faced more and more often with the problem of resource limitations. The most stressful situations reported take place when medical providers are not able to admit a patient who really needs medical help and is entitled to get it. Sometimes there are more patients than beds available in the unit. Then the personnel is forced to choose patients who are all in need of the bed, and this is often perceived as involving ethical dilemmas (Kälvemark et al., 2004). Having to choose among patients may be unethical. It may also be the source of moral distress. As one doctor says,

…that is something that you can feel stressed about and you feel… feel terrible towards the patient because of it. This is when you can't offer someone a hospital bed. … They can be ever so ill and you can't offer them what you really thing they need. (Kälvemark et al., 2004, p. 1079)

One of the nurses continues:

…when a patient arrives here the clinic is often full… and then you suddenly have to prioritise which patient is most fit… to lie somewhere else. Sometimes it will be in the corridor, sometimes in an examination room. But these are often fast decisions that can be stressful. (Kälvemark et al., 2004, p. 1079)

Of course there are always some formal regulations specifying intensive care bed allocation. The regulations typically require the doctors to consider the medical need for the resources in case of a particular patient, the prognosis referring to whether or not the acute problem is likely to reverse, the expected length and quality of life afterwards, and the patient's will, if possible to be stated (Skowronski, 2001).

Some patients arriving to hospitals happen not to belong to social security system. This poses another dilemma, as those patients should not be admitted due to economic reasons. Talking about one of the hospitals in Sweden, Kälvemark and colleagues (2004) state that patients needing help are admitted anyway, even if they are foreigners and do not belong to the structures of Swedish medical care system. Polish hospitals treat patients in a similar way. Those who need urgent help are admitted to hospitals and all the possible means are used to rescue their life, even if the patients do not have health insurance.

It is more than clear that nearly all of the shortages mentioned with reference to institutions providing medical care can be ascribed to economic reasons. Yet, sometimes financial shortages within an institution concern individual patients much more than others. These individual cases often become more noticeable and more bothersome to medical staff members. And they may evoke ethical dilemmas, too. One of the doctors admits:

...some patients do not receive optimal care because of economic reasons. We don't give patients the more expensive medicines they ought to have according to national and international guidelines, because we find them too expensive. This is both right and wrong. It's wrong in relation to that particular patient, not letting the medicine we believe in. But at the same time we are forced to make some sort of economic prioritising, too. We know that if we give too much of this medicine we will have to cut down on something else. (Kälvemark et al., 2004, p. 1079)

As can be seen in this example, economy often stands in opposition to ethics. Financial restrictions often reduce patients' access to the most effective and least detrimental medical procedures. Though, the decisions here are really difficult as, due to financial shortages, providing one patient with what he or she needs may negatively influence the welfare of others. The mere calculations of costs, however, cannot be by itself a response to the moral and ethical dilemma that appears here.

Other Dilemmas: Privacy and Dignity of the Patient

The patient has the right for the respect for of his or her privacy and dignity. Patient's right to privacy refers to confidentiality of all personal information that the medical staff gets during the treatment. It may be both: medical data and other non-medical information that in some way gets revealed to medical staff. The information may concern for example the patient's family relationships, personal contacts, sexual preferences, his or her sterility, etc. Privacy and dignity also imply that only the medically necessary staff (and students doing their apprenticeship in academic or university hospitals) may be present during medical examinations and interventions. Participation of any other people requires the patient's consent. As Nesterowicz (2013) admits, if the patient's objects to the presence of students, his or her wishes should be also taken into account or at least the number of students should be limited. The European Court of Human Rights in Strasbourg stated that human dignity is violated when the patient is being treated in a way that awakens in him the feeling of being frightened and humiliated (Nesterowicz, 2013), which can lead him to physical and psychical breakdown.

In everyday clinical situations it is quite easy to ignore and breach the patient's rights to privacy, even without any intention of doing so. An example here could be the situation taking place in a pharmacy, when the names of required medicines are repeated aloud to other members of the staff, and others can also hear them. This could be intimidating or sometimes humiliating for the patient. Still in certain circumstances the situations appear earlier than one realises they might be inappropriate. And so one pharmacist admits:

Later on in the afternoon it is quite noisy in here and we talk louder during the day, and in the end... Maybe we shout to someone: "Can you get me some Bensodiazepine?" And that's not nice, really. We disregard our professional secrecy. ... And I can feel a bit bad because I may reveal more than the customer would like the others to know. (Kälvemark et al., 2004, p. 1081)

One needs to be very careful in order to avoid similar situations as they may be perceived as invading the patient's rights to privacy and dignity. The right to privacy implies that all medical information concerning a patient should be kept confidential. And so for example in Poland it is forbidden to display any personal data on hospital beds. Several decades ago it was quite obvious that each patient had a paper label on which the nurse put important medical data (depending on the unit, it might have been information concerning the temperature, physiological functions, the information about viral hepatitis and other similar). Labels including such information are no longer allowed, yet medical staff needs to be able to identify patients quickly. And so they develop different strategies for coping with that. One of the possible strategies is the usage of some kind of codes. Which means that the labels still stay on the patients' beds but instead of charts and words they include some coded information, comprehensible only to medical staff.

The regulations also say that intensive care units may give the information concerning patient's condition only to the closest family (wife, husband, mother, father, adult son or adult daughter). In case of further family or friends, the information can be given only to those who had been earlier formally designated by the patient. Cohabitation does not give per se the right to be informed. Still, as ICU doctors admit, they cannot be so cruel. Even if it is against the law, they often give the most general and basic information to cohabitants, telling them, for example, to stay calm when there is no serious danger for the patient. Yet, some people, as one of the doctors notices, are completely alone and have no family.

That happens. And there comes the patient's neighbour as the closest person. We are normally not entitled to give any information in this case. Though, we cannot be inhuman. So, if the patient died and there is no family, we provide the neighbour only with death certificate, just to make it possible for him or her to organize the funeral. (Doctor Y)

Within the Staff

Within their work experience, the medical staff not only deals with the patients, but also cooperates with the colleagues, who often expect loyalty and availability. Medical staff normally agrees with the statement that in clinical situations, especially those involving examination or intervention, the physician is expected to focus his or her attention on the patient and the problems related to the patient. It may be considered unprofessional and invading the patient's dignity if the doctor performing one action is clearly concerned with something else. Yet, as it appears in practice, the presence of newest technology and modern world social demands are likely to provoke behaviours that break these rules. One of the problems here is being "loyal' to your professional colleagues even at the cost of patient's discomfort. The modern professional milieu expects us to be available whenever needed (Kälvemark et al., 2004). The use of modern telecommunication technology allows for one's availability all the time. It is often informally accepted that professional colleagues call one another during the working time and expect to be answered immediately. This may put a physician in an uncomfortable situation, where he or she needs to choose between this up-to-date 'loyalty' to colleagues and respect for the patient. The problem was mentioned by one of the physicians interviewed by Kälvemark and colleagues (2004).

People may be upset [...] you haven't answered. And you may have been sitting with a patient, telling him that he has a lethal disease or something like that. You can't run away from that, even though you have tendency to do that, I'm sorry to say, too often. (p. 1082)

The values that come into conflict in this and similar situations are the loyalty to those who may be of equal or superior status versus respect for the patient, who, as has been mentioned earlier, most often stays at a subordinate role. In such situation the physician needs to assess the circumstances and choose between the two options. The choice will probably depend on particular medical circumstances but also on the values the doctor lives by and enacts.

CONCLUSION

Members of one health care staff may not always agree about what constitutes a moral dilemma (Kälvemark et al., 2004). That is due to differences not only in moral convictions but also in the level of knowledge and in the access to facts concerning particular patient's situation. It may happen that members of the medical staff share the same moral values but prioritize them differently. It is also possible that people agree on values and their ranking in theory, but they differ in the practical implication of their beliefs. One way or another, in everyday clinical situation human rights, being exemplified in the rights of the patients (and also in the rights and duties of the doctors), are challenged to the extremes. The daily routine, demands of the up-to-day fast living society, development of technology, higher expectations of patients and their families as well as the shortages in finances, medical equipment, and in medical human resources are problems which accumulate and intensify. The human rights of the participants of clinical situations may somehow disappear in the chaos of the surrounding problems. Still, they are more likely to come to the fore when the situation becomes critical. As a result of the development of advanced biomedical techniques, health care has become more complex but also ethical issues concerned with the treatment have become more complicated. And so intensive care units, were critically or terminally ill patients are treated, create a space for controversies and sometimes fierce moral discussions. The end-of-life situations evoke numerous ethical dilemmas and doubts. They provoke conflicts within the patients' families and within the medical staff. It is at this point when, due to different interpretations of what is more or less ethical, the human rights of a patient are most likely to be violated. The atmosphere of intensive care units has been described as 'hidden drama' not only due to the poor condition of the patients there, also due to the overwhelming tension rising from the conflict of values and beliefs. Frequent exposure to this tension may contribute to emotional and professional burnout of medical staff. Moral distress is one other affliction concerning health care personnel. It develops as a result of the conflict appearing between one's ethical beliefs and the formal regulations influencing one's professional behaviour. Moral distress is a very serious problem and it concerns almost all clinical situations. The cases reported in the chapter and probably our own life experience make it quite clear that what seems right, noble, clear and widely accepted in theory often appears to be hardly possible to follow in reality. We all believe in the validity of patients human rights, though we tend to differ in our beliefs concerning their enactment. Authors of publications dealing with ethical problems in medical care practice are not very likely to offer easy and ready-made solutions to be applied. These problems are always idiosyncratic and personal. They can be perused and seriously discussed only basing on a substantial knowledge of ethics. That is why probably the first suggestion to follow would be to provide hospitals and medical organizations with groups offering ethical help, not only to the patients, but also to medical staff. In case of intensive care units, ethical help is very important. It should be provided not only to patients and their families, but also to health care providers at every level (to both physicians and nurses). Kälvemark and colleagues (2004) notice that even though the need for ethical help has recently increased, medical care organizations often miss appropriate structures dealing with ethical support, especially if the support for medical staff is concerned. Kälvemark and colleagues (2004) investigated in their research the facility to obtain ethical support in a workplace. As it appears in the research, medical institutions in Sweden have hardly any form of support for medical staff. There was no organized ethical support in the workplace described and no organized way to discuss the important issues. The problems were only mentioned when medical staff met during coffee breaks in an informal way. Meetings were not formalized and not organized on a regular basis. The situation in Poland looks quite similar. Hospitals do offer psychological help to patients, but there are no organized structures that would provide ethical and psychological support for the medical staff within their workplaces. Members of the medical staff are as if expected to deal with what are supposedly their problems on their own. Yet, as the authors notice, "the reducing of moral distress is closely connected to work organization and its provision of support structures for ethical discussions" (Kälvemark et al., 2004, p. 1083). Kälvemark and colleagues (2004) emphasize the fact that nowadays there is an increased need for support resources, education in ethics and discussion forums for discussing ethically difficult everyday clinical situations. The authors strongly recommend organizing ethic rounds - regular meetings with interdisciplinary participation which hopefully could help staff members learn to identify and analyse ethical problems and which could possibly help to foster tolerance and respect for the values represented by others (Kälvemark et al, 2004). The need for more intensive education in ethics and for ethical discussion forums for both hospital and pharmacy staff is emphasized in various publications concerning health care dilemmas. Improving communication between all the participants of clinical situations seems pivotal here. And so Chow (2014) advocates close cooperation of ethics, palliative care teams and ICU staff. She also suggests fostering better communication to deal with the problem of futile care. She suggests that meeting sessions should be arranged, involving members of the ethics, palliative care, attending physicians, and nurses. She also strongly emphasizes the fact that in a futile terminal care situation it is the family who strongly needs help of the ethics and who should be provided with unambiguous information coming from the specialists concerned with the case. The danger of ambiguous or differing messages coming from different specialists or different care givers can impair effective communication and foster the feeling of mistrust for the medial staff. Thus the author recommends frequent meetings including all the parties involved and avoiding medical jargon in order to make the message comprehensible to everybody (Chow, 2014).

Communication and ethical rounds will possibly not solve all the problems we face but they are likely to help us understand the intricacy of ethical issues involved in the everyday clinical situations. They are also very likely to make us more sensitive to the values and ideas professed by other people. This, hopefully, would be of benefit to us and our patients. And it is probably here where the circle of the discussion closes and comes back to its beginning, namely to the earlier quoted words of the Hippocratic Oath: "I will remember that there is art to medicine as well as science, and that warmth, sympathy, and understanding may outweigh the surgeon's knife or the chemist's drug" (Tyson, 2001). These words have been repeated here in order to emphasize the fact that understanding, and so effective communication, may help us resolve many of the problems we face, even if the problems appear serious and ethically challenging.

REFERENCES

Bresnahan, J. F. (1990). Ethical dilemmas in critical care medicine. In R. D. Cane, B. A. Shapiro, & R. Davidson (Eds.), *Case studies in critical care medicine* (pp. 412–426). Chicago: Year Book Medical Publishers.

Bunch, E. H. (2000). Ethical dilemmas in the context of ambiguity on a critical care unit in Norway. *Eubios Journal of Asian and International Bioethics; EJAIB, 10*, 37–40.

Chow, K. (2014). Ethical dilemmas in the intensive care unit. *Journal of Hospice and Palliative Nursing, 16*(5), 256–260. doi:10.1097/NJH.0000000000000069

Convention for the Protection of Human Rights and Fundamental Freedoms as amended by Protocols No. 11 and No. 14. (1950). Retrieved March 18, 2015, from http://conventions.coe.int/treaty/en/treaties/html/005.htm

Curran, C. A. (1977). *Counseling-learning: a whole person model for education.* Apple River, IL: Apple River Press.

European Consultation on the Rights of Patients. (1994). *A Declaration on the Promotion of Patients' Rights in Europe.* Amsterdam: World Health Organization. Retrieved March 20, 2015, from www.who.int/genomics/.../eu_declaration1994.pdf

Goffam, E. (2000). *Człowiek w teatrze życia codziennego.* Warszawa, KR.

Jeffery, M. E., Lanken, P. N., & Taichman, D. B. (2004). Ethical issues in the intensive care unit. *Hospital Physician Pulmonary Disease Board Review Manual, 11*(3), 2–12.

Kälvemark, S., Höglund, A. T., Hansson, M. G., Westerholm, P., & Arnetz, B. (2004). Living with conflicts-ethical dilemmas and moral distress in the health care system. *Social Science & Medicine, 58*(6), 1075–1084. doi:10.1016/S0277-9536(03)00279-X PMID:14723903

Kodeks Etyki Lekarskiej (KEL). (2003). Retrieved March 20, 2015, from http://www.nil.org.pl/dokumenty/kodeks-etyki-lekarskiej

Kübler, A. (2015, April). *Wytyczne postępowania wobec braku skuteczności podtrzymywania funnkcji narządów.* Paper presented at the conference Intensywna Terapia – wyzwania i możliwości w leczeniu chorych w stanach krytycznych, Kraków.

Nesterowicz, M. (2013). *Prawo medyczne.* Toruń: Dom Organizatora.

Skowronski, G. A. (2001). Bed rationing and allocation in the intensive care unit. *Current Opinion in Critical Care, 7*(6), 480–484. doi:10.1097/00075198-200112000-00020 PMID:11805556

Tyson, P. (2001). *The Hippocratic Oath Today.* Retrieved March 10, 2015, from http://www.pbs.org/wgbh/nova/body/hippocratic-oath-today.html

Universal Declaration of Human Rights. (1948). Retrieved March 15, 2015, from http://www.un.org/en/documents/udhr/

Weinberg, S. L. (1985). DRG dilemmas in intensive care. Financial and medical. *Chest Journal, 87*(2), 141. doi:10.1378/chest.87.2.141 PMID:3917891

Zajdel, J. (2008). Ryzyko zdrowotne implikowane błędami lekarskimi. In M. Gałuszka (Ed.), *Zdrowie i choroba w społeczeństwie ryzyka biomedycznego* (pp. 349–386). Łódź: Wydawnictwa Uniwersytetu Medycznego.

ENDNOTES

[1] From the point of view of the social roles theory of Erving Goffman (2000), the relationship between a patient and a doctor can be perceived as one involving a kind of imbalance. In most of the cases it will be perceived as involving two parties of unequal status. This inequality of status is brought by the mere fact that it is the patient who is in need and the doctor who is likely to provide help. This dependence may of course be weaker or stronger depending on the patients' characteristics: their social status, their individual traits and health condition. Still, as it is the patients who tend to be in the 'subordinate' role, they are more vulnerable and more likely to suffer in some way due to possible maltreatment in the relationship. That is possibly why the rights of patients have been discussed in so many different documents proclaimed all over the world.

[2] See the theory of Charles A. Curran (1977).

[3] The name Medical Code of Ethics refers to the Polish document called Kodeks Etyki Lekarskiej (KEL). Further in the text the acronym KEL is used to stand for this particular code of ethics.

[4] Elements of informed consent for interventions in a sample intensive care unit, according to Jeffery, Lanken, & Taichman (2004) should include responses to the following questions: "What are the patient's relevant medical diagnoses? What is the intervention proposed? What is the purpose of the intervention and its benefits, risks, and burdens? What are the likely or important consequences of withholding it? What are the alternatives to forgoing it? What are the likely or important consequences of these alternatives? Is the patient free of coercion?"

This research was previously published in Organizational Culture and Ethics in Modern Medicine edited by Anna Rosiek and Krzysztof Leksowski, pages 255-281, copyright year 2016 by Medical Information Science Reference (an imprint of IGI Global).

Chapter 62

Is Artificial Intelligence (AI) Friend or Foe to Patients in Healthcare?
On Virtues of Dynamic Consent – How to Build a Business Case for Digital Health Applications

Veronika Litinski
MaRS Discovery, Canada

ABSTRACT

Failure to appropriately measure Value is one of the reasons for slow reform in health. Value brings together quality and cost, both defined around the patient. With technology we can measure value in the new ways: commercially developed algorithms are capable of mining large, connected data sets to present accurate information for patients and providers. But how do we align these new capabilities with clinical and operational realities, and further with individual privacy? The right amount of information, shared at the right time, can improve practitioners' ability to choose treatments, and patients' motivation to provide consent and follow the treatment. Dynamic Consent, where IT is used to determine just what patients are consenting to share, can address the inherent conflict between the demand from AI for access to data and patients' privacy principles. This chapter describes a pragmatic Commercial Development framework for building digital health tool. It overlays Value Model for healthcare IT investments with Patient Activation Measures and innovation management techniques.

ARTIFICIAL INTELLIGENCE (AI): THE PATIENT'S FRIEND OR FOE?

Where can AI improve health services? The short answer is, wherever Big Data lives. Policy makers and healthcare administrators are grappling with the recent emergence of Big Data in healthcare. These can include large linked data (from electronic patient records,) streams of real-time geo-located health

DOI: 10.4018/978-1-5225-3926-1.ch062

data (collected by personal wearable devices, etc.) and open data (from shared datasets.) Together these form Big Data, a realm rich in new research opportunities and avenues for commercial exploitation. (Kostkova, 2015)

AI in Health Systems

It is nearly impossible for doctors to stay abreast of all the new and changing rules governing their fields, on top of the constant innovations taking place therein.

In the paper, Analysis of Questions Asked by Family Doctors Regarding Patient Care, (Ely, J. W. et al. 1999) observed 103 physicians over one workday. Those physicians asked 1,101 clinical questions during the day. The majority of those questions (64%) were never answered. Among questions that did get answered, the physicians spent less than two minutes looking for their answers.

Obviously, providing quick answers to clinical questions will always improve the quality of healthcare. No wonder the Chief Health Officer at IBM Corporation, Rhee Kyi, a physician earlier in his career, recognizes the role IBM Watson will play in healthcare delivery. Watson, and other commercial solutions, promise to provide insights, reveal patterns and relationships across data sets. The allure of Watson lies in its being designed to work with unstructured data, such as genetic data and the free text portions of electronic health records.

The expectation is that research on large, shared medical datasets will provide radically new pathways for improving health systems as well as individual care. Facilitating personalized or "stratified medicine," such open data can shed light on causes of disease, and the effects of treatment.

Some of the most powerful applications can be found in Public Health, where data sets from communities of practice, social networks, and wearable devices can be mined for a wide spectrum of public health monitoring, and launch of persuasive technologies for public health interventions. However, these fascinating opportunities develop against a backdrop of decades of under-investment in public health systems, which lack the resources to tackle the full range of health threats, from potential chemical or biological attacks, to serious chronic disease epidemics, or emerging infectious diseases like Zika. (*Trust For America's Health*, 2016)

The allure of analytics here is obvious. It can help health systems crunch data to improve care quality and reduce costs, especially for organizations that aim to profit under shared savings or financial risk contracts. How can we balance cost, value and liability in a regulated healthcare industry?

Me, My Health Care Circle, and AI

Another area where AI can be hugely helpful is in presenting data and helping patients make sense of it. After all, they are confronted with the same challenge as their doctors: quantities of specialized information that can be life saving, or just the opposite. The patient's informed consent is required in every aspect of care – from their contributing biological samples preparing for complex surgeries, to accepting a given course of treatment. How do we empower patients to make truly informed decisions, while allowing developers access to the streams of data?

Respect for a patient's individual autonomy is an established principle in modern medicine. In the past half century, the concept of autonomy has promoted patients from passive recipients of care to partners in planning their own treatments.

The notion of patient empowerment is reflected by developments in regulation and guidance. Think of phrases such as "patient led care," "patient engagement" and "shared treatment decision-making".

The new strategy of patient involvement in health services is emerging in conjunction with initiatives for deepening inter-professional collaboration, all with the further aim of providing team-based care. Policy-makers envision some non-physician providers' expanding scope of practice going hand-in-hand with this increased focus on patient-centered care. Can AI help deepen the trust between patients and the professionals in their care circle?

Research shows that high-performing teams are not built piecemeal. They achieve superior levels of cooperation because their members trust one another. Trust and a strong sense of group identity build confidence in their effectiveness as a team. In other words, such teams possess high levels of group EI (emotional intelligence).

The right amount of information, shared at the right time, can promote significant improvement in patients' ability to choose the right treatments.

In a randomized controlled trial at two hospitals in Boston researchers studied the impact of a video-based decisions support tool for patients in the hospital. Decisions about cardiopulmonary resuscitation (CPR) and intubation are core parts of advance care planning, particularly for seriously ill, hospitalized patients. However, these discussions are often avoided. Seriously ill patients who viewed a video about CPR and intubation were less likely to want these treatments. Better informed about their options, they gave orders to forgo CPR/ intubation, and discussed their preferences with providers. This study brings into question what represents Informed Consent in the emerging world of AI and Big data? (El-Jawahri, et al., 2015)

Anonymizing data is a recognized pre-condition for its collection. It allows access to health data without compromising the patient's right to privacy or security. Sayo, founder of Self-Care Catalysts, makes a compelling case for codifying trust between the givers and the gatherers of data: patients who give their health data should have greater access to it themselves. They should be able to track it, and see how their data is being used. There should also be an available, clearly delineated process of opting out of data sharing. (*Nuffield Council on Bioethics,* 2015)

Researchers in the United Kingdom have tested the concept of Dynamic Consent. (Spencer, K. et al., 2016). Here, information technology is used to determine just what patients are consenting to share. A succession of digital interface screens is presented to the patient. Information and choices about data gathering, and its potential uses, are delineated. Patients are thus enabled to tailor consent according to their own preferences.

However, this concept is bound to come into conflict with the demand from AI for access to large pools of patient data. This is useful in training AI's predictive function, which is not always related to a specific patient's care. These secondary uses of identifiable patients' data, (e.g. to develop commercial products,) represent unchartered waters for public payers, patient advocates and commercial vendors. Google's company, DeepMind, launched several projects with large health systems that bring out important questions about the commercial exploitation of individuals' data and publicly funded health systems. These systems are fertile ground for "schooling" AI programs owned by powerful global corporations. (techcrunch.com, 2016)

There is great potential to be realized by combining data with analytics, and technology with expertise. Many ills can be more efficiently cured, once value is understood and paid for. However, a patient centric, value-defining framework – one capable of informing data-sharing in the new healthcare sphere – does not yet exist.

The Office of the National Coordinator for Health Information Technology, United States Government Health and Human Services (ONC) has identified patient-generated health data (PGHD) as an important issue for advancing patient engagement. It has initiated a series of activities to gain more information about PGHD's value, and the various approaches to its implementation. The PGHD policy framework project is integral to Stage 3 of the Meaningful Use Rule, and the U.S. administration's Precision Medicine Initiative. (HealthIT.gov, 2016)

Institutional View: Focus Areas and Investment

While value dimensions are known, (Institute for Healthcare Improvement, 2016) decision-makers' perspectives still vary widely. And the ways organizations are structured to gather data and make decisions are equally diverse.

The problem of establishing connections between processes of care and their outcomes is not trivial either. However, a number of frameworks have been evaluated (Dwamena et al, 2012; Ryan et al, 2012; Scott, et al, 2011; Bircher, 2016). Furthermore, there is the widely acknowledged need for meaningful measures: feasible, affordable, and embedded in the care delivery system (Beck, 2013).

Digital tools create opportunities to advance the quality of measurements, integrate them with electronic medical records, and allow healthcare practitioners to focus attention where it is needed most.

In practice, the issue of measurement arises at the point of introducing a process redesign. Each new idea within such redesigns has its own story of relative risks and advantages.

Finally, most innovative projects in health care will bring together a diverse set of perspectives, expertise and expectations. The diversity of language and approaches to framing problems make development and evaluation of new products complex. This in turn slows down development and adoption by users.

Can we develop a business case for engaging, game-like applications in Health? We shall describe processes, parameters and methodologies for doing just that.

APPROACH

The Lean Start-up Methodology (Ries, 2011) is a widely used framework for developing new software products. Thinking about process redesign as "validated learning" prepares foundations for Growth Mindset among all participants, from builders to the business managers involved in any given project.

Through decades of research on achievement and success, Stanford University psychologist, Carol Dweck (Dweck C, 2007) discovered what she has termed, "growth mindset". It is an approach to problem-solving that stimulates the resilience essential to getting things done. It also plays an especially important role in long development and implementation projects, which are typical for healthcare. Most take 18-24 months to move from Pilot to Project, to System-wide deployment.

Creating and launching digital tools for health are no simple tasks. Perhaps only one thing is certain: your team will go through multiple iterations of the Build-Learn-Measure cycle on its path to developing a relevant value proposition for users, and demonstrating value to business managers. Resilience is key. In short, your team will reach new heights if all members learn to embrace the occasional tumble.

Who Is at the Table?

To succeed while introducing innovation in a multi-stakeholder environment, it is important to map out priorities for each stakeholder, and make sure that all relevant points of view are considered.

Developers of innovative solutions face the significant challenge of carving a path that both defines and measures success. Typically, the path will address at least these 4 perspectives:

1. Describing an IT development project, it is usual to focus on the tactical elements of delivery: meeting specifications, working within time and budget constraints, and developing the robust architecture necessary to meeting expected levels of quality and scalability.
2. Talking about successful management, the focus is on strategic achievements: meeting an organization's business goals, contributing to competitive advantage, generating financial results, and allocating resources wisely.
3. Discussing quality in healthcare, we must involve measures specific to certain care settings: for example, in rehabilitation, the FIM® instrument helps care providers assess patients' physical and cognitive status.
4. Patients confronting a new interface within the care system will seek simplicity and support on their journey towards self-management and improved health.

Payer's Perspective: Value Dials to Understand Benefits

Healthcare payers – whether these are private insurers, sickness funds or, as is the case in many parts of the world, governments – have the responsibility to provide health care to a pre-defined population within a fixed spending envelope. In this environment some form of priority setting must occur (Mitton & Donaldson, 2004). In the recent past, it was not uncommon to allocate resources in health organizations on the basis of historical or political patterns. Although a lot of work is underway in outcomes research (Pincus, 2016), connections between processes of care and outcomes remain imperfectly understood.

Such connections represent information important in the determining of values obtained from health care investments of any kind. Some of information technology's brightest thinkers have long advocated use of the Value Model when discussing health IT investments. It is an industry-tested approach to discussing and measuring the benefits of such investments, and it focuses upon quantifiable benefits that produce financial impact. The Value Model asks two simple questions:

- Where are we going?
- How will we know we've arrived?

Developed by Intel, the model expresses the "where to" question as a value dial, a starting point for specifying what you want to achieve. Intel's 'value dials' are broad categories of benefits through which an IT investment may deliver strategic value.

The value dials mirror quality indicators defined by the healthcare system, such as patient safety and access, cost optimization, and staff satisfaction. We see some of the significant benefits from applying a value dials framework when we discuss which performance indicators are most relevant to specific HIT-enabled projects, to patient priorities, to organizational goals, and/or to the culture as a whole.

Once value dials are established, the next step is to associate each value dial with a set of observable, quantifiable metrics ('Key Performance Indicators' in Intel's parlance). Each KPI is usually derived from an underlying calculation. The calculation is derived from metrics already collected by a healthcare institution.

With the advent of digital tools put in the hands of patients, there is now an opportunity to add metrics that truly reflect their experiences throughout the care process. Thus, digital tools make it possible for patients to become efficient 'reporters' to the healthcare provider. This in turn supports clinical decision-making and leads to improved outcomes.

Measuring the impact of such patient engagement in health care outcomes is not yet well understood. It may be that solutions will be found at the intersection of system-generated measures and psychometric methods for data collection and analysis. Psychometrics offers quantitative models for psychological phenomena, such as patient engagement. (Dubbels, 2016).

Thus, psychometrics can contribute key elements for ROI analyses of digital health interventions. All this helps diminish the risk and uncertainty associated with the costs of development. In this way, serious games may serve as practice innovations, helping to make care more efficient, effective, and satisfying to patients and providers.

What Represents "Engagement" in the Health Context?

As shown in the 2010 editorial (Nash D, 2010) there is a growing body of evidence demonstrates that patients who are more actively involved in their health care experience better health outcomes and incur lower costs.

'The insider perspective of the illness experience' (Thorne and Paterson, 2000) is gaining more central consideration within service redesign debates. While there are examples of tools improving communications at the bedside, such as the Interactive Patient Whiteboard™, there are many fewer tools suited to community and home care settings.

The efforts of Judith Hibbard and her colleagues (Hibbard, 2004; Hibbard 2013) have helped to create the Patient Activation Measure (PAM), a tool that quantifies an individual's level of activation, or engagement, in their care.

Patients' scores are assigned to one of four stages of activation:

Stage 1: The patient does not yet understand that an active role is important.
Stage 2: The patient lacks the knowledge and/or confidence to take action.
Stage 3: The patient is beginning to take action.
Stage 4: The patient is maintaining behaviors (e.g. 30 minutes of aerobic exercise daily) over time.

High PAM scores correlate positively with self-management behaviors, the use of self-directed services, and high rates of adherence to medication regimens.

"Patient Activation" refers to a patient's knowledge, skills, ability, and willingness to manage his or her own health and care. "Patient engagement" is a broader concept that combines patient activation with interventions designed to increase activation and promote positive patient behavior.

By combining PAM with an understanding of the components of motivation the developers of patient engagement tools can begin designing better interventions.

Case Study

In the case of the Home Assessment Tool (HAT) developed at Cogniciti, (www.cogniciti.com) the team started with very simple, pragmatic questions: How would our target users find HAT amid the clutter of web applications? What words would they use for searches? What would make them try the assessment and trust the results? In order to develop meaningful health interventions that could drive behavior change we needed to understand consumers' day-to-day experiences, ie. the full complexity of their decisions regarding aging-related cognitive change.

The Patient Journey is a practical tool for garnering these insights. Patient decision conflicts arise when values, beliefs, and knowledge associated with their "normal" selves conflict with their experience of the new health environment faced in illness.

Uncertainties associated with choosing a healthcare intervention represent barriers. Often, a treatment is rejected based on fears, not of side effects, but of associated losses of physical freedom, connectedness to family and friends, or a general decline in quality of life. Understanding the conflicts underlying their decisions is crucial to influencing patients to adopt or adhere to an intervention.

Commercial Development Framework

Successful innovative projects in digital health typically go through the milestones defined by the "3 Ps":

1. Identify and understand Problems that the customers, (patients and healthcare providers) actually have and care about.
2. Construct a Path to success for customers to investigate, compare, test and purchase. This includes building a demo or a prototype technology, developing a revenue model, and gathering early indications of the marketing equation (i.e. cost of customer acquisition and customer lifetime value).
3. Develop Proof that the healthcare outcomes and value are real.

Once an application has reached the 3rd milestone it represents the complete package of information required for scaling up across the healthcare landscape. The opposite is also true: without such a package it is very difficult to secure the financial and human resources to implement an innovative solution at a meaningful scale.

Process Map

The process map serves three purposes:

First, it is a shared "sand box" where each stakeholder – users, buyers, and developers – can see how their individual perspectives and objectives fit together. Every time a new idea for a feature comes up the team can decide whether it aligns with the overall plan.

Second, it identifies building blocks for a project plan.

Third, it establishes the foundation for an investment pitch. Whether you are pitching to an internal audience or outside investment, it is important to create a narrative that addresses emotional, rational, and financial considerations. The Process Map (Table 1) contains key points that make explicit how the innovative application will deliver on each level.

Table 1. Process map

Target Audience
• Understand user's motivations • Patient Journey • Clinical flow • Business drivers
Define What You Want to Do for the Target Audience
• Audience pain points • Business drivers, e.g. enhancement/brand loyalty; alignment with audience expectations, alignment with the current business model, value dials defined in the strategic plan • Alignment with the business objectives of a sponsor/buyer
Desired Functionality
Where and how the application will be used
Technology Resources
• Scalability across platforms, screens, privacy and security requirements, integration and inter-operability • Clinical validation: meaningful improvement vs. treatment as usual • Workflow integration
Speed to Market
Define metrics early to make decisions through launch and ongoing support; e.g. Efficacy vs. Uptake; utility across the care pathway.

Table 2. Sample budget

	Activities	Range
Milestone 1: Problem	• Interviews with clinical users • Primary research with patients • Patient journey mapping • Mock-ups and models	$30K-$100K
	• Market segmentation • Test business model with a short list of prospective partners • Establish path to pilots.	$30K-$50K
Milestone 2: Path	Stand alone application/treatment/intervention, validated with patients in a controlled setting	$100K-$300K
	Direct market research with consumers to develop messaging and pricing, and to understand perceived trust-worthiness of various channels (e.g. pharmacies, insurance, social media, primary care)	$50K-$100K
	Complete solution designed to integrate with clinical systems and ensure compliance with data security and privacy regulations	$100K-$300K
	Front end UX and dashboards, with inputs from users, buyers and business partners	$100K-$200K
Milestone 3: Proof	• Design measures to assess business and clinical outcomes • Structure and run a pilot implementation • Collaborate with independent clinical users to collect data.	$100K-$500K

This case study demonstrates utilization of the Commercial Development Framework described above for development of an online memory self-assessment for older adults by Cogniciti (www.cogniciti.com). The assessment was developed in collaboration with clinicians and researchers from Baycrest Hospital for Geriatric Care.

The tool is based on existing in-hospital tests that the research team rated as most sensitive for age-related brain health issues, including memory loss, attention loss, and decline in executive function. The self-assessment can be completed anonymously and in the privacy of home settings, and without the assistance of a health care professional All of which helps to lessen bias and provide a better picture of cognitive and mood health. Cogniciti's customers can determine how their cognitive function compares to population norms, and they are offered coping tools to support overall wellness and brain health.

Identifying brain health issues earlier supports earlier intervention, which may improve both quality of life and brain health outcomes. Anonymized and aggregated data are available to companies developing treatments for Mild Cognitive Impairment and Alzheimer.

Cogniciti's Assessment Tool generates a clinically relevant report based on population norms. The assessment report addresses an important communication gap in brain health monitoring.

- For those with health issues beyond what is expected in normal aging, combining a timely visit to the doctor's office with a means to clearly explain specific areas of difficulty helps doctors decide whether or not further investigation is warranted.
- For members of the inter-professional healthcare team the assessment report is a tool to triage patients in an expedient manner and gather all relevant information (meds, lifestyle, history, etc.) into a convenient format.
- For R&D groups developing interventions for mild cognitive impairment, these assessment data represent a rich resource for better targeting treatments.

CONCLUSION

Ways to reduce cost, improve quality, and improve customer engagement are top of mind for healthcare leaders. The health care delivery system that we are so familiar with was built in the 60's for a model focused upon hospitals and providers. As we transition care to lower cost centres, and put more focus on the wellness of individuals, we are in effect shifting our attention (and corresponding investments) away from institutional care, upstream towards prevention and better quality of life for consumers.

We can now build economical and powerful apps that deliver succinct, task oriented user experiences, thereby supporting patient-centred and collaborative care. By shifting some of the clinical responsibilities to lower cost settings, and powering clinical decisions with AI-mediated analytics, healthcare administrators aim to solve acute operational, economic and clinical problems.

However, to get the full economic potential and quality benefit from this Shift, healthcare is also going through a business re-design - realigning roles and accountabilities for providers, and developing entirely new ways of engaging empowered and informed consumers. The value chain of a $10 trillion global healthcare industry is changing, causing disruptions in established business models and opening myriad opportunities for innovation.

In his 2010, *Value In Health Care* framework, Michael E. Porter (2010) explains that Value brings together quality and cost, both defined around the patient. In his view, our system's failures to measure this Value – and to adopt it as the central goal in health care – have hobbled true innovation, allowing instead pseudo-innovations without meaningful value benefits. It has also resulted in ill-advised strategies for cost containment, including the micromanagement of physician practices, which imposes significant costs of its own. Failure to appropriately measure Value is one of the principal reasons that reform in health care has proven so problematic, as compared with reforms in other fields.

With advances in technology, we are now able to measure value in ways unachievable in the past. This journey has seen the introduction of an entirely new set of players, digital players. Commercially developed algorithms are capable of mining large, connected data sets and applications to present accurate information for patients and providers when they need it.

But how do we align these new digital capabilities with clinical and operational priorities, and further with individual privacy? Value exchanges in traditional consumer markets are not always altogether private. A lot more may be at stake for individuals choosing among surgeries vs. those choosing among brands of computer.

While technology tools – pervasive cloud technologies, mobility and analytics – have become readily, commercially available, an ethical value framework for their uses is as yet ill defined at best.

Healthcare systems around the world are reaching out for solutions. The trick is to re-engineer these health care systems to improve population health and provide quality care, all while confronted with persistent structural and cost pressures.

We need to empower quality and regulatory agencies to develop guidelines for data sharing that balance commercial innovation, the economics of a publicly funded healthcare sector, and individuals' ownership of their health data.

ACKNOWLEDGMENT

Lee Gotham: Editor, Corporate Communications, Konona Health

REFERENCES

Beck, S. L., Weiss, M. E., Ryan-Wenger, N., Donaldson, N. E., Aydin, C., Towsley, G. L., & Gardner, W. (2013, Apr). *Measuring nurses' impact on health care quality: Progress, challenges, and future directions.* Retrieved from http://www.ncbi.nlm.nih.gov/pubmed/23502913

Bircher, J., & Hahn, E. G. (2016, Feb 12) *Understanding the nature of health: New perspectives for medicine and public health. Improved wellbeing at lower costs.* Retrieved from http://www.ncbi.nlm.nih.gov/pmc/articles/PMC4837984/

Consumer e-Health: Patient-Generated Health Data. (n.d.). Retrieved from https://www.healthit.gov/policy-researchers-implementers/patient-generated-health-data

Dubbels, B. (2016). *The Vegas Effect: Serious Games Can Ensure Serious Learning.* Retrieved from https://www.academia.edu/9816169/The_Vegas_Effect_Serious_Games_Can_Ensure_Serious_Learning

Dwamena, F., Holmes-Rovner, M., Gaulden, C. M., Jorgenson, S., Sadigh, G., Sikorskii, A., & Olomu, A. et al. (2012, December 12). Interventions for providers to promote a patient-centred approach in clinical consultations. *Cochrane Database of Systematic Reviews.* Retrieved from http://www.ncbi.nlm.nih.gov/pubmed/23235595 PMID:23235595

Dweck, C. (2007). *Mindset: The New Psychology of Success.* New York: Ballantine Books.

El-Jawahri, A., Mitchell, S. L., Paasche-Orlow, M. K., Temel, J. S., Jackson, V. A., Rutledge, R. R., & Gillick, M. R. et al. (2015, August). A Randomized Controlled Trial of a CPR and Intubation Video Decision Support Tool for Hospitalized Patients. *Journal of General Internal Medicine.*

Ely, J. W., Osheroff, J. A., Ebell, M. H., Bergus, G. R., Levy, B. T., Chambliss, M. L., & Evans, E. R. (1999, August 7). Analysis of questions asked by family doctors regarding patient care. *BMJ (Clinical Research Ed.).*

Hibbard, J. H. (2013). *Patient Engagement, Health Policy Briefs.* Retrieved from http://www.healthaffairs.org/healthpolicybriefs/brief.php?brief_id=86

Hibbard, J. H., Stockard, J., Mahoney, E. R., & Tusler, M. (2004, August). Development of the Patient Activation Measure (PAM): Conceptualizing and Measuring Activation in Patients and Consumers. *Health Services Research.*

Institute for Healthcare Improvement. (2016). Retrieved from http://www.ihi.org/Engage/Initiatives/TripleAim/Pages/MeasuresResults.aspx

Investing in America's Health: A State-by-State Look at Public Health Funding and Key Health Facts. (2016, Apr). Trust for America's Health. Retrieved from http://healthyamericans.org/report/126/

Kostkova, P. (2015, May 5). *Frontiers in Public Health.* ubh.2015.0013410.3389/fp

Lomas, N. (2016, May 18). *Reporting for techcrunch.com, UK's MHRA (medicines and healthcare devices regulator) spokesperson in talks with Google/DeepMind over its Streams app.* Retrieved from https://techcrunch.com/2016/05/18/uk-healthcare-products-regulator-in-talks-with-googledeepmind-over-its-streams-app/

Mitton, C., & Donaldson, C. (2004). *Health care priority setting: Principles, Practice and Challenges, Cost Effectiveness and Resource Allocation* Retrieved from http://www.ncbi.nlm.nih.gov/pmc/articles/PMC411060/

Nash, D. (2010). *P & T: a Peer-reviewed Journal for Formulary Management.* Retrieved from http://europepmc.org/abstract/PMC/PMC2873722

Pincus, H. A., Hudson Scholle, S., Spaeth-Rublee, B., Hepner, K. A., & Brown, J. (2016, June 24). *Quality Measures For Mental Health And Substance Use: Gaps, Opportunities, And Challenges.* Retrieved from http://content.healthaffairs.org/content/35/6/1000.abstract?=right

Porter, M. E. (2010). What Is Value in Health Care? *The New England Journal of Medicine, 363*(26), 2477–2481. doi:10.1056/NEJMp1011024 PMID:21142528

Ries, E. (2011The Lean Startup. *Crown Publishing Group.*

Ryan, A. M., & Doran, T. (2012, Mar). *The effect of improving processes of care on patient outcomes: evidence from the United Kingdom's quality and outcomes framework.* Med Care. Retrieved from http://www.ncbi.nlm.nih.gov/pubmed/22329994

Scott, A., Sivey, P., Ait Ouakrim, D., Willenberg, L., Naccarella, L., Furler, J., & Young, D. (2011, September 7). The effect of financial incentives on the quality of health care provided by primary care physicians. *Cochrane Database of Systematic Reviews.* doi:10.1002/14651858.CD008451.pub2 PMID:21901722

Spencer, K., Sanders, C., Whitley, E. A., Lund, D., Kaye, J., & Dixon, W. G. (2016). Patient Perspectives on Sharing Anonymized Personal Health Data Using a Digital System for Dynamic Consent and Research Feedback: A Qualitative Study. *Journal of Medical Internet Research, 18*(4), e66. doi:10.2196/jmir.5011 PMID:27083521

The Collection, Linking and Use of Data in Biomedical Research and Health Care: Ethical Issues. (2015). Nuffield Council on Bioethics. Retrieved from http://nuffieldbioethics.org/project/biological-health-data/

Thorne, S. E., & Paterson, B. L. (2000). Two decades of insider research: What we know and don't know about chronic illness experience. *Annual Review of Nursing Research.*

This research was previously published in Transforming Gaming and Computer Simulation Technologies across Industries edited by Brock Dubbels, pages 246-257, copyright year 2017 by Information Science Reference (an imprint of IGI Global).

Chapter 63

A Stepped Care mHealth–Based Approach for Promoting Patient Engagement in Chronic Care Management of Obesity With Type 2 Diabetes

Gianluca Castelnuovo
Catholic University of the Sacred Heart, Italy

Emanuele Maria Giusti
Catholic University of the Sacred Heart, Italy

Giada Pietrabissa
Catholic University of the Sacred Heart, Italy

Francesco Borgia
Istituto Auxologico Italiano IRCCS, Italy

Gian Mauro Manzoni
Catholic University of the Sacred Heart, Italy

Enrico Molinari
Catholic University of the Sacred Heart, Italy

Stefania Corti
Istituto Auxologico Italiano IRCCS, Italy

Nicole Ann Middleton
University of South Australia, Australia

Margherita Novelli
Istituto Auxologico Italiano IRCCS, Italy

Roberto Cattivelli
Istituto Auxologico Italiano IRCCS, Italy

Maria Borrello
University of Bergamo, Italy

Susan Simpson
University of South Australia, Australia

ABSTRACT

Diabesity could be defined as a new global epidemic of obesity and being overweight with many complications and chronic conditions. The financial direct and indirect burden of diabesity is a real challenge in many Western health-care systems. Even if multidisciplinary protocols have been implemented, significant limitations in the chronic care management of obesity with type 2 diabetes concern costs and long-term adherence and efficacy. mHealth approach could overcome limitations linked with the traditional, restricted and highly expensive in-patient treatment of diabesity. The mHealth approach could help clinicians by motivating patients in remote settings to develop healthier lifestyles and could be implemented in the Chronic Care Model. A practical stepped-care model for diabesity, including mhealth approach and psychological treatments with different intensity, is discussed.

DOI: 10.4018/978-1-5225-3926-1.ch063

FACING DIABESITY WITH A CHRONIC CARE MANAGEMENT APPROACH: REDUCING COSTS AND IMPROVING LONG-TERM ADHERENCE AND EFFICACY

Francine Kaufman coined the term "diabesity" (diabetes + obesity) to describe the dangerous combination of obesity, insulin resistance, metabolic syndrome and type 2 diabetes (Jones, 2006; Kresser, 2014a, 2014b; Leiter et al., 2013).

Diabesity could be defined as a new global epidemic of obesity and being overweight with many complications and chronic conditions. Such conditions include not only type 2 diabetes, but also cardiovascular diseases, hypertension, dyslipidemia, hypercholesterolemia, cancer, and various psychosocial and psychopathological disorders (Byrne, Cooper, & Fairburn, 2004; Castelnuovo et al., 2014; Flegal, Graubard, Williamson, & Gail, 2005; Wadden, Brownell, & Foster, 2002; Whitlock et al., 2009).

The etiology of diabesity is universally recognized as multifactorial with a complex interaction between genetic, individual, and environmental factors (Marcus & Wildes, 2009). Genetics plays an important role, but behavioral factors, such as a dysfunctional diet and low physical activity, are among the main modifiable and proximal causes strictly connected to obesity and obesity-related complications (Dombrowski et al., 2012).

Diabetes is emerging as a relevant chronic disease in the USA, particularly among children. The financial direct and indirect burden (considering also the clinical resources involved and the loss of productivity) is a real challenge in many Western health-care systems (Malvey & Slovensky, 2014). The total costs of diagnosed diabetes grew from US$ 174 billion in 2007 to US$ 245 billion in 2012 with an increasing of 41 (American Diabetes Association [ADA], 2013).

With respect to the significant health care costs associated with treating obesity and type 2 diabetes, recently the Lancet journal defined diabetes as a 21st-century challenge: "the economic effect of diabetes is enormous. In 2010, global health expenditure attributable to diabetes was estimated to be US$376 billion—that is, 12% of all global health expenditure. In the USA in 2012, the direct medical cost of diabetes was $176 billion" (McCormick & Stone, 2007, p. 60; Zimmet, Magliano, Herman, & Shaw, 2014).

About obesity, different opportunities for prevention and treatment approaches targeting a part of or the entire population have been studied and are well described in (Rothberg, Peeters, & Herman, 2014): "Obesity may be viewed as a continuum with at least three opportunities for intervention... Primary prevention targets the entire population. Indeed, almost everyone in the population is at risk for obesity... Delaying the onset of obesity or limiting its severity may reduce its comorbidities and complications. Interventions for primary prevention focus on decreasing energy intake, increasing energy expenditure, or both. They may include health-care, community, or environmental measures to encourage people to eat less, be more active, and maintain a healthy weight.

Secondary interventions target people with obesity at high risk for complications, such as those with glucose intolerance at risk for type 2 diabetes or those with hypertension or dyslipidemia at risk for cardiovascular disease. Targeted lifestyle interventions and medications may produce and maintain weight loss, improve risk factors, and delay or prevent complications.

Tertiary interventions target people with severe obesity and its attendant complications, such as type 2 diabetes and coronary artery disease. For such individuals, bariatric surgery can induce weight loss and delay or prevent the development of additional complications including diabetic microvascular and neuropathic complications, myocardial infarction, and death. All interventions have the potential to delay comorbidities and complications, reduce costs, and improve quality of life and survival" (pp. 453-454).

In order to promote patient engagement and compliance in diabesity treatment while reducing costs, evidence-based interventions to improve weight-loss, maintain a healthy weight, and reduce related comorbidities combine different treatment approaches: dietetic, nutritional, physical, behavioral, psychological, and, in some situations, pharmacological and surgical. Moreover new technologies can provide useful solutions in this multidisciplinary approach.

Even if multidisciplinary protocols have been implemented, significant limitations in the chronic care management of obesity with type 2 diabetes concern costs and long-term adherence and efficacy.

Another limitation is the difficulty associated with maintaining long-term compliance and adherence in order to ensure clinical efficacy. "In fact, most overweight and obese individuals regain about one third of the weight lost with treatment within one year and they will typically come back to baseline in three to five years" (Pietrabissa et al., 2012, p. 317). Specifically in relation to diabetes, "Lifestyle intervention has been effective in several countries, but its success depends on uptake of intervention programmes and on compliance ... An urgent priority is to identify ways to effectively engage people at risk of diabetes. Long-term sustainability is also a concern" (Zimmet et al., 2014, pp. 61-62).

THE KEY ROLE OF PSYCHOLOGICAL INTERVENTIONS TO IMPROVE MOTIVATION, COMPLIANCE AND ENGAGEMENT IN DIABESITY TREATMENT

Assessment of patients' motivation, compliance, and engagement is a key factor of treatment for obesity with type 2 diabetes (Barello, Graffigna, & Vegni, 2012; Waller, Stringer, & Meyer, 2012).

Psychological therapies with diet and exercise plans could better help patients in achieving weight loss outcomes, both inside hospitals and clinical centers and during out-patient follow-up sessions (Swencionis & Rendell, 2012; Wing, 2002).

Some psychological skills should be implemented for functional chronic care management of obesity and its complications. Such skills include determining the client's ability to self-monitor (e.g., using diaries), assistance with stimulus control through restricting quantities of food, and behavioral modification strategies (e.g., chewing slowly, taking time to enjoy food, and increasing awareness of the pleasure associated with taste and food) (Foster, Makris, & Bailer, 2005; Swencionis & Rendell, 2012; Wing, 2002). Specific psychological actions are also required in order to maintain goals that have initially been achieved, manage possible relapses, and learn strategies to cope with critical situations (Capodaglio et al., 2013; Dombrowski, Avenell, & Sniehott, 2011; Dombrowski et al., 2012; Manzoni et al., 2010; Manzoni et al., 2011b).

In the management of chronic diseases clinical psychology plays a key role (Castelnuovo, 2010a, 2010b), due to the need of working on psychological conditions of patients, their families and their caregivers (de Ridder, Geenen, Kuijer, & van Middendorp, 2008; Levy, Nocerini, & Grazier, 2007; Pagnini et al., 2012; Pagnini et al., 2011; Pagnini et al., 2010), particularly with cardiovascular diseases where psychological variables (anxiety, stress, depression, etc.) have a significant impact in the organic worsening and demanding caregiving with developed case management skills is requested, even if relatives and caregivers are not well trained in accomplishing healthcare tasks (Hemingway & Marmot, 1999a, 1999b; Manzoni, Castelnuovo, & Proietti, 2011; Rozanski, Blumenthal, & Kaplan, 1999). About chronic disease management programs focused on containing costs and improve health outcomes (Villagra, 2004; Villagra & Ahmed, 2004), Mercer noted that "What emerged from these early programs was an understanding that quality improvement and cost reductions could be achieved through enhancing disease process understanding and attending to the psychological aspects of health and illness (Levy et al., 2007; Schneiderman, Antoni, Saab, & Ironson, 2001)" (Mercer, 2011, p. 151).

THE MHEALTH OPPORTUNITY

eHealth could be traditionally defined as a growing field of health services provided through the Internet and other new technologies (Eysenbach, 2001). mHealth (also m-health, mhealth, or mobile health) could be considered an evolution of eHealth and could be defined as the practice of medicine and public health supported by mobile communication devices, such as mobile phones, tablet computers, and PDAs, for health services and information (Castelnuovo et al., 2014; Cipresso et al., 2012; Eysenbach, 2011; Fiordelli, Diviani, & Schulz, 2013; Riper et al., 2010; Whittaker, 2012). Another interesting definition of mHealth, provided in an engineering field, defines it as "the practice of eHealth supported by mobile devices and smartphones, which are used to capture, analyze, store, and transmit health-related information from various sources including personal inputs, sensors, and other biomedical acquisition systems" (Adibi, 2015, p. 2).

mHealth approach could overcome limitations linked with the traditional, restricted and highly expensive in-patient treatment of many chronic pathologies: one of the best up-to-date application is the management of obesity with type 2 diabetes, where mHealth solutions can provide remote opportunities for enhancing weight reduction and reducing complications from clinical, organizational and economic perspectives (Castelnuovo et al., 2015b; Khaylis, Yiaslas, Bergstrom, & Gore-Felton, 2010; Manzoni, Castelnuovo, & Molinari, 2008; Manzoni, Pagnini, Corti, Molinari, & Castelnuovo, 2011a; Rao et al., 2011). Specifically for diabetes management Chomutare, Fernandez-Luque, Arsand and Hartvigsen (2011) reported more than 260 different diabetes applications (for Nokia Symbian, BlackBerry, Apple iPhone and Google Android), able to manage many features of the diabetes management, self-monitoring, blood glucose, weight, physical activity, diet, insulin and medication, blood pressure, education, disease-related alerts and reminders, integration of social media functions (Santoro, 2013; Santoro, Caldarola, & Villella, 2011; Santoro & Quintaliani, 2013), disease-related data export and communication, synchronization with personal health record (PHR) systems, and patient portals (Chomutare et al., 2011).

Programs with mHealth, defined as the practice of medicine and public health supported by mobile communication devices (Castelnuovo et al., 2014; Cipresso et al., 2012; Eysenbach, 2001, 2011; Fiordelli et al., 2013; Riper et al., 2010; Whittaker, 2012), could overcome limitations connected to the traditional in-patient chronic care management of obesity with type 2 diabetes by providing promising opportunities for enhancing weight reduction and reducing complications in terms of long-term efficacy and effectiveness across clinical, organizational, and economic perspectives (Khaylis et al., 2010; Manzoni et al., 2011a; Rao et al., 2011). These technology-based strategies provided in out-patient settings are based on a collaborative approach derived from central planning and grounded in chronic care logic (Rao et al., 2011).

Applications have also been shown to increase participation, compliance, and engagement (Graffigna, Barello, & Riva, 2013; Graffigna, Barello, Wiederhold, Bosio, & Riva, 2013).

Khaylis et al. (2010) underlined five psychological components (Self-monitoring, Counselor feedback and communication, Social support, Structured program, Individually-tailored program) necessary for functional necessary for functional mHealth-based chronic case management in order to facilitate weight loss and a reduction of comorbidities such as type 2 diabetes.

There is a critical need for scientific research to evaluate the specific outcomes of collaborative approaches for weight management that utilize the Internet and mobile-based tools (Turner-McGrievy et al., 2013).

The mHealth approach could help clinicians by motivating patients in remote settings to develop healthier lifestyles (Castelnuovo, 2010a; Pietrabissa et al., 2012), to accept more intrusive medical treatments, and to cope with chronic conditions by reducing complications (such as type 2 diabetes, hypertension, and cardiovascular disease) (Nguyen & Lau, 2012). In order to deal with lifestyle diseases and to prevent chronic medical conditions, mobile applications are able to measure the physical activity of a patient or user, also in a free-living monitoring environment (Torres-Huitzil & Alvarez-Landero, 2015).

The mHealth approach could be implemented in the Chronic Care Model, developed by Wagner (Glasgow, Orleans, & Wagner, 2001; Wagner et al., 2001a; Wagner et al., 2001b), that is based on the collaboration between a well coordinated team of clinicians-providers and an activated-engaged patient, promoting self-management skills, tracking and sharing information about patient health status and treatment programs, focusing on the family, social and community networks (O'Donnell, 2011).

mHealth provides the possibility to monitor oneself or for a clinician to monitor a patient through a mobile platform or device accessing to important information in real time. The smartphone applications can also deliver "education about diet, exercises, health reminders, community resources, and local healthcare providers" (Moss Richins, 2015, p. 24). These opportunities are very important above all for seniors and for people living alone and dealing with diabetes (Javitt, 2014), encouraging the elderly to carry on a healthy lifestyle.

Different clinical applications have been developed about the utility of mobile phones in promoting weight loss behaviors, healthy lifestyle and comorbidities reduction (Bacigalupo et al., 2013; Burke et al., 2012; Cafazzo, Casselman, Hamming, Katzman, & Palmert, 2012; Castelnuovo et al., 2010; Chomutare et al., 2011; Fiordelli et al., 2013; Hebden et al., 2013; Manzoni et al., 2011a; Martinez-Perez, de la Torre-Diez, & Lopez-Coronado, 2013; Park & Kim, 2012; Pellegrini et al., 2012; Rao et al., 2011; Rodrigues, Lopes, Silva, & Torre Ide, 2013; Schiel, Kaps, & Bieber, 2012; Schoffman, Turner-McGrievy, Jones, & Wilcox, 2013; Sharifi et al., 2013; Shaw et al., 2013; Simpson & Slowey, 2011; Turner-McGrievy et al., 2013)

Even if 1 million mobile device applications have been developed (Chouffani, 2013), up to date diabesity monitoring methods do not satisfy patients' requirements and are not so effective in helping people control the disease. As noted by (Shaheen, Mohammed, & Grbic, 2015), results performed for e-health in Finland (Ekroos & Jalonen, 2007) expressed the potential to provide interactive devices useful to engage diabetic patients in the self-management and to improve communications between patients and healthcare providers, but mobile services and biosensors are lacking in encouraging physical activities for diabetic patients in community settings for achieving a better lifestyle. "What is needed is an effective self-management wireless solution that collects, stores, and transmits these important parameters in real time to the health professionals and receives a feedback correspondingly" (Shaheen et al., 2015, p. 52).

THE STEPPED-CARE OPPORTUNITY

In the pioneering book *Stepped Care and e-Health Practical Applications to Behavioral Disorders*, O'Donohue and Draper (2011b, pp. 5-6) proposed a practical stepped-care model for many pathologies, including chronic conditions. A list of the health care "steps" is indicated below:

1. **Assessment and Triage:** This information can be used to determine which step is the best step for an individual in beginning treatment... also consider*ing* how there can be a stepped-care model within the assessment process. For example... consider*ing* more and less intense screening and assessment modules and those that can be used with and without a trained therapist or varying degrees of using therapist time.

2. **Watchful Waiting:** This information can be used to determine which disorders may show a natural return to baseline and disappear without specific intervention... *considering* the idea that immediate treatment after the incident may actually be iatrogenic and... when an individual may want to seek the next level of care.

3. **Psychoeducation:** This type of low-intensity intervention includes several modalities of providing simple information about disorders, treatment for disorders, or other expectations. This can be delivered via web sites, books, pamphlets, groups and classes, or any other mode of information delivery.

4. **Bibliotherapy:** Bibliotherapy, or self-help, is broadly the use of text to implement behavior change or to see movement on a given disorder. The most widely used form of bibliotherapy is self-help books, but *there are also* non interactive web sites and occasionally even videos. Bibliotherapy generally provides consumers with an active intervention including homework (usually in the form of workbooks).

5. **E-Health:** E-health is a broad term, which in this text refers to the use of technology to provide tailored or interactive modules in addition to the treatment that may be used in bibliotherapy. This includes both computer-based interventions (CBIs), in which there is little or no therapist contact, and computer-assisted interventions (CAIs), in which a therapist plays a role in the treatment, although the treatment is delivered largely via computer and may also include adjuncts including the use of electronics such as palm devices or text messaging to enhance other modalities of treatment.

6. **Group Therapy:** This form of therapy may vary greatly in where it falls in the stepped-care model, depending on the structure and purpose of the group. Groups can range from support groups led by non therapists to psychoeducational groups delivered between one or several meetings, to treatments similar to individual treatments, but minimizing therapist time by providing the same information and intervention for multiple people at once.

7. **Individual Therapy:** This step is what we usually would refer to as simply "therapy" and is the portion in the model that has received by far the most research. This step is commonly among the first step for most people who seek treatment (along with medication), and many practitioners accept this and do not triage to lower levels when indicated... This norm is not necessarily the most practical and does not necessarily provide better outcomes.

8. **Medical and Medication:** This step is, for some disorders, often found to be the first line of treatment even when this is counter-indicated by current research. In the treatment of many disorders, this may actually be considered among the last steps of a fail-forward attempt, generally due to side effects and often showing higher cost in the long-term.

9. **Inpatient Treatment:** This step is widely seen as the highest step in the treatment of any disorder and is often only indicated in the event of failures of previous steps.

New technologies play an important role in this model (point 5), even if mHealth does not express all its potentiality in the O'Donohue and Draper model (2011b).

Working out the previous Von Korff and Tiemens's proposal (Von Korff & Tiemans, 2000), a strong model of stepped care based on mhealth is proposed by O'Donnell (2011, p. 265): "The stepped care model is based on the acknowledgement that (1) different patients require different levels of care; (2) the most appropriate level of care is based on closely monitoring outcomes; and (3) moving from lower to more intensive levels of care based on patient response can increase the effectiveness of care while lowering overall costs". Stepped care is "potentially much more consistent with the ethical imperative of choosing the least intrusive intervention for one's patient" (O'Donohue & Draper, 2011a, p. 3). Using this approach, many efforts in the research field have to be focused not only on the development of new clinical protocols or therapies, but in the validation of new health-care delivery model, measuring its reliability, affordability, safety, efficiency and user satisfaction (where users are patients, professionals, stakeholders, etc.) and demonstrating that this model can improve the quality of care and reduce costs (Mercer, 2011; Neumeyer-Gromen, Lampert, Stark, & Kallischnigg, 2004; O'Donohue & Draper, 2011a; Ofman et al., 2004; Weingarten et al., 2002).

According to Bower and Gilbody (2005), psychological treatments with different intensity are necessary in a stepped care approach and they can offer less intensive treatments, such as brief therapies, group approaches, self-help opportunities (bibliotherapy, pc-based treatments). Moreover the stepped care framework could provide significant benefits: minimal interventions can ensure health gains equivalent or similar to that of traditional psychotherapies, reduce costs optimizing healthcare resources in an efficient way, be recognized and considered acceptable for both patients and clinicians.

About a possible economic evaluation of stepped care models in diabesity management, unfortunately empirical data from long term randomized controlled clinical trials are lacking, above all in providing few years of follow-up (less than 4 years and 1 or 2 years of reliable empirical data (Rothberg et al., 2014).

A deep and interesting economic analysis for the US situation is reported by Rothberg et al. (2014, p. 468): "Although lifestyle, pharmacologic, and surgical interventions to prevent and treat obesity appear to be cost-effective, they may have very different cost implications to a health system or society. To understand the cost of an intervention, one must consider the size of the target population and the cost of the intervention... The normal weight and overweight population (66% of U.S. adults $\geq$20 years of age) is large compared to the population with obesity (28% of U.S. adults) and those populations are large compared to the population with severe obesity (6% of U.S. adults). Conversely, the per person cost of a mass media campaign, a new tax, or a regulatory policy, or even a healthy lifestyle intervention for the general population, is low compared to that of a targeted intensive lifestyle intervention, pharmacotherapy, or bariatric surgery. The total costs of an intervention are the product of the number of people in the target population and the per person cost of the intervention. An inexpensive intervention applied to many people may incur total costs as large as those of an expensive intervention applied to a few people. For this reason, even inexpensive interventions applied to large populations may have a substantial cost burden, while very expensive interventions, targeted to small subsets of people, may have smaller cost burdens. At the same time, a less effective intervention broadly applied may result in a greater improvement in the health of the population than a very effective (and expensive) intervention applied to a few people. It is likely that a combination of effective and cost-effective approaches will be needed to address the epidemic of obesity. A range of cost-effective interventions appropriate for each stage of prevention and treatment, from childhood to adulthood, should be implemented".

A STEPPED CARE MHEALTH-BASED APPROACH AS A PERSPECTIVE IN CHRONIC CARE MANAGEMENT OF OBESITY WITH TYPE 2 DIABETES

This section will discuss the feasibility of a stepped care mHealth-based approach as a perspective in chronic care management of obesity with type 2 diabetes. One promising future direction could be treating obesity, considered as a chronic multifactorial disease, using a stepped-care approach (Castelnuovo et al., 2015b; Organization, 2011) as well described in Castelnuovo et al. (2015a):

- The lower level of treatment could be simply a *mhealth or traditional based lifestyle psychoeducational and nutritional approach* to weight management. This step could be also considered as a prevention phase at the population level.
- The following step, useful in moderate conditions, could be represented by the inclusion in *health professionals-driven multidisciplinary protocols* tailored for each patient. The mhealth approach could be useful for providing many parts of the clinical program reducing costs and limiting hospitalizations.
- Another step of care, useful in severe conditions, could be the *inpatient approach with the inclusion of drug therapies and other multidisciplinary treatments* if necessary. The mhealth contribution could be useful for monitoring and motivating patients after the inpatient phase and for reducing costs above all in the follow-up steps.
- Another step, in more severe conditions, needs the solution of *bariatric surgery* and with this option the mhealth approach could be useful for monitoring eating attitudes, motivating patients in changing dysfunctional behaviors and for reducing costs above all in the follow-up steps.

In the chronic care management of globesity mhealth solutions cannot substitute traditional approaches, but they can supplement some steps in obesity prevention and weight loss management, above all in the follow-up phase where the mobile technology can ensure a continuity of care saving costs and avoiding long term lack of connections between patients-citizens and the health care team. (Castelnuovo et al., 2015b, p. 4).

A similar scenario will be possible, from a technological point of view, with the growing development of biomedical devices, sensors and smartphone applications, as well described in (Torres-Huitzil & Alvarez-Landero, 2015): "Micro electromechanical systems (MEMS) sensors have already enable smartphones to provide services that deeply affect the user style of life. For instance, through embedded inertial sensors, smartphones are able to respond to hand gestures, support virtual reality applications, or provide information about physical activities that a user performs and infer knowledge about health status. Currently smartphones are able to hear, see, touch, feel and smell and truly act as sensor hubs and their derived services increasingly rely on how well they know the user and user context. Such smartphone perceptual capabilities are possible thanks to the seamless integration of sensors, at hardware level, into the smartphone complex software stack... In spite of the continuous advance of mobile multicore processors, the resources demands and bandwidths of new and future sensors will become so significant that current mobile operating systems, such as Android, for sensor-streams handling will not be enough. Sensors with high bandwidth demands will require additional processing power that can only be provided by additional hardware working closely to the sensor chip... Thus, developing industry standards for sensor integration in smartphone platforms coupled with the almost unlimited computing capabilities from the cloud is required so as to meet the sensor-processing demand of future cognitive smartphones. With the advance of sensing technology for gathering data about human health and the environment integrated in smartphones it is possible to envisage a great impact in mHealth for the next years" (pp. 165-166).

If the technological component is ready to sustain a stepped care mhealth-based approach, the ideal management and organization of stepped care is not so clear (Bower & Gilbody, 2005). "Although there is some supportive evidence for the use of stepped care, rigorous evaluations of the underlying assumptions are scarce, and a significant research agenda remains. Modelling may be a useful research method in the shorter term" (Bower & Gilbody, 2005, p. 15).

HOW A MHEALTH-BASED APPROACH CAN ENHANCE THE PATIENT ENGAGEMENT IN OBESITY WITH TYPE 2 DIABETES

According to Rodriguez (2013), patients with obesity and diabetes could have different abilities and engaging motivations about the necessary self-management behaviors: these differences are due to several intrinsic and extrinsic factors, such as health beliefs, self-efficacy, level of diabetes knowledge and technical skills, functional health literacy and medication adherence.

About health beliefs, patients with diabesity usually think that a good parameter to evaluate their health status could be the presence/absence of symptoms, whereas obesity with diabetes is a silent condition "until hypoglycemia occurs or the development of a complication arises" (Rodriguez, 2013, p. 172). So engaging patients using the long term risk of complications is not successful. The most motivating approach is to show short-term gains working on day-to-day challenges patients face in managing their diabetes. Mobile health solutions can foster the achievement of these results providing progressive feedbacks where and when necessary, even in everyday life situations.

About self-efficacy mhealth can improve the self-perceived coping skills of each patient in keeping on diabetes self-management activities. Providing real-time and on-line feedbacks about patients' actions, mhealth solutions can foster the active participation of clients (and caregivers) in their own care.

About knowledge-technical skills and functional health literacy, new technologies could create useful solutions in providing up-to-date reliable clinical knowledge in real time that can enhance functional self-management approaches. Moreover mhealth-based clinical records and social media could improve documentation sharing and communication between patients, parents, caregivers, health care professionals, researchers, and stakeholders (Santoro, 2015; Santoro, Castelnuovo, Zoppis, Mauri, & Sicurello, 2015).

CONCLUSION

In diabesity, a key role for a successful chronic care management is to engage patients in healthy behaviors, such as a diet and physical exercise. mhealth approach can provide good solutions such as smartphone-based apps that can create or receive from a server a daily list of things to do, a system to track patients' exercises and reminders to take their medications (Brimmer, 2014; Moss Richins, 2015).

REFERENCES

Adibi, S. (2015). Introduction. In S. Adibi (Ed.), *mHealth Multidisciplinary Verticals* (pp. 1–10). London: CRC Press, Taylor & Francis Group.

American Diabetes Association. (2013). American Diabetes Association releases new research estimating annual cost of diabetes at $ 245 billion. Retrieved from http://www.diabetes.org/for-media/2013/annual-costs-of-diabetes-2013.html?loc=cost-of-diabetes

Bacigalupo, R., Cudd, P., Littlewood, C., Bissell, P., Hawley, M. S., & Buckley Woods, H. (2013). Interventions employing mobile technology for overweight and obesity: An early systematic review of randomized controlled trials. *Obesity Reviews*, *14*(4), 279–291. doi:10.1111/obr.12006 PMID:23167478

Barello, S., Graffigna, G., & Vegni, E. (2012). Patient engagement as an emerging challenge for healthcare services: Mapping the literature. *Nursing Research and Practice*, *2012*, 905934. doi:10.1155/2012/905934 PMID:23213497

Bower, P., & Gilbody, S. (2005). Stepped care in psychological therapies: Access, effectiveness and efficiency. Narrative literature review. *The British Journal of Psychiatry*, *186*(1), 11–17. doi:10.1192/bjp.186.1.11 PMID:15630118

Brimmer, K. (2014, June 2). New technologies, hospital strategies promote patient engagement. *Healthcare Finance News*.

Burke, L. E., Styn, M. A., Sereika, S. M., Conroy, M. B., Ye, L., Glanz, K., & Ewing, L. J. et al. (2012). Using mHealth technology to enhance self-monitoring for weight loss: A randomized trial. *American Journal of Preventive Medicine*, *43*(1), 20–26. doi:10.1016/j.amepre.2012.03.016 PMID:22704741

Byrne, S. M., Cooper, Z., & Fairburn, C. G. (2004). Psychological predictors of weight regain in obesity. *Behaviour Research and Therapy*, *42*(11), 1341–1356. doi:10.1016/j.brat.2003.09.004 PMID:15381442

Cafazzo, J. A., Casselman, M., Hamming, N., Katzman, D. K., & Palmert, M. R. (2012). Design of an mHealth app for the self-management of adolescent type 1 diabetes: A pilot study. *Journal of Medical Internet Research*, *14*(3), e70. doi:10.2196/jmir.2058 PMID:22564332

Capodaglio, P., Lafortuna, C., Petroni, M. L., Salvadori, A., Gondoni, L., Castelnuovo, G., & Brunani, A. (2013). Rationale for hospital-based rehabilitation in obesity with comorbidities. *European Journal of Physical and Rehabilitation Medicine*, *49*(3), 399–417. PMID:23736902

Castelnuovo, G. (2010a). Empirically supported treatments in psychotherapy: Towards an evidence-based or evidence-biased psychology in clinical settings? *Frontiers in Psychology*, *1*, 27. PMID:21833197

Castelnuovo, G. (2010b). No medicine without psychology: The key role of psychological contribution in clinical settings. *Frontiers in Psychology*, *1*, 4. doi:10.3389/fpsyg.2010.00004 PMID:21833187

Castelnuovo, G., Manzoni, G. M., Cuzziol, P., Cesa, G. L., Tuzzi, C., Villa, V., & Molinari, E. et al. (2010). TECNOB: Study design of a randomized controlled trial of a multidisciplinary telecare intervention for obese patients with type-2 diabetes. *BMC Public Health*, *10*(1), 204. doi:10.1186/1471-2458-10-204 PMID:20416042

Castelnuovo, G., Manzoni, G. M., Pietrabissa, G., Corti, S., Giusti, E. M., Molinari, E., & Simpson, S. (2014). Obesity and outpatient rehabilitation using mobile technologies: The potential mHealth approach. *Frontiers in Psychology, 5*, 559. doi:10.3389/fpsyg.2014.00559 PMID:24959157

Castelnuovo, G., Pietrabissa, G., Manzoni, G. M., Corti, S., Ceccarini, M., Borrello, M., & Molinari, E. et al. (2015a). Chronic care management of globesity: Promoting healthier lifestyles in traditional and mHealth based settings. *Frontiers in Psychology*, October. PMID:26528215

Castelnuovo, G., Zoppis, I., Santoro, E., Ceccarini, M., Pietrabissa, G., Manzoni, G. M., & Sicurello, F. et al. (2015b). Managing chronic pathologies with a stepped mHealth-based approach in clinical psychology and medicine. *Frontiers in Psychology, 6*, 407. doi:10.3389/fpsyg.2015.00407 PMID:25926801

Chomutare, T., Fernandez-Luque, L., Arsand, E., & Hartvigsen, G. (2011). Features of mobile diabetes applications: Review of the literature and analysis of current applications compared against evidence-based guidelines. *Journal of Medical Internet Research, 13*(3), e65. doi:10.2196/jmir.1874 PMID:21979293

Chouffani, R. (2013). mHealth clinical apps impacting care, not just with consumers. *TechTarget*. Retrieved from http://searchhealthit.techtarget.com/opinion/MHealth-clinical-apps-impacting-care-not-just-with-consumers?asrc=EM_ERU_27369471&utm_medium=EM&utm_source=ERU&utm_campaign=20140320_ERU%20Transmission%20for%2003/20/2014%20(UserUniverse:%20732731)_myka-reports@techtarget.com&src=5223540

Cipresso, P., Serino, S., Villani, D., Repetto, C., Selitti, L., Albani, G., & Riva, G. et al. (2012). Is your phone so smart to affect your states? An exploratory study based on psychophysiological measures. *Neurocomputing, 84*, 23–30. doi:10.1016/j.neucom.2011.12.027

de Ridder, D., Geenen, R., Kuijer, R., & van Middendorp, H. (2008). Psychological adjustment to chronic disease. *Lancet, 372*(9634), 246–255. doi:10.1016/S0140-6736(08)61078-8 PMID:18640461

Dombrowski, S. U., Avenell, A., & Sniehott, F. F. (2011). Behavioural interventions for obese adults with additional risk factors for morbidity: Systematic review of effects on behaviour, weight and disease risk factors. *Obes Facts, 3*(6), 377–396. doi:10.1159/000323076 PMID:21196792

Dombrowski, S. U., Sniehotta, F. F., Avenell, A., Johnston, M., MacLennan, G., & Ara, Ã. (2012). Identifying active ingredients in complex behavioural interventions for obese adults with obesity-related co-morbidities or additional risk factors for co-morbidities: A systematic review. *Health Psychology Review, 6*(1), 7–32. doi:10.1080/17437199.2010.513298

Ekroos, N., & Jalonen, K. (2007). E-Health and diabetes care. *Journal of Telemedicine and Telecare, 13*(1), 22–23. doi:10.1258/135763307781645013

Eysenbach, G. (2001). What is e-health? *Journal of Medical Internet Research, 3*(2), e20. doi:10.2196/jmir.3.2.e20 PMID:11720962

Eysenbach, G. (2011). Can tweets predict citations? Metrics of social impact based on Twitter and correlation with traditional metrics of scientific impact. *Journal of Medical Internet Research, 13*(4), e123. doi:10.2196/jmir.2012 PMID:22173204

Fiordelli, M., Diviani, N., & Schulz, P. J. (2013). Mapping mHealth research: A decade of evolution. *Journal of Medical Internet Research, 15*(5), e95. doi:10.2196/jmir.2430 PMID:23697600

Flegal, K. M., Graubard, B. I., Williamson, D. F., & Gail, M. H. (2005). Excess deaths associated with underweight, overweight, and obesity. *Journal of the American Medical Association, 293*(15), 1861–1867. doi:10.1001/jama.293.15.1861 PMID:15840860

Foster, G. D., Makris, A. P., & Bailer, B. A. (2005). Behavioral treatment of obesity. *The American Journal of Clinical Nutrition, 82*(Suppl. 1), 230S–235S. PMID:16002827

Glasgow, R. E., Orleans, C. T., & Wagner, E. H. (2001). Does the chronic care model serve also as a template for improving prevention? *The Milbank Quarterly, 79*(4), 579–612. doi:10.1111/1468-0009.00222 PMID:11789118

Graffigna, G., Barello, S., & Riva, G. (2013). Technologies for patient engagement. *Health Affairs (Project Hope), 32*(6), 1172. doi:10.1377/hlthaff.2013.0279 PMID:23733998

Graffigna, G., Barello, S., Wiederhold, B. K., Bosio, A. C., & Riva, G. (2013). Positive technology as a driver for health engagement. *Studies in Health Technology and Informatics, 191*, 9–17. PMID:23792833

Hebden, L., Balestracci, K., McGeechan, K., Denney-Wilson, E., Harris, M., Bauman, A., & Allman-Farinelli, M. (2013). 'TXT2BFiT' a mobile phone-based healthy lifestyle program for preventing unhealthy weight gain in young adults: Study protocol for a randomized controlled trial. *Trials, 14*(1), 75. doi:10.1186/1745-6215-14-75 PMID:23506013

Hemingway, H., & Marmot, M. (1999a). Clinical Evidence: Psychosocial factors in the etiology and prognosis of coronary heart disease: systematic review of prospective cohort studies. *The Western Journal of Medicine, 171*(5-6), 342–350. PMID:18751201

Hemingway, H., & Marmot, M. (1999b). Evidence based cardiology: Psychosocial factors in the aetiology and prognosis of coronary heart disease. Systematic review of prospective cohort studies. *BMJ (Clinical Research Ed.), 318*(7196), 1460–1467. doi:10.1136/bmj.318.7196.1460 PMID:10346775

Javitt, J. (2014). Case study: Using mHealth to manage diabetes. *mHealth News*. Retrieved from http://www.mhealthnews.com/print/24916

Jones, V. (2006). The "Diabesity" Epidemic: Let's Rehabilitate America. *Medscape General Medicine, 8*(2), 34–34. PMID:16926773

Khaylis, A., Yiaslas, T., Bergstrom, J., & Gore-Felton, C. (2010). A review of efficacious technology-based weight-loss interventions: Five key components. *Telemedicine Journal and e-Health, 16*(9), 931–938. doi:10.1089/tmj.2010.0065 PMID:21091286

Kresser, C. (2014a). Diabesity Retrieved from http://chriskresser.com/diabesity#

Kresser, C. (2014b). Diabesity: the #1 cause of death and disease? Retrieved from http://chriskresser.com/diabesity-the-1-cause-of-death-and-disease

Leiter, E. H., Strobel, M., O'Neill, A., Schultz, D., Schile, A., & Reifsnyder, P. C. (2013). Comparison of Two New Mouse Models of Polygenic Type 2 Diabetes at the Jackson Laboratory, NONcNZO10Lt/J and TALLYHO/JngJ. *J Diabetes Res*, *2013*, 165327. doi:10.1155/2013/165327 PMID:23671854

Levy, P., Nocerini, R., & Grazier, K. (2007). Paying for disease management. *Disease Management*, *10*(4), 235–244. doi:10.1089/dis.2007.104646 PMID:17718662

Malvey, D., & Slovensky, D. J. (2014). mHealth. Transforming Healthcare. New York: Springer.

Manzoni, G. M., Castelnuovo, G., & Molinari, E. (2008). Weight loss with a low-carbohydrate, Mediterranean, or low-fat diet. *The New England Journal of Medicine*, *359*(20), 2170, author reply 2171–2172. PMID:19009669

Manzoni, G. M., Castelnuovo, G., & Proietti, R. (2011). Assessment of psychosocial risk factors is missing in the 2010 ACCF/AHA guideline for assessment of cardiovascular risk in asymptomatic adults. *Journal of the American College of Cardiology*, *57*(14), 1569–1570. doi:10.1016/j.jacc.2010.12.015 PMID:21453841

Manzoni, G. M., Cribbie, R. A., Villa, V., Arpin-Cribbie, C. A., Gondoni, L., & Castelnuovo, G. (2010). Psychological well-being in obese inpatients with ischemic heart disease at entry and at discharge from a four-week cardiac rehabilitation program. *Frontiers in Psychology*, *1*, 38. PMID:21833207

Manzoni, G. M., Pagnini, F., Corti, S., Molinari, E., & Castelnuovo, G. (2011a). Internet-based behavioral interventions for obesity: An updated systematic review. *Clinical Practice and Epidemiology in Mental Health*, *7*(1), 19–28. doi:10.2174/1745017901107010019 PMID:21552423

Manzoni, G. M., Villa, V., Compare, A., Castelnuovo, G., Nibbio, F., Titon, A. M., & Gondoni, L. A. et al. (2011b). Short-term effects of a multi-disciplinary cardiac rehabilitation programme on psychological well-being, exercise capacity and weight in a sample of obese in-patients with coronary heart disease: A practice-level study. *Psychology Health and Medicine*, *16*(2), 178–189. doi:10.1080/135485 06.2010.542167 PMID:21328146

Marcus, M. D., & Wildes, J. E. (2009). Obesity: Is it a mental disorder? *International Journal of Eating Disorders*, *42*(8), 739–753. doi:10.1002/eat.20725 PMID:19610015

Martinez-Perez, B., de la Torre-Diez, I., & Lopez-Coronado, M. (2013). Mobile health applications for the most prevalent conditions by the World Health Organization: Review and analysis. *Journal of Medical Internet Research*, *15*(6), e120. doi:10.2196/jmir.2600 PMID:23770578

McCormick, B., & Stone, I. (2007). Economic costs of obesity and the case for government intervention. *Obesity Reviews*, *8*(Suppl. 1), 161–164. doi:10.1111/j.1467-789X.2007.00337.x PMID:17316321

Mercer, V. (2011). Chronic Disease Management. In W. T. O'Donohue & C. Draper (Eds.), *Stepped Care and e-Health: Practical Applications to Behavioral Disorders* (pp. 151–179). New York: Springer. doi:10.1007/978-1-4419-6510-3_9

Moss Richins, S. (2015). *Emerging Technologies in Healthcare*. London: CRC Press, Taylor & Francis Group. doi:10.1201/b18431

Neumeyer-Gromen, A., Lampert, T., Stark, K., & Kallischnigg, G. (2004). Disease management programs for depression: A systematic review and meta-analysis of randomized controlled trials. *Medical Care*, *42*(12), 1211–1221. doi:10.1097/00005650-200412000-00008 PMID:15550801

Nguyen, T., & Lau, D. C. (2012). The obesity epidemic and its impact on hypertension. *The Canadian Journal of Cardiology*, *28*(3), 326–333. doi:10.1016/j.cjca.2012.01.001 PMID:22595448

O'Donnell, R. R. (2011). Stepped Care and E-Health in Behavioral Managed Care. In W. T. O'Donohue & C. Draper (Eds.), *Stepped Care and e-Health: Practical Applications to Behavioral Disorders* (pp. 263–282). New York: Springer. doi:10.1007/978-1-4419-6510-3_14

O'Donohue, W. T., & Draper, C. (2011a). The Case for Evidence-Based Stepped Care as Part of a Reformed Delivery System. In W. T. O'Donohue & C. Draper (Eds.), *Stepped Care and e-Health: Practical Applications to Behavioral Disorders* (pp. 1–16). New York: Springer. doi:10.1007/978-1-4419-6510-3_1

O'Donohue, W. T., & Draper, C. (Eds.). (2011b). *Stepped Care and e-Health: Practical Applications to Behavioral Disorders*. New York: Springer.

Ofman, J. J., Badamgarav, E., Henning, J. M., Knight, K., Gano, A. D. Jr, Levan, R. K., & Weingarten, S. R. et al. (2004). Does disease management improve clinical and economic outcomes in patients with chronic diseases? A systematic review. *The American Journal of Medicine*, *117*(3), 182–192. doi:10.1016/j.amjmed.2004.03.018 PMID:15300966

Organization, W. H. (2011). mHealth: New horizons for health through mobile technologies: Second global survey on eHealth. Global observatory for eHealth series (Vol. 3). Retrieved from http://www.who.int/goe/publications/goe_mhealth_web.pdf

Pagnini, F., Banfi, P., Lunetta, C., Rossi, G., Castelnuovo, G., Marconi, A., & Molinari, E. et al. (2012). Respiratory function of people with amyotrophic lateral sclerosis and caregiver distress level: A correlational study. *BioPsychoSocial Medicine*, *6*(1), 14. doi:10.1186/1751-0759-6-14 PMID:22721255

Pagnini, F., Lunetta, C., Rossi, G., Banfi, P., Gorni, K., Cellotto, N., & Corbo, M. et al. (2011). Existential well-being and spirituality of individuals with amyotrophic lateral sclerosis is related to psychological well-being of their caregivers. *Amyotrophic Lateral Sclerosis; Official Publication of the World Federation of Neurology Research Group on Motor Neuron Diseases*, *12*(2), 105–108. doi:10.3109/17482968.2010.502941 PMID:20653520

Pagnini, F., Rossi, G., Lunetta, C., Banfi, P., Castelnuovo, G., Corbo, M., & Molinari, E. (2010). Burden, depression, and anxiety in caregivers of people with amyotrophic lateral sclerosis. *Psychology Health and Medicine*, *15*(6), 685–693. doi:10.1080/13548506.2010.507773 PMID:21154021

Park, M. J., & Kim, H. S. (2012). Evaluation of mobile phone and Internet intervention on waist circumference and blood pressure in post-menopausal women with abdominal obesity. *International Journal of Medical Informatics*, *81*(6), 388–394. doi:10.1016/j.ijmedinf.2011.12.011 PMID:22265810

Pellegrini, C. A., Duncan, J. M., Moller, A. C., Buscemi, J., Sularz, A., DeMott, A., & Spring, B. et al. (2012). A smartphone-supported weight loss program: Design of the ENGAGED randomized controlled trial. *BMC Public Health*, *12*, 1041. PMID:23194256

Pietrabissa, G., Manzoni, G. M., Corti, S., Vegliante, N., Molinari, E., & Castelnuovo, G. (2012). Addressing motivation in globesity treatment: A new challenge for clinical psychology. *Frontiers in Psychology, 3*, 317. doi:10.3389/fpsyg.2012.00317 PMID:22969744

Rao, G., Burke, L. E., Spring, B. J., Ewing, L. J., Turk, M., Lichtenstein, A. H., & Coons, M. et al. (2011). New and emerging weight management strategies for busy ambulatory settings: A scientific statement from the American Heart Association endorsed by the Society of Behavioral Medicine. *Circulation, 124*(10), 1182–1203. doi:10.1161/CIR.0b013e31822b9543 PMID:21824925

Riper, H., Andersson, G., Christensen, H., Cuijpers, P., Lange, A., & Eysenbach, G. (2010). Theme issue on e-mental health: A growing field in internet research. *Journal of Medical Internet Research, 12*(5), e74. doi:10.2196/jmir.1713 PMID:21169177

Rodrigues, J. J., Lopes, I. M., Silva, B. M., & Torre Ide, L. (2013). A new mobile ubiquitous computing application to control obesity: SapoFit. *Informatics for Health & Social Care, 38*(1), 37–53. doi:10.3109/17538157.2012.674586 PMID:22657250

Rodriguez, K. M. (2013). Intrinsic and extrinsic factors affecting patient engagement in diabetes self-management: Perspectives of a certified diabetes educator. *Clinical Therapeutics, 35*(2), 170–178. doi:10.1016/j.clinthera.2013.01.002 PMID:23411000

Rothberg, A. E., Peeters, A., & Herman, W. H. (2014). Cost-Effectiveness of Obesity Prevention and Treatment. In A. G. Bray & C. Bouchard (Eds.), *Handbook of Obesity. Clinical Applications* (pp. 453–470). London: CRC Press, Taylor & Francis Group.

Rozanski, A., Blumenthal, J. A., & Kaplan, J. (1999). Impact of psychological factors on the pathogenesis of cardiovascular disease and implications for therapy. *Circulation, 99*(16), 2192–2217. doi:10.1161/01.CIR.99.16.2192 PMID:10217662

Santoro, E. (2013). [Social media and medical apps: how they can change health communication, education and care]. *Recenti Progressi in Medicina, 104*(5), 179–180. PMID:23748682

Santoro, E. (2015). [Social media and health communication: do we need rules?]. *Recenti Progressi in Medicina, 106*(1), 15–16. PMID:25621774

Santoro, E., Caldarola, P., & Villella, A. (2011). [Using Web 2.0 technologies and social media for the cardiologist's education and update]. *Giornale Italiano di Cardiologia, 12*(3), 174–181. PMID:21560473

Santoro, E., Castelnuovo, G., Zoppis, I., Mauri, G., & Sicurello, F. (2015). Social media and mobile applications in chronic disease prevention and management. *Frontiers in Psychology, 6*, 567. doi:10.3389/fpsyg.2015.00567 PMID:25999884

Santoro, E., & Quintaliani, G. (2013). [Using web 2.0 technologies and social media for the nephrologist]. *Giornale Italiano di Nefrologia, 30*(1). PMID:23832442

Schiel, R., Kaps, A., & Bieber, G. (2012). Electronic health technology for the assessment of physical activity and eating habits in children and adolescents with overweight and obesity IDA. *Appetite, 58*(2), 432–437. doi:10.1016/j.appet.2011.11.021 PMID:22155072

Schneiderman, N., Antoni, M. H., Saab, P. G., & Ironson, G. (2001). Health psychology: Psychosocial and biobehavioral aspects of chronic disease management. *Annual Review of Psychology, 52*(1), 555–580. doi:10.1146/annurev.psych.52.1.555 PMID:11148317

Schoffman, D. E., Turner-McGrievy, G., Jones, S. J., & Wilcox, S. (2013). Mobile apps for pediatric obesity prevention and treatment, healthy eating, and physical activity promotion: Just fun and games? *Translational Behavioral Medicine, 3*(3), 320–325. doi:10.1007/s13142-013-0206-3 PMID:24073184

Shaheen, S., Mohammed, A., & Grbic, N. (2015). Mobile Services for Diabetic Patients' Sustainable Lifestyle. In S. Adibi (Ed.), *mHealth Multidisciplinary Verticals* (pp. 51–61). London: CRC Press, Taylor & Francis Group.

Sharifi, M., Dryden, E. M., Horan, C. M., Price, S., Marshall, R., Hacker, K., & Taveras, E. M. et al. (2013). Leveraging text messaging and mobile technology to support pediatric obesity-related behavior change: A qualitative study using parent focus groups and interviews. *Journal of Medical Internet Research, 15*(12), e272. doi:10.2196/jmir.2780 PMID:24317406

Shaw, R. J., Bosworth, H. B., Silva, S. S., Lipkus, I. M., Davis, L. L., Sha, R. S., & Johnson, C. M. (2013). Mobile health messages help sustain recent weight loss. *The American Journal of Medicine, 126*(11), 1002–1009. doi:10.1016/j.amjmed.2013.07.001 PMID:24050486

Simpson, S. G., & Slowey, L. (2011). Video therapy for atypical eating disorder and obesity: A case study. *Clinical Practice and Epidemiology in Mental Health, 7*(1), 38–43. doi:10.2174/1745017901107010038 PMID:21559235

Swencionis, C., & Rendell, S. L. (2012). The psychology of obesity. *Abdominal Imaging, 37*(5), 733–737. doi:10.1007/s00261-012-9863-9 PMID:22392131

Torres-Huitzil, C., & Alvarez-Landero, A. (2015). Accelerometer-Based Human Activity Recognition in Smartphones for Healthcare Services. In S. Adibi (Ed.), *Mobile Health: A Technology Road Map* (pp. 147–170). Berlin: Springer. doi:10.1007/978-3-319-12817-7_7

Turner-McGrievy, G. M., Beets, M. W., Moore, J. B., Kaczynski, A. T., Barr-Anderson, D. J., & Tate, D. F. (2013). Comparison of traditional versus mobile app self-monitoring of physical activity and dietary intake among overweight adults participating in an mHealth weight loss program. *Journal of the American Medical Informatics Association, 20*(3), 513–518. doi:10.1136/amiajnl-2012-001510 PMID:23429637

Villagra, V. G. (2004). Integrating disease management into the outpatient delivery system during and after managed care. *Health Affairs (Project Hope)*, (Suppl. Web Exclusives), W4-281–283. PMID:15451998

Villagra, V. G., & Ahmed, T. (2004). Effectiveness of a disease management program for patients with diabetes. *Health Affairs (Project Hope), 23*(4), 255–266. doi:10.1377/hlthaff.23.4.255 PMID:15318587

Von Korff, M., & Tiemans, B. (2000). Individualized stepped care of chronic illness. *The Western Journal of Medicine, 172*(2), 133–137. doi:10.1136/ewjm.172.2.133 PMID:10693379

Wadden, T. A., Brownell, K. D., & Foster, G. D. (2002). Obesity: Responding to the global epidemic. *Journal of Consulting and Clinical Psychology, 70*(3), 510–525. doi:10.1037/0022-006X.70.3.510 PMID:12090366

Wagner, E. H., Austin, B. T., Davis, C., Hindmarsh, M., Schaefer, J., & Bonomi, A. (2001a). Improving chronic illness care: Translating evidence into action. *Health Affairs (Project Hope)*, *20*(6), 64–78. doi:10.1377/hlthaff.20.6.64 PMID:11816692

Wagner, E. H., Glasgow, R. E., Davis, C., Bonomi, A. E., Provost, L., McCulloch, D., & Sixta, C. et al. (2001b). Quality improvement in chronic illness care: A collaborative approach. *The Joint Commission Journal on Quality Improvement*, *27*(2), 63–80. PMID:11221012

Waller, G., Stringer, H., & Meyer, C. (2012). What cognitive behavioral techniques do therapists report using when delivering cognitive behavioral therapy for the eating disorders? *Journal of Consulting and Clinical Psychology*, *80*(1), 171–175. doi:10.1037/a0026559 PMID:22141595

Weingarten, S. R., Henning, J. M., Badamgarav, E., Knight, K., Hasselblad, V., Gano, A. Jr, & Ofman, J. J. (2002). Interventions used in disease management programmes for patients with chronic illness-which ones work? Meta-analysis of published reports. *BMJ (Clinical Research Ed.)*, *325*(7370), 925. doi:10.1136/bmj.325.7370.925 PMID:12399340

Whitlock, G., Lewington, S., Sherliker, P., Clarke, R., Emberson, J., Halsey, J., & Peto, R. et al.Prospective Studies Collaboration. (2009). Body-mass index and cause-specific mortality in 900 000 adults: Collaborative analyses of 57 prospective studies. *Lancet*, *373*(9669), 1083–1096. doi:10.1016/S0140-6736(09)60318-4 PMID:19299006

Whittaker, R. (2012). Issues in mHealth: Findings from key informant interviews. *Journal of Medical Internet Research*, *14*(5), e129. doi:10.2196/jmir.1989 PMID:23032424

Wing, R. R. (2002). Behavioral weight control. In T. A. Wadden & A. J. Stunkard (Eds.), *Handbook of obesity treatment* (pp. 301–316). New York: Guilford Press.

Zimmet, P. Z., Magliano, D. J., Herman, W. H., & Shaw, J. E. (2014). Diabetes: A 21st century challenge. *The Lancet Diabetes & Endocrinology*, *2*(1), 56–64. doi:10.1016/S2213-8587(13)70112-8 PMID:24622669

KEY TERMS AND DEFINITIONS

Bariatric Surgery: Surgery on the stomach and-or intestines to help patients with extreme obesity lose weight (traditionally it is an option for people who have a body mass index-BMI above 40).

Chronic Care Management: The comprehensive activities of education, prevention, monitoring and treatment conducted by health care professionals to help patients with chronic diseases and health conditions motivating patients to persist in necessary interventions to protect achieve a reasonable quality of life.

eHealth: A growing field of health services provided through the Internet and other new technologies.

mHealth: The practice of medicine and public health supported by mobile communication devices, such as mobile phones, tablet computers, and PDAs, for health services and information (it is an evolution of eHealth).

Obesity: A condition with a BMI (Body Mass Index, a person's weight in kilograms-kg divided by their height in meters-m squared) of 30 and above.

Social Media: Advanced forms of electronic communication through which users create online communities to share information, ideas, personal messages, and other content (as videos).

Stepped Care: Treatment that follows a predetermined sequence with a care approach adjusted in steps according to the failure or lack of effect of lower intensity interventions. The simplest and most affordable treatment regimen is used first: if that fails, other options are employed one after another until an endpoint is reached.

Type 2 Diabetes: A form of diabetes mellitus that is present especially in obese subjects with a condition of hyperglycemia resulting from impaired insulin utilization and with the body's inability to compensate with increased insulin production.

Chapter 64
Knowledge Sharing for Healthcare and Medicine in Developing Countries:
Opportunities, Issues, and Experiences

Kgomotso H. Moahi
University of Botswana, Botswana

Kelvin J. Bwalya
University of Johannesburg, South Africa

ABSTRACT

Knowledge sharing has always been used as a platform for cross-pollination of ideas and innovations in a bid to improve and enhance performance thereby increasing competitiveness and responsiveness both in organizations and individual levels. Healthcare systems are not an exception. However, for knowledge sharing to take place there is need for certain factors to be noted and addressed such as the individual, organizational and technological. Further, knowledge sharing goes hand in hand with knowledge management and must become part of the strategic fabric of organizations. This chapter focuses on knowledge sharing by health professionals in healthcare and medicine in developing countries. The chapter covers knowledge management and its link with knowledge sharing; the various methods of knowledge sharing in healthcare; factors that make knowledge sharing an important strategic move for healthcare organizations; and factors and issues that affect or determine knowledge sharing behavior. Finally, a literature search for examples of knowledge sharing in developing or low and middle-income countries was conducted and the results are presented. The chapter shows that developing countries have recognized the value of knowledge sharing in healthcare systems and there are tangible signs that this is going to shape cross-pollination of ideas and innovations in the health systems in the foreseeable future.

DOI: 10.4018/978-1-5225-3926-1.ch064

INTRODUCTION

Healthcare is information and knowledge intensive. It is characterized by rapid developments in medical knowledge that are generated as new conditions and diseases arise. It is not a secret that research and development in the pharmaceutical and in the biomedical fields yields vast amounts of information and knowledge. To deliver high quality, cost-effective services, healthcare professionals must have access to and use this knowledge. Healthcare organizations such as hospitals have turned to knowledge management to enable knowledge access, translation, sharing, and use. To be able to keep up-to-date, professionals must engage in robust knowledge sharing activities – which can only happen if knowledge itself is adequately managed. Whilst it is recognized that knowledge is important and valuable, Lefika and Mearns (2014) make the point that without sharing, knowledge has no value – it must be shared for its value to be fully recognized. Apart from value, sharing of knowledge ensures that knowledge is peer-reviewed culminating into added inferences and interpretations given different contextual settings. Sharing of knowledge practices and approaches is very important for replication and cross-pollination of knowledge translating into improved medical practice.

Healthcare professionals in developing countries are faced with a litany of problems that affect their ability to effectively share knowledge. They are invariably overworked with large patient loads due to a shortage of doctors, nurses, and other auxilliary health workers. Attending to patients leaves very little time for knowledge sharing, let alone even updating what they know on their own. Further, the infrastructure that might enable knowledge sharing – such as computing, Internet connectivity, and other modes of communication is in most cases obsolete and not adequate. Many healthcare workers in such countries find themselves in rural areas where the infrastructure is not as developed as in urban areas, and have been reported to feel isolated and away from current practices in the field (Pakenham-Walsh & Bukachi, 2009). Pakenham-Walsh & Bukachi (2009) conducted a review of the literature on the information needs of healthcare workers in Africa. They noted that most healthcare workers face isolation because they are mostly operating in rural areas that have limited information infrastructure, and they are swamped by huge workloads due to the shortage of healthcare workers in general. They identified the dire consequences to patient safety when healthcare workers' needs are unmet; their research identified issues such as a sizeable lack of knowledge of the basics of how to diagnose and manage common diseases. Not only do healthcare professionals not get the most recent and up-to-date research findings that would be useful in their work, but a gap between scientific evidence and its use in developing countries has been identified (Dagenais et al (2015).

This chapter focuses on knowledge sharing by health professionals in healthcare and medicine in developing countries and explores other prerequisite conditions for effective knowledge sharing. The chapter covers knowledge management and its link with knowledge sharing; the various methods of knowledge sharing in healthcare; factors that make knowledge sharing an important strategic move for healthcare organizations; and factors and issues that affect or determine knowledge sharing behavior. Finally, a literature search for examples of knowledge sharing in developing or low and middle-income countries was conducted and the results are presented. The search for literature was carried out on the following databases: PubMed, CINAHL, Library Information & Technology Abstracts, ERIC, Academic Search Premier, Africa-Wide Information, SocINDEX – all of them on EBSCOhost.

BACKGROUND

Knowledge Management and Knowledge Sharing

There is no one standard definition of knowledge management. At the heart of the definitional problem lies the lack of a clear distinction between information and knowledge and the tendency of many writers to use them interchangeably. Davenport et al. (1998) provided a definition of knowledge that distinguishes the two concepts of knowledge and information. To them, *knowledge is information amplified by context, experience, interpretation, and reflection.* Thus, knowledge management according to them is the management of information to enable its re-use. A way of thinking clearly about information and knowledge is to recognize that knowledge is largely tacit – it is embodied in the ways that people view the world, in how they address situations, solve problems and achieve their goals; it is a combination of prior experience, information processing, cognitive ability, and ability to apply all these to both familiar and new circumstances. However, knowledge can be made explicit by being vocalized, or codified and recorded. In this case, someone's knowledge becomes information that may be used by others to generate knowledge for achieving some goal.

The aim of knowledge management in organizations therefore is to ensure that knowledge within the organization is generated, codified, organized and managed to facilitate its sharing and harnessing for improved processes, procedures, and problem-solving. Knowledge management and knowledge sharing are very closely linked. Some researchers maintain that knowledge management facilitates knowledge sharing (Rowley & Farrow, 2000; Chennamaneni, 2012). To others such as Noor et al (2014), knowledge sharing is a key enabler of knowledge management, and as Lee et al (2014) point out, the success of knowledge management is determined by how effectively organizational members share and use their knowledge. Knowledge sharing enables the sharing of skills, knowledge, experiences and information between individuals and organizations. It also facilitates mutual learning, promotes best practice, reduces costs, and facilitates knowledge creation and reuse at both individual and organizational levels (Chennamaneni, 2012:1097).

Rahman (2011) describes knowledge sharing as the communication of both tacit and explicit knowledge. This communication especially for tacit knowledge would entail face to face interaction and is done through observation, imitation, practice and interaction with the environment (Rahman, 2011:213). The knowledge management literature indicates that tacit knowledge is generally difficult to articulate and requires trust for it to be shared; it is also difficult to acquire for mastery, it requires time; further, it makes sense only to those within a particular context – it is situated/bounded or local (Williams, 2011). Nonaka and Takeuchi (1995) advanced the Socialization, Externalization, Combination, and Internalization (SECI) model - which includes four (4) processes at play that in the author's view are at the heart of knowledge sharing. The first stage of socialization describes how knowledge is transmitted from tacit to tacit (understanding the knowledge traits by repeating the practical processes experienced during knowledge generation and creation under the guidance of the knowledge owner); the second stage of externalization describes how knowledge can be transformed from tacit to explicit (knowledge is transformed into a tangible resource so that it can visibly be added to the organizational or community knowledge inventory as intellectual capital and easily used as reference for further improving organizational business processes); the third stage describes how knowledge can be transformed from explicit to explicit; and the fourth stage describes how knowledge can be transformed from explicit to tacit (understanding and learning). This model offers a blueprint for turning tacit knowledge into explicit knowledge, and vice versa (Williams, 2011).

Knowledge sharing is important within organizations because organizations are essentially about the collective knowledge that lies in its people, as well as in various knowledge artifacts. Organizations create knowledge; they use it, transmit it and communicate it. It should be understood that for organizational effectiveness and for competitive advantage, knowledge must flow unhindered within the organization (Niels-Ingvar Boer, 2005) and that every actor in the organization's business process and value chain should be able to access knowledge instantaneously when needed for ad hoc decision-making, but this is often not the case. The reasons for this include a number of factors that have been identified by a plethora of researchers and can be classified as individual, organizational, and technology related (Noor et al., 2014). There are many methods and ways that are used or have been used to facilitate knowledge sharing, but more has to be done to ensure that knowledge sharing does indeed happen.

Methods of Knowledge Sharing

Knowledge sharing may be explicit or implicit (Navimipour, 2016), it can occur through face-to-face interactions and teamwork, as well as in the documentation of knowledge that can be availed to others (Wang & Noe, 2010). Knowledge sharing can also be technology assisted (Lefika & Mearns (2014) using, amongst others, knowledge management systems (KMS) (Chennamaneni et al., 2012). KMS have been used to support ad hoc sharing of knowledge; anonymous sharing through Wikipedia and open source software; community based implicit sharing where users benefit from the feedback or evaluation of others; and social networking based sharing (Chennamaneni et al 2012). Noor et al (2014) emphasize the importance of IT and an enabling technology infrastructure for knowledge sharing.

Lefika & Mearns (2014) have identified a number of methods of knowledge sharing that include knowledge cafes; peer assist; after action review; knowledge fairs, knowledge networks, mentoring/coaching; formal group-based knowledge sharing; storytelling, Weblogs, and communities of practice (CoP). Cudney et al (2015) reported on the use of gamification for knowledge sharing for continuous improvement in healthcare. Knowledge brokering is another strategy for bringing scientific evidence to health workers for practice (Dragonais et al (2015). According to Waring et al (2013) knowledge brokering has been a strategy to foster learning and innovation in healthcare for some time now. The role of informal networks or communities of practice (CoP) has been highlighted as being preferred by clinicians. However, for knowledge sharing to be part of a strategy of improvement and competitive advantage, there is need for formalization of networks and CoPs in order to entrench knowledge sharing within organizations (Bordoloi & Islam, 2012). Other ways that knowledge may be shared include the use of electronic medical records (EMRs) which facilitate knowledge sharing between physicians and other caregivers and contribute to continuing healthcare; clinical decision support systems (CDSS) also provide a platform for knowledge sharing, containing clinical guidelines, diagnosis tools, drug information, etc. (Bordoloi & Islam, 2012).

The use of social media for knowledge sharing in various healthcare settings, especially in developed countries has been a subject of particular interest (Chou et al 2009; Grajales et al (2014); Ratib et al, 2011; Kaufman, 2010; Huang et al, 2010; Rolls et al., 2016). Nattestad (2012) considered the use of social media such as Facebook and Twitter as examples of knowledge management systems that facilitated organizing and collaboration between health professionals in both developing and developed countries.

Rolls et al., (2016) point out that there are polarized views about the benefits and negative aspects of social media use by healthcare professionals. A study by Ali et al (2012) found that healthcare providers in New Zealand were using ICTs more for sharing explicit than tacit knowledge. However a review of the literature on social media use for virtual CoPs found that there was modest use of social media (Web 2.0) to establish virtual CoPs for exchanging experience based knowledge (tacit knowledge). Panahi et al (2012) conducted research that considered the potential of social media for tacit knowledge sharing among physicians and found that social media could contribute to tacit knowledge sharing and identified the following contributions as expressed by participants in their study:

- Ability to socialize online – talk to others, seeking second opinions, question and answer sessions, etc.;
- Best practice demonstrations through videos and podcasts;
- Networking with other colleagues;
- Interactive storytelling to share tips and lessons; and case reporting and dissemination;
- Increasing visibility of information;
- Openness – allowing everyone to have a voice;
- Trust;
- Archiving articulated knowledge.

Whilst it is very important to share scientific knowledge to engender evidence based practice, the sharing of knowledge at a local level, emanating from practice and experience in a particular context shared by the source and the recipient is also just as important (Ali et al (2012). In fact, research has shown that tacit knowledge is linked with context and situation, and that this is the knowledge mostly likely to be useful to individuals (e.g. healthcare professionals) in a given context (Williams, 2011). Abidi (2005) quoted by Panahi et al (2012) acknowledges the fact that tacit knowledge in healthcare is built through experience as clinicians and other healthcare workers deliver healthcare, and therefore should be an important part of knowledge sharing. Panahi et al, (2012:1) distil tacit knowledge sharing among physicians to include the sharing of clinical experience, skills, know-how and know-who; and that this sharing enhances clinical diagnosis and treatment outcomes. However, unlike explicit knowledge, this type of individual specific knowledge has been a challenge to tap into. The challenge is exacerbated by educational, professional, and organizational factors – as illustrated by Weller et al (2014); power relations among health professionals can inhibit knowledge sharing (Williams, 2011).

Why Knowledge Sharing in Healthcare

Knowledge management and in particular, knowledge sharing has been promoted extensively in developed countries as a means of improving patient safety, efficiency of healthcare, and to enhance the quality of delivered care (Nor'ashikin et al (2012). Knowledge sharing in healthcare has been studied widely (Abidi, 2007; Zhou & Nunes, 2016). This is because healthcare is knowledge rich (Abidi, 2007); and knowledge sharing is critical if high quality healthcare and outcomes are to be achieved. Knowledge sharing is defined as *systematically planned and managed activity involving a group of like-minded individuals engaged in sharing their knowledge resources, insights and experiences for a defined* objective (Abidi, 2007:67).

Healthcare by nature is a knowledge rich enterprise facing an avalanche of new knowledge and information at all times. This knowledge comes in the form of scientific research, drug trials, information about new conditions and diseases; new ways and technology of diagnosing and treating diseases; new protocols and care pathways, etc. For this reason, health professionals are in need of such knowledge to keep their knowledge up-to-date and to improve their competencies to provide safe and quality healthcare. Managing knowledge in healthcare settings is a complex task due to the sheer amount of knowledge that is generated as well as its fragmentation and compartmentalization (Gagnon et al, 2015). Bordoloi & Islam (2012) describe the state of healthcare as characterized by professionals who are overwhelmed by the amount of knowledge relevant to their clinical practice, but also by a lack of a central clearinghouse where such knowledge can be located and accessed.

Healthcare professionals should strive at all time to provide quality healthcare, better health outcomes and decreased costs. This can be achieved if knowledge is shared. Healthcare is also a highly collaborative endeavor involving people from different scientific fields and educational backgrounds who need to have effective knowledge sharing mechanisms (Boateng et al., 2016). In addition there are many actors involved such as patients, their families, doctors, nurses, students, auxiliary personnel, administrators, policy makers, etc., and as such knowledge sharing amongst them is a sure way of ensuring quality healthcare (Mansingh et al (2014) citing Wahle & Grooithuis, 2005). Such knowledge can be found in what has been termed knowledge retainers - human and codified knowledge retainers. Knowledge in healthcare can further be classified as declarative knowledge (know what), procedural knowledge (know how); social knowledge (know who), and contextual knowledge (know why) (Mansingh et al (2014).

Knowledge sharing is undertaken for a number of purposes that may include organizational learning, collaborative problem solving, peer support, and capacity building (Abidi, 2007). Gagnon et al (2015) identify Peter Senge's concept of the learning organization for advancing knowledge management and sharing. The learning organization can contribute to a culture of sharing and learning for adaptability, innovation, and continuing education. Organizational learning is facilitated by converting individual memory/knowledge into organizational memory, and ensuring that this organizational memory is usable. Waring et al (2013) explore the role of knowledge brokers in advancing knowledge sharing for patient safety, and articulate a further role in the diffusion of research into clinical practice. Another critical outcome of knowledge sharing is also the generation of new knowledge and innovation for improved organizational performance (Rahman, 2011). Rahman's (2011) case study at Malaysia's Healthcare Research Institute identified a number of perceived benefits that included: improvement in knowledge, skills and competencies; improvement in group productivity; better decision-making, increase in individual productivity; increase in job motivation; creativity and motivation. However motivating factors include effective communication channels; improved work processes; and recognition and promotion.

Ensuring patient safety has been identified as one of the primary reasons knowledge sharing has to be encouraged in healthcare settings. Pakenham-Walsh & Bukachi (2009) brought to the fore the issues that make knowledge sharing in healthcare a must. They identified a number of issues faced by healthcare workers in Africa as being a lack of basic knowledge on how to diagnose common conditions; feelings of being professionally isolated; problems of cognition where guidelines have been prepared. Thus, a more intentional knowledge sharing process is required that will enable rural health workers in particular to interact with peers wherever the need arises. In developing countries, knowledge sharing is at a premium given the context that healthcare providers find themselves in – of large caseloads; varied life threatening conditions, an increase in infectious and non-communicable diseases; and less than adequate information/knowledge resources etc. Knowledge sharing in healthcare is critical also for ensuring best practices and continuity in healthcare delivery (Boateng, et al 2016).

Issues and Challenges of Knowledge Sharing

There are many factors or issues that affect knowledge sharing in organizations in general, and in healthcare organizations in particular. Many attempts at knowledge management and knowledge sharing have assumed that once the structures and technologies are in place to implement KM, knowledge sharing will occur. However there is need to pay close attention to individual, social and organizational factors for knowledge sharing to succeed. Noor et al (2014) developed a conceptual framework that focused on organizational, individual, and technological factors that affect the success of knowledge sharing. Similarly, Wong & Noe (2010) identified the organizational context, interpersonal and team characteristics, cultural context, individual characteristics, and motivational factors. Chennamaneni (2012) points out that even when knowledge management is practiced and systems are in place, there is no guarantee that knowledge sharing will occur – there are certain factors that include the psychological, social, cultural, and organizational that may affect how knowledge sharing is carried out or whether it is in fact practiced. According to Rahman (2011:213) and others, it is difficult to get people to share knowledge largely because of the very nature of knowledge itself – that it is personal (tacit), mobile and portable and knows no boundaries.

Knowledge sharing can be hindered by a lack of teamwork spirit, poor communication channels, and lack of trust for peers and management. Although healthcare is known to be knowledge rich, that knowledge is underutilized for a variety of reasons (Abidi, 2007). One of the reasons is the effect of professional silos on communication between healthcare stakeholders. This lack of communication has been linked with compromised patient safety and increased medical errors (Weller et al, 2014). The communication issues are a result of educational, psychological and organizational factors (Weller et al, 2014).

Establishment of a knowledge sharing culture is paramount, and a change in corporate culture is even more critical for knowledge sharing to become practice (Rahman, 2011). According to the writer, culture has been stated as the real concern behind knowledge sharing initiatives. The willingness to share knowledge depends on the social capital (social interaction, trust and shared vision) (Navimipour, 2016; Chang et al., 2011), more than it does on the technologies used to facilitate knowledge sharing (Wang & Noe, 2010). The relationships and social networks that obtain in an organization will also affect knowledge sharing because relationships between people influence trust (Boh & Wong, 2014). Chang et al (2011) report that trust and a shared vision for nurses in Taiwan is positively linked with knowledge sharing. They explain the importance of knowledge sharing in order to ensure patient safety. Nurses should be provided with the knowledge, as well as the platform to share knowledge in a number of instances – when they detect human error on the part of other healthcare providers; when they detect changes in patients that require certain interventions, etc. Williams (2012) has indicated that in the sharing of tacit knowledge in particular, trust and interpersonal relations play a major role. Zhou & Nunes (2016) identified interpersonal trust barriers as a factor affecting knowledge sharing. The social network structures in an organization influence the flow of information and access to it; the social relationships will also influence the reciprocity and obligations that people may feel towards each other (Boh & Wong, 2014).

It has been stated that knowledge sharing can be inhibited by professional boundaries because professionals will not share knowledge with those not perceived to be members of a profession for fear of threatening their status or identity (Waring et al, citing Currie & White, 2012 and Warring & Currie,

2009). While healthcare professionals were found to use social media to create virtual CoPs they tended to do so along what Rolls et al (2016) call "tribal" lines, that is, along professional demarcations. Power asymmetry is a factor that can inhibit knowledge sharing (Currie, 2007). Intuitively, there is expectation that in organizations knowledge should be shared towards attainment of organizational goals. This is not the case as political issues come into play and must be addressed first if there is to be knowledge sharing. The politics of knowledge adversely affect sharing across organizational and professional boundaries. Thus there are challenges of knowledge sharing between specialists and general practitioners; doctors and nurses; and doctors and administrators. Knowledge sharing can also be affected by different knowledge bases and background (Tjoflat et al, 2012). This is especially so between people of different cultural background who do not take time to open up a communication process that allows a bi-directional flow. Tjoflat et al focus on knowledge sharing between people from diverse cultural contexts and the effect of a one-way communication that does not try to engage in order to understand and learn from others perceived as "inferior" in terms of experience, knowledge and perspective.

Knowledge sharing is positively linked with leadership and whether it is open and democratic and therefore influences behavior towards the sharing of knowledge. Leaders and managers are therefore seen to play a critical role in influencing knowledge sharing within the organization (Boh & Wong, 2014; Zhou & Nunes, 2016). The lack of knowledge sharing policies is also an issue and it has been found that many hospitals/health facilities in developing countries do not have them (Boateng, 2016). Reasons for sharing knowledge were distilled by Wang & Noe (2010), who identified research possibilities into the uptake or lack of – of knowledge sharing. These included, amongst others, understanding the difference between interpersonal and technology aided knowledge sharing; and the influence of organizational and national culture on knowledge sharing.

KNOWLEDGE SHARING IN DEVELOPING COUNTRIES

A form of knowledge sharing between healthcare professionals in developing countries has always been in practice through professional communication on cases, requests for second opinions, and sharing information regarding scientific evidence between peers; knowledge would also be shared in official settings such as meetings and briefings. With healthcare being knowledge intensive, it is expected that knowledge would be generated and communicated as necessary. However, this expectation is not formalized to become part of an articulated strategy to ensure that knowledge, skills and experiences of the people in organizations is intentionally managed to enable achievement of entrenched knowledge sharing in order to enhance healthcare processes, improve patient safety and achieve quality healthcare.

Over and above that, given the challenges faced by the healthcare sectors in developing countries, health professionals are faced with access challenges to the latest, cutting edge health research to use in handling the complexity of healthcare delivery. In addition, literature has shown that despite the existence of knowledge management and its application in many domains inclusive of the healthcare sector in developed countries, knowledge management practice has been and is still a concept that is difficult to implement for a variety of reasons, chiefly, being the lack of capacity and requisite resources. Knowledge sharing generally requires that knowledge is managed to facilitate its sharing. However, not many healthcare industries and sectors in developing countries have paid attention to instituting formal knowledge management activities, such as how to capture existing knowledge (Mansingh et al, 2014).

Over the years many initiatives were put in place to address this lack of access to knowledge and information, chief amongst them, SatelLife and its HealthNet news service. The aim of HealthNet was to provide the much needed information to healthcare professionals from well-resourced institutions in developed countries to those in developing countries; as well as foster communication between professionals in developing countries and from professionals in developing countries to those in developed countries. The service was satellite based requiring that participating centers use a personal computer and a ham radio that would be used to upload questions and any other communication from professionals which would be 'picked up and delivered' through low earth orbiting satellite. HealthNet was able to deliver scientific knowledge that professionals in developing countries would never have had access to, but as well provided HIV and AIDS related information, and provided a channel through which health professionals could engage each other on cases (McCullough & Royall, 2015). As technology developed and the Internet became widely available, the system took advantage of this and communication was effected through mobile hand-held devices. The services ceased in 2014 with the last issue of Healthnet News delivered on 2nd May 2014 (McCullough & Royall, 2015). Another notable program for providing access to biomedical and health literature is HINARI – a World Health Organization (WHO) project to provide access to national universities, teaching hospitals, research institutions, and professional schools in developing countries. WHO has entered into agreement with major publishers to enable access to a vast amount of health related literature (WHO). HINARI has proven to be an important lifeline to many healthcare institutions.

Both these services while providing access to scientific knowledge did not necessarily guarantee knowledge sharing to address the knowledge gaps faced by health professionals in developing countries. Receiving scientific knowledge is a good thing, but for colleagues within an organization it is also critical to share contextualized knowledge based on similar environments and experiences with health problems and challenges. Knowledge sharing is critical in developing countries especially because of the challenges healthcare professionals face in the delivery of medical and healthcare. Boateng et al (2016) mention challenges such as poor management of patient records, delays experienced by patients to get healthcare delivery, financing of healthcare, quality of healthcare delivered, and the shortage of health professionals in Ghana, West Africa. Other challenges include inequality of the public and private healthcare systems in South Africa, resulting in poorly resourced public health system, servicing the majority of the population with poor infrastructure, and low health professional and patient ratios (Badimo & Buckley, 2014). In Ethiopia, Gebretsadik et al. (2014) articulated a major cause of the problems facing the healthcare sector being the high turnover of healthcare workers.

The digital divide that persists between urban and rural centers in developing countries impacts on knowledge sharing. According to Pakenham-Walsh & Bukachi (2009) infrastructural disparities limit the ability of health workers to use technology for information and knowledge sharing. Vital Waves Consulting (2009) concluded that because of limited ICT infrastructure and information literacy, many healthcare workers in Africa rely on mobile phones to share knowledge.

Knowledge sharing initiatives in developed countries such as the US indicate that complex information systems for knowledge sharing have not been easy to implement (Ali et al., 2012). The writers suggest instead the use of commonly available ICTs for knowledge sharing as a much simpler and more workable approach. They studied the use of common ICTs in secondary healthcare organizations in New Zealand. Such challenges have given some impetus to a number of studies of knowledge sharing in developing countries, which are discussed below.

Studies on Knowledge Sharing in Developing Countries

The literature review for knowledge sharing by healthcare professionals in developing countries unearthed a relatively small number of papers when compared with papers focusing on developed countries. Overall 28 papers were found to be relevant and used for this chapter. Developing countries were identified from the World Bank list of such countries using the level of income (low and middle income economies).

Knowledge sharing in many developing countries is still to a large extent ad hoc in nature and reliant on individuals' predisposition and perspective on knowledge sharing. The study of knowledge sharing in 3 hospitals in Ghana found that there were no knowledge management systems where health professionals could capture, find and share knowledge, leaving them to rely on informal channels such as clinical meetings, verbal communication with colleagues. Nevertheless, healthcare professionals expressed an interest in sharing knowledge for various reasons – to update themselves with current medical knowledge, to prevent patient harm, achieve desired results, as well as ensure there is continuity of care when one is not available. Their constraints though included lack of time – given the large workloads, lack of trust, complacency, and network failures when using mobile phones (Boateng et al., 2016). The same authors attribute the challenges to knowledge sharing in Ghana hospitals to a lack of an IT platform for knowledge sharing. They therefore recommend that municipalities should put in place knowledge management stems such as an intranet or e-mail system. They advocate for management/leadership intervention to make knowledge sharing possible. Badimo and Buckley (2014) also found a lack of formalized knowledge management and sharing system in South African health system, The study revealed that even though most participants felt the environment was conducive for knowledge sharing, many felt that knowledge belonged to individuals and that issues such as lack of trust and open-mindedness, lack of awareness of other people's knowledge need, lack of an IT platform, and lack of a centralized information repository for documenting knowledge and sharing it constrained effective knowledge sharing.

Dagenais et al (2015) report the development of a knowledge brokering program in Burkina Faso to promote research use. The idea of knowledge brokering arose out of recognition that even when research results are made available to healthcare practitioners, there is no guarantee that they will be translated into practice. There may be any number of reasons for this: it could be that the information is articulated in ways that are too technical to understand, and requires repackaging to understand contextualized knowledge, and it could be that the value of such knowledge is not immediately clear. The project was implemented for a year and then evaluated. The evaluation showed a positive response to having a knowledge broker break down/repackage research to facilitate application. It also underscored the need for collaboration and community involvement when introducing an innovation such as knowledge brokering as a way of encouraging knowledge sharing.

As indicated earlier, cultural factors, specifically intercultural literacy do affect knowledge sharing, and Tjoflat & Karlsten (2012) illustrated through a case study, how cross-cultural factors affected knowledge sharing between an expert from a developed country and nurses in a South Sudanese hospital. Knowledge sharing, between individuals from very different cultures was reportedly fraught with problems, especially where no effort was made on the part of the "expert" to first reach or negotiate an understanding of the context of the person to share knowledge with, or even a lack of appreciation that knowledge sharing is not a one way communication. Knowledge sharing is a social activity and requires some amount of interaction beyond the establishment of IT platforms and other knowledge management systems. Hence, use of knowledge networks and communities of practice (CoPs) should form a pillar of knowledge sharing activities (Bordoloi & Islam, 2012). Meessen et al (2011) acknowledge the challenges of knowledge management implementation in low income countries and posit that the CoP strategy is the missing link that could address the implementation challenges, they state that *the strength of CoP as a knowledge management strategy is to fully recognize the importance of sharing both explicit and implicit knowledge* (Meessen et al, 2011:1011).

Hamel & Schrecker (2011) studied the knowledge translation of a public health professional association to influence health policy in Burkina-Faso. Knowledge translation or research utilization is not necessarily the same as knowledge sharing – but in this case is considered as an example of efforts towards using knowledge to improve performance. Professional associations in the medical and healthcare fields are actually very powerful and command the allegiance and commitment of their members even much more than of their employers as they advocate, they educate, but they also license and can levy sanctions. Knowledge translation is also the main feature in the study by Yazdizadeh et al (2014). To them knowledge networks represent one way of furthering the ambitions of knowledge sharing, in particular, ensuring that the results of scientific research are fed into healthcare practice (Yazdizadeh, et al, 2014). The researchers present lessons learnt from an attempt at establishing knowledge networks in Iran's health system – a total of 10 medical research networks. This case is presented here to suggest the possibility of using knowledge networks in healthcare settings to engender knowledge sharing.

Another way that knowledge sharing might be enhanced is through practitioner research approach, reported on by Singh (2011). The specific project that was carried out using this approach was the implementation of an e-mentoring program to support healthcare professionals in developing countries. The practitioner research approach had the effect of building "intentional networks" that linked practitioners and contributed to knowledge sharing.

Motivation is one of the factors contributing to knowledge sharing in organizations identified in the literature. As such Singh et al (2016) conducted a study of the factors that motivate knowledge sharing by community health volunteers in rural Uganda. The volunteers were brought in to relieve the burden to healthcare workers and community health workers and revealed they were motivated more by the knowledge they gained whilst being trained than the prospects of transport allowance or possible employment. They stated that gaining and sharing knowledge with members of the community was an important factor in their retention.

Esmaeilzadeh et al (2015) studied the factors influencing physicians' intention to adopt clinical decision support systems (CDSS) in Malaysia. They specifically considered the role of physicians' attitude towards knowledge sharing and interactivity perception about CDSS. They also considered the effect of the physicians' involvement in decision-making, their computer efficacy and effort expectancy. They found that physicians' intentions to adopt CDSS was linked to perceived threat to their professional autonomy, performance expectancy and their involvement in making decisions about CDSS. Secondly, that the physicians' attitudes towards knowledge sharing, interactivity perspective, and computer efficacy played a role in influencing their perceived threats on professional autonomy. Also that social networks, shared goals and helping behavior impact physicians' attitude towards knowledge sharing.

Gorry (2008) explored the role of libraries, specifically virtual libraries in facilitating knowledge sharing in Cuba. Cuba healthcare system, like many other developing country systems is characterized by significant disease burdens, lack of requisite infrastructure and resource scarcity.

The use of mobile phones in healthcare in developing countries is a growing trend given the growing ubiquity of mobile devices in these settings. Tuijin et al (2011) report a project that experimented with using mobile phones to strengthen microscopy-based diagnostic services in low and middle-income countries' laboratories. The images are uploaded to a central web site using mobile phones, and once in the web site, they are evaluated and feedback sent by text to their originators. A feasibility study was carried out in Uganda, and was well received.

Knowledge sharing on a global scale is also one way that developing countries are assisted to improve healthcare delivery. Ramaswamy et al (2016) wrote on building a multi-national collaboration for the improvement of maternal and neonatal health. They posit that international funding alone will not build lasting solutions in developing countries, but rather a global commitment of sharing knowledge and resources through international partnerships. As such, they report on a partnership building model of an international NGO.

One of the challenges of healthcare systems in developing countries is the shortage of qualified healthcare workers. The prospect of task sharing between qualified healthcare workers and community health extension workers (CHEW) to detect early signs of preeclampsia in was explored in Ogun State, Nigeria. This task sharing obviously entails training and knowledge sharing which is critical in a low resource environment (Akeju et al 2016).

Telemedicine has been described as a way of addressing the shortage of healthcare practitioners in developing countries. Besides availing access to expertise that would not available at the local level, knowledge sharing opportunities are possible through telemedicine implementation. Brauchli et al (2005) describe iPath (an internet based telemedicine platform) designed to support healthcare providers in developing countries. Two case studies are presented, a teledermatology project in South Africa, and a telepathology project in the Solomon Islands. Farshidi et al (2011) also discuss the implementation of teledermatology as a possibility to effect amongst others, knowledge sharing. Reported in this volume by Ndlovu et al., (2017) is the use of technology to facilitate knowledge sharing between tuberculosis (TB) clinicians and medical officers in Botswana's public health system – on multi drug resistant TB (MDR-TB). The medical officers are provided with a tablet loaded with resources such as MDR-TB guidelines for the prevention, monitoring and treatment of TB.

Healthcare in developing countries is provided through two systems – western based and indigenous health care system. Most jurisdictions have recognized the need for collaboration between these two systems to leverage on their synergies. Knowledge sharing is critical to ensure that these synergies are leveraged, but it must be preceded by efforts to document, preserve and disseminate traditional medical knowledge. Affue-Arthur & Kwame (2016) explore how Ghanain university libraries can play a role in implementing knowledge management in indigenous medicine.

Health information portals for health professionals are available on the Internet, including those that are targeted at users in developing countries such as the volunteer driven Global Healthnews at Global Health Hub, WHO's HINARI providing biomedical and health information to developing countries, the Directory of Open Access Journals, Health Science Online, and Pubmed Central. Many of these are developed and maintained in developed countries, with only a few having the input of users in the developing countries. Zambia Health Information portal is one such, involving a partnership between two universities (University of Alabama at Birmingham and the University of Iowa eGranary Digital Library) in the US and a health institute in Zambia to produce a digital library of health information resources. Khanna (2013) reports a home grown repository on maternal and child health in India meant to serve professionals involved in healthcare either as policy makers, administrators, planners, and academics and researchers. The portal was launched in July 2010 and evaluated in 2013; it was created to enable knowledge sharing, noting the dearth of such knowledge in the healthcare system of India.

CONCLUSION

The purpose of this chapter was to establish the opportunities, challenges and experiences of knowledge sharing in developing countries. Clearly, knowledge sharing would enable healthcare professionals and organizations to leverage on their knowledge resources in order to deliver effective and efficient healthcare delivery, patient safety, creativity, and innovation. However, there are a number of issues and factors that challenge the implementation of knowledge sharing in both developed and developing countries. These can be categorized as individual, organizational, and technological. The literature has revealed that there have been efforts to study as well as implement knowledge sharing in healthcare settings in developing countries. There has been recognition of the need to move away from making assumptions that knowledge sharing is happening or should be happening, to investigating how it could be formalized to become part of strategic directions. Examples of formalized knowledge sharing are provided that include the establishment of research networks, communities of practice, telemedicine, knowledge brokers, the use of mobile phones, the role of librarians, and use of social networks or Web 2.0 technologies. Given that most of the developing world countries in Africa have jumped onto the bandwagon for putting in place effective knowledge sharing in healthcare systems, the future is bright for paramedical knowledge sharing.

REFERENCES

Abidi, S. S. R. (2007). Healthcare knowledge sharing: practice and prospects. In R. K. Bali & A. N. Dwivedi (Eds.), *Healthcare Knowledge Management: Issues, Advances and Successes*. New York: Springer-Verlag. doi:10.1007/978-0-387-49009-0_6

Abidi, S. S. R., Cheah, Y. N., & Curran, J. (2005). A knowledge creation information structure to acquire and crystallize tacit knowledge of healthcare experts. *IEE Transactions on IT in Biomedicine, 9*(2), 193–204. doi:10.1109/TITB.2005.847188

Afful-Arthur, P., & Filson, C. K. (2016). Knowledge management in indigenous medicine: The expected role of Ghanaian university libraries. *Library Philosophy and Practice, 2016*, 1–22.

Akeju, D. (2016, September). Human resource constraints and the prospect of task-sharing among community health workers for the detection of early signs of preeclampsia in Ogun state, Nigeria. *Reproductive Health, 13*(2), 115–122. PMID:27766973

Ali, N., Whiddett, D., Tretiakov, A., & Hunter, I. (2012). The use of information technologies for knowledge sharing by secondary healthcare organizations in New Zealand. *International Journal of Medical Informatics, 81*(7), 500–506. doi:10.1016/j.ijmedinf.2012.02.011 PMID:22460023

Badimo, K. H., & Buckley, S. (2014). Improving knowledge management practices in the South African healthcare system. *International Scholarly and Scientific Research and Innovation, 8*(11), 3449–3455.

Boateng P & Pabbi K.A. (2016). Knowledge sharing among healthcare professionals in Ghana. *Vine Journal of Information and Knowledge Management Systems, 46*(4), 479-491.

Boer Niels-Ingvar. (2005). *Knowledge sharing within organizations: A situated and relational perspective.* PhD Thesis. Accessed on 27/05/2016 from: http://repub.eur.nl/pub/6770/eps2005060lis_9058920860_boer.PDF

Boh, W. F., & Wong, S. (2014). Managers versus workers as referents: Comparing social influence effects on within and outside subsidiary knowledge sharing. *Organizational Behavior and Human Decision Processes, 2015*(126), 1–17.

Bordoloi, P., & Islam, N. (2012). Knowledge management practices and healthcare delivery: A contingency framework. *Electronic Journal of Knowledge Management, 10*(2), 110–120.

Brauchli, K., O'mahony, D., Banach, L., & Oberholzer, M. (2005). Article. *Studies in Health Technology and Informatics, 14*, 7–11.

Chang, C., Huang, H., Chiang, C., Hsu, C., & Chang, C. (2011, September). Social capital for knowledge sharing: Effect on patient safety. *Journal of Advanced Nursing, 68*(8), 1793–1803. doi:10.1111/j.1365-2648.2011.05871.x PMID:22077142

Chennamaneni, A., Teng, J. T. C., & Raja, M. K. (2012, November). A unified model of knowledge sharing behaviours: Theoretical development and empirical test. *Behaviour & Information Technology, 31*(1), 1097–1115. doi:10.1080/0144929X.2011.624637

Cudney, E.A., Murray, S.L., Sprague, C.M., Byrd, L.M., Morris, F., Merwin, N., & Warner, D. (2015). Engaging healthcare users through gamification in knowledge sharing for continuous improvements in healthcare. *Procedural Manufacturing, 3,* 3416-3421.

Currie, G., Finn, R., & Martin, G. (2007). Spanning boundaries in pursuit of effective knowledge sharing within networks in the National Health Service (NHS). *Journal of Health Organization and Management, 21*(415), 406–417. doi:10.1108/14777260710778934 PMID:17933372

Currie, G., & White, L. (2012). Inter-professional barriers and knowledge brokering in an organizational context: the case of healthcare. *Organization Studies, 33*(10), 1333e1361.

Dagenais, C., Some, T.D., Boilleau-Falardeau, M., Mcsween-Cadieux, E., & Ridde, V. (2015). Collaborative development and implementation of a knowledge brokering program to promote research use in Burkina Faso, West Africa. *Global Health Action, 8*(26004). 10.3402/gha.v8.26004

Davenport, T. H., & Prusak, L. (1998). *Working Knowledge: How Organizations Manage What They Know.* Boston: Harvard Business Press.

Esmaeilzadeh, P., Sambasivan, M., Kumar, N., & Nezakati, H. (2015, August). Adoption of clinical decision support systems in a developing country: Antecedents and outcomes of physicians threat to perceived professional autonomy. *International Journal of Medical Informatics, 84*(8), 548–560. doi:10.1016/j.ijmedinf.2015.03.007 PMID:25920928

Farshidi, D., Craft, N., & Ochoa, M. T. (2011). Mobile teledermatology: As doctors and patients are increasingly mobile, technology keeps us connected. *Skinmed, 9*(4), 231–238. PMID:21980708

Gagnon, M., Payne-Gagnon, J., Fortin, J., Pare, G., Cote, J., & Courcy, F. (2015). A Learning organization in the service of knowledge management among nurses: A case study. *International Journal of Information Management, 35*(5), 636–642. doi:10.1016/j.ijinfomgt.2015.05.001

Gebretsadik, I., Mirutse, G., Tadesse, K., & Terefe, W. (2014). Knowledge sharing practice and its associated factors of healthcare professionals of public hospitals, Mekelle, Northern Ethiopia. *American Journal of Health Research, 2*(5), 241–246. doi:10.11648/j.ajhr.20140205.14

Gorry, C. (2008, January). Cuba's virtual libraries: Knowledge sharing for developing world. *MEDICC Review, 10*(1), 9–12. PMID:21483349

Grajales, F. J., Sheps, S., Ho, K., Novak-Lauscher, H., & Eysenbach, G. (2014). Social media: A review and tutorial of application in medicine and healthcare. *Journal of Medical Internet Research, 16*(2). PMID:24518354

Hamel, N., & Schrecker, T. (2011, January). Unpacking capacity to utilize research: A tale of the Burkina Faso public health association. *Social Science & Medicine, 72*(1), 31–38. doi:10.1016/j.socscimed.2010.09.051 PMID:21074923

Khanna, R., Karikalan, N., Mishra, A. K., Agwaral, A., & Bhattacharya, M. (2013). Repository on maternal child health: Health portal to improve access to information on maternal and child health in India. *BMC Public Health, 13*(2), 1–20. PMID:23281735

Lee, H. S., & Hong, S. A. (2014). Factors affecting hospital employees knowledge sharing intention and behavior. *Osong Public Health Research Perspective, 5*(3), 148–155. doi:10.1016/j.phrp.2014.04.006 PMID:25180147

Lefika, P.T., & Mearns, M.A. (2014). Adding knowledge cafes to the repertoire of knowledge sharing techniques. *International Journal of Information Management, 35*(1), 26-32.

Liu, F. C., Cheng, K. L., Chao, M., & Tseng, H. M. (2012). Team innovation climate and knowledge sharing among healthcare managers' mediating effects of altruistic intention. *Chang Gung Medical Journal, 35*(3), 408–415. PMID:23127346

Maiga G. & Mutuwa P.L. (2015). An integrating model of knowledge management for improved pedriatic healthcare practice. *Journal of Information and knowledge Management, 14*(2), 1-15.

Mansingh, G., Osei-Brynson, K.-M., & Reinchgelt, H. (2014). Knowledge sharing in the health sector in Jamaica: the barriers and the enablers. In K.-M. Osei-Bryson, G. Mansigh, & L. Rao (Eds.), *Knowledge Management for Development: domains, strategies and technologies for developing countries.* New York: Springer. doi:10.1007/978-1-4899-7392-4_12

McCullough, L., & Royall, J. (2015). *SatelLife and Healthnet News.* Retrieved on 4/12/2016 from: http://juliaroyall.com/wp-content/uploads/2015/04/SatelLife-HNN-for-NLM.pdf

Meessen, B., Kouanda, S., Musango, L., Richard, F., Ridde, V., & Soucat, A. (2011, August). Communities of practice: The missing link for knowledge management on implementation issues in low-income countries? *Tropical Medicine & International Health, 16*(8), 1007–1014. doi:10.1111/j.1365-3156.2011.02794.x PMID:21564426

Nattesdat, A. (2012). Knowledge management systems for oral health in developing and developed countries. *Periodontology 2000, 60*(1), 156–161. doi:10.1111/j.1600-0757.2011.00403.x PMID:22909113

Navimipour, N. J., & Charband, Y. (2016). Knowledge sharing mechanisms and techniques in project teams: Literature review, classification, and current trends. *Computers in Human Behavior, 62*(September), 730–742. doi:10.1016/j.chb.2016.05.003

Nonaka, I., & Takeuchi, H. (1995). *The knowledge creating company: how Japanese companies create the dynasties of innovation.* Oxford, UK: Oxford University Press.

Noor, A. D., Hashim, H. S., & Ali, N. (2014, September). Factors influencing knowledge sharing in organizations: A literature review. *International Journal of Science and Research, 3*(9), 1314–1319.

Ohkubo, S., Harlan, S., Ahmed, N., & Salem, R. M. (2015). Conceptualising a new knowledge management logic model for global health: a case study approach. Journal of Information and Knowledge Management, 14(2).

Pakenham-Walsh, N., & Bukachi, F. (2009). Information needs of healthcare workers in developing countries: a literature review with a focus on Africa. Human Resources for Health, 7(30).

Panahi, S., Watson, J., & Partridge, H. (2012). Potentials of social media for tacit knowledge sharing amongst physicians: preliminary findings. *23rd Australian conference on Information Systems.*

Rahman, R. A. (2011). Knowledge sharing practices: A case study at Malaysias healthcare research institution. *The International Information & Library Review, 43*(4), 207–214. doi:10.1080/10572317. 2011.10762902

Ramaswamy, R., Kallam, B., Kopic, D., Pujic, B., & Owen, M. D. (2016). Global health partnerships: Building multi-national collaborations to achieve lasting improvements in maternal and neonatal health. *Globalization and Health, 12*(1), 1–8. doi:10.1186/s12992-016-0159-7 PMID:27206731

Rolls, K., Hansen, M., Jackson, D., & Elliott, D. (2016, June). Jackson d. & Elliot D. (2016). How health care professionals use social media to create virtual communities: An integrative review. *Journal of Medical Internet Research, 18*(6), 29p. doi:10.2196/jmir.5312 PMID:27328967

Rowley, J., & Farrow, J. (2000). *Organizing knowledge: an introduction to managing access to information.* Aldershot, UK: Gower.

Singh, D., Cumming, R., Mohajer, N., & Negin, J. (2016, July). Motivator of community health volunteers in rural Uganda: The interconnectedness of knowledge, relationship and action. *Public Health, 136*, 166–171. doi:10.1016/j.puhe.2016.01.010 PMID:26877064

Singh, G. (2013). Disrupting the implementation gap with digital technology in healthcare distance education: Critical insights from an e-mentoring intensional network practitioner research project. *European Journal of Open, Distance and E-learning, 16*(1), 67–77.

Suppiah, V., & Sandhu, M. S. (2011). Organizational cultures influence on tacit knowledge sharing behavior. *Journal of Knowledge Management, 15*(3), 462–477. doi:10.1108/13673271111137439

Tjoflat I. & Karlsen B. (2012). Challenges in sharing knowledge: reflections from the perspective of an expatriate nurse working in a South Sudanese hospital. *The International Nursing Review,* 489-493.

Tuijn, C. J., Hoefman, B. J., van Beijma, H., Oskam, L., & Chevrollier, N. (2011). Data and image transfer using mobile phones to strengthen microscopy-based diagnostic services in low and middle income laboratories. *PLoS ONE, 6*(12), 1–8. doi:10.1371/journal.pone.0028348 PMID:22194829

Vital Waves Consulting. (2009). *Health information systems in developing countries: a landscape analysis.* Accessed on 15/12/2016 from: http://vitalwave.com

Wahle, A. E., & Grooithuis, W. A. (2005). How to handle knowledge management in healthcare: a description of a model to deal with the current and ideal situation. In N. Wickranasinghe, J. N. D. Gupta, & S. K. Sharma (Eds.), *Creating Knowledge-based healthcare organizations.* Hershey, PA: IDEA Group. doi:10.4018/978-1-59140-459-0.ch003

Wang, S., & Noe, R. A. (2010). Knowledge sharing: A review and directions for future research. *Human Resource Management Review, 20*(2), 115–131. doi:10.1016/j.hrmr.2009.10.001

Waring, J., & Currie, G. (2009). Managing expert knowledge: organisational challenges and managerial futures for the UK medical profession. *Organization Studies, 30*(7), 755-778.

Waring, K., Currie, G., Crompton, A., & Bishop, S. (2013). An exploratory study of knowledge brokering in hospital settings: Facilitating knowledge sharing and learning for patient safety? *Social Science & Medicine, 98*, 79–86. doi:10.1016/j.socscimed.2013.08.037 PMID:24331885

Weller, J., Boyd, M., & Cumin, D. (2014). Teams, tribes and patient safety: Overcoming barriers to effective teamwork in healthcare. *Postgraduate Medical Journal, 90*(1061), 149–154. doi:10.1136/postgradmedj-2012-131168 PMID:24398594

Williams, F. (2011). *Knowledge management in the National Health Service: an empirical study of organisational and professional antecedents to knowledge transfer in knowledge management initiatives* (PhD thesis). University of Nottingham. Access from the University of Nottingham repository: http://eprints.nottingham.ac.uk/12026/1/Fabrice_Williams_phd_thesis.pdf

Williams, P. M. (2012). Integration of health and social care: A case of learning and knowledge management. *Health & Social Care in the Community, 20*(5), 550–560. doi:10.1111/j.1365-2524.2012.01076.x PMID:22741611

Yazdizadeh, B., Majdzadeh, R., Alami, A., & Amrolalael, S. (2014). How can we establish more successful knowledge networks in developing countries? Lessons learnt from knowledge networks in Iran. Health Research Policy and Systems, 12(63).

Zhou, L., & Nunes, M. B. (2016). Barriers to knowledge sharing in Chinese healthcare referral services: An emergent theoretical model. *Global Health Action, 2016*, 9. PMID:26895146

ADDITIONAL READING

Dixon, B. E., Hook, J. M., & McGowan, J. J. (2008). Using Telehealth to Improve Quality and Safety: Findings from the AHRQ Portfolio (Prepared by the AHRQ National Resource Center for Health IT under Contract No. 290-04-0016). AHRQ Publication No. 09-0012-EF. Rockville, MD: Agency for Healthcare Research and Quality. December 2008.

Karamitri I.; Talias M. A. & Bellali T. (2015). Knowledge management practices in healthcare settings: a systematic review. *Int J Health Plann Mgmt (2015)*. Published online in Wiley Online Library (wileyonlinelibrary.com) DOI: .10.1002/hpm.2303

Kim, Y.-M., Newby-Bennett, D., & Song, H.-J. (2012). Knowledge sharing and institutionalism in the healthcare industry. *Journal of Knowledge Management, 16*(3), 480–494. doi:10.1108/13673271211238788

Simonyan, D., Gagnon, M.-P., Duchesne, T., & Roos-Weil, A. (2013). Effects of a tele-health programme using mobile data transmission on primary healthcare utilisation among children in Bamako, Mali. *Journal of Telemedicine and Telecare, 19*(6), 302–306. doi:10.1177/1357633X13503429 PMID:24163292

Watts, C., & Ibegbulam, I. (2006). Access to Electronic Healthcare Information Resources in Developing Countries: Experiences from the Medical Library, College of Medicine, University of Nigeria. *IFLA Journal, 32*(1), 54–61. doi:10.1177/0340035206063903

Wilkesmann, M. (2016). Ignorance management in hospitals. *VINE Journal of Information and Knowledge Management Systems, 46*(4), 430–449. doi:10.1108/VJIKMS-08-2016-0046

KEY TERMS AND DEFINITIONS

Developing Countries: Countries with less developed human resource base, healthcare systems, socio-economic infrastructure, industrial base and a low Gross Domestic Product (GDP).

Healthcare: Mechanisms and processes put in place in a given place to cure or mitigate human being's physical or mental discomfort.

Knowledge Management: The management of knowledge resources in an organization in support of knowledge generation, translation and sharing. Also, the management of information to facilitate sharing and re-use given a specific contextual setting.

Knowledge Sharing: The sharing of task based knowledge between co-workers or professionals in within or across organizations. Knowledge sharing is the communication of both tacit and explicit knowledge.

This research was previously published in Health Information Systems and the Advancement of Medical Practice in Developing Countries edited by Kgomotso H. Moahi, Kelvin Joseph Bwalya and Peter Mazebe II Sebina, pages 60-77, copyright year 2017 by Medical Information Science Reference (an imprint of IGI Global).

Chapter 65
Human Interaction in the Use of Health Information Systems:
A Case of a Developing Country

Irja N. Shaanika
Namibia University of Science and Technology, Namibia

ABSTRACT

In developing countries, Health Information Systems (HISs) are increasingly used to enable and support both clinical and administrative processes for healthcare services. The use of the HISs in developing countries' healthcare centres is influenced and impacted by humans' interactions which manifests from culture and traditions. Due to the diverse nature of culture and traditions, it is near impossible to have single formula in addressing the patients' needs. As a result, the aim to improve quality of healthcare through HISs is challenged, and many stakeholders do not seem to understand the problem. The challenge continues to significantly contribute to poor service delivery, as the need for healthcare services increases. This study focused on the interaction between the healthcare professionals and the HISs, to understand how and why the challenges of using the ICT systems exist. This includes examining the implication, and how the challenges impact the recipients of healthcare services.

INTRODUCTION

In developing countries, Health Information Systems (HISs) are increasingly used to enable and support both clinical and administrative processes for healthcare services. To this extend, McDonald (2006) explored limitations to opportunities that are offered by ICTs in developing countries. This includes infrastructure availability and lack of skill among health workers, in the use of ICT tools. Due to the number of patients on the increase on daily basis and the sensitive of patients' records, healthcare services providers requires a more adequate, reliable, and accurate information. This is to support and enable healthcare workers to deliver improved services to their patients. Rodrigues (2010) argued that HISs is an ICT-based tool, to make healthcare delivery more effective and efficient.

DOI: 10.4018/978-1-5225-3926-1.ch065

Health Information Systems (HISs) is considered to be a functional computerised system, to execute healthcare related processes and activities. According to Lippeveld (2001), HIS provides specific information primarily to enable and support the processes of health organisations. In one of World Health Organization' (WHO) document of 2003, it is stated that HIS is an integrated effort to collect, process, report, and use health information and knowledge, in order to influence policy making, programme action, and research (WHO, 2003).

The use of HIS requires interaction between people, process, and technology, to support operations and management in delivering of essential information in order to improve the quality of healthcare services (Cleverley, 2009). Similar to other industries, the nature of healthcare industry has changed over time, from a relatively stable conservative industry to a dynamic one. This is attributed to the role of people, in the innovation and management of activities. The dynamism is based on the interactions with technology that people bring in from their different culture and traditions. This includes the types of technologies that are available and how they are used and managed to provide services. As stated by McDonald (2006) exploring the limitations to opportunities offered by IS in developing countries such as inadequate basic physical infrastructure availability and lack of skill among health workers for using information technology tools.

Reporting on the current states of HIS, the World Health Organisation noted that the current status of HIS varies among countries. Most developed countries have fully utilized HIS in their systems as they have the resources, expertise, and capital to implement them. While developing countries HIS are not being fully utilized yet (WHO, 2011). This could be attributed to factors such as lack of computer infrastructure, funding, technical know-how, and how culture and traditions are employed in the use and management of HISs to address health services.

This study therefore examined the impact of human interaction on HISs in a natural setting. The following questions were formulated in order to guide and collect data, to addressing the objectives of the study: (1) what are the factors which impact Human Interaction in the use of health information systems; and (2) What are the roles of Human actors in the healthcare service delivery.

The remainder of the paper is divided into five main sections. The first section presents literature review. The second section discusses the methodology used. In the third sections data analysis is presented and based on the findings the implications for the Human Interaction in the HIS are discussed.

LITERATURE REVIEW

The power of ICT is dramatically changing the ways in which the healthcare organisations operate. Istepanian (2006) explains that, networking technologies and database management systems are able to incorporate better healthcare service, faster in response, and easier to meet increasing demands for the system integration. According to Keenan et al., (2006), the implementation of information systems in hospitals has helped healthcare professionals to improve the efficiency and effectiveness of their services. Health information systems (HIS) that can record and locate important information quickly have become a standard practice in many hospital organisations. The vision of a paperless hospital is delineated as the embodiment of the future health information systems with the hope that it brings an improved promise of more reliable effectiveness and efficiency to the environment (Leppeveld, 2000).

HIS comprises of different computing applications that support the needs of healthcare organisations, clinicians, patients, and policy makers in collecting and managing all data that are related to both clinical and administrative processes (Rada, 2008). Advances in HIS are vital for our society, in that the technologies guide everyday lives, and without them life had been more difficult (Mukama, 2003). Along the same line of argument, Winter (2006) argued that the traditional recording methods of healthcare activities are limited because the captured data and information can only be kept largely in a "physical" form, and are not easily accessible, transportable, or available digitally to other expert clinicians. This makes the use of such data difficult or impossible for human interactions, in carrying out healthcare services to the needy, of different cultural and traditional affiliations.

For health information systems to provide information at the right time and when required, certain factors must be considered and understood. Sinha (2010) argued that such factors include what to collect, where to collect, whom to report to, and how the information will be used and by whom. The results of these factors are manifestations of human interactions. A poorly planned system that ignores user needs, fails to understand organisation capacities, neglects cultural constraints and ignores the local knowledge base will only result in failure for health technologies (Rodrigues & Risk, 2003). This has impact on providing services through human interaction. HIS require a process of learning and adaption from the people and systems that will use them (Steinmueller, 2001). Furthermore, technology rarely stands independently; it is rather embedded in a system of complementary technologies and capabilities and requires three key elements for success, people, process, and technology (Cleverley, 2009). The interaction between people, process and technology supports operation and management in delivering essentials information in order to improve the quality of healthcare service delivery.

Rob (2009) reported that effective use of information technologies has become a critical success factor in modern society. Yet, success is not easily achieved, hence the work in progress in many environments. John (2002) stated that many of the failures occur not in the technology, but in how technology is used in the context of the application domain and settings. This is influenced by the organisational culture and its role in IS organisational (Robey, 2007). According to Mylopoulus (2006), IS changing the social structures of the environment in which people work. In performing some aspects of work that would otherwise be performed by people, they change how tasks are allocated to individuals and groups. From the perspectives of human interactions, Lyytinen(2007) added, by his argument that each time a system is introduced or modified; responsibilities and relationships are reallocated, possibly contested and renegotiated.

The importance of social factors in information systems has long been recognised (Anshari & Almunawar, 2009). Anshari and Almunawar further argued that many systems fail or fall into disuse not because of technical failure, but in how the technology is matched to the social environment. Each time an information system is introduced within an organisational context, the corporate agenda of the target system dominates. Kahn, Aulakh and Bosworth (2006) argued that in such a case the new system is intended to improve productivity and profitability while users who are employees are expected to fit their work practices to the new system (Kahn, Aulakh, & Bosworth, 2006).

RESEARCH METHODOLOGY

The qualitative research method was adopted as the strategy for the study. The qualitative method was selected primary because it allows subjects or objects to be studied in their natural setting (Myers, 2009). Also, the qualitative method focuses on human behaviour which is considered to significantly influenced and be influenced by the setting of the environment. According to Atieno (2009), individuals and groups interpret their thoughts, feelings and actions within the qualitaive paradigm.

The case study approach was employed within the qualitaive paradigm to elicit specific answer to the problem as stated above. According to Yin (2003), a case study is an empirical inquiry that investigates a contemporary phenomenon within its real-life context. Windhoek central hospital in Namibia was used as a case. The Windhoek Central hospital in Windhoek was selected because at the time of the study it was the only public hospital in Namibia that has implemented HIS.

The semi-structured interview technique was used for the data collection. Semi structured interview implies that the researcher will have questions to guide the interview but can possibly ask any other question for clarity or to enhance data gathering process. This means that the interview questions are generally organised around a set of predetermined open-ended questions, with other questions emerging from the dialogue between interviewer and interviewees. In this way, respondents can elaborate on their responses and possibly connect them with other matters of relevance. The interviews conversations were recorded using a tape recorder and were later transcribed. A total of ten people were interviewed. The respondents included a pharmacist (1), nurses (3), network administrators (2), payroll administrator (1), administrative assistant (2) and the system administrators (1). The respondents were selected because of their lengthy years of services and their more frequent daily interaction with the HIS at the Windhoek Central hospital.

The transcribed data was analysed using a thematic analysis approach, as discussed below. The approach includes identification of patterns and themes in the data. Braun and Clarke (2006) elaborated that thematic analysis is a method for identifying, analysing, and reporting patterns (themes) within data. It is also noted by Rice and Azzy (1999) that thematic analysis process involves the identification of themes through the careful reading and re-reading of the data. According to Braun and Clarke (2006), a theme captures something important about the data in relation to the research question, and represents some level of patterned response or meaning within the data set. The thematic analysis process involved six stages as follows:

Step 1: The researcher prepared the data which was recorded data transcribed, in a summative way.

Step 2: Data classification. The data was classified in accordance to the questions, following respondents' responses as expressed in a form of single words, phrases, sentences or paragraphs.

Step 3: Develop categories and a coding scheme. In this study categories were established based on the research questions. Different colours were used in interview transcripts to identify phrases, words or statement that describes each category.

Step 4: Coded all text through sampling of data. This was done to check for consistency and revise coding rule as an interactive process. While new data continue to be analysed it was likely that new themes emerge. Step four was repeated as new themes emerged from the interviews (example: challenges).

Step 5: Draw conclusion from the coded data. "This step involves making sense of the themes or categories identified and their properties".

Step 6: report your methods of findings. Step six suggests that the researcher should report practices concerning the coding process supported by the descriptions and interpretations to provide the reader with an understanding of the phenomenon (Zhang & Wildemuth, 2009).

Table 1. Elaboration and implication of colour coding

Theme (s)	Categories	Colour Coding
ICT	Other Systems	Green
	HIS	Red
	Medical data collection	Grey
	mediation technology between offices	Purple
	Challenges on daily operations	Blue
	Service delivery	Pink

Data coding is based on the research questions in this study. Sub themes further emerged as the data analysis continues and thematic analysis steps outlined above were repeated. To determine the implication of responses, additional descriptions in different colours were pertinent.

ANALYSIS OF THE IDENTIFIED CATEGORIES

In a complementary fashion, the thematic and interpretive techniques were used in the data analysis. Thus, six categories were identified. The selection of the categories was guided by the study objectives of the study. The interpretive technique was used to analyse and better understand the categories as follows.

I. HIS and Other Systems

At the time of this study, various information systems (IS) were implemented at the hospital, in addition to the HIS. This includes the Financial Integrated System (IFMS) and the Human Resource Management Systems (HRMS).

The IFMS was used by the finance employees to carry out the hospital financial related activities. According to the payroll administrator *"the system is the same one used in all the government public services accounting activities (RS005, p5, 140-141)"*. The system is an integrated system with various financial modules. One of the respondents, an accountant stated that *"the system is working by categories, it have a payroll, SNTies and suppliers payments"* (RS0011, p9, 265-267). Additionally the system *collaborates with the IFMS system at the Ministry of Health, so whatever captured in the system, can be viewed at the Ministry of finance* (RS005, p5, 154-157).

HRMS is another information system that was used in the organisation. The system was used for supporting and enabling some activities and processes of the human resource (HR). One of the respondents shared her views as follows" *We only use the system to list employees wellness program and advertise vacancies internally but we have store room called registry where we manually keep all our employees files"*(RS001, p1,11-15).

Both the IFMS and HRMS were of importance to the hospital as they supported and enabled automation of processes and activities. The employees interacted with the systems. Also, they made use of the systems to interaction with other actors. The interactions were based on their interest as well as their technical know-how skills. As such depending on the level of expertise about the systems, employees either fully interacted with the system or were reluctant (or limited) in their use and interaction with the systems. The limited use of the systems made them white elephants in the organisation. At the hospital, skills were acquired through systems training or via previous educational background. It was the responsibility of the human resource business unit to ensure that all employees are technical know-how competent.

II. Health Information System (HIS)

The health Information system implemented at the Windhoek Central hospital is called Integrated Health Care Information Management System (IHCIMS). The system has been operating for the last two years. The system is part of The Ministry of Health and Social Services (MoHSS) initiatives to eradicate manual process and to improve healthcare service delivery. According to Suresh (personal communication, September 4, 2013) *the IHCIMS is a comprehensive web based enterprise-wide application that covers all aspects of management and day-to-day operations of a hospital.* The application modules include (i) admission - for administering patients contact details; (ii) pharmacy - for management and allocation of prescribed medications; and (iii) inpatient and outpatient – for managing patient's circulations within the hospital. The various modules are integrated and able to communicate. A pharmacist illustrated this stating that" *The doctors enter the details about the prescribed medication and when the patients collect medicine at the pharmacy, we retrieve the record using the Medical Record(MR)number in order to hand out medicines* "(RS004,p32, 115-117)

III. Medical Data Collection

The hospital did realise that they do needs reliable and accurate data in order to deliver effective and efficient services to patients. However, they employed two different systems namely (1) paper-based (2) computer-based (IHCIMS) for their activities and processes.

A. Paper-Based System

The paper-based system was the main form that was used to store and manage patients' data at the hospital. Patient data are recorded in health passport (small green and yellow booklet) that is provided by the public hospitals and clinics country wide. It is mandatory that each time a patient visit the hospital he/she is expected to have their health passport in order to receive treatment. In case a patient loses the health passport, provision for a new health passport is made. However, one of the challenges that was experienced with the use of the paper-based system was that there are no backup od patients' medical treatment, hence when a patients loses their health passport, healthcare professionals have nowhere to follow up on the patient treatments. As a result this often leads to repetition of efforts, and therefore slows down the treatment process.

B. Computer-Based System

The hospital regards this method to be the future method for data collection. With this method on the first encounter with the hospital patients are first assigned a medical record (MR) number. The record number which is automatically generated by the IHCIMS is unique henceforth it uniquely identify each patient. With this method all patients' data are recorded on the computerised system with real-time backup data available. Henceforth the system eradicates data redundancy and provides healthcare professionals with real time data required for effective service delivery. An administrative nurse shared her views stating that *"The system works with internet and each patient is allocated medical record number and then all details are being entered on the computer system and this make it easier to retrieve the in formation"(RS156,pg5,187-191).*

IV. Mediation Technology between Offices

Technologies in healthcare environment are primarily implemented to support and enable efficient and effective healthcare service delivery. Various technologies existed in the hospital environment at the time of this study. The technologies included software and hardware such as printers, scanners, servers and desktops. Technology mediation between the offices was enabled due to some of the integrated systems and systems internet connectivity. However the application of such technologies was dependent on the level of technical know-how among the employees. As such the technologies implementation, usage and maintenance depend on human interpretation and understanding. .

V. Challenges on Daily Operations

Healthcare professionals encountered challenges as they carry out their daily activities. These challenges are both technical and non-technical challenges. Both challenges hinder quality service delivery.

A. Technical Challenges

Healthcare professionals encountered technical challenges such as slow internet connectivity and system downtimes. Majority of the respondents viewed their frustration about the slow internet. As a result most of the activities were delayed due to the slow internet connectivity. Systems downtime was also a main concern among the health professionals. Most of the time the system was down due to maintenance. One of the respondents shared her dissatisfaction *"the system is not yet fully implemented"* (RS006, pg6, 195). When system is down the healthcare professionals perform their responsibilities manually. For example the doctors would write down the medicine prescription in the health passport whereby the patients will than take their passport to the pharmacist for medicines collection. In both instances there is no data recorded on the system. Also the various systems were not integrated making it difficult or impossible for employees to collaborate.

B. Non-Technical Challenges

In the organisation non-technical challenges included lack of technical know-how and lack of communication among the healthcare professionals. Most of the healthcare professionals were not able to utilise computers due to the lack of computer user skills. The use of HIS requires awareness and technical know-how. Unfortunately this was lacking among the healthcare professionals especially among the nurses. Stating her views a registers nurse said*" most of the people are not computer literate especially the nurses and then they don't have enough skills to do that"* (RS006, pg5, 193-194). As a result majority healthcare professionals preferred carrying out their activities manually. Therefore most of the computer systems were not used or rather employees found them hard to use.

Lack of sufficient training about the systems and technologies implemented at the hospital was the main factor that attributed to the lack of technical know-how. In most cases trainings are conducted but are not adequate enough for the employees to acquire the necessary skills.

There were also communication challenges within the organisation. The systems down times were most of the time not communicated on time." *When the system is being updated we are not actually informed*" stating (RS005, pg4, 144). This was attributed to the lack communication between technical people and healthcare professionals.

VI. Service Delivery

Many actors are involved in healthcare service delivery. These actors are either human or non-human. The human actors include the healthcare professionals, (such as nurses, doctors and pharmacist), administrative workers, patients and other stakeholders (Ministry of Health). The non-human actors were the ICT artefacts, medical tools and the processes used to deliver service.

Service delivery was influenced by the actors' interaction. The interaction involved human-to-human, human-to-non-human and non-human-to-non-human. The interactions were guided by rules and regulations as defined in the organisation. Based on the various interactions, it became clear that not all actors involved in the service delivery were satisfied with the processes of service delivery. For example some actors were dissatisfied with the paper based forms as most of the times files would get missing resulting in the repetition of activities that had been performed .This caused delay and response time in service delivery.

FINDINGS AND DISCUSSION

Based on the analysis of the qualitative data as presented above, there were findings from the study. This includes communicative scheme, infrastructure obsolete, system integration, systems parallel, and lack of technical know-how, data omission, and trivial use of the IHCIMS. The findings are discussed below. The discussion should be read with the Figure 1 so as to gain better understanding of how human interaction influence and impact the HIS (IHCIMS) in Windhoek Central hospital. The arrows indicates a bidirectional link among the various components

I. Communicative Scheme

The communicative scheme in the context of this study is viewed as a form of interaction among actors. Callon (1986) defined actors as both human and non-human linked together in this network by common interest. The communicative scheme enacts the interaction between actors: human-to-human, human-to-nonhuman (such as technology), and nonhuman-to-nonhuman. The use and management of the HIS in Windhoek Central hospital is influenced by many factors as depicted in Figure 1. The outcomes of the use and management of the HIS is as a result of the reproductive interaction among those factors.

The infrastructures enabling and supporting the HIS were left, or remained obsolete primarily because of limited communication among the actors. There were lapses in the collaboration of the systems due

Figure 1. Human Interaction with HIS

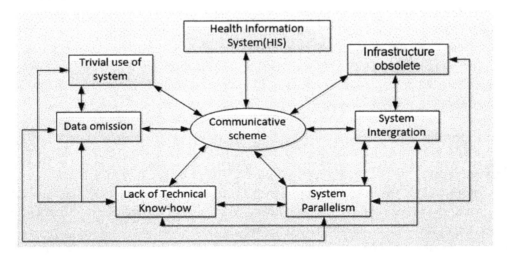

to lack of technology-to-technology communication. Also, a more robust interaction among the actors would have eradicated parallel systems in the environment. From a more non-technical perspective, the communicative scheme facilitates, in addressing factors such as trivial use of the IHCIMS, data omission by the medical professionals, and the lack of technical know-how among the medical professionals.

II. Infrastructure Obsolete

The integrated health care information management system (IHCIMS) was web enabled, meaning the system could be accessed through the internet. This necessitated reasonable support and maintenance of the infrastructures. However, as revealed from the data, the infrastructures that were deployed to enable and support the IHCIMS were obsolete. This hampered some of the services as there was reliance on the system. For example, the -Internet connectivity was often slow, delaying services including data retrieval.

III. Systems Integration

The systems (IHCIMS, HRMS, IFMS) used at the Windhoek Central hospital to support the administration of employees' activities were not integrated, for their activities rather they were stand-alone systems. This leads to lack of collaboration among employees as they could not share and access real-time data. This hindered response time in providing services to co-employees as well as patients For example, during Practitioner-to-Practitioner referrals within the hospital, it becomes difficult to identify and allocate individual (as per their specialisation and availability. It gets more challenging for new practitioners who are still trying to understand the environment. Systems integration enables effective human interaction of the HIS as it minimises systems parallelism that causes implications, such as data duplications of functions. The development and implementation of integrated systems requires resources, such as personnel with technical know-how.

IV. Systems "Parallelism"

As it was revealed from data analysis, both paper-based and the IHCIMS systems were used at the Windhoek Central hospital. The use of parallel systems created data inconsistencies as some data were being recorded on the IHCIMS system and others on paper-based (manual) system. Also, the parallelism of the systems leads to implications, such as duplication of processes and activities resulting in inefficient use of resources. Integration of the systems will address the problems and challenges caused by parallelism. Otherwise, service delivery will continue be jeopardised at the Windhoek Central hospital.

V. Lack of Technical Know-How

As with other areas of expertise, technical know-how was paramount in the use of the hospital's HIS (IHCIMS). The know-how is a set of skill acquired from training and education. However, this was lacking at Windhoek Central Hospital. In the study, it was revealed that not all the system users were trained or did receive productive training to be able to use the systems to support their daily activities. Some employees were requested and expected to familiarise themselves with the functionality of the system. Thus, they lost productive time while navigating around the system. What was even more challenging was that majority of the nurses were not computer literate. As a result, they were more comfortable following the manual processes. The lack of technical know-how plays significant in human interaction with the IHCIMS, in that it contributed to data omission. Also, this contributed to trivial use of the IHCIMS in the hospital, which affected efficiency of service delivering.

VI. Data Omission

Data is an important aspect of every organisation primary because it can enable or constrain activities through its use for decision making. In lure of this, we gathered from our analysis of the data that not all patients that visit the hospital are registered on the HIS. This was because the HIS was trivially used, which was caused by lack of technical know-how. As such, some patients (or visitors) were registered manually on the paper-based forms (system). The paper-based practise contributed to patients' data incompleteness or omission. This process negatively impact service delivery due to lack of insufficient data required to make informed decisions.

VII. Trivial Use of System

At the Windhoek Central hospital, the systems, such as the HRMS were hardly used, or reluctantly used as empirically revealed. At the hospital, the HRMS was only used for internal vacancies advertisement. What was even more trivial was that the workers could not make use of the systems (HRMS) to apply for the jobs that were advertised through the system. One of the implications of this is that the system does not support online application processing. As a result, the departments mainly use manually paper forms to perform their daily activities. For example with the leave processing employees fill in their forms manually. After forms have been processed they are manually stored in cabinets in the registry. The implication is that the documentation are vulnerable to threat and disaster, such as fire and theft.

CONCLUSION

It is now hard to imagine the survival of a hospital without information and communication technologies. As known and revealed in this study, the use of HIS is critically influenced by human interaction. This means that how human interact determines the success or failure of the HIS in providing healthcare services in the Namibia. The Ministry of Health and Social Services of the Republic of Namibia thus requires a comprehensive modern Integrated Health Care Information Management System (IHCIMS) to improve the quality and effectiveness of health care for all Namibians.

The challenges of transitioning from a paper environment to an electronic environment must involve rethinking of factors, such as workflow, staff skills, availability of resources, habits and the organisational culture. Acknowledgement of this has led to a need for understanding the match between IHCIMS and existing IT infrastructure, organisational structure, and established routines. This means that the decision-making process leading to the implementation and use of ICT-based applications at the hospital has to improve generally. It should be noted that technology is an enabler and requires support from the people using it to be affective, thus the need for hospital employees to be trained and be well informed of the technology in place.

REFERENCES

Anshari, M., & Almunawar, M. N. (2009). *Health Information Systems (HIS): Concept and Technology.* Academic Press.

Atieno, O. (2009). An analysis of the strengths and limitation of qualitative and quantitative research paradigms. *Problems of Education in the 21st Century, 13,* 13-18.

Braun, V., & Clarke, V. (2006). Using thematic analysis in pyschology. *Qualitative Research in Psychology, 3*(2), 77–101. doi:10.1191/1478088706qp063oa

Callon, M. (1986). Some elements of the sociology of translation: Domestication of the scallops and the fisherman of St Brieuc Bay. In J. Law (Ed.), *A New Sociology of Knowledge, power, action and belief* (pp. 196–233). London: Routledge.

Cleverley, M. (2009). How ICT advances might help developing nations. *Communications of the ACM, 52*(9), 30–32. doi:10.1145/1562164.1562177

Goldschmidt, P. G. (2005). Implications of health information technology and medical information systems. *Communications of the ACM, 48*(10), 69–74.

Istepanian. (2006). Design and Implementation of a Mobile Diabetes Management System. *Journal of Mobile Multimedia, 1*(4), 273-284.

John, T. G. (2002). *Requirements Engineering:Social and Technical Issues.* London: Academic Press.

Kahn, J. S., Aulakh, V., & Bosworth, A. (2006). What it takes: Characteristics of the ideal personal health record. *Health Affairs, 28*(2), 369–376. doi:10.1377/hlthaff.28.2.369 PMID:19275992

Keenan, C. R., Nguyen, H. H., & Srinivasan, M. (2006). Electronic medical records and their impact on residents and medical student education. *Academic Psychiatry*, *30*(6), 522–527. doi:10.1176/appi.ap.30.6.522 PMID:17139024

Lippeveld, T. (2001). Routine health information systems:the glue of a unified health system. *The RHINO Workshop on Issues and Innovation in Routine Health In Information in Developing Countries*.Arlington, VA: JSI Research and Training Institute.

McDonald, M. (2006). Public Health Informatics: How Information Age Technology Can Strengthen Public Health. *Annual Review of Public Health*, *4*(2), 239–252. PMID:7639873

Mukama, F. (2003). *A study of health information systems at local levels in Tanzania and Mozambique.* (MSc thesis). University of Oslo.

Myers, M. D. (2009). *Qualitative Research in Business & Management.* New Zealand: SAGE Publications Ltd.

Mylopoulus, J. (2006). Representing Knowledge About Information Systems. *ACM Transactions on Information Systems*, *3*(2), 131–140.

Rada, R. (2008). *Information Systems and Healthcare Enterprises.* Hershey, PA: IGI Publishing. doi:10.4018/978-1-59904-651-8

Rice, P., & Azzy, D. (1999). *Qualitative research methods: A health focus.* Melbourne: Oxford University Press.

Robey, D. (2007). Cultural Analysis and the Organizational Consequences of I.T. *Accounting. Management and Information Technologies*, *3*(1), 23–24.

Rodrigues, R., & Risk, A. (2003). eHealth in Latin America and the Caribbean:Development and policy issues. *Journal of Medical Internet Research*, *5*(1), 4–22. doi:10.2196/jmir.5.1.e4 PMID:12746209

Sauerborn, R., & Lippeveld, T. (2000). *What is wrong with current health information systems?* Geneva: WHO.

Sinha, R. (2010). Impact of health information technology in public health. *Sri Lanka Journal of Bio-Medical Informatics*, *1*(4), 223–236. doi:10.4038/sljbmi.v1i4.2239

Steinmueller, W. (2001). ICTs and the possibilities for leapfrogging by developing countries. *International Labour Review*, *140*(2), 193–210. doi:10.1111/j.1564-913X.2001.tb00220.x

Yin, R. (2003). *Case Study Research: Design and Methods* (3rd ed.). Sage.

KEY TERMS AND DEFINITIONS

Health Information System: A computer system used to store and process health related information.
Healthcare: The services and products offered by the hospital to the communities.

Human Interaction: The communication between the humans and computer systems as they carry out the activities and processes.

Information Systems: A computer system used to store and processes organisational information.

This research was previously published in Maximizing Healthcare Delivery and Management through Technology Integration edited by Tiko Iyamu, Arthur Tatnall, pages 257-269, copyright year 2016 by Medical Information Science Reference (an imprint of IGI Global).

Chapter 66

Unobtrusive Smart Environments for Independent Living and the Role of Mixed Methods in Elderly Healthcare Delivery:
The USEFIL Approach

Alexander Astaras
Aristotle University of Thessaloniki, Greece & American College of Thessaloniki, Greece

Hadas Lewy
Maccabi Healthcare, Israel

Christopher James
University of Warwick, UK

Artem Katasonov
VTT Technical Research Center, Finland

Detlef Ruschin
Fraunhofer Heinrich Hertz Institute, Germany

Panagiotis D. Bamidis
Aristotle University of Thessaloniki, Greece

ABSTRACT

In this chapter the authors describe a novel approach to healthcare delivery for the elderly as adopted by USEFIL, a research project which uses unobtrusive, multi-parametric sensor data collection to support seniors. The system is based on everyday devices such as an in-mirror camera, smart TV, wrist-mountable personal communicator and a tablet computer strategically distributed around the house. It exploits sensor data fusion, intelligent decision support for carers, remote alerting, secure data communications and

DOI: 10.4018/978-1-5225-3926-1.ch066

storage. A combined quantitative and qualitative knowledgebase was established and analysed, target groups were established among elderly prospective users and scenarios were built around each group. Use cases have been prioritised according to quantitative functional and non-functional criteria. Our research findings suggest that an unobtrusive system such as USEFIL could potentially make a significant difference in the quality of life of elderly people, improve the focus of provided healthcare and support their daily independent living activities.

INTRODUCTION

The increasing strain placed by an ageing global population on healthcare systems needs to be addressed, immediately in the case of certain nations such as Japan, Germany, Italy and Greece. Planning for maximisation of an elder's capability to live independently could be part of a technological solution, as would the next step, assisted living. The USEFIL project performs research on smart assistive and monitoring environments for this purpose, involving research and pilot study sites in Germany and Greece, two countries which are particularly affected by this global trend.

BACKGROUND

Population ageing is a global trend, primarily driven by an increase in life expectancy and decreasing fertility. The phenomenon is reflected in an increase of the population's mean and median ages, as a consequence of a rising proportion of the elderly population, defined as all people over 65 years of age. It is a phenomenon without parallel in human history, has pervasive characteristics affecting every person on the planet and is expected to be enduring: we are unlikely to ever return to the young populations that our ancestors knew (UN, 2001).

AGEING POPULATION: A EUROPEAN PERSPECTIVE

Seniors over the age of 65 are the fastest growing demographic group globally, expected to reach 1.5 billion by the year 2050, out of a total of approximately 9 billion people. Statistical data show that three out of the top four most aged populations in the world are the citizens of European countries (Beard J. R et al., 2012). In 2010 Japan had the most aged society with 23% of its population being over 65m while Italy, Germany and Greece follow it in the global ranking. Seniors in these European countries account for 21%, 20% and 19% of the total population, respectively. At the other end of the European spectrum, Slovakia, Cyprus and Ireland are the least aged European countries with an elderly percentage of 13%, 12% and 11% respectively.

By comparison the USA, the world's largest economy, has a ratio of 13% elderly citizens. The three largest emerging economies, China, India and Brazil, are among the world's least aged countries: seniors account for 8%, 5% and 7% of the population, respectively. (UK Office for National Statistics, 2011)

The implications of a rapidly ageing population are socioeconomically significant: a proportionally smaller workforce has to sustain increasing numbers of pensioners, while medical and social insurance infrastructures need to adjust towards more emphasis on diseases of old age. Part of the solution to these and future aging-related social challenges will likely involve empowering senior citizens to continue living independently, within the community (Bovenschulte M & Huch M, 2010). Apart from the obvious benefits of better targeted healthcare delivery, the required technological developments and infrastructure changes can be combined to help provide more efficient personalised healthcare for elderly citizens (Codagnone, 2009).

This paper presents the work undertaken so far by the USEFIL project (USEFIL, 2011) specifically following such a service-oriented and technologically innovative approach. The project involves planning, technology development of a novel system and associated services, data collection, as well as final pilot studies validation (USEFIL Consortium, 2011). The three countries selected by the project consortium to host the pilot studies are Greece, the UK and Israel. Elderly citizens in these countries represent a proportion of 19%, 17% and 10%, as compared to an overall European Union average of 16%. Moreover, the EU average is expected to increase by 3% during the 2010-2020 decade, double the rate of increase of the past two decades (UN, 2001).

Comparative research performed by USEFIL scientists based on demographic literature produced the following common observations among the three pilot study host countries:

- The population in all three countries follows the global trend and is thus ageing.
- It is ageing at an increasing pace, due to diminishing fertility rates and increasing life expectancy.
- The difference in the percentages of elderly males and elderly females over the entire population is decreasing.

In Greece, intergenerational co-residence has been a traditional form of support within the family structure. As in most industrialised countries, this form of domestic arrangement has been on the decline throughout the 20th century. Detailed demographic data is sparse and elusive in the literature, however there is clear evidence that this decline had been dramatic during the latter half of the century: the percentage of elderly people living alone or in couples was 46% in 1974 and increased to 68% in 1999. Following the same trend, the number of independent households consisting exclusively of elderly residents increased by 41% between 1991 and 2001. Over the same time period, the number of households consisting of a single elderly occupant increased by 36%. Independent living among the elderly is clearly becoming more common at a quick pace in Greece. These senior citizens are often supported by family relatives or social day care centres, the latter being less common in rural areas (Hellenic Statistical Authority, 2009).

In the UK, 2009 demographic data indicate that 32% of women aged 65-74 lived alone, as compared to 22% of men in the same age group. For seniors aged 75 and over the proportion of those living alone increases to 60% for women and 36% for men. The effect of family structure changes to people living separately remains unchanged as divorce rates have remained fairly constant for the population of over 65+ (UK Office for National Statistics, 2011).

In Israel, 25% of the elderly population live alone, having increased from 12% as reported by a 1961 census. The proportion increases with age and -significantly for project USEFIL- the proportion of elderly women living alone is more than three times that of men. There is also some variation related to ethnic background: 94% of elderly Jews versus 71% of elderly Arabs live in households of up to two persons— usually with a spouse and less commonly with a son or daughter (Israeli Central Bureau of Statistics, 2012).

Common Trends and Implications for National Policy

Overall, the demographic literature research within USEFIL for the three countries where the pilot site hosts are located –Greece, the UK and Israel- showed the following common trends:

- A growing percentage of elderly citizens are living independently, alone or with a spouse. Multigenerational co-residence households are increasingly rare, with adult children more likely to be living at ever greater geographic distance from their parents. Older people value their independence and express a preference for living in the community rather than in institutional facilities.
- A growing percentage of seniors live alone. In all three countries, the majority of elderly living alone are females because women tend to outlive men. Increasing numbers of elderly who live alone have no relatives living nearby, while some have no family at all.
- Providing the psychological support and safety for elderly people who are willing to live independently in their houses for longer is as much a political and socioeconomic challenge as it is technological.

A system which can provide discrete safety monitoring and alert generation without violating privacy may help improve quality of life, focus human resources on non-repetitive tasks as well as reduce costs to public health and social care systems. The USEFIL consortium made the choice to involve all stakeholders in the system design and evaluation phase: gerontology psychiatrists, professional carers, social security planners, the elderly themselves and their relatives.

Much like other industrialised countries, population aging of the U.S. is forecast to be unprecedented and will "present societal and economic challenges unlike anything the US society has ever seen," while health care costs are expected to skyrocket during the following decades (US Senate Commitee Hearing on Aging, 2003). Simply increasing the amount of resources poured into support for the elderly is unlikely to be the most efficient response to the growing pressure of an ageing population. As in other countries, adaptation of existing healthcare delivery models and introduction of additional ones will be necessary (Inst. of Medicine of the National Academies, 2008).

A consumer-directed orientation of publicly funded support has been successfully employed in several European countries and thirty states in the USA (Benjamin, 2001). This model is particularly amenable to combination with technologies that can extend independent for the elderly in the USA, where studies have shown that elders strongly prefer independent living (Kasper, Shore, & Penninx, 2000) and are highly averse to nursing-home placement (Mattimore, Wenger, Desbiens, & Teno, 1997).

Systems that support and extend the duration of independent living are particularly beneficial for sparsely populated countries as well as countries where family members tend to live geographically distant from each other, such as in the United States. Early warning and electronic alerting are practically important for healthcare coordinators and psychologically reassuring for beneficiaries, especially in areas where ambulances need considerable time to reach remote residential areas. Technologies such as USEFIL provide added value to national healthcare systems and private-public partnerships aiming to support elders in the community rather than institutional care (Mukamel et al., 2006); (Gross, Temkin-Greener, Kunitz, & Mukamel, 2004). Prime candidates to benefit from such added value would be pioneering and successful initiatives such as such as *Programs of All-Inclusive Care for the Elderly (PACE)* already operating in several states in the USA (National PACE Association, 2007).

The USEFIL Approach: Mixed Method Research Into Independent Living Support

The USEFIL project employs mixed methods in both the system design and operational phases. The project's main objectives include:

- To support elderly people who are willing to live independently to do so for longer, in a safer fashion, with increased or sustained social interaction and improved quality of life.
- To integrate lifestyle data collection, notifications for carers and relatives, alerts towards emergency services, motivational recommendations for the elderly and electronic health record logging into a single, unobtrusive and transparent system.
- To provide technological solutions which improve data access for carers, drive costs down and increase safety without requiring retrofitting the elderly participants' residences.

The USEFIL consortium comprises eight institutions, including three European universities, three research institutes and two multinational companies. Three of the partners include or have access to clinical facilities and are in charge of performing pilot trials of the system under development. The project kicked off in November 2011 and has a duration of three years.

Expertise within the consortium spans several business and scientific disciplines: medicine, clinical psychology, electrical and biomedical engineering, computer science, medical services, ubiquitous computing and instrumentation. One of the companies in the USEFIL consortium, the Israeli company Maccabi Healthcare, already operates a nearly-automated healthcare data flow. The University of Thessaloniki Medical School has research experience with home automations supporting elderly individuals living alone.

Sociological Study Into Independent Living

The first few months of the USEFIL project involved a systematic review of the literature and census data on the capacity for elders to live independently in the three pilot study host countries. In addition to the information already presented in this section, the study also concluded:

- Preventing the strain placed by an ageing population on social and healthcare systems can be partly alleviated by encouraging independent living.
- Expecting more elderly people to live independently for longer will inevitably require pre-emptive investment in supportive care services and technologies.
- The elders who are likely to benefit most from improved services are those with health-related problems that occur as a person ages and which threaten their independence.
- Such medical conditions threatening independent living include.
- A range of co-morbidities (e.g. cerebrovascular and heart disease).
- Risk of cognitive decline and functional deterioration.
- Fall related injuries.
- Urinary incontinence.
- Infections.

- Musculoskeletal conditions limiting mobility.
- Sensory loss and depression.
- Different target groups should be selected for the three pilot sites in order to research the effect of the USEFIL system on a variety of these factors.

METHODS

Qualitative Research at Three Pilot Sites: Greece, the UK, and Israel

During the design phase of the USEFIL system, the application of qualitative methodology commenced with focus group sessions in each of the three pilot sites in Greece, Israel and the UK. The data flow subsequently involved semi-structured interviews with elderly USEFIL users, technical observations collected from the users' houses, a second round of focus group sessions and final processing of the data by the USEFIL partner institutions. The results formed the basis for consequent extraction of functional and non-functional system design requirements.

The methodology employed mixed quantitative and qualitative research technique on various levels. The interviews covered both explicit quantitative questions as well as more subjective qualitative material. Technical observations provided exclusively quantitative content to the focus groups. Finally, focus group transcripts were processed using standard qualitative analysis methods, so as to extract generalised conclusions and expert opinions in a detached and methodical fashion. Figure 1 depicts a diagram showing qualitative and quantitative data flow during the USEFIL design phase.

Focus Group Meetings

Two focus group sessions took place in each of the 3 pilot sites, involving 39 professionals: physicians, clinicians, clinical psychologists, geriatric nurses, biomedical engineers, electrical engineers and informaticians. Input from elderly participants and their relatives was taken into account through inclusion of the pre-pilot interview data.

The first sessions processed the project's objectives, raised questions that need to be answered during the system design phase, planned pre-pilot mixed method interviews with prospective elderly users, drafted a path to system design requirements and proposed relevant actions for the USEFIL consortium. The second focus group sessions processed the interview results and technical observations made at the senior participants' homes, and created use case scenarios from which the system design requirements would later be extracted.

The participants for the focus group sessions were selected and by the research team leaders in the participating institutions, aiming to cover all stakeholders. They included clinical psychologists, geriatric care professionals, electrical and biomedical engineers, informatics and artificial intelligence scientists, as well as businessmen from the medical services sector.

Each focus group session contained both semi-structured and open discussion intervals, held in the local language. Transcripts translated in English were later produced from audio recordings, keeping the translation as faithful as possible. The translated transcripts were re-circulated among focus group members who had a chance to check that their opinions were accurately presented.

There were slight variations among the three pilot sites in the methodology used, however all focus group transcripts were processed using a mix of phenomenology and ground theory, so as to be able to account for the multi-faceted nature of the input data.

Pre-Pilot Semi-Structured Interviews with Elderly Participants

The first focus group session drafted a questionnaire for interviews with elderly people living alone, aimed at determining their needs, wishes and habits from the point of view of project USEFIL's objectives. A total of 18 seniors were interviewed, 8 men and 10 women. Seven of the interviewees were from Greece (2 men, 5 women, mean age = 76.0, st. dev. = 7.4), six were from the UK (3 men, 3 women, mean age = 76, st. dev. = 6.26) and five from Israel (3 men, 2 women, mean age = 71.8, st. dev. = 9.1).

Interviews were semi-structured and involved questions drafted during the first focus group session. Audio was recorded in all cases. In Greece, the interview visit included obtaining technical observations from the interviewee's house, as well as a brief open discussion during which the elderly person was allowed to ask questions and express their opinion on the USEFIL system being designed.

Planning for Sensor Data Fusion and a Decision Support System

As mentioned in earlier sections, the USEFIL system being developed utilises data originating from a variety of sensors and transceivers: cameras, microphones, gyroscopic accelerometers, GPS receivers and radio frequency transceivers. Landline telecommunication is also logged but not monitored. The aforementioned sensors are unobtrusively embedded in several USEFIL devices:

- A wrist-mounted smart watch.
- A mirror concealing an embedded camera.
- A tablet touch-screen communicator.
- A smart, networked television set.
- Camera domes in rooms (depending on system configuration).

The sensors and transceivers provide the USEFIL system with multi-parametric data which needs to be processed inside the house, in order to secure privacy. Pre-processing the data involves filtering, extracting higher level signal characteristics in real time and redirecting the results to software algorithms which subsequently perform thresholding and feature extraction functions. This signal filtering and sensor data fusion takes place inside the house, leading to the extraction of higher level information which can be securely communicated to the USEFIL database outside. For instance, camera footage of an elderly person getting dressed in the morning is never retained on the USEFIL system, however associated logged time stamps may be securely communicated and stored in the USEFIL database outside the house.

The output of the sensor data fusion algorithm module is subsequently handled by decision support software developed specifically for the USEFIL system. This software includes trend detection, further feature extraction and artificial intelligence classification algorithms. It is currently under development and expected to have access to data both inside the house and on the USEFIL server outside, while its output will be securely communicated and stored outside. This module generates events and associated content for the alert module, a piece of software running outside the house and handling user recommendations, alerts for carers and emergency alerts. Figure 1 depicts an indicative outline of sensor, device and database distribution within and around a house supported by the USEFIL system and services.

Definition of Pilot Study Target Groups

The USEFIL consortium and steering committee evaluated the conclusions and recommendations originating from the focus group sessions, the sociological study on independent living, the project's stated objectives and the technological and financial restrictions. Taking all these factors into account, the consortium decided to steer the pilot study towards the following target groups for the three partner sites:

1. Aristotle University Medical School, Greece
    a. Seniors aged 60 or older -ideally older than 65 (required)
    b. Living alone independently or with a partner-carer (required)
    c. Healthy individuals who wish to improve or extend their capacity for independent living
    d. Patients with mild cognitive impairment
    e. Seniors with a propensity for sporadic bouts of mild depression.
2. Warwick University Institute of Digital Healthcare, UK
    a. Seniors aged 65 or older (required)
    b. Living alone independently or with a spouse (required)
    c. Who are cognitively well functioning (required)
    d. Chronic condition sufferers (co-morbidities included) excluding any form of dementia
    e. Participants with a range of conditions including: Parkinson's, Multiple Sclerosis, Prostate Cancer, hypertension/cardiovascular conditions, history of falls

Figure 1. Qualitative assessment data flow during USEFIL system design

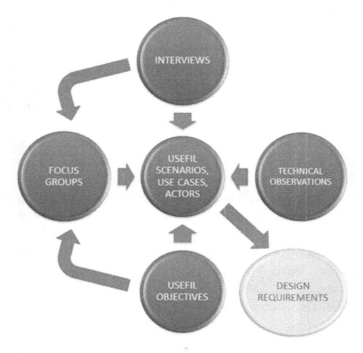

3.   Maccabi Healthcare, Israel
    a.   Seniors aged 65-80 years (required)
    b.   Who are living at home independently or with limited assistance for some daily operations (required)
    c.   Who are functional on a cognitive and linguistic basis (required)
    d.   Patients who have suffered a mild to moderate level stroke
    e.   Who receive occasional treatment at home (e.g. physiotherapy)

The pilot studies will cover 30-60 USEFIL system installations in the three pilot sites during the third year of the project. Each installation will involve unobtrusively placed hardware placed inside the house, containing the sensors required for USEFIL data collection.

Semi-Structured Interviews With Prospective Elderly Users

The interviews were designed to obtain data regarding:

- Daily patterns of behaviour of the seniors.
- Acceptance of USEFIL technologies.
- Social, medical, security and privacy needs on behalf of the seniors.
- Physical limitations and difficulties related to old age.
  ◦ Type of assistance required.
  ◦ Types of service is not suitable for elderly people.
- Expectations from the USEFIL service.
- List of wishes of what the seniors would like to receive from USEFIL.

The results show that although the interviews were conducted in 3 different countries, with different target populations, there were significant similarities with respect to the needs, expectations and patterns of behaviour among senior interviewees. Table 1 summarises the overall results and conclusions from the 3 prospective pilot sites.

Use Case Scenarios

Results obtained from the focus group sessions and semi-structured interviews were processed in order to provide insights, conclusions and theories from which design requirements would eventually be extracted (Figure 2). Based on the processed material, scenarios were generated based on stakeholders and actors defined during a collective consortium meeting. These scenarios are mock storylines, that is realistic brief descriptions of foreseen daily interaction of the users with the USEFIL system. The scenarios facilitate the identification of the functional and non-functional requirements needed for the system to fulfil its intended purpose, ultimately leading to the extraction of the final technical requirements for hardware and software development.

Eleven use case scenarios were developed, covering all project objectives, the target groups recommended by the focus groups and even moving beyond these targets:

Table 1. Main conclusions and recommendations based on interviews with senior prospective USEFIL users

	STROKE PATIENTS: OBSERVATIONS & CONCLUSIONS
1	Participants that had survived a stroke event had the following aspects of their lives most affected: daily function, mobility, speech ability and short term memory.
2	Most significant difficulty due to stroke event: speech, walking long distances, fear (general), and fear to be alone.
3	The stroke event affected self-confidence of some of the interviewees (fear) even if there was no actual loss of consciousness or control.
4	Women, especially those living alone, tend to fear more than men with the same medical condition.
5	Long-range vision over a few meters, such as reading TV subtitles, is problematic for several senior interviewees. Arm-reach short range eyesight is considerably better overall.
6	Most patients have a TV set in the bedroom or living room and watch regularly each day, for several hours.
7	Four out of five interviewees have expressed interest in a smart TV.
8	Most interviewees don't use a computer at all.
9	Most patients envision themselves communicating through technology with younger relatives and healthcare professionals, but not with their friends.
10	Younger patients and those in relatively good physical condition do not see a need for the watch/bracelet. Those in poor physical condition, and/or with fear of falls and loss of control are interested in this device.
11	The place where they spend most of their time is the bedroom. During the day, they spend time in the living room or outside the house.
12	The camera is perceived by the interviewees as the component with the most potential benefit, since it can alert about problems in an emergency in which they lose consciousness.
13	The camera addresses a psychological need regarding the fear of stroke patients of experiencing another event or losing consciousness.
14	The service as a whole is perceived as needed for several reasons: monitor and identify problems at an early stage (prevention) medical information and alerts delivered to authorized carer regardless of the patient's condition emergency alerting can sped up the arrival of assistance (treatment).
15	Most common expectations after signing up to the service: reasonable cost training on how to use the system improved personal safety.
16	Interviewees did not express any concern about privacy issues since it was explained to them that it will keep their privacy.
17	The interviewees in the best physical condition (which were younger), didn't like the monitoring devices such as: bracelet, camera and clock. However, the interviewees with more physical limitations showed interest in all monitoring elements – watch/bracelet" camera.
	SMART TV: MAIN RECOMMENDATIONS
18	It should maintain a bright, clear image, large icons\ buttons easy to operate, large fonts, audio and image contrast, short and clear instructions, large display.
19	It is recommended that the TV control application have a "look and feel "of cell phone applications rather than a Web site. Use large, intuitive icons.
20	The touch-screen tablet device is less familiar to seniors. It may be more difficult to convince them to use it than the smart TV.
21	The elderly participants would prefer to have a range of channels that they can switch between to bring up relevant apps/functions.
22	Participants indicated the possibility that the video-conferencing facility while having benefit would not work if the people at the other side viz. clinicians, family, friends –were not suitably trained, involved or if they lacked the right equipment. They preferred using a phone or meeting in person.
	TABLET PC: MAIN RECOMMENDATIONS
23	The use of a Tablet PC is appropriate mostly for seniors that have prior experience using a computer.
24	Participants liked the form factor of the tablet.
25	Participants like the fact that the tablet is light and portable, unlike desktop computers.
26	While some interviewees liked the touch-screen aspect at least one participant mentioned having difficulty using touch screens preferring buttons.
27	The size of the tablets needs to be optimized – a larger screen size was not necessarily attractive.

continued on following page

Table 1. Continued

CAMERA MIRROR: MAIN RECOMMENDATIONS	
28	To have full coverage of the patients, it is recommended to install one camera in the living room, one in the bedroom
29	The patients sees the camera as the most important part of the system that can alert events (even when they are not aware of it)
30	The analyzing system should have reliable predictive and alerting capabilities
31	They were however concerned about installation and wiring issues.
32	The emotion tracking aspect raised concerns because it is subjective
WRIST WATCH: MAIN RECOMMENDATIONS	
33	Patients in a deteriorated physical condition are afraid of falls and loss of control, and would like to use watch/bracelet.
34	There is a correlation between physical condition and willingness to use the bracelet
35	Participants liked the wrist-watch as it suited an independent and active lifestyle.
36	They also found it to be an unobtrusive way of continuous monitoring.
37	The GPS feature – was cited as being useful if they were lost or if they found themselves needing to be tracked in an emergency.
38	The Fall detection feature is highly desired.
39	The potential of the wrist device to place emergency calls or receive updates was highly desired. Say in the case of a fall to talk to emergency services
40	The wrist watch needs to meet the rigours of daily life – being water-proof to use in the shower(high fall risk area)
41	The strap and the dial need to be of a form-factor and material that is comfortable to wear all day long and to even sleep with without being uncomfortable.
USEFIL SYSTEM OVERALL: MAIN RECOMMENDATIONS	
42	Perceived need and willingness to use the USEFIL system depends on physical condition and fears (sense of control, events)
43	The main perceived advantage of the service is prevention and treatment: Prevention: monitoring the patient automatically without the involvement of the patient and alerting Treatment: response to the alert by Health Care professionals and relatives (Falls, stoke, heart-attacks).
44	The most common expectations from the USEFIL system are: low cost clear instructions training on how to operate the system a system responsive to their problems and needs a system that addresses safety rapid alerting and quick response in case of medical emergency
45	Most interviewed seniors have had no prior exposure to computers or the internet and thus need training on basic computing skills.
46	The interviewees enjoyed the experience overall and would be keen to try the USEFIL system. They were sceptical if that adequate technology currently exists and whether they would be able to see it implemented in their life-time.
47	Most of them indicated that they wish to see the developed system before offering their opinion and deciding whether to participate in the pilot study.
48	Almost half of the participants have programmed the channels on their TV. None ever tried to program a DVD recording. VCR programming is rare.
49	Privacy issues: In Israel, no fears were expressed regarding the system as long as it will keep their privacy. In the UK some concerns were raised regarding privacy and data security. In Greece, some Greek elderly interviewees turned out to be particularly sensitive to privacy protection.
50	Privacy concerns focused mainly on the use of cameras inside the house, with the monitoring of phone call data (caller ID, etc) being the secondary focus of concerns
51	Strategically placed microphones and the wrist-watch accelerometers could help make up for some of the data from cameras that have not been installed.
52	Some seniors expressed concern regarding the monitoring of their phone call activity. This concern persisted even after the USEFIL researchers explained that no conversation contents would be recorded: one subject expressed concern that even revealing being in contact with a person was a potential liability to them.

Figure 2. Data collection and processing at the AUTH pilot study site

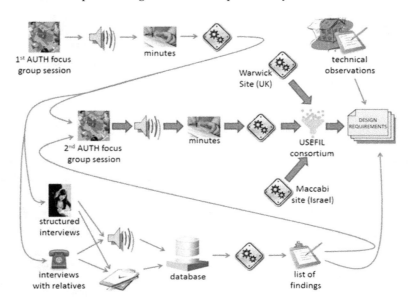

- Activities of Daily Living (ADL) assessment.
- Gait and balance assessment.
- Unobtrusive clinical parameter extraction (e.g. temperature, blood pressure).
- Detecting and preventing sporadic bouts of depression.
- Early detection of signs of Mild Cognitive Impairment (MCI).
- Engagement of the decision support system (DSS), alert generation.
- Outdoor monitoring and social wellbeing.
- Midnight waking / change of activity signature.
- Social interaction facilitated by the USEFIL system.
- Physical, social and cultural environment awareness demo.
- Family support for an elderly person living alone.

Prioritized Use Case List Generation

The term "use cases" is the terminology used in informatics to describe a list of steps followed in order to achieve a specific goal: typically these steps are interactions between an actor and the system being designed, comprising mock storyline scenarios. For instance, use cases considered essential for the USEFIL system are titled "Detect user's time of awakening and their sleep-wake cycle" and "Determine body posture: supine, sitting or standing".

A total of 70 use cases were extracted from the USEFIL scenarios, covering all project objectives and pilot study target groups. The use cases were subsequently processed using quantitative assessment methodologies. Relevant experts from all USEFIL partner institutions agreed to provide clinical, social and risk of unsuccessful development values. Each USEFIL partner institution had one vote and had to assign values to all parameters for all use cases.

A weighted summation of the value ratings was calculated and subsequently normalised to be inversely proportional to the risk rating, according to the following formula

$$I = \frac{O \cdot \left[\left(2 \cdot C + S \right) - 3 \right]}{6 \cdot R}$$

where O = [0, 1] is the truth value with respect to the existence of an associated project objective, C = [1, 2, 3] be the clinical value of a uses case with a higher number indicating higher value, S = [1, 2, 3] be the social value of a uses case with a higher number indicating higher value, R = [1, 2, 3] be the risk of failure to realize a use case with a higher number indicating a higher risk. I is the final ranking score for each use case (0 < I < 1), denoting prioritisation urgency: a use case with a higher number has a higher priority.

Some use cases needed to be considered as a cluster due to interdependencies and were thus ranked collectively. Table 2 presents a sample of the prioritized use case list. Top priorities are considered critical for the project and will certainly be implemented. Bottom priorities may not all be implemented, depending on available resources. Partners agreed on a minimum of mandatory top-ranked use cases which are needed to ensure function of the USEFIL system.

Table 2. Indicative list of project USEFIL use cases. Values in the risk of development column correspond to "Low = 1", "Medium = 2" and "High = 3". In the clinical and social value columns values correspond to "Mandatory = 3", "Important = 2" and "Nice to have = 1".

#	Use Case Description	Risk of Development (L/M/H)	Clinical Value (M/I/N)	Social Value (M/I/N)
1	Detect time of awakening and sleep-wake cycle.	L	M	M
2	Detect and analyze body posture: supine, sitting, standing.	M	M	M
4	Detect independent eating and drinking capacity while eating.	H	M	M
5	Detect & analyze dressing ability (upper body, lower body, socks, shoes)	H	M	M
7	Enable duplex video telecommunication between healthcare organization and participant.	L	M	M
8	Determine gait pattern while walking.	H	M	M
9	Determine length of steps.	L	M	M
11	Measure gait velocity during walking.	M	M	I
14	Measure feet elevation during walking	H	I,M	I
15	Detect near-miss almost falling events.	M	M, I	M, I
16	Measure physiological parameters: heart rate, body temperature, blood pressure.	L,M	M,I	M, I
18	Measure eye pupil equality	M	M	I

Discussion

- A primary objective for project USEFIL is to develop a system and associated services to support elderly citizens living independently in the community for as long as possible. We aim to achieve this and several additional objectives by designing, developing and deploying a flexible and adaptable technological solution which can fit the needs of seniors and their carers, even when they are of diverse cultural, socioeconomic, demographic and housing backgrounds.
- Current information systems adoption theory (Davis, Bagozzi, & Warshaw, 1989; Venkatesh, Morris, Davis, & Davis, 2003) states that the main determinants for adoption are ease of use and utility. Consequently, project USEFIL's main objectives are:
- To generate ease of use systems and services by:
  - Developing a simplified approach using ease of use unobtrusive low cost ICT solutions.
  - Providing services more adaptable to individual needs and preferences (personalization)
  - Promoting practicality developing systems and services that their installation will not require retrofitting of the residence of the elderly people, no new skills.
- And to generate useful systems and services (for end users and main stakeholders) by:
  - Supporting the elderly in maintaining their social activities
  - Supporting mobility
  - Providing a new health care paradigm redefining the way of treating elderly people and managing health care services
  - Promoting cost and time effective health care solutions for end users and carers

Part of the challenge for project USEFIL is to design and develop a system for a wide range of populations operating in different regulatory environments and different healthcare organization's structure.

Mixed Methods for Healthcare Delivery in Independent Living

Researchers in projects which employ both qualitative and quantitative analysis do not always integrate data and conclusions from different components of their study. On occasion qualitative components are not published at all, or each component may be published in separate journals, sometimes with inadequate reference to each other. This breaking up of a study into its methodological pieces makes it hard for health professionals, policy makers and patients to identify what can be learnt from a single research project (Lewin, Glenton, & Oxman, 2009).

In some research projects, different teams work separately on qualitative and quantitative directions, in a multidisciplinary but segregated fashion which leads to a lack of integration between components later. In other cases, research teams meet frequently to share findings and interpretations in an interdisciplinary way which can lead to publication of knowledge accessed through integration of components. Even given the tight focus and stringent word limits of most science and engineering journals, a successful approach can be the publication of one component of a study first and then the publication of the second component can draw on findings from the first publication. This link can be presented in the introduction, results or discussion sections of the second publication in order to aid analysis or interpretation (O'Cathain, Murphy, & Nicholl, 2010).

The USEFIL consortium aims to maximise the benefits of mixed methods, integrating these factors into its research and design plan from the beginning. This paper presents the work performed during the beginning of the project, which is inevitably more qualitative in nature: a sociological study needed to be performed, theories had to be developed and the opinions of prospective users and experts had to be pooled in order to extract the optimum system design requirements. The quantitative aspects of the project however, will gradually become stronger and dominate towards its conclusion as objective sensor data starts being collected and processed.

Even at this stage however, the project has so far benefited from mixed lists of questions used to conduct the semi-structured interviews (see earlier Methodology section). Moreover, the use cases described in the same section were generated through a long qualitative process and prioritised using discrete quantitative techniques. This has been a strategic choice, in order to exploit the diverse collective knowledge base possessed by the consortium, and optimally fuse it with the opinions and expectations of senior prospective users, their relatives and carers.

CONCLUSION

There are currently numerous research and development projects in several countries that provide some level of home tele-monitoring for elderly residents, using sensors that transmit to a clinical caregiver or dedicated call Centre. Some provide for communication with the older person using video conferencing. The USEFIL project goes beyond the current state of the art by bringing together, in one integrated platform, a number of different technologies that will provide unobtrusive monitoring of the older person, both in and outside of his home as well as enhancing his ability to communicate with caregivers and others, and providing input to his caregivers in order to enable them to provide more timely and appropriate care. An unobtrusive, user friendly and integrated system such as this can make a dramatic change in the quality of life of elderly people, as well as significantly improve the focus and quality of the provided care and support for their daily independent living activities.

The project is about to conclude its first year of operations, out of a total duration of 3 years. It involves using sensors in multiple unobtrusive devices around a senior's house to monitor their activities of daily living, assess their health and mood and provide notifications, recommendations and emergency alerts. Mixed methodologies combining quantitative and qualitative analysis have been used during the design phase of the system and will be used even more extensively during the following pilot studies phase.

By October 2012 the USEFIL consortium had undertaken a sociological study on European seniors living independently, held expert focus groups sessions, conducted semi-structured interviews with prospective users and carers, composed mock scenarios and used them to produce a prioritised list of use cases. Functional and non-functional requirements have been drafted, technical requirements and specifications have been assembled and software development has started. System validation and user acceptance surveys will take place through pilot studies planned at the three host sites in Greece, the UK and Israel.

ACKNOWLEDGMENT

The "USEFIL: An Unobtrusive Smart Environments for Independent Living" project (www.usefil.eu) is under a funding scheme of Small or medium scale focused research project (STREP) by FP7-ICT-2011-7. The partners of USEFIL are: National Center for Scientific Research "Demokritos" (Greece), VALTION

TEKNILLINEN TUTKIMUSKESKUS (Finland), Universität Bremen (Germany), University of Warwick - IDH (UK), Aristotle University of Thessaloniki (Greece), FRAUNHOFER-GESELLSCHAFT ZUR FOERDERUNG DER ANGEWANDTEN FORSCHUNG E.V Fraunhofer –HHI (Germany), T.P. Vision (Netherlands) and MACCABI Healthcare (Israel). The authors would like to thank the project partners for their contribution and fruitful collaboration.

REFERENCES

Beard, J. R., Biggs, S., Bloom, D. E., Fried, L. P., Hogan, P., Kalache, A., & Olshansky, S. J. (2012). *Global Population Ageing: Peril or Promise?* (Global Agenda Council, Trans.). World Economic Forum.

Benjamin, A. E. (2001). Consumer-directed services at home: A new model for persons with disabilities. *Health Affairs, 20*(6), 80–95. doi:10.1377/hlthaff.20.6.80 PMID:11816693

Bovenschulte, M., & Huch, M. (2010). More Years, Better Lives: The Potentials and Challenges of Demographic Change. In Joint Programming Initiative: German Federal Ministry of Education and Research (BMBF).

Codagnone, C. (2009). *Reconstructing the whole: present and future of Personal Health Systems.*

Davis, F. D., Bagozzi, R. P., & Warshaw, P. R. (1989). User acceptance of computer technology: A comparison of two theoretical models. *Management Science, 35*(8), 982–1003. doi:10.1287/mnsc.35.8.982

Gross, D. L., Temkin-Greener, H., Kunitz, S., & Mukamel, D. B. (2004). The growing pains of integrated health care for the elderly: Lessons from the expansion of PACE. *The Milbank Quarterly, 82*(2), 257–282. doi:10.1111/j.0887-378X.2004.00310.x PMID:15225330

Hellenic Statistical Authority. (2009). *Demographic data - Population - Statistical Database.* Retrieved Oct 2012, from Hellenic Statistical Authority (EL. STAT.) http://www.statistics.gr/portal/page/portal/ESYE

Inst. of Medicine of the National Academies. (2008). *Retooling for an aging America: Building the health care workforce*: National Academy Press.

Israeli Central Bureau of Statistics. (2012). Aged 65 and Over in Households, by Type of Household, Size of Household and Population. Statistical Abstract of Israel (2011 ed., pp. 263).

Kasper, J., Shore, A., & Penninx, B. (2000). Caregiving arrangements of older disabled women, caregiving preferences, and views on adequacy of care. *Aging , 12*(2), 141–153. PMID:10902055

Lewin, S., Glenton, C., & Oxman, A. D. (2009). Use of qualitative methods alongside randomised controlled trials of complex healthcare interventions: methodological study. *BMJ: British Medical Journal, 339.*

Mattimore, T. J., Wenger, N. S., Desbiens, N. A., & Teno, J. M. (1997). Surrogate and physician understanding of patients' preferences for living permanently in a nursing home. *Journal of the American Geriatrics Society.* PMID:9215332

Mukamel, D. B., Temkin-Greener, H., Delavan, R., Peterson, D. R., Gross, D., Kunitz, S., & Williams, T. F. (2006). Team performance and risk-adjusted health outcomes in the program of all-inclusive care for the elderly (PACE). *The Gerontologist, 46*(2), 227–237. doi:10.1093/geront/46.2.227 PMID:16581887

National PACE Association. (2007). What is PACE? Retrieved 21/10/2012, 2012, from www.npaonline. org/website/article.asp?id=12

O'Cathain, A., Murphy, E., & Nicholl, J. (2010). Three techniques for integrating data in mixed methods studies. *BMJ (Clinical Research Ed.)*, 341. PMID:20851841

UK Office for National Statistics. (2011). Older People's Day 2011: Statistical Bulletin (pp. 1-17).

UN. (2001). World population ageing 1950-2050. In Population Division (Ed.): UN Dept. of Economic and Social Affairs.

US Senate Commitee Hearing on Aging. (2003). *Ageism in the health care system: short shrifting seniors?* (Vol. 4). Washington, D.C.: USGPO.

USEFIL. (2011). Unobstrusive smart enviroments for independent living. Retrieved 22 Oct, 2012, from www.usefil.eu

USEFIL Consortium. (2011). *Description of Work*. Brussels: EC Framework Programme 7.

Venkatesh, V., Morris, M. G., Davis, G. B., & Davis, F. D. (2003). User acceptance of information technology: Toward a unified view. *Management Information Systems Quarterly*, 425–478.

KEY TERMS AND DEFINITIONS

Ageing Population: A global demographic trend according to which the elderly (senior citizens over 65 years of age) constitute a consistently increasing share of the general population.

Biomedical Engineering: The application of engineering principles and design concepts to medicine and biology for healthcare purposes (e.g. diagnostic, therapeutic or both).

Decision Support System: A computer-based information system that supports procedural or organizational decision-making activities. Decision support systems are used in healthcare to increase the speed, efficiency and reliability of health-related decisions.

Elderly: For statistical and public administrative purposes, old age is frequently defined as 65 years of age or older. This is not consistent in international literature: a 60 year threshold is occasionally used.

Independent Living: Living without the need of support from other people or from medical equipment that requires frequent human supervision. In the context of eldercare, independent living is seen as a step in the continuum of care, with assisted living being the next step.

Smart Environment: A physical world interwoven with invisible sensors, actuators, displays, and computational elements. These computing elements are generally embedded seamlessly in everyday objects and networked to each other and beyond (the internet, usually).

Ubiquitous Computing: A concept in informatics and engineering where computing can occur everywhere and anywhere. In contrast to desktop computing, ubiquitous computing can occur using any device, based on data obtained by sensors present in any location, in any format.

Unobtrusive Research: Science research based on data collection which does not involve direct elicitation of data from the research subjects. An example would be the extraction of a subject's sleeping schedule based on examination of a log containing the setting and snoozing times of the mobile phone alarm clock. A counter-example (obtrusive research) would be to directly interview the subject and ask them for this information or to dispatch a researcher to the subject's residence to monitor and log the occupant's daily habits.

This research was previously published in the Handbook of Research on Innovations in the Diagnosis and Treatment of Dementia edited by Panagiotis D. Bamidis, Ioannis Tarnanas, Leontios Hadjileontiadis, and Magda Tsolaki, pages 290-305, copyright year 2015 by Medical Information Science Reference (an imprint of IGI Global).

Chapter 67

Impact of Trust and Technology on Interprofessional Collaboration in Healthcare Settings:
An Empirical Analysis

Ramaraj Palanisamy
St. Francis Xavier University, Canada

Nazim Taskin
Massey University, New Zealand

Jacques Verville
SKEMA Business School, USA

ABSTRACT

The increases in complexity of patient care, healthcare costs, and technological advancements shifted the healthcare delivery to interprofessional collaborative care. The study aims for identifying the factors influencing the quality of team collaboration. The study examines the impact of trust and technology orientation on collaboration with the mediating effects of communication, coordination and cooperation. A questionnaire survey was conducted to gather data from healthcare professionals (N=216). Statistical analysis conducted for this study include correlations, factor analysis with reliability and validity tests and Partial Least Squares (PLS) method. The results of the study validate that (i) collaboration has positive and significant relationship with coordination, and cooperation; (ii) trust has positive and significant relationship with communication, coordination, and cooperation; and (iii) technology orientation has positive and significant relationship with cooperation but not with communication and coordination. The research and managerial implications of these factors are given in discussion. As with most empiri

DOI: 10.4018/978-1-5225-3926-1.ch067

cal studies, the subjectivity of the opinion of respondents present some limitations to generalization. Other limitations include the lack of availability and use of standard measures for various constructs in the research model. The results can be used by healthcare professionals and managers to advance their understanding on the impact of trust and technology on collaboration mediating communication, coordination and cooperation practices. The significant value of this study is the identification of the factors influencing the quality of team collaboration in healthcare industry.

1. INTRODUCTION

In the modern healthcare system, healthcare provision has shifted from that of autonomous practice to interprofessional team based approach which involves multiple professionals with different educational background, training and expertise, working on behalf of patients, sharing a common goal (Woods et al., 2011). Interprofessional team approach enhances healthcare access, efficiency of services, resource utilization, health knowledge, skills and more satisfaction for the patients (Barrett et al., 2007; Safran, 2003).

Patients receive safer and higher-quality care when healthcare professionals work as a team and collaborate effectively while they practice. The increases in complexity of patient care, healthcare costs for medical specialization and technological advancements shifted the way the healthcare is delivered to interprofessional collaborative care (Gaboury et al., 2009; Smith et al., 2002; Welton et al., 1997). The increasing complexity of health problems inevitably makes professionals interdependent in a collaborative manner foregoing a competitive approach (D'Amour, 1999). In the complex healthcare environment, poor collaboration among health professionals significantly increases the possibilities of mistakes occurring in the delivery of patient-care, medication-error-related deaths, wrong-site surgeries and increased staff turnover (Woods et al., 2011). Interprofessional collaborative practice meets current demands of the healthcare system reducing errors and costs and thereby improving quality of patient care (Canadian Health Services Research Foundation, 2006; Lemieux-Charles & McGuire, 2006).

High degree of interprofessional collaboration is essential for team success. The task of improving interprofessional collaboration has received considerable attention as it is a key factor to increase the effectiveness of healthcare services. Nonetheless, effective team functioning in a collaborative manner is challenging and difficult to achieve (Bailey et al., 2006; Sicotte et al., 2002). The literature provides conceptual definitions and frameworks of interprofessional collaboration and indicates about limited knowledge of this complex phenomenon. Specifically, the vast majority of published work on the influence of determinants of interprofessional collaboration relies on conceptual approaches rather than empirical data (Rodri´Guez et al., 2005). The knowledge on the factors influencing quality of team collaboration and the linkages between the elements in the complex interprofessional relationships is limited (Gocan et al., 2014; Baerg et al., 2012; D'Amour et al., 2005; Zwarenstein, Reeves & Perrier, 2004). As effective collaboration does not emerge merely by grouping the professionals together, very few studies have investigated the influence of interactional determinants for effective collaboration.

Based on a qualitative study, communication, coordination, cooperation, and trust were found to be the factors for communication-based-collaborative practice (Palanisamy & Verville, 2015). In general, successful collaborative practice in healthcare requires coordination and cooperation (Williams et al., 2010; Apker et al., 2006; Way et al., 2000). Way et al. (2000) emphasize on communication and coordination mechanisms as they play a key role for developing collaborative relationship among team members. The complexity of healthcare problems could be addressed by different interprofessional cooperation types (Molleman et al., 2008). The collaboration of healthcare professionals requires mentoring and constantly communicating with team members to clarify the roles and responsibilities of team members, which is an important characteristic of cooperation (Apker et al., 2006). In providing high-quality care to patients, professionals have to interact and collaboratively work together with a number of other healthcare professionals cultivating relationships using best communication practices ensuring better patient outcomes (Haeuser & Preston, 2005; Thomas et al., 2004).

The professionals interact in a collaborative environment, which provides opportunities as well as constraints thereby increase in complexities for effective collaboration. In the complex environment, trust is another determinant of collaboration and enables communication, coordination and cooperation of healthcare professionals (Jacobsen, 1999; Mechanic, 1998; San Martin-Rodriguez et al., 2005). Trust enables communication and enhances the quality of interactions (Jacobsen, 1999); mutual trust is emphasized for coordinated behavior among the team members and using coordination mechanisms (San Martin-Rodriguez et al., 2005). Furthermore, trust is a facilitator for having smooth cooperative interprofessional relationships (Misztal, 1996). As patient care is provided by multidisciplinary healthcare professionals, the technology orientation facilitates communication among healthcare professionals by improving information flows, coordinates the common goal of enhanced health outcome by caring the patients, and accomplishes cooperation among professionals to seek healthcare solutions (Weaver et al., 2012; InfoDev, 2006; Henault et al., 2002).

The study examines the question of what are the factors improving the quality of interprofessional collaboration among healthcare professionals in healthcare industry in North American settings? The paper aims to advance our understanding of current practices of interprofessional collaboration by empirically testing the impact of trust and technology orientation on collaboration in association with communication, coordination and collaboration having mediating effects with trust and collaboration as well as technology orientation and collaboration. In particular, the study aims for empirically examining (i) the impact of trust on communication, coordination and cooperation; (ii) the impact of technology orientation on communication, coordination and cooperation; and (iii) the impact of communication, coordination and cooperation on collaboration. The study results enable to find the factors influencing collaboration and provide guidelines for implementing communication, coordination and cooperation of healthcare practices.

The remaining part of the paper is organized as follows. Section 2 evolves the research model based on a review of literature; Section 3 documents the research methodology followed for this study; Section 4 shows the data analysis and findings; Section 5 discusses the managerial implications of this study followed by areas of future research; and Section 6 gives the limitations and concluding remarks.

2. RESEARCH MODEL

This section gives the conceptual definitions of the various constructs of the model. The hypotheses are evolved based on a review of literature.

2.1. Collaboration

Collaboration, defined as the relationships and interactions between professionals, seen as a process comprised of dynamic, interactive, interpersonal, transformational and evolving nature of processes (D'Amour, Ferrada-Videla, San Martin, & Beaulieu, 2005; Hanson, et al., 2000; Sullivan, 1998; D'Amour, Sicotte, & Le´vy, 1999). Collaboration in healthcare is the process by which interdependent professionals structure a collective action towards patient's care (D'Amour, 1997). Working with other professionals in a collaborative manner leads to enhanced healthcare outcomes that are not achievable individually. The two key elements of collaboration are: (i) the team's collective action for addressing the complexity of patient needs; and (ii) integrating the perspectives of each professional into a team in which trusting relationships are built (D'Amour et al., 2005).

Interprofessional collaboration is characterized by interdependence between multiple stakeholders including physicians, nurses, pharmacists, clients, community partners and health educators among many other health professionals working side by side in clinical practice to develop a cohesive plan that meets clients' needs (Careau et al., 2011). Way et al. (2000, p3) define collaborative practice as "an inter-professional process for communication and decision making that enables the separate and shared knowledge and skills of care providers to synergistically influence the client/ patient care provided". The effective interprofessional collaboration is the engagement of multiple different professionals working together from different disciplines as a team sharing a common goal (of optimal/ improved patient care), sharing the knowledge/ skills/ expertise of other professionals for creative outcomes by understanding other professionals' roles in a team, having multiple interactions over time by showing symmetrical power, and showing interdependence among professionals in a supportive organizational environment (Broers et al., 2009). The concept of power refers to the professional's power based on knowledge and experience recognized by team members (Henneman, 1995).

The 'collaboration' construct is not yet fully understood and operationalized; in the literature, it is commonly defined through five underlying concepts: sharing, partnership, power, interdependency and process (D'Amour et al., 2005). As collaboration is more likely to occur when professionals share similar interests and the following facets of sharing can be seen in a collaborative undertaking: shared responsibilities, shared decision-making, shared values, shared data, sharing different professional perspective, shared planning and intervention (Wagner, 2004; Arslanian-Engoren, 1995; D'Amour, 1997). In a collaborative learning setting, the influences can be Individual to Group (I-to-G) and Group to Individual (G-to-I) (Papanikolaou & Gouli, 2013). In collaborative relationships, extensive efforts are taken to avoid conflicts concerning the sharing of tasks and responsibilities. The concept of partnership implies that two or more actors join in a collaborative task characterized by a collegial like relationship that is constructive and authentic (Hanson, Carr, & Spross, 2000). Interdependency implies mutual dependence of professionals who depend on one another for addressing the patient's needs (D'Amour, 1997). The skills required for interprofessional collaboration are: rapport building, effectively communicating skill, leadership, and conflict management (Baerg et al., 2012).

2.2. Communication

Communication is defined as the process of transmitting/ exchanging message(s), formal as well as informal sharing of meaningful and timely information for common understanding between the sender and receiver (Keyton, 2011; Sharma et al., 2013; Khan, 2014). The various aspects of communication are share and receive information, express or perceive feelings, define and clarify issues, present or understand views or opinions (Merriman-Webster, 2009). When there is no common understanding, there is no effective communication. The key elements of communication process are sender, receiver, message, medium, noise and feedback (Cheney, 2011). Sender initiates the communication with a desire to convey a(n) idea/ concept/ opinion to receiver to whom the message is sent. The idea is encoded in the form of message by selecting words, symbols, or gestures. The message takes the form of verbal, nonverbal, written or electronic. The message is sent through a medium or channel (say face-to-face, telephone, email, or written document). The receiver gets meaningful information out of decoding the message. Any distortion in the communication process is the noise (say barriers or interruptions). The receiver's response to the message is the feedback, which ensures the receiver understands the sender's intended message. These elements in the communication process determine the effectiveness of communication. The effectiveness is hampered if there is any problem in any one of these elements. Effective communication is a two-way interactive mutual process based on human emotions demanding efforts and skills from both sender and receiver (Alshatnawi, 2014).

Formal communication is motivated by the need to overcome the difference with other professional and to achieve common ground for productive exchange (Lingard et al., 2002). Besides, each professional in the healthcare team needs to clearly articulate his/ her contribution to the team by effectively delegating the work and directing other team members (Suter et al., 2009). Lingard et al. (2006) give two types of formal communicative utilities: informational and functional. In interprofessional communication informational utility occurs when there is a visible improvement of team's awareness or knowledge by exchanging new information, explicit confirmation, reminders and education. Here, the formal communicator makes use of negotiating skills to overcome differences in viewpoints and enhances the team-understanding of the issue. Functional utility occurs when formal communication prompts decision-making, follow-up actions, problem identification, and other work-related connections. Lingard et al. (2008) give examples of variety of communication failures in healthcare settings with and without visible consequences. The key failures are content and occasion (timing or frequency of exchange). When relevant information is not exchanged among the team members, the issues are not resolved resulting in delays in providing healthcare. Late or less frequent information exchange results into inefficiency, tension and repetition of work.

2.3. Communication and Collaboration

Formal and informal communications among healthcare professionals are the key to collaborative care (Kripalani et al., 2007). Communication is an interactional element that influences the degree of collaboration and communication skills of health professionals play a key role for developing collaborative relationship among team members (Way et al., 2000). The reasons for communication to be key determinants of collaboration are: help the professionals to understand how their work contributes to team goals, allows constructive negotiations with other professionals, and drives other determinants of collaboration, such as trust (Lindeke & Block, 1998; Henneman et al., 1995).

The collaborative practice requires appropriate communication and coordination mechanisms, such as sessions, forums, formal meeting structures involving all team members (Way, Jones & Busing, 2000). The capabilities for collaborative practice include communication of sharing of professional knowledge (mentoring) and reflection (e.g., problem solving, feedback) (Walsh, Gordon, Marshall, & Hunt, 2005). Lack of communication on how each professional contributes to the team, delegating work and directing team members hamper collaboration (Brown, Crawford, & Darongkamas, 2000; Hall, 2005). Improving communication among health professionals can improve collaboration in terms of knowledge sharing and collaborative decision making (Vazirani et al., 2005). Stein et al. (1990) noted that more communication makes use of professional's observational and intellectual skills and thereby improves the ability to contribute to patients' care in a collaborative manner. Furthermore, the collaboration aspects include communication in analyzing patient's information for applying to treatment decisions (Hansen et al., 1999). For collaborative management of healthcare, the most heavily used communication methods are face-to-face, telephone, electronic communication of which regular meetings (both electronic and non-electronic) improves collaboration and access to information to support decision making (Batt & Purchase, 2004; Safran et al., 1998). The above discussion leads to Hypothesis H1.

Hypothesis 1: The degree of collaboration is positively related with the level of communication.

2.4. Coordination

Coordination means the regulation of diverse professionals into an integrated and harmonious operation with a goal and plan to support patient for receiving effective healthcare (Stille et al., 2005). Bodenheimer (2007) defined coordination as a function for meeting patient's needs for health services achieving by sharing information across professionals. Alter & Hage (1993) defined coordination as "the articulation of elements in a service delivery system so that comprehensiveness, accessibility and compatibility among elements are maximized". In the context of interprofessional coordination, "comprehensiveness" means the extensive involvement of the team members; "accessibility" means access to information or resources needed for patient care; and "compatibility" means professionals working together in a coherent manner. The studies on healthcare coordination have been grounded on this coordination framework (e.g., Axelsson & Bihari-Axelsson, 2005; Brazil et al., 2004; Gulzar & Henry, 2005). Shortell et al. (1994) defined coordination as "the extent to which functions and activities both within the unit and between units are brought together in a way that promotes cost-effective continuous care". This "bringing together" refers to the coordination of activities of healthcare professionals as a team. In general, coordination is achieved by vertically integrating the team using a management hierarchy (Meyer, 1985). The team coordination results into value added services/ activities for achieving goals and plans for the patient care using complementary expertise and resources that could not be delivered by each professional separately. Starfield et al. (1998) describes coordination in healthcare as "the availability of information about prior problems and services and the recognition of that information as it bears on needs for current care."

Interprofessional coordination is typically established by standardizing healthcare practice so as to avoid conflicts and reducing replicated activities as well as an efficient flow of knowledge and information among team members (Brazil et al., 2004). Team coordination encourages inputs that may be needed to improve planning of patient outcomes (with more knowledge about patients and procedures) from team members and acknowledges them for their contribution and thereby participate in decision making regarding patient care. In a coordinated environment, professionals interact with colleagues with more freedom to be different and to disagree.

2.5. Collaboration and Coordination

Collaboration is the act of working together and coordination means regulating the team for higher order functioning (Stille et al., 2005). Team coordination means team members' shared and organized understanding of relevant knowledge for performance (Burtscher & Manser, 2012) and it makes team members to feel "on the same page" with respect to the common task to be performed (Mohammed et al., 2010). Apker et al. (2006) give the following skill set required for collaboration: identifying solutions to problems, participate decision making, actively listening to team members, seeking clarification, solve patient care problems, and presenting information in a precise and concise manner. The skill set for coordination are: collaborative skills regarding patient goals and plans, conflict resolution skills, committing to work together, delegating tasks to team members, sharing updated information, mentoring team members, and serving as liaison between team members who have limited contact with each other (Apker et al., 2006). For patient-centered collaborative practice, competencies most commonly emphasized are communication, understanding roles of other health professionals, effective team working skills including understanding group norms, conflict resolution and the ability to tolerate differences, the ability to contribute to shared care plans and goal setting, a willingness to collaborate with mutual trust and respect (Suter et al., 2009; Canadian Health Services Research Foundation [CHSRF], 2006; San Martin-Rodriguez, Beaulieu, D'Amour, & Ferrada-Videla, 2005). Information sharing which is a characteristic of coordination has been found to be related to collaboration (Williams et al., 2010). Thus, having a shared understanding regarding team member's knowledge and skills facilitates collaboration. Based on this discussion, this study derives Hypothesis H2.

Hypothesis 2: The degree of collaboration is positively related with the level of coordination.

2.6. Cooperation

The Merriam Webster dictionary defines cooperation as "a situation in which people work together to do something". Our particular interest is interprofessional cooperation in healthcare settings. Cooperation is the actions of individuals, committing to work together as a team of healthcare professional in a complementary mode rather than competing mode, which is being helpful by doing what is wanted or asked for improving the care of the patients. The cooperative professional shares a common vision of patient's care that asks and provides opinion from other professionals, who is straightforward when sharing information, who discusses and plans joint strategies for patient-care, who understands (her) his roles and shares decision-making responsibilities. Cooperation in healthcare setting is the assistance provided by different professionals by frequently communicating with colleagues from other disciplines to include their views, to give consistent feedback and thereby fulfilling the expectations of other professionals (Davies, 1996; Krogstad et al., 2004). In a cooperative environment, the professionals have a good understanding of the distinction between their roles and support the role of other colleagues (Verschuren & Masselink, 1997). This way each professional works to the expectation of the other by often seeking patient information and providing feedback.

The cooperation of professionals varies along a continuum ranging from low to high degree of cooperation (Doherty, 1995). 'Consultation' occurs in the lower end where providing information and support to another on request happens; and in the other extreme, high degree of cooperation refers to 'multidisciplinary teamwork' (MTW), where professionals with different backgrounds, collectively discussing for decision-making and action to enhance the quality of healthcare (Molleman et al., 2008). The team work creates opportunities for more dialogues and creative problem-solving by integrating expertise from different professions. Depending on the complexity of patients' health problems, the degree of cooperation varies. For simple problems, less intensive cooperation, such as 'consultation' is needed and more complex problems require a high degree of cooperation, such as 'multidisciplinary teamwork'.

2.7. Cooperation and Collaboration

In the last two decades, the complexity of healthcare problems has increased due to multiple and inter-related problems (Hudson, 2002). On the healthcare provider side, there is a growth in advanced and comprehensive technologies for evidence-based knowledge and treatment. The knowledge expansion has demanded an increased specialization of functions with different professional backgrounds (Heinemann & Zeiss, 2002). Molleman et al. (2008) analyzed the complexity of healthcare problems to cooperation types and concluded that the complexity could be addressed by interprofessional cooperation and collaboration. Barimani & Hylander (2008) explore healthcare professionals' cooperation to conceptualize barriers and facilitators of cooperation to generate a comprehensive theoretical model. The past research emphasize the main barriers as tendency to professional ethnocentricity (Schofield & Amodeo, 1999), ignorance about the other professional's area of competence and a tendency among professionals to regard their profession as superior to the others (Waskett, 1996). In general, the intensity of collaboration depends upon the roles and relationships of healthcare professionals which are the characteristics of cooperation (Hojat et al., 2001). Healthcare professional (e.g., physician or a nurse) collaborates by serving as team leader/ member who exhibits leadership role, assigns responsibilities, organize team member roles, frequently communicate, providing consistent feedback, support the role of colleagues and serve as the communicative hub of their healthcare teams (Apker et al., 2006). For patient-centered collaborative practice, competencies most commonly emphasized are communication, providing consistent feedback and understanding roles of other health professionals (Suter et al., 2009; Canadian Health Services Research Foundation [CHSRF], 2006; San Martin-Rodriguez, Beaulieu, D'Amour, & Ferrada-Videla, 2005). Collaboration means mentoring and constantly communicating with team members to ensure clarity on individual roles and responsibilities. This discussion provides the basis for Hypothesis H3.

Hypothesis 3: The degree of collaboration is positively related with the level of cooperation.

2.8. Trust

Trust is essentially a psychological state seen as important in its own right involving an element of vulnerability where an individual who places trust on other party is vulnerable irrespective of the ability to control over the actions or inactions of the other party. Trust is defined as "the willingness of a party to be vulnerable to the actions of another party based on the expectation that the other will perform a particular action important to the trust or, irrespective of the ability to monitor or control that other party" (Mayer, Davis, & Schoorman, 1995) or, more briefly, "accepted vulnerability to another's possible but not expected ill will (or lack of good will)" (Baier, 1986). Trust is the reliance by one individual, or group, or firm (or trustor) upon a voluntarily or non-voluntarily accepted duty on the part of the other individual, or group, or firm (or trustee) to recognize and protect the rights and interests of all others engaged in a joint endeavor, information exchange or economic exchange (Culnan & Bies, 2003; Hosmer, 1995). In general, trusting someone refers to voluntary action based on expectations of behaviors in relation to oneself. When the expectations are disappointed, then trust decays and generates negative outcomes (Brockner & Siegel, 1996; Luhmann, 2000). Therefore, trust has an element of risk based on trustee's uncertain future actions.

Interprofessional trust characterizes a relationship between two or more professionals known to each other (Goold, 1998). This has been conceptualized with the following overlapping domains: caring for the patients interests and avoiding conflicts of interest; competence for interpersonal skills, decision-making (trusting patient-care decisions), and avoiding mistakes; honesty, avoiding intentional falsehoods by telling the truth; and confidentiality, privacy maintenance of sensitive information (Mechanic & Meyer, 2000). In the early treatment process, interprofessional trust is more likely to build and as the interprofessional relationship continues, results build trust and members learn more about each other keeping informed about events or changes that affect them (Hall et al., 2002). Since learning is important to the development of trust, trust decays when interprofessionals do not deliver on their promises and underperform (Berwick, 2003).

Trust enables communication among the professionals to understand how their contribution helps to achieve team goals and thereby drives determinants of collaboration (Henneman et al., 1995). Trust in terms of emotional bonds facilitates repeated interactions in the interprofessional relationships (Newman, 1998). Past experience of each other and communicative behaviors form expectation of trusting behavior. Prevalence of trusted relationship among professionals enhances the quality of their interactions lead to quality decisions in treatment (Mechanic, 1998). Therefore, trust encourages communication and information flows (Jacobsen, 1999). The care decision-making approaches allow engagement and dialogue among health care professionals and thereby facilitate the process of building trust. The above discussion leads to the following Hypothesis H4.

Hypothesis 4: The level of trust is positively related with the level of communication.

Interprofessional interactions take place by using coordination mechanisms, such as sessions, forums, and formal meeting structures where mutual trust is commonly emphasized for collaborative practice (San Martin-Rodriguez, Beaulieu, D'Amour, & Ferrada-Videla, 2005; Cabello, 2002). Trust facilitates smooth interpersonal relationships among team members and thereby enables coordinated behavior. Building trust requires confidence in one's own abilities, coordinated efforts for collaborative practice, patience, and previous positive experiences with others (Henneman et al., 1995). Trust is indispensable for establishing coordinated and collaborative working relationships (Baggs & Schmitt, 1997; D'Amour, 1997). In the context of healthcare settings, the term coordination conveys the idea of sharing (knowledge, tasks and responsibilities) implies collective action oriented towards a common goal in a spirit of trust (D'Amour et al., 2005). Trust facilitates and underpins coordination, which is collective action to achieve common goals and plan quality care of patients (Gilson, 2003). Trust-based coordination makes an important contribution to building value in patient-care and work through conflicts in efforts to resolve them. Continuance in trusted interactions with different professionals creates opportunities for working together with freedom to be different and disagree. This discussion provides the basis for Hypothesis H5.

Hypothesis 5: The level of trust is positively related with the level of coordination.

Trust is a facilitator for smooth running of cooperative interprofessional relationships, helps to reconcile professionals' own interests with others, and secures open communication and dialogue (Misztal, 1996). The types of expected behaviors underlie trust are technical competence, openness, and concern (Davies, 1999; Mechanic, 1996). Trust breaks down the constraints of the cooperative behavior. Trust catalyses cooperative behavior for payoff/ benefits in healthcare, which is rooted in risk and expectations about how another professional will behave in case of uncertainties in healthcare related decisions (Gambetta, 2000). When other professional's future actions are beneficial rather than harmful, cooperation is advantageous outweighing the costs and risks involved in cooperation. Therefore, trust provides a context in which healthcare professionals work cooperatively for setting care objectives and seek ways of achieving them (Perry et al., 1999). Mutual trust between colleagues establishes a platform for knowledge sharing by consistently asking/ giving feedback/ opinion to members of the team, and keeps each other informed about events or changes that affect them by frequent communication (D'Amour et al., 2005). Trust enables frequent communication with colleagues from other disciplines and incorporates views of treatment thereby improves the ability to meet patient needs. Trust protects the interests of professionals for running smooth cooperative relations in caring patients (Misztal, 1996). The above discussion leads to Hypothesis H6.

Hypothesis 6: The level of trust is positively related with the level of cooperation.

2.9. Technology Orientation

In general, technology orientation reflects the philosophy of "technology push" where state-of-the-art technology is acquired and applied (Gatignon & Xuereb, 1997). Lee & Meuter (2010, p.357) define technology orientation as "an organizational-wide engagement of technology-oriented practices in developing policies, practices and procedures, and sensing and responding to technology opportunities. These activities will lead to technology adoption and utilization." In the healthcare settings, the technology orientation (adoption and use) transforms the healthcare delivery for improved efficiency and coordination (Senate Finance Committee, 2009). In the healthcare context, technology orientation is the adoption and use of technology in day-to-day operation, which requires healthcare professional's propensity and analytical skills for using it to perform tasks relevant to healthcare. In healthcare, the reliance of individual communication technologies is ever increasing.

Personal technology orientation is how an individual perceives the technology in terms of the details and use by analyzing the technology (Manaikkamakl, 2007). The healthcare professionals with technology orientation perceive the use of sophisticated communication technology for gaining personal productivity, effectiveness and efficiency in healthcare delivery. The technology oriented professional rapidly adopt and use technology for communication advantage among team members for enhancing the work effectiveness.

In general, technology is utilized to lower transaction costs, increase in decision quality and speed of decision making, improved productivity and elimination of routine tasks (Srinivasan, 1985; Byrd, 1992). A variety of models has been applied in the past research for understanding technology usage. IS investigators have suggested models for determinants of technology usage (e.g., the TRA model by Ajzen & Fishbein (1980) and Ajzen's (1991) the planned behavior model). Subsequently, Davis et al.

(1989) suggested technology acceptance model (TAM) suggesting two antecedents of technology usage: perceived ease of use (PEOU) and perceived usefulness (PU) of a technology. Perceived usefulness is the user's subjective probability that using a technology will increase his or her job performance. Perceived ease of use is the degree to which the user expects the target technology to be free of efforts. An unused technology provides no value and technology usage is measured by daily use (duration of use), frequency of use, number of applications used, and the number of tasks supported (Igbaria, Guimaraes, & Davis, 1995). Technology adoption by an individual is to be determined by his or her voluntary intentions towards using the technology. The intention is determined by the person's attitude towards using the technology and perception of its usefulness. Attitudes are formed from evaluating beliefs about the use of the technology.

Information and communication technologies (ICT) facilitate communication of information and sharing of knowledge by electronic means. In a broader sense, ICT tools are comprised of the range of digital and analog ICTs, from radio and television to telephones (landline and mobile), computers, Internet, audio-video recording, social networking and web-based communities (GAID, 2010). ICT usage facilitates professionals to work in an innovative manner, positive attitude and commitment for networked environment with global thinking (Open Clinical, 2011). Effective usage of ICT improves information flows and enhances the dissemination of evidence-based knowledge for improving health outcome (InfoDev, 2006).

2.10. Technology Orientation and Communication

Usage of electronic communication technologies, such as email, text messaging, and social media are increasing for enhanced outcomes, improving efficiency, decreasing costs and seek solutions in healthcare (Weaver et al., 2012). Email is the e-communication technology used in healthcare, which does not require the presence of both parties at the same time, and allows continuous access and participation (Mann et al., 2006). Though email communication becomes part of patient's health record, it cannot be used for communicating urgent or time-sensitive information. Text messaging provides one-to-one exchanges of short messages or distributes to a larger audience (Terry, 2008). This type of e-communication is convenient, immediate and can be used for monitoring/ reporting symptoms. Introduction of e-messaging enhances connections among healthcare professionals and made easy access of information (Lyngstad, 2013). The availability of social media tools, such as Facebook, YouTube, Twitter, etc. are used to disseminate health messages and enable the professionals to connect with each other (Fox, 2011).

Information and Communication Technology (ICT) tools can enhance productivity and support interprofessional communication even when the group is multilingual (Aiken et al., 2011) and virtual (working in a geographically distributed environment) (Duranti & de Almeida, 2012). Early adoption of e-communication technologies increases the flow of information. Methods of e-communications are changing from email to short messaging (SMS) to social networking (Weaver et al., 2012). The use of email facilitates communication among healthcare professionals within the medication system related to care of patients. For electronic communication, the messages are exchanged using personal computers (PC) and many wireless, non-PC options including personal digital assistants (PDAs), pagers, and telephones. The electronic communication among team members is easy, efficient and has several advantages: often less costly, less disruptive than face-to-face communication (Nardi & Whittaker, 2002); has boundary spanning capability to cross geographical and even status boundaries (Sproull & Kiesler, 1991); team members can communicate with a variety of professionals even when members are not able to exchange immediately (Cummings & Ghosh, 2005; Kraut et al., 2002). In a group environment, e-brainstorming generates a large number of quality ideas; and e-decision making produces more personal disclosure and uncertainty reduction (Tidwell & Walther, 2002).

In the healthcare settings, the barriers for using technology for communication are: preference of face-to-face communication for richer interaction, privacy/ security concerns, and the potential increase in efforts to learn and use new technologies (Healthcare News, 2001). Specifically, web messaging is preferred to the telephone if the information to be exchanged is not time-sensitive (Liederman et al., 2005); healthcare professionals use secured web-based portals for administrative tasks, such as refill requests and scheduling appointments (Kittler et al., 2004). The above discussion leads to the following Hypothesis H7:

Hypothesis 7: The degree of communication is positively related with the degree of technology orientation.

2.11. Technology Orientation for Coordination

E-communication technology creates and sustains interprofessional connections that improve outcomes and accomplishes common goal of patient-care (Weaver, 2012). The electronic communication tools, such as mobile devices are used by healthcare professionals to change prescription, symptom control and so on thereby to achieve the common goal of caring the patients. As patient care is provided by a 'team of care' comprised of multidisciplinary healthcare professionals, communication technology enables coordination among the professionals. The team members work together using e-communication and that use of technology orientation occurs ranging from low to high use for each member (Hinds & Kiesler, 2002). Electronic interaction is often motivated by goals and plans, such as collaboration, conflict resolution, and commitment to work together (Tiegland & Wasko, 2003). Healthcare professionals use email for communication and to better coordinate care of patients (Henault et al., 2002). Technology enables for sharing information across professionals and thereby helps professional coordination. For instance, radiologists in one country may read x-rays, MRIs, or mammograms transmitted from other country (Leonhardt, 2006). Professionals with questions can have audiovisual contact with others to diagnose the problems quickly, to track the use of a variety of medications, and monitor the health conditions (Boden et al., 2006).

Communication tools and technologies, such as PDAs are used routinely by healthcare professionals who are separately responsible for providing care to a patient can share health information, such as drug references, prescriptions and simultaneous view of patient data (Baumgart, 2005). Furthermore, communication technology supports the creation, coordination and management of virtual medical teams for treating patients. Email affords a written record of information exchange and enables professionals to focus on questions to be asked and follow-up questions, which can be reviewed at any time for the purpose of coordination (Ball & Lillis, 2006). Social networks can be a source of learning for health professionals as the social media tools disseminate health messages. This can provide effective forum to interact, share information and concerns, and even manage healthcare. Besides, social media facilitates interactive communication and empower professionals to make decisions. As the network continues to trend upward and provides frequent and topic-specific updates, this can be an excellent source of professional networking and education. The above discussion leads to Hypothesis H8.

Hypothesis 8: The degree of coordination is positively related with the degree of technology orientation.

2.12. Technology Orientation for Cooperation

Communication technology enables cooperation of multidisciplinary healthcare professionals by incorporating views of treatment held by colleagues in order to meet patient needs. Electronic communication facilitates the healthcare professionals for consistently giving feedback and for special advice to caring for a patient. For instance, telemedicine networks provide consultations in specialties, such as oncology, radiology, pathology, surgery, pharmacy, psychiatry, and behavioral health (Blanchet, 2005). Health professionals use today's e-communication tools, such as email, invited Facebook groups, text messages, websites and more to effectively manage patients' connection, health and support. In the healthcare environment, providing timely and consistent feedback is important in correcting misunderstandings about the treatment (Armstrong & Cole, 2002). The inconsistency in giving feedback between team members may end up with errors in treatment. Use of communication technology is related with higher levels of message feedback lead to enhanced level of mutual knowledge and ability to meet patient needs (Cramton, 2001).

Providing high quality care demands secure and timely exchange of information in a cooperative manner. Through the usage of communication technology better cooperation is achieved in terms of frequent communication among the professionals; and to understand the distinction between the roles of professionals. Team members are better acquainted with each other's roles and support the roles of colleagues by using electronic communication technology (Bradner et al., 2005). Tools, such as Short Message Service (SMS) enables push and pull of data and alerts affecting the entire team of care. The communication technologies, specifically social media tools introduce substantial and ubiquitous changes to communication between individuals replacing face-to-face interactions (Kietzmann et al., 2011). Social media technologies facilitate joint interaction with different professionals and establish a communicative environment with open and interoperable systems in which individuals share, discuss, and modify opinions/ contents (Franchi, Poggi, & Tomaiuolo, 2013). Social media tools facilitate conversations among individuals, sharing of information and foster engagement for effectively cooperate in a multidisciplinary work environment (Kaplan & Haenlein, 2010). This discussion provides the basis for Hypothesis H9.

Hypothesis 9: The degree of cooperation is positively related with the degree of technology orientation.

The research model is shown in Figure 1 demonstrates the hypotheses of the current study.

3. RESEARCH METHODOLOGY

Questionnaire survey was the data collection method adopted for this study. For data collection purpose, mail surveys were sent to Healthcare Professionals in North America. The survey questions were adopted mainly from previously tested and validated instrument originally developed by Bronstein (2002; 2003). Some questions were modified or designed based on the literature on collaboration in healthcare system as well as through some structured interviews with healthcare professionals while majority of them were used as in the original form. The survey instrument had 74 questions organized in two sections. The first section focuses on measuring the degree of agreement with each featured factors. Items agreed were measured using a five-point Likert scale. The second section focuses with demographic information about the respondents. The survey instrument was refined with a small pilot study and a pretest (N=30)

Figure 1. Conceptual model with hypothesis

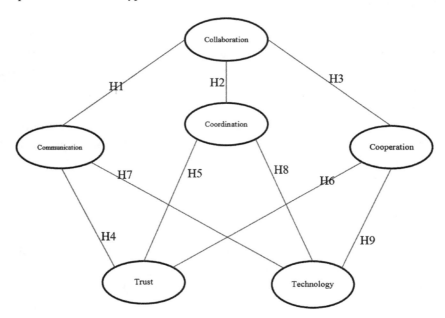

that aimed to identify any ambiguities with wording and structure as well as other potential problems with the instrument.

The finalized questionnaire survey with a cover letter was mailed to a random group of 1800 healthcare professionals in North America. The healthcare institutions that the data were collected were chosen among North American healthcare companies. The contact information was gathered from online databases that the University had access to. In order to enhance the response rate, pre-addresses and pre-stamped envelopes were attached with the questionnaire. The response rate was about 12% with the total returned survey as 216. The responders were from a wide range of areas including medical doctors, nurses and nurse practitioners, etc.

In general, one concern about the survey questionnaires is that they are based on perceptions; so they are prone to errors of measurement through bias (Hair et al., 2006). A robust solution to that matter is using multiple indicators for the variables. This method is called structural equation modeling (SEM) (Kline, 1998). In this study, we utilized SPSS version 20 and WarpPLS 4, an SEM based analysis, for the analysis of the data. There are several reasons of using a Partial Least Squares (PLS) method in this study. PLS, which is a second generation multivariate method (Fornell, 1987), evaluates both the measurement model and the theoretical or structural model simultaneously (Urbach & Ahlemann, 2010). The required adjustments for the relationships among constructs are handled by the method (Chin et al., 2003; Fornell, 1987). Other characteristics, such as ability to run with smaller sample sizes (Cassel et al. 1999; Urbach & Ahlemann, 2010) unlike covariance based structural equation modeling (SEM) methods and calculate the estimates for each latent variable makes PLS methods are robust and highly used. In addition, PLS can be used for both theory development and confirming a theory (Chin, 1998b; Urbach & Ahlemann, 2010). On the other hand, PLS is considered to be more appropriate for exploratory model analysis. The last but not the least, PLS method does not require data to be normally distributed.

Non-response bias is another measurement that researchers control to determine with survey data to test the representativeness of the selected sample (Rogelberg & Stanton, 2007). Non-response bias can be tested by comparing the means of early wave of respondents and late wave of respondents (Lambert & Harrington, 1990; Armstrong & Overton, 1977). The reasoning behind this is that late respondents in a study tend to act as non-respondents (Armstrong & Overton, 1977). The sample sizes for the two groups were 175 as early respondents, who returned the survey within 2 weeks and 41 as late respondents, whose data were received between the second and the fourth week. The results on randomly selected variables revealed no significant differences between the two groups of respondents. Therefore, non-response bias was considered not to be an issue in this study.

4. DATA ANALYSIS AND RESULTS

Tests on measurement model are required before testing the structural model in PLS and SEM analysis. In order to test the measurement model validity and reliability tests were conducted. There are three common tests for validity, namely, content validity, criterion-related validity, and construct validity. Content validity refers to "...the degree to which an instrument has an appropriate sample of items for the construct being measured" (Polit & Beck, 2004, p. 423). Content analysis may include both quantitative and qualitative processes (Haynes et al., 1995). Expert opinion is the common way used for testing content validity (Lynn, 1986). Literature provides different approaches for quantifying the expert or judge opinion. These approaches include, but not limited to averaging the experts' ratings and using "pre-established criterion of acceptability" (Polit & Beck, 2006, p.490; Beck & Gable, 2001). Content validity was tested by a group of 4 expert/ judges for this study. The instrument was refined after the first round of expert opinions. In the second round, the required threshold value for scale-level content validity index (S-CVI) (Polit & Beck, 2006) is reached and measured as 0.8.

"Criterion validity is demonstrated by finding a statistically significant relationship between a measure and a criterion" (Nunnally & Bernstein, 1994; Rubio et al., 2003). Correlation is the most common way to test the criterion validity.

Construct validity is "...the degree to which an assessment instrument measures the targeted construct (i.e., the degree to which variance in obtained measures from an assessment instrument is consistent with predictions from the construct targeted by the instrument" (Haynes et al., 1995, p. 239). One way to test the construct validity to use confirmatory factor analysis (CFA) through structural equation modeling (SEM) (Rubio et al., 2003). In this study, we used CFA (see Table 1). In factor analysis the acceptable values of factor loadings are 0.5 or higher (Hair et al., 2006). After the first round of analysis, a few indicators were removed or replaced with another indicator if they were cross-loading with another factor. Table 1 shows that all variables in the second round are loading to expected factors and their loading is above 0.5, ranging between 0.519 and 0.886.

Common methods for testing reliability or internal consistency include Cronbach's Alpha and composite reliability measures (Fornell & Larcker, 1981; Nunnaly, 1978). Although in general Cronbach's Alpha value of 0.7 is considered as acceptable, values over 0.6 are considered as marginally acceptable (Gliner & Morgan, 2000). The Cronbach's alpha values are 0.634 for collaboration, 0.682 for communication, 0.759 for coordination, 0.724 for cooperation, 0.632 for trust, and 0.807 for technology orientation. Therefore, our results indicate that (see Table 1) all of the constructs are within acceptable or marginally acceptable range in terms of reliability. We also checked whether reliabilities of the con-

Table 1. Factor analysis and loadings

Factors	Coll	Comm	Coord	Coop	Trust	Techn	Alpha	CR
Coll1	0.869	-0.189	0.117	0.110	-0.109	-0.018	0.634	0.805
Coll2	0.866	-0.051	-0.114	-0.006	-0.109	-0.002		
Coll3	0.519	0.402	-0.005	-0.174	0.365	0.034		
Comm1	0.145	0.757	-0.002	-0.079	-0.176	-0.064	0.682	0.808
Comm2	-0.035	0.765	0.206	-0.045	-0.054	0.058		
Comm3	0.079	0.622	-0.369	0.119	0.199	0.006		
Comm4	-0.184	0.715	0.102	0.029	0.071	0.001		
Coord1	0.152	0.094	0.826	0.093	-0.024	-0.073	0.759	0.848
Coord2	0.158	-0.255	0.766	-0.007	-0.148	0.063		
Coord3	-0.087	0.116	0.802	-0.149	0.058	0.061		
Coord4	-0.270	0.038	0.651	0.074	0.133	-0.056		
Coop1	0.276	0.101	-0.213	0.685	-0.141	0.024	0.724	0.813
Coop2	-0.211	-0.136	-0.049	0.654	0.338	0.047		
Coop3	-0.162	0.039	0.278	0.584	0.137	0.057		
Coop4	0.156	-0.141	-0.119	0.698	-0.107	0.078		
Coop5	-0.149	0.117	0.457	0.618	-0.139	-0.161		
Coop6	0.042	0.036	-0.284	0.648	-0.069	-0.054		
Trust1	-0.008	0.100	0.145	-0.101	0.835	0.060	0.632	0.803
Trust2	-0.021	-0.092	-0.115	0.243	0.747	-0.036		
Trust3	0.033	-0.021	-0.051	-0.140	0.693	-0.034		
Tech1	-0.039	-0.126	0.101	-0.040	0.044	0.875	0.807	0.886
Tech2	-0.020	-0.031	0.031	0.114	-0.093	0.886		
Tech3	0.067	0.175	-0.147	-0.084	0.056	0.786		

Notes: Coll: Collaboration Comm: Communication Coord: Coordination Coop: Cooperation Trust: Trust Techn: Technology Orientation

structs are acceptable through composite reliability, especially for those that are in marginally acceptable portion. The composite reliabilities for collaboration, communication, coordination, cooperation, trust, and technology orientation are 0.805, 0.808, 0.848, 0.813, 0.803, and 0.886, respectively. These results indicate that reliabilities of our constructs are acceptable.

We tested discriminant validity through inter-item correlations. Table 2 reveals the correlations among the constructs as well as square root of average variance extracted (AVE) values in diagonal. Based on these results, the constructs are positively and significantly correlated with each other. One exception for that significant relationship is the one between technology orientation and coordination. In addition, an indication of acceptable discriminant validity is the case where square roots of AVE values are greater than the correlations for that construct with other constructs. In this case, square root of AVEs would have higher scores than the values on the same column and row for that construct. Table 2 indicates that discriminant validity is acceptable for our model.

Variance Inflation Factors (VIF) is a measure for identifying the threat of multicollinearity. VIF values of 5 and above are considered to have risk of multicollinearity. Our results indicate that (see Table 3)

Table 2. Correlations and square roots of Average Variance Extracted (AVE) values

Constructs	Collaboration	Communication	Coordination	Cooperation	Trust	Techn
Collaboration	(0.769)					
Communication	0.451**	(0.717)				
Coordination	0.588**	0.700**	(0.764)			
Cooperation	0.569**	0.636**	0.628**	(0.649)		
Trust	0.415**	0.593**	0.675**	0.587**	(0.760)	
Tech. Orientation	0.155*	0.181**	0.077	0.219**	0.170*	(0.850)

*. Correlation is significant at the 0.05 level (2-tailed).
**. Correlation is significant at the 0.01 level (2-tailed).

Table 3. Model fit and quality indices (as defined in WarpPLS Output)

Constructs	Collab	Commun	Coordi	Cooper	Trust	TechO
Collinearity VIF	1.722	2.314	2.991	2.238	2.064	1.086
Average full collinearity VIF (AFVIF)	2.069			acceptable if <= 5, ideally <= 3.3		
Average path coefficient (APC)	0.324**					
Average R-squared (ARS)	0.454**					
Average block VIF (AVIF)	1.543			acceptable if <= 5, ideally <= 3.3		
Sympson's paradox ratio (SPR)	1.000			acceptable if >= 0.7, ideally = 1		
R-squared contribution ratio (RSCR)	1.000			acceptable if >= 0.9, ideally = 1		
Statistical suppression ratio (SSR)	1.000			acceptable if >= 0.7		

multicollinearity may not be a threat for our study since all VIF values are lower than 5, the threshold value. Although there is no globally accepted goodness of fit values for PLS analysis, Average Path Coefficient, and Average block VIF, and Averaged R-Squared are commonly used model fit indices for PLS (Moqbel et al., 2013). Model fit and quality indices, such as Average Path Coefficient (0.324, p<0.01), Average Root Square (0.454, p<0.01), Average Variance Inflation Factors (1.543), Sympson's paradox ratio (1, the ideal score), R-squared contribution ratio (1, the ideal score), and Statistical suppression ratio (1) show no evidence of problem regarding the fit; therefore, the results indicate that our model has a good fit (see Table 3).

Common method bias (CMB) is considered a type of measurement method problem (Kock, 2015) for studies collecting data via survey questionnaires (Podsakoff et al., 2003). Among different ways to measure CMB, such as Harman's single factor test (Podsakoff & Organ, 1986), marker variable (Lindell & Whitney, 2001), and full collinearity variance inflation factors (VIFs), the last method is considered as a more conservative approach. In addition, VIFs approach is recommended for variance-based SEM analysis (Kock, 2015; Kock & Lynn, 2012). Therefore, in this study we adopt this approach to test CMB. The results of the study reveals that all of the collinearity VIF values are smaller than the recommended threshold of 3.3 (Kock, 2015) and varies between 1.086 for Technology Orientation and 2.991 for Coordination as seen in Table 3. Therefore, threat of CMB can be considered minimal for the study.

Table 4 and Figure 2 show the coefficients of paths among the constructs as well as the R square values for the model developed for this study. In addition to this model, we have tested alternative models as well. However, the proposed model provided the highest R-square and model fit among all the tested models. Therefore, we explain the proposed and the most robust model in this study. Table 4 suggests that collaboration has a positive and significant relationship with coordination ($\beta=0.413$, $p<0.01$), and cooperation ($\beta=0.325$, $p<0.01$). As suggested by Figure 2, trust has positive and significant relationship with communication ($\beta=0.582$, $p<0.01$), coordination ($\beta=0.705$, $p<0.01$), and cooperation ($\beta=0.651$, $p<0.01$). Finally, technology has similar relationship with cooperation ($\beta=0.107$, $p<0.01$). However, our results did not indicate any significant relationship between collaboration and communication, as well as between technology orientation and communication and coordination.

Table 5 shows the hypotheses tested in this study and their status regarding whether they are rejected or not.

Table 4. R square value, path coefficients and their significances

Constructs	Collab	Commun	Coordi	Cooper	Trust	TechO	R^2	Adj. R^2
Collaboration		0.012	0.413**	0.325**			0.482	0.474
Communication					0.582**	0.081	0.368	0.362
Coordination					0.705**	0.037	0.495	0.491
Cooperation					0.651**	0.107*	0.470	0.465
Trust								
Tech.Orientation								

*. P-Value is significant at the 0.05 level.

**. P-Value is significant at the 0.01 level.

Figure 2. Estimated parameters in the model

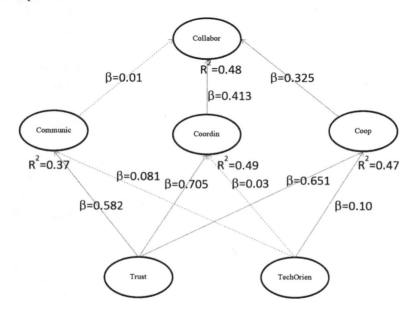

Table 5. Hypotheses and their status

Hypotheses	Status
H1: The degree of collaboration is positively related with the level of communication.	Not Supported
H2: The degree of collaboration is positively related with the level of coordination.	Supported
H3: The degree of collaboration is positively related with the level of cooperation.	Supported
H4: The level of trust is positively related with the level of communication.	Supported
H5: The level of trust is positively related with the level of coordination.	Supported
H6: The level of trust is positively related with the level of cooperation.	Supported
H7: The degree of communication is positively related with the degree of technology orientation.	Not Supported
H8: The degree of coordination is positively related with the degree of technology orientation.	Not Supported
H9: The degree of cooperation is positively related with the degree of technology orientation.	Supported

5. DISCUSSION

To advance our understandings of current practices of interprofessional collaboration, this research aims for empirically examining the impact of trust and technology on collaboration in association with mediating effects of communication, coordination and collaboration. In particular, the study finds the factors influencing interprofessional collaboration in healthcare settings. The study results shown in Figure 2 and Table 4 indicate that collaboration has positive and significant relationship with coordination and cooperation but not with communication. On the other hand, the study results validate that trust has positive and significant relationship with communication, coordination, and cooperation. Furthermore, the study results (shown in Figure 2 and Table 4) indicate technology orientation has positive and significant relationship with cooperation but not with communication and coordination. Table 4 indicates that the constructs are positively and significantly correlated except collaboration-communication, technology-communication, and technology-coordination. Therefore, the study finds coordination and cooperation as the factors significantly influencing interprofessional collaboration. In other words, the study finds positive impact of trust on collaboration with mediating effects of coordination and cooperation; and positive impact of technology orientation on collaboration with mediating effect of cooperation. The discussion on the managerial implications of these findings is given in this section.

5.1. Factors for Collaboration

The primary research question is to find the factors influencing the quality of interprofessional collaboration. The study results indicate coordination and cooperation are the factors influencing interprofessional collaboration but not the communication. Table 4 and Figure 2 show high degrees of correlations for collaboration with the following constructs: coordination and cooperation.

The finding of collaboration and coordination having positive and significant relationship is consistent with analytical framework of interdisciplinary collaboration developed by Sicotte et al. (2002), in which intensity of collaboration was found to be related with the degree of interprofessional coordination in community health centers. In studying healthcare teamwork behaviors, Williams et al. (2010) found positive relationship between coordination and collaboration. These findings validate the results of the study reported in this paper. D'Amour (1997) developed a model, which has been tested with empirical data to understand interprofessional collaboration (Echaquan, 2003). The key dimension of the model is appropriating a common goal and plan for the patient care. Creative outcomes emerge when multiple different professionals work together sharing a common goal, plan, and decision-making (Woods et al., 2011). For effective collaboration, the interprofessional team efforts are to be coordinated toward a common goal and plan. The significant outcome of coordination is the emergence of creative care and optimal care of patients, which is difficult to achieve individually. Working through conflicts concerning the sharing of tasks and responsibilities is considered to be a key skill for effective interprofessional collaboration (Baerg et al., 2012). The beliefs and values of diverse professionals foster conflicts and put constraints for effective collaboration. The conflicts are to be approached without hindering the freedom to be different and disagree. Formalizing the tasks and responsibilities offer a collaborative environment for professionals to commit for working together.

Accordingly, the healthcare professionals need to effectively coordinate for achieving effective collaboration in patient care delivery. For effective coordination of healthcare delivery efforts, the professionals need to function as the communicative hub of their healthcare teams, perform as team leaders, direct/mentor the team members, assign tasks and responsibilities. Effective collaboration requires processing of needed information for successful delivery of patient care. The effective coordination requires a plan integrating inputs of various professionals toward a common goal of delivering care to the patient. It implies encouraging inputs from other professionals and acknowledging their contributions. Coordination ensures that the patient's needs for health services are met over time. Actively listening to ideas makes the team members feel valued and increases their participation in collaborative decision making for patient care. Similarly, effective coordination requires offering ideas and opinion to others. In general, having a shared understanding of each team member's knowledge and skills facilitate effective coordination and thereby collaboration. The essence of effective coordination requires shared understanding about prior problems and services as it needs for current care, interaction and collaboration.

Working with colleagues in a collaborative practice requires cooperation in terms of frequent communication for sharing knowledge/ skills, incorporating views of others, providing consistent feedback, and clarity of roles influencing creative outcomes in providing quality care to the patients (Barrett et al., 2007; San Martin-Rodriguez et al., 2005; Way et al., 2000). Frequent communication enables the professionals to understand each other's perspective and one another's contributions so that quality decisions are made for improved patient care. Effective cooperation leads to effective collaboration. In the healthcare team, the professionals need to work in a complementary mode rather than competing mode by understanding each other's role. There is a range of barriers for effective collaboration including ignorance or insufficient knowledge about other professional's area of competence, inclination more towards professional ethnocentricity regarding one's profession as superior to others. In general, specialists often may have strong sense of independence, and concerns that they may lose their importance and identities in team environment. This tendency restricts the willingness to participate in cooperative activities. To improve the levels of cooperation aiming at better quality of care, professionals must clarify their position, roles and responsibilities to others in a healthcare team. In general, the complexity of healthcare problems relate to the degree of cooperation. More complex problems need multidisciplinary teamwork (high degree of cooperation) and less complex problems require consultation (low degree of cooperation). The cooperative behaviors of professionals build effective relationships and structure a collective action towards patient care. The intensity of cooperation indicates a positive collaboration resulting in team integration, and joint decision making for enhanced healthcare.

The study finds that the impact of communication on collaboration is not significant. Frequent and formal communication becomes ineffective and unproductive when the required information is not communicated. As a result, it may not lead to any collaborative outcome. When collaboration takes place, there is an accomplishment of tangible outcomes, such as conflict resolution and creative outcomes. Though the communication enables the professionals' capacity to work together, when the capacity is not effectively utilized, then the professional works on separate silos and the collaborative approach become fragmented.

5.2. Impact of Trust

Another research objective is to find the impact of trust on communication, coordination and cooperation. The study results given in Figure 2 and Table 4 show high degrees of correlations and path coefficients indicating trust has positive and significant impact on communication, coordination and cooperation.

Trust has significant influence on communication. This is convincing as the literature says trust encourages communication and thereby positive information flows (Tyler & Kramer, 1996; Veenstra & Lomas, 1999). Trust keeps the individuals' mind open to ideas and secures more dialogue and communication (Misztal, 1996). The professionals consider the trust beliefs based on their past communication with others and develop a good or bad attitude towards multi-disciplinary team work. When mutual trust between the colleagues is high, building relations in a communicative environment becomes easier. The frequency of information exchange among professionals increases and leads to more formal and informal communication. Trust facilitates more interprofessional communication for both patient understanding and the capacity to work with members of the teams. Mutual trust in healthcare encourages more face-to-face interactions, email communications, messaging, team meetings, interprofessional committees, team retreats, hallway conversations, and mini-conferences for engaging and sharing information for optimized care of patients and decision-making. Building trust is so important for lessening the impact of negative attitude and continuance interactions among professionals. As professionals get more experienced in working with the team in a complex multidisciplinary environment, the risk perception of distrust may change over time. In a multidisciplinary environment, professionals need to keep each other informed about events or changes that affect them. The professionals have to ensure the patient care decisions are always trusted/ supported by their colleagues. Thereby, professionals get more confidence in interactions as the communicative experience is positive. Winning trust at the beginning is important as initial trust could be a starting point for continuance participation in interactive decision making aiming quality care of patients.

Trust has significant influence on coordination. Trust facilitates collective action leading to cooperation among professionals to achieve common goal of quality care of patients (D'Amour et al., 2005; Gilson, 2003). As trust protects the professionals' interests in a multi-disciplinary environment, trust-based coordination contributes to build more value in patient-care (Gilson, 2003). Mutual trust between the colleagues enables the professionals to collaborate regarding patient goals and plans. Besides, the existence of trust among professionals keeps each other informed about events or changes that affect them, it provides a basis for their coordination by creating strong personal bonds, conflicts concerning the sharing of responsibilities are resolved without much difficulty. On the contrary, the distrusting environment may create conflicts concerning the sharing of tasks and responsibilities. These conflicts make the professionals to stick rigidly to their job descriptions and generate negative outcomes in delivering patient care. Also, the trusted environment provides more freedom to be different and to disagree, more comfort to ask questions in meetings, and provides ability to express ideas openly without fear of any misunderstandings. When mutual trust between the professionals is high, the element of risk in expected behavior is nullified. As a result, decisions about approaches to treatment are made unilaterally. As a trusted environment keeps the professionals informed about events or changes in the treatment that affect them, it improves their ability to meet patient's needs. When patient care decisions are trusted by other members of the team, the trust facilitates dialogues between professionals from different disciplines. With the mutual trust in the background, professionals accomplish the coordinated activities, such as showing leadership by directing and supervising team members, mentoring others, assigning responsibilities, and delegating tasks to others. Trust facilitates information sharing and organized understanding of relevant knowledge and thereby improves individual's contribution for delivering quality care for patients. Mutual trust between multi-disciplinary professionals underpins the coordination by committing them for working together.

Trust has significant positive impact on cooperation. As trust protects the interests of professionals engaged in a joint endeavor, it can be silent background for running smooth cooperative relations in caring patients (Misztal, 1996). Trust enables the professionals to have autonomy in their own contribution, reconciles their own interests with those of others, and supports cooperative problem solving. Trust establishes a platform for knowledge sharing by consistently asking/ giving feedback/ opinion to members of the team, and for discussing strategies to improve working relationships. As trust is essentially a psychological state rooted in risk, trust or distrust creates expectations of how others will behave (in a cooperative or non-cooperative way). Trust among professionals enables the members better understand the work of other health professionals. In particular, trust plays a key role in distinguishing between roles and responsibilities. In a trusted environment, more support for each other's roles and responsibilities are provided as part of cooperation. As trust is essentially a calculation that the other professional's future action will be beneficial for enhancing the quality of patient-care, in case of necessities, trust motivates the individual to support the tasks outside his/ her job description, which indicates cooperation. Trust breaks down the barriers for cooperative behavior and develops a good understanding of mutual responsibilities.

The impact of mutual trust on collaboration mediating coordination and cooperation is emphasized in the literature (D'Amour et al., 2005; Stichler, 1995; Siegler & Whitney, 1994). D'Amour (1997) developed a model for understanding interprofessional collaboration in which 'trusting relationships' among professionals is considered to be a key dimension. Mutual trust is required for two or more professionals to join in a collaborative task, which demands coordination and cooperation among them. For collaboration, professionals are expected to be aware of contributions made by members, develop an understanding of each other's roles/ responsibilities and keep each other informed about events or changes that affect them. This trusted environment is favorable for collaborative undertaking in which members exchange ideas and opinion for delivering quality care for the patients. So, for establishing a collaborative process, professionals have to develop trust among them. On the other hand, simply bringing professionals together in teams will not lead to any sort of collaboration. When mutual trust between professionals is high, collaboration generates creative outcomes as treatment decisions are coordinated and made unilaterally by professionals from other disciplines. Trust enables the professionals to work through conflicts for resolving them through coordination by creating formal procedures/ mechanisms for facilitating dialogue between professionals from different disciplines.

5.3. Impact of Technology Orientation

The research question associated with technology orientation is to identify the ways in which technology can be used for enhancing communication, coordination and cooperation of healthcare professionals. The study results show positive and significant relationship with cooperation but not with communication and coordination. The impact of technology orientation on collaboration mediating cooperation is significant and positive.

This study suggests that technology orientation plays a large role for cooperation with colleagues in healthcare setting, to incorporate views of treatment of other professionals, to provide consistent feedback to team members, and to support the role of other professionals in the healthcare team. The health professionals use technology for better cooperation. Leonhardt (2006) emphasize the usage of technology beyond communication especially for cooperation. The study findings suggest for professionals to adopt and use technology for enhancing cooperation. As the healthcare team members may not always present in the same location, relying on e-communication technology is increased for information exchange, interaction, and knowledge access for each individual in the team. Technology oriented organizations relying on e-communication technology for accomplishing work is very common and considered to be a substitute for face-to-face interaction (Hinds & Kiesler, 2002). Technology orientation has several advantages including enhanced capability for frequent communication of quality content and resources (Rice & Gattiker, 2001). Furthermore, technology enables the team members to access the expertise of other professional and incorporate views of treatment. Thereby, technology improves the ability of team members to meet patient needs. Of course, the usage of technology for cooperation for each team member occurs along a continuum from low to high use. As an information-seeking activity to understand the distinction between roles, technology enables the team members to engage in information exchange in a timely manner. Encouraging a culture of technology enabled cooperation facilitates improved quality care of patients.

Besides, communication technology is used to bring diverse professionals from areas, such as pathology, oncology, pharmacy, surgery, psychiatry, and behavioral health for frequent communication and consistent feedback. Technology enables the professionals to identify problems quickly and helps to make timely adjustments of therapy. Technology facilitates sharing of personal health information of patients across professionals for providing quality care to a specific patient. Complex and chronic illnesses demand the use of sophisticated technologies by multidisciplinary team of professionals. As the complexity of illness requires providers from diverse areas, technology plays a key role in incorporating views (expertise) of treatment of different professionals and enables for secure, easy and timely exchange of information for the enhanced quality care. Thereby, professionals are powered with e-communication technology as a source of learning to create and maintain cooperation with other professionals. The technology engages them to be better partners in providing care with improved outcomes. Technology enables for more collaborative outcomes as technology contributes for effective cooperation in implementing treatment decisions.

The usage of technology for communication has undergone dramatic changes and continues to evolve over time. Technology facilitates communication among the professionals within a given health care system. Technology enables health professionals to consult with others or can seek "specialty" consults for the benefit of patient care. The communication technology devices allow for "always immediate access" with the exception of out of coverage areas. Though the technology limits face-to-face communication, the usage in terms of daily use (duration), frequency of use, and the number of applications used are ever increasing among healthcare professionals. Since the perceived usefulness and ease of use of these technologies are realized for accomplishing the tasks and the job performance, the acceptance rate of the communication technologies is exponentially increasing. Despite the presence of privacy/ security concerns in using the technology for communication, the usage has increased for communicating sensitive and no time-sensitive issues (Liederman & Morefield, 2003; Liederman et al., 2005).

The study finds that the impact of technology orientation on communication is not significant. This may be because of having more face-to-face communication in healthcare instead of using technology for communication. In the healthcare settings, face-to-face communication has several advantages including richer communication. Non-verbal cues with face-to-face communication make the professional to prefer it compare to the e-communication especially in communicating sensitive information about the patients. Besides, the study finds that the impact of technology orientation on coordination is not significant. This implies that coordinated activities, such as conflict resolution and collaboration regarding patient goals and plans can take place without much use of technology. For instance, face-to-face communication may be more preferred in health-care settings rather than e-communication for coordination especially for handling sensitive, difficult, unanalyzable and non-routine tasks in healthcare.

5.4. Example for Implementable Ideas from an Industry Perspective

Healthcare is one of the highest growing industries, in which professionals including physicians, nurses, pharmacists, clients, community partners and health educators work together to provide medical care to patients. The modern healthcare is divided into several sectors and depends on interdisciplinary teams of trained healthcare professionals to meet healthcare needs of patients. In the industry perspective, the rising cost of healthcare largely from chronic disease is unmanageable. The healthcare providers are committed to address the increasing cost in healthcare spending. Another trend is shared decision making on treatment decisions for which effective inter-professional collaboration becomes necessary. This section provides an example illustrating how the ideas in the paper could be implemented from an industry perspective.

Consider patients with Diabetes, Heart Disease, Kidney Disease, and other heath related problems. Multi-disciplinary teams of professionals are required for treating such diseases. Each team-member learns from each other's discipline as the disease demands cross-disciplinary knowledge and expertise. The team has to build up the treatment process by knitting and sharing the different pieces from different disciplines and perspectives. Thereby, working with colleagues from other professions becomes necessary as individuals can achieve only limited outcomes. Besides, the collaborative outcomes are more creative and unpredictable compared to that of individuals. Bringing the team together to work on may be a challenging task as the members come from varying experience and background. In the practitioner's perspective, for improving the quality of collaboration this research emphasizes cooperation and coordination of professionals.

5.5. Enhance the Quality of Collaboration

When diverse professionals work together for a common goal, conflicts are common. The health professionals have to work through the conflicts and resolve them to prevent the ongoing impact. Extensive efforts are to be taken to avoid conflicts concerning the sharing of tasks and responsibilities. To cultivate collaborative culture, encourage open communication and allow colleagues openly represent the professional perspectives about patient's healthcare needs. In day-to-day program functioning, collaborative behaviors, such as collaborative treatments are to be encouraged. Contextual strategies/ approaches are to be evolved to bring the team together. Structuring a collective action and joint decision making on treatment enable the team to work in an integrated manner towards patient care. Also, collaboration nurtures the process of sharing knowledge and skills; evolves approaches for engaging multiple different professionals to work together as a team sharing a common goal of improved care for the patients; and creates collaborative culture among the professionals by sharing responsibilities, decision-making, values, data, and intervention.

5.6. Understand on How Best to Cooperate

Cooperation creates a work environment in which professionals frequently communicate with colleagues from other professional disciplines. It encourages developments of mechanisms electronically (such as web portal, mobile apps and other electronic access) to incorporate views of treatment held by colleagues from other disciplines. These mechanisms could be used to provide constant feedback to colleagues. Instead of sticking to one's own job description, extending the boundaries by understanding the distinction between each other's roles avoid the professionals to work in silos. In other words, the professionals need to understand that supporting the role of colleagues is also part of their job description. Sometimes, a professional has to sacrifice some degree of his/ her autonomy to support cooperative problem solving. Often, strategies (such as retreats, annual/ semi-annual meetings) are to be discussed to improve working relationships of professionals. These activities usually encourage the colleagues to ask for opinion from other professionals and often refer them for consultations. Hierarchical barriers (if any) are to be removed in these kind of opinion seeking activities (e.g., physicians seeking opinion from nurses). Similarly, work evaluations are to be carried out jointly.

5.7. Create a Coordinated Environment

The professionals are to be brought together as a team, which can be achieved by vertically integrating the team using a management hierarchy. Coordination regulates the diverse professionals into an integrated and harmonious operational team with a common goal of providing effective healthcare to patients. It involves the team members by providing access (for both within and between units) to information or resources needed for patient care. A better coordination is achieved when the information about prior problems and treatments (e.g., medical history of patients) are available for current care. Coordination not only standardizes healthcare practices in order to reduce duplicated activities in patient-care, but also emphasizes on the coordinated activities, such as: mentoring the team members, showing leadership by assigning tasks and responsibilities, acknowledging the contribution of other professionals, providing the care in time/ budget, offering/ seeking ideas to/ from others, and developing a shared understanding of the patient's care. Overall, coordination creates a coordinated environment where there is freedom to be different and to disagree.

5.8. Effective Communication

Interprofessional communication has to be emphasized for both patient understanding and the capacity to work with members of teams. Most common methods of communication, such as face-to-face, telephone, computer/ mobile (email, social media, or specific mobile app) are to be followed. Education and providing several communication toolkits may enhance effective communication among inter-disciplinary professionals. During formal and informal meetings, each team member should feel free to share his/ her opinions openly without fear of being misunderstood. In other words, participants should feel good comfort level to say what is on their mind (i.e., work related issues, information sharing, etc.). Providing feedback makes communication more effective. The professionals are to be engaged electronically in an interactive manner. For achieving this, an effective web site portal (with access to desktop and mobile) needs to be maintained where announcements, schedules, policies, procedures, and other materials can be posted. Hospitals usually provide the current communication technologies, such as portal, email, phone, blackberry, bulletin board, and specific software systems, which are to be used meaningfully for effective communication.

5.9. Build Trust

The professionals have to rely on other colleagues for understanding the treatment decisions. So, creating a trusted environment becomes mandatory where members can recognize and protect the rights and interests of other team members. The trust can be built by caring for the patient's interests, avoiding conflicts of interests, acknowledging patient-care decisions, avoiding mistakes, showing honesty, avoiding intentional falsehoods, and maintaining confidentiality of sensitive information. Continuous learning facilitates the development of trust. Engage the participants with dialogues regarding treatment decisions; thereby, it facilitates the process of building trust among the healthcare professionals. Having confidence in one's own abilities, coordinated efforts, and having previous positive experience with other colleagues establish trusted working relationships. Securing open communication and dialogue, frequent communication, and consistently asking/ giving feedback/ opinion to members of teams build trust among professionals.

5.10. Use Technology

Use information and communication technologies for sharing information and knowledge to perform healthcare relevant tasks, to gain personal productivity, to increase decision quality, to eliminate routine tasks, to improve information flows, effectiveness, and efficiency in healthcare delivery. E-communication technologies, such as email, text messaging, social media tools, such as Facebook, YouTube, and Twitter are to be used to disseminate health messages and seek solutions in healthcare. Early adoption of e-communication technologies from e-mail to short messaging to social networking facilitates inter-professional collaboration. Use of technology encourages adopting and using personal communication technologies, such as PDAs, pagers, and mobile devices in an individual environment and use group communication technologies (such as video conferencing) in a group environment. It increases the mobile usage for healthcare such as change prescription, symptom control etc.; and use secured web-based portals for administrative tasks, such as scheduling appointments. Using e-communication tools, such as email, invited Facebook groups, text messages, websites help for effectively managing patients' connection, health and support.

6. CONCLUSION, LIMITATIONS, AND AREAS FOR FURTHER RESEARCH

The increases in complexity of patient care, healthcare costs, and technological advancements shifted the healthcare delivery to interprofessional collaborative care. This interdisciplinary team approach inevitably makes professionals interdependent in a collaborative manner by interacting with others cultivating relationships using effective coordination and cooperation. However, collaboration is challenging and difficult to achieve. Though the literature gives conceptual approaches, there is a limited empirical knowledge on factors influencing collaboration.

To fill this gap, the study aimed for understanding current practices of interprofessional collaboration by empirically testing the impact of trust and technology on collaboration in association with communication, coordination and collaboration. Hypotheses were evolved to examine the following: (i) the impact of communication, coordination and cooperation on collaboration (ii) impact of trust on communication, coordination, and cooperation; and (iii) the impact of technology orientation on communication, coordination, and cooperation.

The results of the study validate that collaboration has positive and significant relationship with co-ordination and cooperation but not with communication; similarly, the study found that trust has positive and significant relationship with communication, coordination, and cooperation. Furthermore, the study results have shown technology orientation has positive and significant relationship with cooperation but not with communication and coordination. Besides, the study finds positive impact of trust on collaboration with mediating effects of coordination and cooperation; and positive impact of technology on collaboration with mediating effect of cooperation. The managerial implications of these findings were discussed.

In considering the study results, interprofessional collaboration can be achieved by creating a trusted relationship among the professionals. The team lead/ manager needs to take efforts to create a positive attitude for each member towards collaboration. Such efforts may include: encouraging members to use several modes of communication (e.g., face-to-face, telephone, email, social media, and digital), frequent exchange of information (which is feasible in the era of social media networking), create opportunities for members to express views/ comments through e-messaging, team meetings, committees, team retreats, hallway conversations, and mini-conferences for effective engagement. In expressing opinion, the team member should be given freedom to be different and to disagree. Electronic maintenance of the past communication on treatment decisions and outcomes (e.g., medical history records) enable the members for building mutual trust with colleagues.

The interprofessional team structure plays a key role for better coordination. A clear definition of roles, tasks, and responsibilities avoid any possible conflicts. A better coordinated collaboration occurs when the professionals are informed about events or changes, latest improvements and conditions in the hospital through a web-portal with an access to all kinds of device including desktop and mobile. This establishes platform for knowledge sharing by asking/ giving feedback/ opinion periodically to team members. This information sharing can happen through several other methods including email, bulletin boards, smaller program meetings (e.g., Diabetes Meeting, Renal Meeting, Cardiovascular Meeting, etc.). As team members may not always be in the same location, it becomes imperative to use technology for enhanced cooperation. Diverse professionals from different fields (e.g., pathology, oncology, pharmacy, surgery, psychiatry, and others) are to be linked by communication technology for sharing their expertise towards patient-care. Though the hospitals usually have adequate technological infrastructure, the team members need to be encouraged for meaningful use of technology. Thus, establishing technological culture facilitates easier and effective way of communication.

Surprisingly, this study has a counterintuitive implication; this research didn't support the impact of technology orientation on collaboration with communication as mediating variable. This is different from what one might expect. This implies that using technology for communication alone does not guarantee any effective collaboration. Besides, leadership is important in teams where generally team members prefer an open-door policy where they can discuss any concerns with leaders. When the power and hierarchy of the leader is less, the team members feel more involved in treatment-decision making and this perception leads to a better collaboration.

The previous research contributed conceptual frameworks and this research build upon those conceptual foundations for empirically validating the factors relating to collaboration. The significance of this research is to build collaboration among healthcare professionals, it is imperative to have trust and technology with effectiveness in communication, coordination, and cooperation aiming quality care of the patients. Technology orientation is an important enabler for achieving effective cooperation. There are still many things on collaboration in healthcare setting, which has not been explored. For instance, what are the best practices for coordination and cooperation to achieve effective collaboration? What are the barriers for effective collaboration among healthcare professionals? The future research can design a questionnaire survey to answer these research questions. A descriptive study on trust building strategies for collaboration is a valuable one as trust plays a key role for improved outcomes of healthcare. A case study methodology is suggested to fulfill this objective. Regarding technology orientation, the use of social media for effective collaboration and cooperation has been realized as a key issue. So, a study on acceptance and effective use of social media for collaboration would be an interesting topic for future researchers. Seeing the importance of patient-physician collaboration for enhanced care, another research avenue would be to validate this research model in the context of patient-physician collaboration.

Lack of availability of standard measures for various constructs steered the development of survey questionnaire based on a previous qualitative study and literature on collaboration in healthcare system. The respondents were asked to indicate their degree of agreement with the statements in the questionnaire. Though we made a concerted effort to include a range of healthcare professionals to participate in the study, their opinion on the degree of agreement is highly subjective. Despite these limitations, however, our study makes a noteworthy contribution to healthcare collaboration.

REFERENCES

Aiken, M., Wang, J., Gu, L., & Paolillo, J. (2011). An Exploratory Study of How Technology Supports Communication in Multilingual Groups. *International Journal of e-Collaboration*, 7(1), 17–29. doi:10.4018/jec.2011010102

Ajzen, I. (1991). The theory of planned behavior. *Organizational Behavior and Human Decision Processes*, 50(2), 179–211. doi:10.1016/0749-5978(91)90020-T

Ajzen, I., & Fishbein, M. (1980). *Understanding attitudes and predicting social behavior*. Englewood Cliffs, NJ: Prentice-Hall.

Alter, C., & Hage, J. (1993). *Organizations working together*. Sage Publications, Inc.

Apker, J., Kathleen, M. P., Wendy, S. Z. F., & Hofmeister, N. (2006). Collaboration, credibility, compassion, and coordination: Professional nurse communication. *Journal of Professional Nursing, 22*(3), 180–189. doi:10.1016/j.profnurs.2006.03.002 PMID:16759961

Arslanian-Engoren, C. M. (1995). Lived experiences of CNSs who collaborate with physicians: A phenomenological study. *Clinical Nurse Specialist CNS, 9*(2), 68–74. doi:10.1097/00002800-199503000-00002 PMID:7600484

Armstrong, J. S., & Overton, T. S. (1977). Estimating nonresponse bias in mail surveys. *JMR, Journal of Marketing Research, 14*(3), 396–402. doi:10.2307/3150783

Armstrong, D., & Cole, P. (2002). Managing distances and differences in geographically distributed work groups. In P. Hinds &cS. Kiesler (Ed.), Distributed Work (pp. 167-189). Cambridge, MA: MIT Press.

Axelsson, R., & Bihari-Axelsson, S. (2005). Intersectoral problems in the Russian organization of public health. *Health Policy (Amsterdam), 73*(3), 285–293. doi:10.1016/j.healthpol.2004.11.020 PMID:16039347

Alshatnawi, E. A. R. (2014). Assessing communication skills among Jordanian tour guides: German tourists perceptions. *Journal of Management Research., 6*(1), 1–11. doi:10.5296/jmr.v6i1.4361

Baerg, K., Lake, D., & Paslawski, T. (2012). Learning needs and training interest in health professionals, teachers, and students: An exploratory study. *Journal of Research in Interprofessional Practice and Education., 2*(2), 1–19.

Baggs, J. G., & Schmitt, M. H. (1997). Nurses and resident physicians perceptions of the process of collaboration in an MICU. *Research in Nursing & Health, 20*(1), 71–80. doi:10.1002/(SICI)1098-240X(199702)20:1<71::AID-NUR8>3.0.CO;2-R PMID:9024479

Baier, A. (1986). Trust and antitrust. *Ethics, 96*(2), 231–260. doi:10.1086/292745

Bailey, P., Jones, L., & Way, D. (2006). Family physician/nurse practitioner: Stories of collaboration. *Journal of Advanced Nursing, 53*(4), 381–391. doi:10.1111/j.1365-2648.2006.03734.x PMID:16448481

Ball, M. J., & Lillis, J. (2006). E-health: Transforming the physician/patient relationship. *International Journal of Medical Informatics, 61*(1), 1–10. doi:10.1016/S1386-5056(00)00130-1 PMID:11248599

Barimani, M., & Hylander, I. (2008). Linkage in the chain of care: A grounded theory of professional cooperation between antenatal care, postpartum care and child health care. *International Journal of Integrated Care, 8*(4), 1–13. doi:10.5334/ijic.254 PMID:19209242

Barrett, J., Curran, V., Glynn, L., & Godwin, M. (2007). *CHSRF synthesis: Interprofessional collaboration and quality primary healthcare*. Ottawa, ON: Canadian Health Services Research Foundation.

Batt, P. J., & Purchase, S. (2004). Managing collaboration within networks and relationships. *Industrial Marketing Management, 33*(3), 169–174. doi:10.1016/j.indmarman.2003.11.004

Baumgart, D. C. (2005). Personal digital assistants in health care: Experienced clinicians in the palm of your hand? *Journal of the American Medical Association, 366*(9492), 1210–1222. PMID:16198770

Beck, C. T., & Gable, R. K. (2001). Ensuring content validity: An illustration of the process. *Journal of Nursing Measurement, 9*(2), 201–215. PMID:11696942

Berwick, D. M. (2003). Improvement, trust, and the healthcare workforce. *Quality & Safety in Health Care*, *12*(6), 448–452. doi:10.1136/qhc.12.6.448 PMID:14645761

Blanchet, J. (2005). Innovative programs in telemedicine: The Arizona telemedicine program. *Telemedicine Journal and e-Health*, *11*(2), 116–123. doi:10.1089/tmj.2005.11.116 PMID:15857251

Boden, C., Sit, A., & Weinreb, R. N. (2006). Accuracy of an electronic monitoring and reminder device for use with travoprost eye drops. *Journal of Glaucoma*, *15*(1), 30–34. doi:10.1097/01.ijg.0000196654.77836.61 PMID:16378015

Bodenheime, T. (2007). Coordinating care: A perilous journey through the health care system. *The New England Journal of Medicine*, *358*(10), 1064–1071. doi:10.1056/NEJMhpr0706165 PMID:18322289

Brazil, K., Whelan, T., OBrien, M. A., Sussman, J., Pyette, N., & Bainbridge, D. (2004). Towards improving the co-ordination of supportive cancer care services in the community. *Health Policy (Amsterdam)*, *70*(1), 125–131. doi:10.1016/j.healthpol.2004.02.007 PMID:15312714

Bradner, E., Mark, G., & Hertel, T. (2005). Team size and technology fit: Participation, awareness, and rapport in distributed teams. *IEEE Transactions on Professional Communication*, *48*(1), 68–77. doi:10.1109/TPC.2004.843299

Brockner, J., & Siegel, P. (1996). Understanding the interaction between procedural and distributive justice: The role of trust. In R. M. Kramer & T. R. Tyler (Eds.), *Trust in organizations: Frontiers of theory and research*. Thousand Oaks, CA: Sage. doi:10.4135/9781452243610.n18

Broers, T., Poth, C., & Medeves, J. (2009). What's in a word? Understanding interprofessional collaboration from the students' perspective. *Journal of Research in Interprofessional Practice and Education*, *1*(1), 3–9.

Bronstein, L. R. (2002). Index of interdisciplinary collaboration. *Social Work Research*, *26*(2), 113–126. doi:10.1093/swr/26.2.113

Bronstein, L. R. (2003). A model for interdisciplinary collaboration. *Social Work*, *48*(3), 297–306. doi:10.1093/sw/48.3.297 PMID:12899277

Brown, B., Crawford, P., & Darongkamas, J. (2000). Blurred roles and permeable boundaries: The experience of multidisciplinary working in community mental health. *Health & Social Care in the Community*, *8*(6), 425–435. doi:10.1046/j.1365-2524.2000.00268.x PMID:11560713

Burtscher, M. J., & Manser, T. (2012). Team mental models and their potential to improve teamwork and safety: A review and implications for future research in healthcare. *Safety Science*, *50*(5), 1344–1354. doi:10.1016/j.ssci.2011.12.033

Byrd, T. A. (1992). Implementation and use of expert systems in organizations: Perceptions of knowledge engineers. *Journal of Management Information Systems*, *8*(4), 97–116. doi:10.1080/07421222.1992.11517941

Canadian Health Services Research Foundation. (2006). *Teamwork in healthcare: Promoting effective teamwork in healthcare in Canada. Policy Synthesis and Recommendations.* Ottawa, ON: Canadian Health Services Research Foundation. Retrieved from http://www.chsrf.ca/Migrated/PDF/ResearchReports/CommissionedResearch/teamwork-synthesis-report_e.pdf

Careau, E., Vincent, C., & Swaine, B. R. (2011). Consensus group session of experts to describe interprofessional collaboration processes in team meetings. *Journal of Interprofessional Care*, 25(4), 299–301. doi:10.3109/13561820.2011.566649

Cassel, C., Hackl, P., & Westlund, A. H. (1999). Robustness of Partial Least-Squares Method for Estimating Latent Variable Quality Structures. *Journal of Applied Statistics*, *26*(4), 435–446. doi:10.1080/02664769922322

Cheney, G. (2011). *Organizational communication in an age of globalization: Issues, reflections, practices*. Long Grove, IL: Waveland Press.

Chin, W. W. (1998). The Partial Least Squares Approach to Structural Equation Modeling. In G. A. Marcoulides (Ed.), *Modern Methods for Business Research* (pp. 1295–1336). Mahwah, NJ: Lawrence Erlbaum Associates.

Chin, W. W., Marcolin, B. L., & Newsted, P. R. (2003). A partial least squares latent variable modeling approach for measuring interaction effects: Results from a Monte Carlo simulation study and voice mail emotion/adoption study. *Information Systems Research*, *14*(2), 189–217. doi:10.1287/isre.14.2.189.16018

Cramton, C. (2001). The mutual knowledge problem and its consequences for dispersed collaborations. *Organization Science*, *12*(3), 346–371. doi:10.1287/orsc.12.3.346.10098

Culnan, M. J., & Bies, J. R. (2003). Consumer privacy: Balancing economic and justice considerations. *The Journal of Social Issues*, *59*(2), 323–342. doi:10.1111/1540-4560.00067

Cummings, J., & Ghosh, T. (2005). Teams as Networks in a Connected Organization: The Critical Role of Geographic Distance. *Proceedings of the Academy of Management Conference*, Honolulu.

D'Amour, D. (1997). Structuration de la collaboration interprofessionnelle dans les services de santé de première ligne au Québec. These de doctorat. Montreal: Université de Montréal.

D'Amour, D., Ferrada-Videla, M., Rodriguez, L. S. M., & Beaulieu, M. D. (2005). The conceptual basis for interprofessional collaboration: Core concepts and theoretical frameworks. *Journal of Interprofessional Care*, 19(S1), 116 – 131. doi:10.1080/13561820500082529

DAmour, D., Sicotte, C., & Levy, R. (1999). Laction collective au sein dequipes interprofessionnelles dans les services de santé. *Sciences Sociales et Sante*, *17*(3), 68–94. doi:10.3406/sosan.1999.1468

Daneci-Patrau, D. (2011). Formal communication in organisationfalse. *Economics. Management and Financial Markets*, 6(1) 487–497.

Danermark, B., & Kullberg, C. (1999). *Samverkan: välfärdsstatens nya arbetsform* [Collaboration: The new working methods of the welfare state]. Lund: Studentlitteratur. [in Swedish]

Davies, H. (1994). Falling public trust in health services: Implications for accountability. *Journal of Health Services and Policy Research, 4*(4), 193–194. doi:10.1177/135581969900400401 PMID:10623032

Davies, C. (1996). The sociology of professions and the sociology of gender. *Sociology, 30*(4), 661–678. doi:10.1177/0038038596030004003

Doherty, W. J. (1995). The whys and the levels of collaboration. *Family Systems Medicine, 13*(3), 275–281. doi:10.1037/h0089174

Duranti, C. M., & de Almeida, F. C. (2012). Is More Technology Better for Communication in International Virtual Teams? *International Journal of e-Collaboration, 8*(1), 36–52. doi:10.4018/jec.2012010103

Fornell, C., & Larcker, D. F. (1981). Evaluating structural equation models with unobservable variables and measurement error. *JMR, Journal of Marketing Research, 18*(1), 39–50. doi:10.2307/3151312

Fornell, C. (1987). A Second Generation of Multivariate Analysis: Classification of Methods and Implications for Marketing Research. In M. J. Houston (Ed.), *Review of Marketing* (pp. 1407–1450). Chicago: American Marketing Association.

Fox, S. (2011). The social life of health information, 2011. In *Pew Internet & American Life Project*. Retrieved from http://pewinternet.org/Reports/2011/Social-Life-of-Health-Info.aspx

Franchi, E., Poggi, A., & Tomaiuolo, M. (2013). Open Social Networking for Online Collaboration. *International Journal of e-Collaboration, 9*(3), 50–68. doi:10.4018/jec.2013070104

Gaboury, I., Bujold, M., Boon, H., & Moher, D. (2009). Interprofessional collaboration within Canadian integrative healthcare clinics: Key components. *Social Science & Medicine, 69*(5), 707–715. doi:10.1016/j.socscimed.2009.05.048 PMID:19608320

Gambetta, D. (2000). Can we trust trust? In D. Gambetta (Ed.), Trust: Making and breaking cooperative relations (pp. 213–237). Electronic edition, Department of Sociology, University of Oxford. Retrieved from http://www.sociology.ox.ac.uk/papers/gambetta213-237.pdf

Gatignon, H., & Jean-Marc, X. (1997). Strategic orientation of the firm and new product performance. *JMR, Journal of Marketing Research, 34*(2), 77–90. doi:10.2307/3152066

Gilson, L. (2003). Trust and the development of health care as a social institution. *Social Science & Medicine, 56*(7), 1453–1468. doi:10.1016/S0277-9536(02)00142-9 PMID:12614697

Gliner, J. A., & Morgan, G. A. (2000). *Research Methods in Applied Settings: An Integrated Approach to Design and Analysis*. Lawrence Erlbaum Associates Publishers.

Global Alliance for ICT and Development (GAID). (2010). Information and communication technologies for development: Health (White Paper). Retrieved from http://www.scribd.com/doc/35120854/GAID-White-Paper-on-ICT4D-Health

Gocan, S., Laplante, M. A., & Woodend, A. K. (2014). Interprofessional collaboration in ontario's family health teams: A review of the literature. *Journal of Research in Interprofessional Practice and Education., 3*(3), 1–19.

Goold, S. (1998). Money and trust: Relationships between patients, physicians, and health plans. *Journal of Health Politics, Policy and Law, 23*(5), 688–695. PMID:9718519

Gulzar, L., & Henry, B. (2005). Interorganizational collaboration for health care between nongovernmental organizations (NGOs) in Pakistan. *Social Science & Medicine, 61*(9), 1930–1943. doi:10.1016/j.socscimed.2005.03.045 PMID:15935537

Haeuser, J. L., & Preston, P. (2005). Communication strategies for getting the results you want. *Healthcare Executive, 20*(1), 16–22. PMID:15656222

Hall, M. A., Camacho, F., Dugan, E., & Balkrishnan, R. (2002). Trust in the medical profession: Conceptual and measurement issues. *Health Services Research, 37*(5), 1419–1439. doi:10.1111/1475-6773.01070 PMID:12479504

Hall, P. (2005). Interprofessional teamwork: Professional cultures as barriers. *Journal of Interprofessional Care, 19*(1), 188–196. doi:10.1080/13561820500081745 PMID:16096155

Hair, J. F., Black, W. C., Babin, B. J., Anderson, R. E., & Tatham, R. L. (2006). *Multivariate Data Analysis* (6th ed.). Upper Saddle River, New Jersey: Prentice Hall.

Hanson, C. M., Carr, D. B., & Spross, J. A. (2000). Collaboration. In A. B. Hamric, J. A. Spross, & C. M. Hanson (Eds.), *Advanced nursing practice. An integrative approach* (2nd ed., pp. 315–347). Philadelphia: W. B. Saunders.

Hansen, H. E., Biros, M. H., Delaney, N. M., & Schug, V. L. (1999). Research utilization and interdisciplinary collaboration in emergency care. *Academic Emergency Medicine, 6*(4), 271–279. doi:10.1111/j.1553-2712.1999.tb00388.x PMID:10230977

Haynes, S. N., Richard, D. C. S., & Kubany, E. S. (1995). Content validity in psychological assessment: A functional approach to concepts and methods. *Psychological Assessment, 8*(3), 238–247. doi:10.1037/1040-3590.7.3.238

Humphrey, T. (2001). The increasing impact of eHealth on physician behavior. *Health Care News, 1*(31).

Heinemann, G. D., & Zeiss, A. M. (Eds.). (2002). *Team performance in health care.* New York: Kluwer Academic Publishers. doi:10.1007/978-1-4615-0581-5

Henault, R. G., & Eugenio, K. R., Kelliher, A. F., Alexis, G., & Conlin, P. R. (2002). Transmitting clinical recommendations for diabetes care via e-mail. *American Journal of Health-System Pharmacy, 59*(2), 2166–2169. PMID:12455299

Henneman, E. A. (1995). Nurse-physician collaboration: A poststructuralist view. *Journal of Advanced Nursing, 22*(2), 359–363. doi:10.1046/j.1365-2648.1995.22020359.x PMID:7593958

Henneman, E. A., Lee, J. L., & Cohen, J. I. (1995). Collaboration: A concept analysis. *Journal of Advanced Nursing, 21*(1), 103–109. doi:10.1046/j.1365-2648.1995.21010103.x PMID:7897060

Hinds, P., & Kiesler, S. (2002). *Distributed Work.* Cambridge, MA: MIT Press.

Hojat, M., Nasca, T. J., Cohen, M., Fields, S. K., Rattner, S. L., Griffiths, M., & Garcia, A. et al. (2001). Attitudes toward physician-nurse collaboration: A cross-cultural study of male and female physicians and nurses in the United States and Mexico. *Nursing Research*, *50*(1), 123–128. doi:10.1097/00006199-200103000-00008 PMID:11302292

Hosmer, L. T. (1995). Trust: The connecting link between organizational theory and philosophical ethics. *Academy of Management Review*, *20*(2), 379–403.

Hudson, B. (2002). Interprofessionality in health and social care: The Achilles heel of partnership? *Journal of Interprofessional Care*, *16*(1), 7–17. doi:10.1080/13561820220104122 PMID:11915720

Igbaria, M., Guimaraes, T., & Davis, G. (1995). Testing the determinants of microcomputer usage via a structural equation model. *Journal of Management Information Systems*, *11*(4), 87–114. doi:10.1080/07421222.1995.11518061

*info*Dev. (2006). ICT in Health: The Role of ICTs in the Health Sector in Developing Countries (InfoDev Activity File #1254). Retrieved from: http://www.infodev.org/en/Project.38.html

Jacobsen, D. I. (1999). Trust in political administrative relations: The case of local authorities in Norway and Tanzania. *World Development*, *27*(5), 839–853. doi:10.1016/S0305-750X(99)00032-7

Joint Commission on Accreditation of Healthcare Organizations. (*2006*). *Critical Access Hospital and Hospital National Patient Safety Goals*. Retrieved from http://www.jcaho.org/accredited+organizations/patient+safety/06_npsg/06_npsg_cah_hap.htm

Kahn, W. A. (1990). psychological conditions of personal engagement and disengagement at work. *Academy of Management Journal*, *33*(4), 692–724. doi:10.2307/256287

Kaplan, A., & Haenlein, M. (2010). Users of the world, unite! The challenges and opportunities of social media. *Business Horizons*, *53*(1), 59–68. doi:10.1016/j.bushor.2009.09.003

Keyton, J. (2011). *Communication and organizational culture: A key to understanding work experience*. Thousand Oaks, CA: Sage.

Khan, M. T. (2014). Relationship Marketing - Some Aspects (Review). International Journal of Information. *Business and Management*, *6*(2), 108–122.

Kietzmann, J. H., Hermkens, K., McCarthy, I. P., & Silvestre, B. S. (2011). Social media? Get serious! Understanding the functional building blocks of social media. *Business Horizons*, *54*(4), 241–251. doi:10.1016/j.bushor.2011.01.005

Kline, R. B. (1998). *Principles and Practice of Structural Equation Modeling*. New York, NY: The Guilford Press.

Kittler, A. F., Carlson, B. A., & Harris, C. (2004). Primary care physician attitudes towards using a secure web based portal designed to facilitate electronic communication with patients. *Informatics in Primary Care*, *12*(2), 129–138. PMID:15606985

Kock, N. (2015). Common method bias in PLS-SEM: A full collinearity assessment approach. *International Journal of e-Collaboration*, *11*(4), 1–10. doi:10.4018/ijec.2015100101

Kock, N., & Lynn, G. S. (2012). Lateral collinearity and misleading results in variance-based SEM: An illustration and recommendations. *Journal of the Association for Information Systems, 13*(7), 546–580.

Kraut, R. E., Fussell, S. R., Brennan, S. E., & Siegel, J. (2002). Understanding Effects of Proximity on Collaboration: Implications for Technologies to Support Remote Collaborative Work. In P. Hinds & S. Kiesler (Eds.), *Distributed Work* (pp. 139–162). Cambridge, MA: MIT Press.

Kripalani, S., LeFevre, F., Phillips, C. O., Williams, M. V., Basaviah, P., & Baker, D. (2007). Deficits in Communication and Information Transfer Between Hospital-Based and Primary Care Physicians Implications for Patient Safety and Continuity of Care Coordination. *Journal of the American Medical Association, 297*(8), 831–841. doi:10.1001/jama.297.8.831 PMID:17327525

Krogstad, U., Hofoss, D., & Hjortdahl, P. (2004). Doctor and nurse perception of inter-professional co-operation in hospitals. *International Journal for Quality in Health Care, 16*(6), 491–497. doi:10.1093/intqhc/mzh082 PMID:15557359

Lambert, D. M., & Harrington, T. C. (1990). Measuring Nonresponse Bias in Mail Surveys. *Journal of Business Logistics, 11*(1), 5–25.

Lee, O. F., & Meuter, M. L. (2010). The adoption of technology orientation in healthcare delivery: Case study of a large-scale hospital and healthcare systems electronic health record. *International Journal of Pharmaceutical and Healthcare Marketing, 4*(4), 355–374. doi:10.1108/17506121011095209

Lemieux-Charles, L., & McGuire, W. (2006). What do we know about heath care team effectiveness? A review of the literature. *Medical Care Research and Review, 63*(3), 263–300. doi:10.1177/1077558706287003 PMID:16651394

Leonhardt, P. (2006, April 19). *Political clout in the age of out sourcing. The New York Times.*

Liederman, E. M., Lee, J. C., Baquero, V. H., & Seites, P. G. (2005). Patient-physician web messaging: The impact on message volume and satisfaction. *Journal of General Internal Medicine, 20*(1), 52–57. doi:10.1111/j.1525-1497.2005.40009.x PMID:15693928

Lindell, M. K., & Whitney, D. J. (2001). Accounting for Common Method Variance in Cross-Sectional Research Designs. *The Journal of Applied Psychology, 86*(1), 114–121. doi:10.1037/0021-9010.86.1.114 PMID:11302223

Lindeke, L. L., & Block, D. E. (1998). Maintaining professional integrity in the midst of interdisciplinary collaboration. *Nursing Outlook, 46*(5), 213–218. doi:10.1016/S0029-6554(98)90052-5 PMID:9805340

Lingard, L., Regehr, G., Orser, B., Reznick, R., Baker, G. R., Doran, D., & Whyte, S. et al. (2008). Evaluation of a preoperative checklist and team briefing among surgeons, nurses, and anesthesiologists to reduce failures in communication. *Archives of Surgery (Chicago, Ill.), 143*(1), 12–17. doi:10.1001/archsurg.2007.21 PMID:18209148

Lingard, L., Reznick, R., Espin, S., Regehr, G., & DeVito, I. (2002). Team communications in the operating room: Talk patterns, sites of tension, and implications for novices. *Academic Medicine, 77*(3), 232–237. doi:10.1097/00001888-200203000-00013 PMID:11891163

Lingard, L., Whyte, S., Espin, S., Baker, G. R., Orser, B., & Doran, D. (2006). Towards safer interprofessional communication: Constructing a model of utility from preoperative team briefings. *Journal of Interprofessional Care, 20*(5), 471–483. doi:10.1080/13561820600921865 PMID:17000473

Luhmann, N. (2000). Familiarity, confidence, trust: Problems and alternatives. In D. Gambetta, (Ed.), Trust: making and breaking cooperative relations (Elec. ed., pp. 94–107). Department of Sociology, University of Oxford, Retrieved from http://www.sociology.ox.ac.uk/papers/luhmann94-107.pdf

Lynn, M. R. (1986). Determination and Quantification of Content Validity. *Nursing Research, 35*(4), 382–385. PMID:3640358

Lyngstad, M., Melby, L., Grimsmo, A., & Hellesø, R. (2013). Toward Increased Patient Safety? Electronic Communication of Medication Information Between Nurses in Home Health Care and General Practitioners. *Home Health Care Management & Practice, 25*(5), 203–211. doi:10.1177/1084822313480365

Mann, M. Y., Lloyd-Puryear, M. A., & Lizer, D. (2006). Enhancing communication in the 21st Century. *Pediatrics, 117*(4 Suppl. 3), 315–319. doi:10.1542/peds.2005-2633K PMID:16735258

Manaikkamakl, P. (2007). Personal technology orientation in R&D: A tool to intensify organizational learning. *Development and Learning in Organizations, 21*(6), 18–20.

Mayer, R. C., Davis, J. H., & Schoorman, F. D. (1995). An Integrative Model of Organization Trust.'. *Academy of Management Review, 20*(3), 709–733.

Mckinney, E. H., Barker, J. R., Davis, K. J., & Smith, D. (2005). How swift starting action teams get off the ground. *Management Communication Quarterly, 19*(2), 198–237. doi:10.1177/0893318905278539

Mechanic, D. (1996). Changing medical organization and the erosion of trust. *The Milbank Quarterly, 74*(2), 171–189. doi:10.2307/3350245 PMID:8632733

Mechanic, D. (1998). Trust in the provision of medical care. *Journal of Health Politics, Policy and Law, 23*(411), 661–686. doi:10.1215/03616878-23-4-661 PMID:9718518

Mechanic, D., & Meyer, S. (2000). Concepts of trust among patients with serious illness. *Social Science & Medicine, 51*(5), 657–668. doi:10.1016/S0277-9536(00)00014-9 PMID:10975226

Merriam-Webster OnLine Dictionary. (n. d.). Communication. Retrieved from http://www.merriamwebster.com/dictionary/communication

Meyer, M. W. (1985). *Limits to bureaucratic growth.* New York: De Gruyter. doi:10.1515/9783110865295

Miller, K. (2005). *Communication theories: Perspectives, processes, and contexts* (2nd ed.). New York: McGraw-Hill.

Misztal, B. A. (1996). *Trust in modern societies: The search for the bases of moral order.* Cambridge: Polity Press.

Mohammed, S., Ferzandi, L., & Hamilton, K. (2010). Metaphor no more: A 15-year review of the team mental model construct. *Journal of Management, 36*(4), 876–910. doi:10.1177/0149206309356804

Molleman, E., Broekhuis, M., Stoffels, R., & Jaspers, F. (2008). How health care complexity leads to cooperation and affects the autonomy of health care professionals. Health Care Analysis. An. *International Journal of Health Care Philosophy and Policy, 16*(4), 329–341. doi:10.1007/s10728-007-0080-6

Moqbel, M., Nevo, S., & Kock, N. (2013). Organizational members use of social networking sites and job performance. *Information Technology & People, 26*(3), 240–264. doi:10.1108/ITP-10-2012-0110

Nardi, B. A., & Whittaker, S. (2002). The Place of Face-to-Face Communication in Distributed Work. In P. Hinds & S. Kiesler (Eds.), *Distributed Work* (pp. 83–110). Cambridge, MA: MIT Press.

Newman, J. (1998). The dynamics of trust. In A. Coulson (Ed.), *Trust and contracts: Relationships in local government, health and public services*. Bristol: The Polity Press.

Nunnally, J. C., & Bernstein, I. H. (1994). *Psychometric Theory* (3rd ed.). New York: McGraw-Hill.

Nunnaly, J. (1978). *Psychometric Theory*. New York, NY: McGraw Hill.

Open Clinical. (2011). Open Clinical: Knowledge Management for Medical Care. Retrieved from http://www.openclinical.org/e-Health.html#applications

Palanisamy, R., & Verville, J. (2015). Factors enabling communication based collaboration in interprofessional healthcare practice: A case study. *International Journal of e-Collaboration, 11*(2), 8–27. doi:10.4018/ijec.2015040102

Papanikolaou, K. A., & Gouli, E. (2013). Investigating Influences among individuals and groups in a collaborative learning setting. *International Journal of e-Collaboration, 9*(1), 9–25. doi:10.4018/jec.2013010102

Pearce, W. B. (2003). *The coordinated management of meaning (CMM): Theorizing about communication and culture*. Thousand Oaks, CA: Sage.

Perry, H., Robison, N., Chavez, D., Taja, O. O., Hilari, C., Shanklin, D., & Wyon, J. (1999). Attaining health for all through community partnership: Principles of the census based, impact-oriented (CBIO) approach to primary health care developed in Bolivia, South America. *Social Science & Medicine, 48*(8), 1053–1068. doi:10.1016/S0277-9536(98)00406-7 PMID:10390044

Podsakoff, P. M., MacKenzie, S. B., Lee, J. Y., & Podsakoff, N. P. (2003). Common Method Biases in Behavioral Research: A Critical Review of the Literature and Recommended Remedies. *The Journal of Applied Psychology, 88*(5), 879–903. doi:10.1037/0021-9010.88.5.879 PMID:14516251

Podsakoff, P. M., & Organ, D. W. (1986). Self-reports in Organizational Research: Problems and Prospects. *Journal of Management, 12*(4), 531–544. doi:10.1177/014920638601200408

Polit, D. F., & Beck, C. T. (2004). *Nursing Research: Principles and Methods* (7th ed.). Philadelphia: Lippincott, Williams, & Wilkins.

Polit, D. F., & Beck, C. T. (2006). The Content Validity Index: Are You Sure You Know Whats Being Reported? Critique and Recommendations. *Research in Nursing & Health, 29*(6), 489–497. doi:10.1002/nur.20147 PMID:16977646

Rice, R. E., & Gattiker, U. E. (2001). New Media and Organizational Structuring. In F. M. Jablin & L. L. Putnam (Eds.), *The New Handbook of Organizational Communication* (pp. 544–584). Thousand Oaks, CA: Sage Publications. doi:10.4135/9781412986243.n14

Rodriguez, L. S., Beaulieu, M., DAmour, D., & Ferrada-Videla, M. (2005). The determinants of successful collaboration: A review of theoretical and empirical studies. *Journal of Interprofessional Care*, *19*(1), 132–147. doi:10.1080/13561820500082677 PMID:16096151

Rogelberg, S. G., & Stanton, J. M. (2007). Understanding and dealing with organizational survey non-response. *Organizational Research Methods*, *10*(2), 195–209. doi:10.1177/1094428106294693

Rubio, D. M., Berg-Weger, M., Tebb, S. S., Lee, E. S., & Rauch, S. (2003). Objectifying Content Validity: Conducting a Content Validity Study in Social Work Research. *Social Work Research*, *27*(2), 94–104. doi:10.1093/swr/27.2.94

Safran, D. G. (2003). Defining the future of primary care: What can we learn from patients? *Annals of Internal Medicine*, *138*(3), 248–255. doi:10.7326/0003-4819-138-3-200302040-00033 PMID:12558375

Safran, C., Jones, P., Rind, D., Bush, B., Cytryn, K., & Patel, V. (2004). Electronic communication and collaboration in a health care practice. *Artificial Intelligence in Medicine*, *12*(2), 137–151. PMID:9520221

Schofield, R. F., & Amodeo, M. (1999). Interdisciplinary teams in health care and human services settings: Are they effective? *Health & Social Work*, *24*(3), 210–219. doi:10.1093/hsw/24.3.210 PMID:10505282

Senate Finance Committee. (2009). Transforming the health care delivery system: proposals to improve patient care and reduce health care costs. Retrieved August, 2, 2016 from http://finance.senate.gov/sitepages/leg/LEG%202009/042809%20Health%20Care%20Description%20of%20Policy%20Option.pdf

Sharma, G., Qiang, Y., Wenjun, S., & Qi, L. (2013). Communication in virtual world: Second life and business opportunities. *Information Systems Frontiers*, *15*(7), 677–694. Doi:10.1007/s10796-012-9347-z

Shortell, S. M., Zimmerman, J. E., Rousseau, D. M., Gillies, R. R., Wagner, D. P., Draper, E. A., & Duffy, J. et al. (1994). The performance of intensive care units: Does good management make a difference? *Medical Care*, *32*(5), 508–525. doi:10.1097/00005650-199405000-00009 PMID:8182978

Sicotte, C., DAmour, D., & Moreault, M. (2002). Interdisciplinary collaboration within Quebec community health care centers. *Social Science & Medicine*, *55*(6), 991–1003. doi:10.1016/S0277-9536(01)00232-5 PMID:12220099

Siegler, E. L., & Whitney, F. W. (1994). *Nurse-Physician collaboration. Care of adults and the elderly.* New York: Stringer Publishing Company.

Silen-Lipponen, M., Turunen, H., & Tossavainen, K. (2002). Collaboration in the operating room: The nurses perspective. *The Journal of Nursing Administration*, *32*(1), 16–19. doi:10.1097/00005110-200201000-00006 PMID:11802633

Smith, M., Greene, B. R., & Meeker, W. (2002). The CAM movement and the integration of quality health care: The case of chiropractic. *The Journal of Ambulatory Care Management*, *25*(2), 1–16. doi:10.1097/00004479-200204000-00003 PMID:11995192

Sproull, L., & Kiesler, S. (1986). Reducing social context cues: Electronic mail in organizational communication. *Management Science, 32*(11), 1492–1512. doi:10.1287/mnsc.32.11.1492

Srinivasan, A. (1985). Alternative measures of system effectiveness: Associations and implications. *Management Information Systems Quarterly, 9*(3), 243–253. doi:10.2307/248951

Starfield, B. (1998). *Primary care: Balancing Health Needs, Services, and Technology*. New York: Oxford University Press.

Stein, L. I., Watts, D. T., & Howell, T. (1990). The doctor-nurse game revisited. *The New England Journal of Medicine, 322*(6), 536–549. PMID:2300124

Stichler, J. F. (1995). Professional interdependence: The art of collaboration. *Advanced Practice Nursing Quarterly, 1*(1), 53–61. PMID:9447005

Stille, C. J., Jerant, A., Bell, D., Meltzer, D., & Elmore, J. G. (2005). Coordinating Care across Diseases, Settings, and.: A Key Role for the Generalist in Practice. *Annals of Internal Medicine, 142*(7), 700–708. doi:10.7326/0003-4819-142-8-200504190-00038 PMID:15838089

Suter, E., Arndt, J., Arthur, N., Parboosingh, J., Taylor, E., & Deutschlander, S. (2009). Role understanding and effective communication as core competencies for collaborative practice. *Journal of Interprofessional Care, 23*(1), 41–51. doi:10.1080/13561820802338579 PMID:19142782

Teigland, R., & Wasko, M. (2003). Integrating Knowledge through Information Trading: Examining the Relationship between Boundary Spanning Communication and Individual Performance. *Decision Sciences, 34*(2), 261–286. doi:10.1111/1540-5915.02341

Terry, M. (2008). Text messaging in healthcare: The elephant knocking at the door. *Telemedicine Journal and e-Health, 14*(5), 520–524. doi:10.1089/tmj.2008.8495 PMID:18729749

Thomas, E. J., Sherwood, G. D., Mulhollem, J. L., Sexton, J. B., & Helmreich, R. L. (2004). Working together in the neonatal intensive care unit: Provider perspective. *Journal of Perinatology, 24*(9), 552–559. doi:10.1038/sj.jp.7211136 PMID:15141266

Tidwell, L. C., & Walther, J. B. (2002). Computer-Mediated Communication Effects on Disclosure, Impressions, and Interpersonal Evaluations. *Human Communication Research, 28*(3), 317–348. doi:10.1111/j.1468-2958.2002.tb00811.x

Tyler, T. R., & Kramer, R. M. (1996). Whither trust? In R. M. Kramer & T. R. Tyler (Eds.), *Trust in organizations: Frontiers of theory and research*. Thousand Oaks, CA: Sage. doi:10.4135/9781452243610.n1

Urbach, N., & Ahlemann, F. (2010). Structural Equation Modeling in Information Systems Research Using Partial Least Squares. *Journal of Information Technology Theory and Application, 11*(2), 5–40.

Vazirani, S., Hays, R. D., Shapiro, M. F., & Cowan, M. (2005). Effect of a multidisciplinary intervention on communication and collaboration among physicians and nurses. *American Journal of Critical Care, 14*(1), 71–77. PMID:15608112

Veenstra, G., & Lomas, J. (1999). Home is where the governing is: Social capital and regional health governance. *Health & Place, 5*(1), 1–2. doi:10.1016/S1353-8292(98)00037-9 PMID:10670986

Verschuren, P. J., & Masselink, H. (1997). Role concepts and expectations of physicians and nurses in hospitals. *Social Science & Medicine, 45*(6), 1135–1138. doi:10.1016/S0277-9536(97)00043-9 PMID:9257405

Wagner, E. H. (2004). Effective teamwork and quality of care. *Medical Care, 42*(11), 1037–1039. doi:10.1097/01.mlr.0000145875.60036.ed PMID:15586829

Walsh, C., Gordon, F., Marshall, M., & Hunt, T. (2005). Interprofessional capability: A developing framework for interprofessional education. *Nurse Education in Practice, 5*(4), 230–237. doi:10.1016/j.nepr.2004.12.004 PMID:19038204

Waskett, C. (1996). Multidisciplinary teamwork in primary care: The role of the counsellor. *Counselling Psychology Quarterly, 9*(4), 243–260. doi:10.1080/09515079608258706

Way, D., Jones, L., & Busing, N. (2000). *Implementation strategies: Collaboration in primary care. (Discussion paper).* Ottawa, ON: Ontario College of Family Physicians.

Weaver, B., Lindsay, B., & Gitelman, B. (2012). Communication technology and social media: opportunities and implications for healthcare systems. *OJIN: The Online Journal of Issues in Nursing, 17*(3), 17-24. *Manuscript, 3.* doi:10.3912/OJIN.Vol17No03Man03

Welton, W. E., Kantner, T. A., & Moriber, K. S. (1997). Developing Tomorrows Integrated Community Health Systems: A leadership challenge for public health and primary care. *The Milbank Quarterly, 75*(2), 261–288. doi:10.1111/1468-0009.00054 PMID:9184684

Williams, A. L., Lasky, R. E., Dannemiller, J. L., Andrei, A. M., & Thomas, E. J. (2010). Teamwork behaviours and errors during neonatal resuscitation. *Quality & Safety in Health Care, 19*(1), 60–64. doi:10.1136/qshc.2007.025320 PMID:20172885

Woods, J. A., Jackson, D. J., Ziglar, S., & Alston, G. L. (2011). Interprofessional communication. *Drug Topics, 155*(8), 42–53.

Ye, J. (2006). Deliberate Learning in The Frontlines of Service Organizations [Ph.D. Dissertation]. Department of Marketing and Policy Studies, Case Western Reserve University.

Zwarenstein, M., Reeves, S., & Perrier, L. (2004). Effectiveness of pre-licensure interdisciplinary education and post-licensure interprofessional collaboration interventions. In I. Oandasan, *D. D'Amour, M. Zwarenstein et al.* (Eds.), *Interdisciplinary education for collaborative patient-centred practice* (pp. 38–50). Toronto: Health Canada.

This research was previously published in the International Journal of e-Collaboration (IJeC), 13(2); edited by Ned Kock, pages 10-44, copyright year 2017 by IGI Publishing (an imprint of IGI Global).

Chapter 68
E–Healthcare Disparities Across Cultures:
Infrastructure, Readiness and the Digital Divide

Seema Biswas
Ben Gurion University of the Negev, Israel

Keren Mazuz
Ben Gurion University of the Negev, Israel

Rui Amaral Mendes
Case Western Reserve University, USA

ABSTRACT

As e-healthcare becomes a reality for healthcare service provision across the world, challenges in acceptance, implementation, usage and effectiveness have begun to emerge. The infrastructure, readiness and literacy levels required for the effective delivery of e-healthcare services may be prohibitive in providing access to those most in need. As research brings to light the real effectiveness of e-healthcare programmes across the globe, this paper explores how e-healthcare has been implemented worldwide and how populations have been served by an innovation in Information Technology and healthcare that has sought to bring health services to remote areas, improve access to healthcare and narrow the divide between healthcare providers and patients. While notable achievements have seen real time clinical data captured and medical records digitalised, the very determinants responsible for actual health and social disparities are equally responsible for disparities is access to e-healthcare.

INTRODUCTION

We live in the digital age. There is an app for everything. Every aspect of our lives, from the phones glued to our hands to home-shopping networks, depends on the Internet; why, then, would the manner by which we access healthcare be any different? The potential benefits of applying every advance in telecommunications and online technology to healthcare are enormous. In hospital alone, electronic

DOI: 10.4018/978-1-5225-3926-1.ch068

patient records, radiological images and reports, blood results, endoscopy results and pathology results - even the images of the slides - may be retrieved at the click of a mouse. No clinician with the correct access to this data would want to go back to the days of manual searches for patient files and X-rays.

In community medicine the potential benefits are even more far reaching in terms of monitoring and managing chronic diseases, and reaching patients who live far from specialist services. Body sensors and monitoring devices worn by patients may convey real time data to distant health professionals for immediate analysis or to send automated reminders to patients to take their medication. They may even trigger alarms for emergency response, say, in remote homecare of the elderly or for patients with dementia, with monitors fitted to walking sticks, walking frames or even vital sign body sensors worn on their person. It is reassuring that as we prepare our health services for ageing populations across the world, help for someone who has fallen at home could be on its way in minutes (Center for Technology and Aging, 2009). Clearly, however, the scenarios described above are not applicable in every part of the world, or, indeed, in every part of every nation. This chapter gives examples of e-healthcare in action across the globe, and highlights disparities inherent in the resources necessary to both *provide* e-healthcare and in order to benefit from *access* to this. It is no accident that the determinants of e-healthcare are inexorably linked to the determinants of health itself.

DEFINITIONS

The World Health Organization, WHO, defines e-health as *the transfer of health resources and health care by electronic means*. They explain that e-health comprises three main areas:

- The delivery of health information, for health professionals and health consumers, through the Internet and telecommunications.
- Using the power of information technology and e-commerce to improve public health services, e.g. through the education and training of health workers.
- The use of e-commerce and e-business practices in health systems management. (WHO, 2015)

They describe telehealth as including *surveillance, health promotion and public health functions - a broader definition than telemedicine as it includes computer-assisted telecommunications to support management, surveillance, literature and access to medical knowledge. Telemedicine is the use of telecommunications to diagnose and treat disease and ill-health. Telematics for health is a WHO composite term for both telemedicine and telehealth, or any health-related activities carried out over distance by means of information communication technologies.*

LeRouge asserts that telemedicine is so integral to the development of healthcare services that it "serves as the vital connective tissue for expanding health care organization networks" (LeRouge, 2012). As Kalema (2014) and Ackerman (2010) put it, the opportunity in e-healthcare is to break down barriers to healthcare, improve access for all - especially those underserved by healthcare services - and enable medical personnel to better connect with their patients – especially those remote from healthcare services - in other words, to improve equity in healthcare and access to health care: to improve Global Health. The intention is to do this at a lower cost, while improving efficiency and effectiveness. The importance to both developed and developing world health services is, therefore, clear. The vision, in particular in the developing world, is to harness information technology towards meeting crucial public health needs.

Three priorities emerge from these descriptions: The administrative, educational and clinical applications of e-healthcare are intended from the outset to:

- improve healthcare both in terms of provision and access
- connect distant sites, and, therefore, improve rural access to healthcare
- improve health in both the developed and developing world

In order to implement e-healthcare, however, an infrastructure and health network does need to be in place. Even, telemedicine requires a remote Internet connection that can bridge the developed and developing world in terms of healthcare support.

ETHICAL AND LEGAL ISSUES: GENERAL CONSIDERATIONS AND THE EUROPEAN CASE

The application of information and communication technologies across the whole range of tasks involving the health care sector, e-health, is attracting a growing interest at the European level. In fact, associated with the fact that cross-border activities in health care in the European single market are increasing and many of these cross-border developments are related to e-Health, it has become clear that there is a rather evident need for an appropriate regulatory framework able to ensure its promotion in the European Union, under close scrutiny. The Treaty of the European Union (TFEU) (OJC115/47, 2008), expresses that Member States bear sole responsibility for their health policy and the provision of health care to their citizens.

In 2006, the European Commission identified some of the issues requiring clarification, calling for a Directive that could provide:

- "Minimum (practical) information and (legal) clarification requirements to enable cross-border health care."
- "Identification of competent authorities and related responsibilities in various fields (quality, safety, redress, compensation)."

The latter was regarded was one of the main aspects to be considered, since it would provide the necessary insight into how to address the current uncertainties between national systems, while reducing the uncertainty of the application of case-law principles.

These concerns gave rise to the Directive 2011/24/EU, which provided a greater legal certainty regarding rights and entitlements relating to care obtained in a Member State other than the patient's own Member State.

Other more recent Directives may also be regarded as further steps in this direction. The Data Protection Directive, the E-Commerce Directive, the Medical Device Directive and the Directive on Distance Contracting are some of the most important European legal documents that try to provide some adequate context to e-Health, despite the fact that these directives are not adopted especially for e-health applications.

The Data Protection Directive applies to personal data, which form part of a filing system and contains several important principles that have to be complied with by e-Health actors processing personal data concerning health. The E-commerce Directive, on the other hand, concerns services provided at a distance by electronic means, which clearly targets many of the e-Health applications which are known to fall within this scope. Moreover, the Medical Devices Directive is of importance for the e-Health sector, especially with regard to e.g. the medical software that is used in many e-health applications. Finally, the Directive on Distance Contracting may also be of application, considering that e-health business may actually involve the conclusion of contracts.

Nevertheless, there are still areas characterized by ambiguity. Whereas Directive 2011/24/EU was designed to clarify the rights of EU citizens in evaluating, accessing and obtaining reimbursement for cross-border care, it has yet left out some core qualms related to liability and data protection issues within cross-border health care. Overall, despite all these Directives, more developments are needed at the European level in order to make sure that e-health may play a more important role in health care systems, although placing the rights and the overall global interest of the "global patient" as a core issue.

New e-health applications (e.g. e-health platforms, electronic health records, health grids) and the enhancement of human tissue and genetic data use are a growing matter of concern, leading to new legal challenges.

Several member states are introducing electronic health records or e-health platforms. However, the use of electronic health records containing data of several health actors poses new ethical and deontological risks that may lead to legal consequences. For example, grids recently in use in some ambitious medical and healthcare applications must draw huge amounts of data from disparately located computers in order to be truly effective. Needless is to say that this implies data sharing across jurisdictions and the sharing of responsibilities by a range of different data controllers. Finally, more and clear guidelines on the reimbursement criteria for telemedicine and on liability are mandatory.

E-HEALTH READINESS

It is hard to imagine whether during the 1960's linking computers was seen as the means to link populations and deliver public services, but the success of the expansion of information and telecommunications networks has been to connect us all. Globalization would not have been possible without this. Where the infrastructure does exist, the last fifteen years has witnessed an explosion in telecommunications and the exponential growth of online applications for e-healthcare (Della Mea, 2001). Where infrastructure is lacking, e-healthcare is all the more crucial to support healthcare workers in their access to information as well as sharing of this information. The Russian Federation has used this as an opportunity to expand infrastructure into remote areas, connecting the vast expanse of the federation and preparing for medical emergencies (Eltchiyan 2004, Natenzon 2008). Considering the competing financial priorities in developing countries serving disadvantaged communities, improved healthcare at reduced cost of service delivery and utilization is key.

The WHO, in collaboration with the International Telecommunication Union, has produced the National eHealth Strategy Toolkit (NeHST, 2012) for "countries at every level of development, who seek to adapt and employ the latest information communication technologies in health for the measurable benefit of their citizens." The vision is for health promotion and awareness, medical education, research and e-learning; for disease surveillance, collection and storage of health data and statistics, management of health care service provision and delivery systems; and, finally, the delivery of health care itself: consultation, diagnosis, the analysis of investigations, monitoring of treatment and electronic patient records.

Regardless of the potential benefits, barriers to the implementation of e-healthcare may be considerable, especially in developing countries (Khoja, 2008, Khoja, 2013, Sood, 2004, Li, 2013, Rezai-Rad, 2012). Khoja, Li, and Rezai-Rad, amongst others, have all described the exhaustive infrastructural requirements necessary simply to meet information technology (IT) goals: the identification of suitable, affordable technology in healthcare institutions in developing countries; institutional preparedness to meet the costs of equipment, installation of IT equipment and training, IT support and maintenance; legal and regulatory frameworks for e-healthcare management and, crucially, the establishment of e-healthcare within the milieu of other online frameworks in government and public service (i.e. e-government, e-banking, e-commerce) (Rezai-Rad, 2012). Still larger barriers exist that limit function of the e-healthcare platform itself in country, let alone communication with centres of health expertise and referral outside the country. They include healthcare services themselves (Qureshi, 2012), lack of personnel, training, equipment and good management (Justice, 2012), not to mention the hardships of operating in undeveloped infrastructure, in general: no national electrical grid, no telephone service and no postal service.

Most medical data is still stored in paper form and files retrieved manually. This information is, therefore, inaccessible in terms of e-healthcare (Justice, 2012). Even where computerized data does exist, there may be separate datasets with no interface (Coleman, 2013). This makes e-healthcare difficult even for those medical personnel who do have IT training and some Internet connectivity. These problems are surprisingly common in countries with reasonable technology infrastructure such as South Africa, India and Mexico (Kimaro, 2007, Cline, 2013); how then is e-healthcare achievable in lower income countries?

E-health readiness describes the process by which countries may evaluate their infrastructures in preparation for the implementation of e-healthcare. The model, as shown below, is to assist healthcare decision makers and governments to make informed decisions on how to provide e-healthcare across the nation. Implicit in planning, is e-healthcare delivery to remote and rural areas.

Both in terms of infrastructure and organization, developing countries are still challenged by poor co-ordination of e-health integration, misalignment of the implementation processes, poor e-government and insufficient policies and frameworks to guide technology integration into public services (Odit, 2014, Taneja, 2007). Taneja identified appropriate and innovative government policies and health provider and consumer mind-sets as critical factors for a successful e-healthcare strategy in India – a change in culture and expectations.

Such challenges to support and implementation show the lack of preparedness that necessitates readiness assessment before planning e-healthcare provision (Digital Divide in Asia, 2005). There is some irony in the discovery that the same vulnerable populations who lack equal access to healthcare services, also lack access to the technology designed to mitigate their unmet health needs.

SPECTRUM OF E-HEALTHCARE APPLICATIONS ACROSS THE WORLD

Where e-healthcare can be implemented, chronic diseases like diabetes and asthma may be better monitored. The patients can do this themselves at home, with storage and retrieval of daily blood sugar and peak flow measurements, for example; but technology aside, success in long term health outcomes remains dependent on individual motivation to perform measurements regularly and comply with treatment. The shift in emphasis to healthcare access in the home rather than the consultation room, and personal responsibility in healthcare is, however, by no means complete. Potential applications to modify health behaviours and fundamentally affect the management of chronic disease have so far included the reduction in cardiovascular risk and promotion of healthy lifestyles, education and information about medical treatments, the reporting and monitoring of side effects, monitoring of blood pressure and optimization of treatment, optimization of statin therapy, support for adherence to medication, smoking cessation and nicotine replacement therapy, support and optimization of diet and weight, and monitoring of alcohol consumption (Thomas, 2014).

Diabetes management has seen a particular expansion in e-healthcare with efforts to mitigate individual variations in compliance with monitoring and treatment (Telehealth link, 2015). Accurate blood glucose monitors may be used to collect blood glucose levels regularly and at the patients' convenience, obviating the need for multiple tests (and, therefore, a less painful experience) with the aim to improve glycaemic control and prevent or delay complications. Insulin adjustments at home are made possible through automatic uploads of blood glucose results to e-health servers integrated into the glucose meters. Rapid analysis permits the display of results on secure webpages available to doctors, nurses and even family members so that doses of insulin may be adjusted and these adjustments recorded in real time. Compliance and glycaemic control are, therefore, indelibly charted.

With a burgeoning aged population worldwide, the increasing incidence of diabetes, hypertension and cardiac failure, and the rising costs of global healthcare delivery, the potential benefits of remote monitoring, consultation and treatment are easy to see and a tempting investment (Tamura, 2007). New applications for use have been trialed across the world as we discover what works, what is acceptable to the public and whether these modes of healthcare delivery are truly cost-effective. Innovations in homecare, even robots bathing the elderly in Japan, have shown how cameras in the home may circumvent the need for home nursing. The idea of cameras in the bathroom is not, however, acceptable to everyone, and the success of this technology in impacting the well-being of patients and the public at home is very much dependent on the involvement of patients in the design and implementation of the applications, as well as a respect for individual and cultural perceptions in the invasion of technology into their private lives and personal space.

E-healthcare in automated home dialysis (both peritoneal and haemodialysis) is an example of homecare that patients have found acceptable (Nakamoto, 2000). Since the first applications of e-healthcare in outpatient dialysis units (Mitchell, 1996), applications in the home via telephone, email and video cameras have enabled patients to communicate with healthcare personnel without leaving their homes. Patients far from specialist hospital renal units are able to attend satellite hospitals for occasional routine physical examination, blood tests and prescriptions but continue regular dialysis at home. In time, however, it is foreseeable that even these occasional hospital visits may be circumvented. Plans are already underway to expand applications for elderly patients undergoing home peritoneal dialysis who live alone or cannot attend the hospital by themselves, for patients with disabilities that preclude regular hospital visits and patients who live far from specialist renal units.

In terms of training, the sharing of information and telemedicine for medical advice and diagnosis, several successful programmes exist. The World Health Internetwork Access to Research Initiative (HINARI) provides free or low-cost access to online journals in developing countries (Kwakam, 2004). Online partnerships in medical education, including training for medical students, are increasing and changing all the time in terms of innovation and the breadth of interaction they afford (patient.co.uk, Meducation). Telemedicine connects medical centres in rural areas in the developed world or the developing world with centres of expertise at home or abroad. In many ways, a great equalizer, for areas with limited healthcare infrastructure, telemedicine enables remote diagnosis and advice in effective medical care and the urgent transfer of patients to referral centres when possible (American Telemedicine Association, Operation

Village Health). The basic requirements are Internet access and a digital camera. Connected Health is an organisation in Boston that runs Operation Village Health, providing telemedicine health services in two Cambodian villages using cameras, X-ray, ultrasound and electrocardiogram machines. Doctors in the United States provide free remote consultations for patients in Cambodia (Harvard College).

In Bangalore, India, virtual medical kiosks with phones and web cams allow patients to chat with medical professionals (Biospectrum, 2012). Patients may seek on-demand consultations at any time of the day via a touch screen system with audio-video capabilities, diagnostic equipment, a scanner and medical management software capable of recording personal health data to give a real-life experience. Bangalore has a tech-savvy population linked to e-commerce and IT. This is clearly a mitigating factor.

There are plans in India to help the government towards the implementation of the Universal Health Care programme (UHC) with the help of NGOs in remote places and applications for e-healthcare in India continue to grow as the Indian IT industry thrives. The Ministry of Health and Family Welfare has already prepared the white paper of the "e-health care service". The aim is to reach rural India. An information web portal is to be introduced by the government across rural India in order to raise awareness of which free health services are available. The success of this must surely lie in the existence of actual health services in rural areas and free universal health coverage. This is perhaps where disparities between virtual proposals and actual delivery of healthcare services arise.

PROBLEMS OF DELIVERY LEADING TO DISPARITIES

For those of us who do have reliable online access, computerizing medicine has not always met with success. In his column in the Boston Globe, Joseph B Martin (2007) alludes to the challenges that doctors face in making the most of technology designed to organize and simplify our work and easily retrieve stored information. Instead, however, doctors find themselves communicating with their desktop computers instead of the patient in front of them, tests take minutes to order on seemingly unnecessary complex software where writing on a paper order form was simply a matter of seconds, and little comment is made about the fact that diagnoses now have to fit computer codes rather that the reverse. Doctors are now coders...Heads of department ask for the technology to be removed and doctors seek employment in non-e-healthcare environments. Martin's solution is that doctors need more training in technology and writes that "these technologies let computers do what they do best – collect and disseminate data – while letting doctors do the doctoring". Clearly, there is a long way to go before the doctors can really be left to do the doctoring. Where does this leave doctors in the developing world, where the workload for healthcare workers is far greater?

While describing the obvious benefits of e-healthcare in Australia (increased access to healthcare services and health-related information, improved ability to diagnose and track diseases, timely public health information, and expanded access to ongoing medical education and training) Jolly's research paper for the Australian government (Jolly, 2011) details the difficulties of implementing e-healthcare and the unmet potential of e-healthcare within a relatively well-resourced healthcare service. In Australia and in the developing world, therefore, the problems of e-healthcare are centered on delivery. According to Ojo (2008), in many developing countries, the potential for e-healthcare to revolutionize healthcare and harness computer technology towards equality in healthcare and access for all to quality healthcare has been hindered by the fact that it is actually not possible to deliver e-healthcare across the country, especially to rural populations where the obstacles to delivering actual healthcare in terms of infrastructure are the same in terms of delivery of e-healthcare.

In rural areas, there may be very little development. Rural areas may be economically, politically and geographically disadvantaged, even cut off. Thirty nine million people in India have no access to healthcare – most of them live in the rural areas. How many of these people really stand to benefit from e-healthcare? The population of the African continent is approximately 800 million, but only 4 million people have access to e-mail, and of these, 2 million are based in South Africa. How many Africans, therefore, really stand to benefit for e-healthcare? In the rural areas where socio-economic status is lower, there is more poverty and unemployment, and the population inevitably depends on one state hospital with few trained medical personnel with little functioning equipment. Disadvantaged populations not only trek long distances to reach the state hospitals but also spend considerable time waiting in long queues to see any health officer that they can find. In these, environments where real health care services are not in existence, does telemedicine really reduce physical barriers to care?

Successful e-healthcare interventions need to take into account local geographical and social determinants of health rather than simply assuming that e-healthcare initiatives will address current disparities in health and be delivered and accessed optimally in all regions. Further, this geographical disparity in health is strongly associated with the prevalence of disease, social and economic disadvantage, poor literacy and little or no Internet access and technology skills. Of greatest concern is the possibility that existing health inequalities in socioeconomically disadvantaged areas may actually be exacerbated (not simply in terms of health information but also in terms of access to real healthcare) by inequitable distribution of Internet-based e-health interventions – available only to those who can afford to own or use computers (Han, 2010).

Research in e-healthcare inequalities must focus on identification and discussion of specific disparity issues across all applications of e-healthcare from basic literacy, computer literacy, the effects of poverty and lack of infra-structure and the mitigation of benefits in access to e-healthcare, while there remains a lack in access to actual healthcare. All populations, especially the most vulnerable, must be sampled for a truly accurate representation of disparities that should be addressed not only through critical revision of e-healthcare provision but through wider policies that improve the specific social determinants of health of vulnerable populations (Viswanath, 2007, Van Dijk 2006, Mphidi 2008).

DIGITAL DISPARITIES ACROSS THE GLOBE

Lack of investment in the poor and the underserved and a failure to build infrastructure contribute to disparities in access to healthcare. It was hoped that e-healthcare would go some way to bridging these disparities but the same core reasons are responsible for e-healthcare disparities. The *digital divide* describes disparities in Internet access and is discussed, especially for the developing world, in detail below, but even in the developed world, access to broadband services, though prices are falling, is dependent on local infra-structure and competition amongst different Internet Service Providers (ISPs). If there is no competition, there is no incentive for ISPs to drop the prices thus limiting affordable broadband access to those who live in areas where demand for these services is already high. Is it likely that the current telecommunication policies could leave rural areas, inner-city neighborhoods and the poor behind leading to an exacerbation of "digital divisions" (Visanath, 2007, Pew Research Center, 2013).

The American Library Association's (ALA) Office for Information Technology Policy defines the digital divide as the differences due to geography, race, economic status, gender and physical ability in access to information through the Internet, and other information technologies and services; and in the skills, knowledge, and abilities to use information, the Internet and other technologies (Lor, 2005). The Digital Divide Network (DiMaggio, 2004) defines the concept as the gap between those who have access to communication tools, such as the Internet and those who do not.

Limitations in access to online technology reflect limitations in access to a broader range of commodities in society. In Sub-Saharan Africa and India, for example, women have less access to the Internet than men (Mutula, 2001, Singh, 2004), but while the ALA's definition refers to disparities between groups and individuals within countries, the term "digital divide" refers more broadly to the disparities between societies and nations. This reflects the growing economic disparities between nations, as well as the growing disparity worldwide in access to healthcare in general (Marmot, 2008). The "digital divide", therefore, refers to the unequal and disproportionate pace of development in societies which do have access to a digital infrastructure and services and those which do not.

The overwhelming factors in India in the digital divide remain disparities in language and literacy. There are over 100 languages in India. For Indians who speak little or no English, the Internet, largely in English, is inaccessible. Indian dialects used online are usually the main northern dialects, thus disparity exists not simply between urban English speakers and the rural poor but also amongst different ethnicities within India. Disparities in literacy and education further confound this. According to the 2001 India population census male literacy was 76% while female literacy was as low as 54%. Disparities, remain, however, between urban and rural areas, and in terms of education, of the 23 million children who begin school every year only 15 million continue to secondary education. Only 2.3 million students pursue higher education every year (Agarwal, 2007). While the government has introduced information technology into the school syllabus, there is enormous variation in the standard of education across the country, especially in rural areas - the areas perhaps most in need of the links to healthcare that information technology is designed to provide.

Elsewhere in Asia, literacy, education and Internet access follow the indicators for economic success but disparities do remain. In Japan and South Korea poor Internet access is associated with low income, lack of fluency in English and female gender, while in Singapore, the digital divide mirrors income inequalities (Lim, 2003). In Australia, in 2011, only 59% of people in the lowest income bracket had Internet access (SMH, 2014).

In Turkey, 54% of the population between the ages of 16 and 74 are Internet users. Ninety two percent of the population have a mobile phone subscription. Women use the Internet less than men but the only 3% of the elderly use the Internet at all in Turkey. Sixty percent of households have Internet access – most of whom have a broadband connection. Most Internet use (71%) is within the home but up to 58% access the Internet on a mobile device or smart phone. Half of all Internet users access the government services via the Internet (Turkish Statistical Institute).

South Africa's digital divide is rooted in decades of disparity in access to education and infra-structure. As in India, South Africa is tasked with addressing widespread inequality is access to education and public services before initiatives to bridging the digital divide can really succeed. The challenges are daunting: inequalities in information technology infrastructure across the country (especially in the rural areas) must be addressed, the government is yet to really embrace e-technology and competing priorities on the budget for essential development across a range of public services remain (Mphidi, 2008, Nakamoto 2000). According to the Organization for Economic Co-operation and Development, the economically disadvantaged have the lowest level of access to e-governance (Kroukamp, 2005, Van Themat, 2004, Martin, 2005). Van Themat (2004) argues that although South Africa is ranked 65th in the world and first on the African continent as far as e-governance capacity is concerned, these statistics do not reflect the fact that areas disadvantaged in terms of infrastructure, especially in rural areas, have limited access to electricity and telephone lines and share more in common with the rest of the continent where only 7% of Africans are online (Guardian, 2012). While mobile phone use across Africa is widespread at 72%, this masks regional differences. Eritrea's mobile penetration rate, for example, is just 5%.The Internet's limited reach is compounded further because the language of the web is English and mobile connectivity is limited as only18% of Africa's mobiles are smartphones. In Liberia mobile penetration is 42% and over a third of the country illiterate.

In Mexico only 38% of the population use the Internet. A report by the Economic Commission on Latin America and the Caribbean found that while 60% of urban 15-year-olds in Mexico had access to a computer in 2009, only 20% of rural students had access. The Opportune Breast Cancer Screening and Diagnosis Program (2010) piloted in rural Mexico to send mammograms from rural areas to radiologists in cities via the Internet, reported equipment breakdown and prohibitively slow Internet connections as major impediments to the programme in spite of equipped, ready diagnostic centres capable of over 150 screenings daily. Only one third of the screening target was achieved as a result.

Chile leads South America with 61% Internet uses, while only 27% of the population of Paraguay has access to the Internet. In Honduras and El Salvador, Internet penetration is only 20% (Alvarez, 2014). Brazil launched a new programme to bring low-cost Internet service to 70% of the country's households by 2014, while Panama's government uses free Internet initiatives to get as many people as possible online (Swinhoe, 2012).

The disparities in the USA are according to education and income. Seventy five percent of households in the USA now have Internet access. Of the 25% without Internet, half claim that they simply do not want to use this and a quarter say that the costs are prohibitive (Badger, 2014).

In Russia, Internet use is mainly amongst people ages between 16 and 34 years. Use in Moscow is 2.4 times higher than elsewhere in Russia. In rural Russia Internet use is as low as 17%. Fifty three percent of Russian men use the Internet as opposed to only 34% of women (Russian Longitudinal Monitoring Survey) although more women work with computers. Barriers to use include level of education, language and age (ADOC, 2011). Improving Internet coverage across the Federation is seen as an essential process in the modernization of the nation. Initiatives include the government programme "Information Society 2011 - 2020". In 2010, however, only 43% of Russians reportedly used the Internet (InternetWorldStats, 2010). Russia is ranked 59th out of 70 in terms of digital economy rankings (digital infrastructure and the ability of consumers, commerce and government to use Internet Technology).

In the UK, in 2014, 76% of the population accessed the Internet every day. Access to mobile Internet increased from 24% to 58% between 2010 and 2014. Of those without Internet access, 39% are over the age of 65 – the 'grey divide' and 49% are in the lowest socio-economic groups. Seventy percent of those living in social housing are not online. In spite of this, 80% of all government interactions with the public take place with the poorest 25% of society – the assumption is that this interaction is not online. Digitally excluded households are missing out on £560 each year as a result of not shopping and paying bills online. 15% of people living in deprived areas have used a government online service (21st Century Challenges, 2010, Office of National Statistics, 2013, HM Gov, 2014).

THE DIGITAL DIVIDE IN LONDON: A CASE STUDY

Internet connectivity and the digital divide is much researched in the UK and invites much comment in national newspapers. Although London is one of the most affluent cities in the world, it has some of the UK's poorest communities. Half of the UK's ethnic minority population lives in London and over half of London's population is non-White British (London Census, 2011, Poverty UK, 2015). There are significant social divides according to affluence, literacy, employment and education, all of which contribute to the digital divide. Internet household connectivity in London remains higher than in any other region in the UK but the least connected boroughs in London in 2001 were Barking and Dagenham, Hackney and Islington, where less than a quarter of households were connected. The three most connected boroughs were Kingston upon Thames, Richmond upon Thames and the City of London.

Ethnic minority groups access and use Internet technology considerably less than white ethnic groups. Unemployment, poor literacy, low incomes, poor housing, high crime environments, bad health and family breakdown all contribute to the digital divide (Katz, 1997). Prohibitive costs remain a significant factor in accessing the Internet amongst households with lower levels of disposable income. Unemployment precludes Internet use at the work place. Manual workers have little or no access to the Internet at work. Long-term illness and disabilities are barriers to Internet adoption and use. Technologies are insufficiently adapted for the special needs of disabled or chronically ill individuals even though they have the capability to be adapted.

In an era where social interaction, information, business and social mobility are hugely dependent on the Internet, and the Internet may be used to access health and social services, it is in reviving communities through employment, the provision of public services and through targeting the social determinants of health that local government seeks to improve Internet connectivity. Low education and literacy levels compound computer literacy. Twelve percent of people aged less than 25 years state that they have no information technology skills and are, therefore, excluded from opportunities in education and employment, as well as health and social services easily accessed online.

Fifty percent of people aged over 50 in London claim to have no information technology skills. This potentially excludes them from health and public services available over the internet. Initiatives, therefore, target not simply literacy and access to the Internet, but information technology skills. The elderly affected by the grey divide cite a lack of interest, the perception that they are too old, the fear of new technology and fears about personal data security as reasons that they have not adopted the Internet (Foley, 2002). Bridging the digital divide, therefore, entails much more than the provision of affordable Internet access, efforts must include training in the use of the Internet, building confidence, reviving inner-city communities and the provision of health and public services through Internet technology that communities find acceptable, cost-effective and safe to use.

PORTUGAL CASE STUDY

A recent joint-venture between the Catholic University of Portugal and the Pharmaceutical Industry gave rise to the first Portuguese network aimed to provide timely information about oral healthcare (PSO, 2015).The Oral Health Platform is an innovative project developed with the scientific support of the Catholic University, and aims to be a simple and swift way to connect patients, dentists, clinics and pharmacies. Through this website potential users may not only easily find the nearest oral healthcare provider, but are further given the tools to access a specialized online consultation on a specific topic, in a practical and simplified form, via e-mail. Thus, this platform becomes a means of promoting oral health and providing credible scientific advice on oral hygiene, general information, advice and practical tips in the area of oral health for adults and children, while giving users several tips to help them identify and address several problems. Overall, in addition to providing an aggregate set of resources aimed to achieve a greater and better understanding of the various problems in the field of Oral Health, the platform also allows the development of clinical and scientific discussion forums, thereby promoting the sharing of knowledge.

CONCLUSION

The power of the Web is in its universality. Access by everyone regardless of disability is an essential aspect. (Tim Berners-Lee, Director and inventor of the World Wide Web)

The development of multifunctional e-healthcare platforms should be regarded as a way to offer attractive, up-to-date and easily accessible information and education, while serving not only those in higher education institutions (students, staff, researchers), but also healthcare providers (doctors, nurses), healthcare-related industries, and policy makers and, above all, patients. These platforms should operate in the future as cornerstones aiming to promote the incorporation and integration of *learning, information and research.* Furthermore, by allowing a swifter exchange of information, it will enable the creation of a global database which may be used in epidemiological research.

Building modern, more equal societies depends on the concept of a networked society. The challenge to link communities with access to e-healthcare via free or low-cost portals in their own homes or within their communities is an important precept for the success of e-healthcare. Health organization, governments and key global institutions such as the World Health Organization and World Bank recognize that the digital divide is a problem that public policy must begin to address. The digital divide and inequalities in basic infrastructure contribute to the same disparities in e-healthcare as in access to actual healthcare services. Priorities to improve e-healthcare for all must, therefore, include policies that target infrastructure and the wider determinants of health, not simply Internet connectivity.

REFERENCES

Access to information: bridging the digital divide in Africa. *The Guardian Jan 24, 2014.* Available at http://www.theguardian.com/global-development-professionals-network/2014/jan/24/digital-divide-access-to-information-africa

Ackerman, M. J., Filart, R., Burgess, L. P., Lee, I., & Poropatich, R. K. (2010). Developing Next-Generation Telehealth Tools and Technologies: Patients, Systems, and Data Perspectives. *Telemedicine Journal and e-Health, 16*(1), 93–95. doi:10.1089/tmj.2009.0153 PMID:20043711

ADOC Project. (2011). APEC Digital Opportunity Center. Retrieved from http://www.apecdoc.org/site/pmes/russia-pme/

Agarwal, P. (2007). Higher education in India: Growth, concerns and change agenda. *Higher Education Quarterly*, *61*(2), 197–207. doi:10.1111/j.1468-2273.2007.00346.x

Alvarez, A. L. P. Latin America's Digital Divide. Available from http://latinamericanscience.org/2014/05/latin-americas-digital-divide/

American Telemedicine Association. Available at http://www.americantelemed.org/

Badger, E. The Stubborn Persistence of America's Digital Divide. Available from http://www.citylab.com/work/2014/02/stubborn-persistence-americas-digital-divide/8280

Cline, G. B., & Luiz, J. M. (2013). Information Technology Systems in Public Sector Health Facilities in Developing Countries: The Case of South Africa. *Medical Informatics and Decision Making*, *13*, 1–12. PMID:23347433

Coleman, A., & Coleman, M. F. (2013). Activity Theory Framework: A Basis for E-health Readiness Assessment in Health Institutions. *Journal of Communication*, *4*, 95–100.

Consolidated versions of the Treaty on European Union and the Treaty on the Functioning of the European Union (9 May 2008). *Official Journal of the European Union 51*. Delivering Digital Inclusion: An Action Plan for Consultation, HM Government. Available from http://fm.schmoller.net/2008/10/delivering-digi.html

Della Mea, V. (2001). What is e-Health (2): The death of telemedicine? *Journal of Medical Internet Research*, *3*(2), e22. doi:10.2196/jmir.3.2.e22 PMID:11720964

Digital Divide in East Asia: Evidence from Japan, South Korea and Singapore. Hiroshi Ono Stockholm School of Economics. Working Paper Series Vol. 2005, (26 November 2005) available from http://www.agi.or.jp/user03/832_176_20110622102135.pdf

Digital divide still an issue for low income earners. *The Sydney Morning Herald* (February 26, 2014).

DiMaggio, P., & Hargittai, E. (2004). From Unequal Access to Differentiated Use: A Literature Review and Agenda for Research on Digital Inequality. In K. Neckerman (Ed.), *Social Inequality* (pp. 355–400). New York: Russell Sage Foundation.

Directive 2011/24/EU of the European Parliament and of the Council of 9 March 2011 on the application of patients' rights in cross-border healthcare. Available from http://eur lex.europa.eu/LexUriServ/LexUriServ.do?uri=OJ:L:2011:088:0045:0065:en:PDF

Eltchiyan, R., Emelin, I., Fedorov, V., Mironov, S., & Stoliar, V. (2004). Telemedicine in Russia. Studies in Health Technology and Informatics. E-book. *Medinfo*, *10*, 953–955.

Facts and figures of the digital divide in UK. *21st Century Challenges*. Available from http://www.21stcenturychallenges.org/60-seconds/what-is-the-digital-divide/

First of its kind medical kiosk in India. Available from http://www.biospectrumasia.com/biospectrum/news/122495/first-virtual-medical-kiosk-india

Foley P, Alfonso X, Ghani S. (20 June 2002). The digital divide in a world city. IECRC, Citizens Online for the Greater London Authority, London Connects and the London Development Agency

Han, J. H., Sunderland, N., Kendall, E., Gudes, O., & Henniker, G. (2010). Chronic disease, geographic location and socioeconomic disadvantage as obstacles to equitable access to e-health. *Health Information Management Journal*, *39*(2), 1833–3583. PMID:20577021

Harvard College. Global Health Review. Available from http://www.hcs.harvard.edu/hghr/print/spring-2011/telemedicine-developing/

Internet World Stats. (2010). Internet Usage in Europe. Available from http://www.internetworldstats.com/stats4.htm#europe

Jolly, R. (17 November 2011).The E-health revolution - easier said than done. Social Policy Section, available from http://www.aph.gov.au/About_Parliament/Parliamentary_Departments/Parliamentary_Library/pubs/rp/rp1112/12rp03

Justice, E. O. (2012). E-Healthcare/Telemedicine Readiness Assessment of Some Selected States in Western Nigeria. *IACSIT International Journal of Engineering and Technology*, *2*, 195–201.

Katz, J. E., & Apsden, P. (1997). A nation of strangers. *Communications of the ACM*, *40*(12), 81–86. doi:10.1145/265563.265575

Kelema, B. M., & Kgasi, M. R. (2014). Leveraging e-health for future-oriented healthcare systems in developing countries. *EJISDC*, *65*(8), 1–11.

Khoja, S., Durrani, H., Scott, R. E., Sajwani, A., & Piryani, U. (2013). Conceptual framework for development of comprehensive e-health evaluation tool. *Telemedicine Journal and e-Health*, *19*(1), 48–53. doi:10.1089/tmj.2012.0073 PMID:22957502

Khoja, S., Scott, R., & Gilani, S. (2008). E-health readiness assessment: Promoting "hope" in the healthcare institutions of Pakistan. *World Hospitals and Health Services*, *44*(1), 36–38. PMID:18549033

Kimaro, H. C., & Nhampossa, J. L. (2007). The Challenges of Sustainability of Health Information Systems in Developing Countries: Comparative Case Studies of Mozambique and Tanzania. *Journal of Health Informatics in Developing Countries*, *1*, 1–10.

Kroukamp, H. (2005). E-governance in South Africa: Are we coping. *Acta Academia*, *37*(2), 52–69.

Kwankam, S. Y. (2004). What e-Health can offer. *Bulletin of the World Health Organization*, *82*(10). PMID:15643805

LeRouge, C., Garfield, M. J., & Webb Collins, R. (2012). Telemedicine: Technology mediated service relationship, encounter, or something else? *International Journal of Medical Informatics*, *81*(9), 622–636. doi:10.1016/j.ijmedinf.2012.04.001 PMID:22579395

Li, J., Talaei-Khoei, A., Seale, H., Ray, P., & MacIntyre, C. R. (2013). Healthcare provider adoption of e-health: Systematic literature review. *Interact J Med Res*, *2*(1), e7. PMID:23608679

Lim, S. S., & Tan, Y. L. (2003). Old People and New Media in Wired Societies: Exploring the Socio-Digital Divide in Singapore. *Media Asia*, *30*(2), 95–102.

London Census. 2011. Census Information Scheme. GLA. Available from Intelligencehttp://data.london. gov.uk/census/

Lor, P. J. (2005). Preserving African digital resources: Is there a role for repository libraries? *Library Management, 26*(1/2), 63–72. doi:10.1108/01435120510572888

Marmot, M., Friel, S., Bell, R., Houweling, T. A. J., & Taylor, S. (2008). Closing the gap in a generation: Health equity through action on the social determinants of health. *Lancet, 372*(9650), 1661–1669. doi:10.1016/S0140-6736(08)61690-6 PMID:18994664

Martin, B. (2005). The information society and the digital divide: Some North-South comparisons. *International Journal of Education and Development Using ICT, 1,* 4.

Martin, J. B. (March 29, 2007). Digital Doctoring. *The Boston Globe*, retrieved from http://www.boston. com/news/globe/editorial_opinion/oped/articles/2007/03/29/digital_doctoring/

Meducation, available from www.meducation.net

Mitchell, B. R., Mitchell, J. G., & Disney, A. P. (1996). User adoption issues in renal telemedicine. *Journal of Telemedicine and Telecare, 2*(2), 81–86. doi:10.1258/1357633961929835 PMID:9375067

Mphidi, H. (2008). Digital divide and e-governance in South Africa. *Research, Innovation and Partnerships*, retrieved from http://www.ais.up.ac.za/digi/docs/mphidi_paper.pdf

Mutula, S. M. (2001). Internet access in East Africa: A future outlook. *Library Review, 50*(1), 28–34. doi:10.1108/00242530110365341

Nakamoto, H., Hatta, M., Tanaka, A., Moriwaki, K., Oohama, K., Kagawa, K., & Suzuki, H. et al. (2000). Telemedicine system for home automated peritoneal dialysis. *Advances in Peritoneal Dialysis. Conference on Peritoneal Dialysis, 16,* 191–194. PMID:11045291

Natenzon, M. Y. The National Telemedicine System is effective facility for improvement over health services to population in the Russian Federation. *National Telemedicine Agency Research-and-Production Union.* TANA Group National e-health Strategy Toolkit, available from http://www.itu.int/pub/D-STR-E_HEALTH.05-2012

Odit, M. C. A., Rwashana, A. S., & Kituyi, G. M. (2014). Antecedents and Dynamics for Strategic Alignment of Health Information Systems in Uganda. *The Electronic Journal of Information Systems in Developing Countries, 64*(6), 1–20.

Office for National Statistics. retrieved from http://www.ons.gov.uk/ons/rel/rdit2/internet-access---households-and-individuals/2014/stb-ia-2014.html

Ojo, S. O., Olugbara, O. O., Ditsa, G., Adigun, M. O., & Xulu, S. S. (2008). Formal Model for EHealthcare Readiness Assessment in Developing Country Context, retrieved from IEEE: http://limu.edu.ly/pub/34-21286-final.pdf

Operation Village Health. retrieved from http://connectedhealth.partners.org/patient-programs/virtual-care/operation-village-health.aspx

Opportune Breast Cancer Screening and Diagnosis Program, retrieved from http://en.esacproject.net/project/opportune-breast-cancer-screening-and-diagnosis-program-mexico-obcsdp

Patient.co.uk http://www.patient.co.uk

Pew Research Center. who's not online and why? (2013) retrieved from http://www.pewinternet.org/2013/09/25/whos-not-online-and-why/

Plataforma Saude Oral. retrieved from http://www.plataformasaudeoral.pt/

Professor in telemedicine: Don't forget to involve the users! Retrieved from http://www.alexandra.dk/uk/right_now/news/news-2014/apr-jun/pages/husk-at-faa-brugerne-med.aspx

Qureshi, Q. A., Ahmad, I., & Nawaz, A. (2012). Readiness for E-health in the Developing Countries like Pakistan. *Gomal Journal of Medical Sciences*, *10*, 160–163.

Rezai-Rad, R., Vaezi, R., & Nattagh, F. (2012). E-Health Readiness Assessment Framework in Iran. *Iranian Journal of Public Health*, *41*(10), 43–51. PMID:23304661

Russian Longitudinal Monitoring Survey, retrieved from http://www.cpc.edu/projects/rlms-hse

Singh, N. (2004). Information technology and rural development in India, *UC Santa Cruz Economics* Working Paper 56

Sood, S. P. (2004). Implementing telemedicine technology: Lessons from India. *World Hospitals and Health Services*, *40*(3), 29–30, 41–43. PMID:15566276

Swinhoe, D. (November 27, 2012 South America). The Digital Divide and its Impact in Latin America, retrieved from http://www.idgconnect.com/blog-abstract/688/dan-swinhoe-south-america-the-digital-divide-and-its-impact-in-latin-america

Tamura, T., Kawarada, A., Nambu, M., Tsukada, A., Sasaki, K., & Yamakoshi, K. (2007). E-healthcare at an experimental welfare techno house in Japan. *Open Med Inform J*, *1*(1), 1–7. doi:10.2174/1874431100701010001 PMID:19415129

Taneja, U, Sushil. (2007). E-Healthcare in India: Critical Success Factors for Sustainable Health Systems. *Studies in Health Technology and Informatics*, *129*(Pt 1), 257–261. PMID:17911718

Technologies for remote patient monitoring in older adults. Position paper. Discuss Draft. (2009). Available from http://www.techandaging.org/RPMpositionpaperDraft.pdf

Telehealth Link. retrieved from http://www.telehealthlink.com/Telehealth/PkgDiabetes.aspx

Thomas, C. L., Man, M.-S., O'Cathain, A., Hollinghurst, S., Large, S., Edwards, L., & Salisbury, C. et al. (2014). Effectiveness and cost-effectiveness of a telehealth intervention to support the management of long-term conditions: Study protocol for two linked randomized controlled trials. *Trials*, *15*(1), 36. doi:10.1186/1745-6215-15-36 PMID:24460845

Turkish Statistical Institute. (22 August 2014). Available from http://www.turkstat.gov.tr

United Kingdom Low Income and Ethnicity. retrieved from http://www.poverty.org.uk/06/index.shtml

Van Dijk, J. A. G. M. (2006). Digital divide research, achievements and shortcomings. *Poetics, 34*(4), 221–235. doi:10.1016/j.poetic.2006.05.004

Verloran Van Themat, C. (2004). The digital divide: Implications for South Africa. *South African Journal of Information Management, 6*(3), 12–19.

Viswanath, K., & Kreuter, M. W. (2007). Health disparities, communication inequalities, and eHealth. *American Journal of Preventive Medicine, 32*(5Suppl), S131–S133. doi:10.1016/j.amepre.2007.02.012 PMID:17466818

World Health Organization. E-health retrieved from http://www.who.int/trade/glossary/story021/en/

This research was previously published in the International Journal of User-Driven Healthcare (IJUDH), 4(4); edited by Ashok Kumar Biswas, pages 1-16, copyright year 2014 by IGI Publishing (an imprint of IGI Global).

Chapter 69

Enhancing the Reach of Health Care Through Telemedicine:
Status and New Possibilities in Developing Countries

Surya Bali
All India Institute of Medical Sciences Bhopal, India

ABSTRACT

Healthcare sector is now using telemedicine solutions to increase the reach of its services to population. Target areas are highly sparsely distributed devoid of basic amenities which makes the job of Governments difficult. Further people don't have enough disposable income to travel long distances and take preventive health care from urban areas. Problems are uniformly the same across the developing countries. The mindboggling developments in Information and Communication Technologies (ICT) particularly the web based technologies have opened up exciting new possibilities for health care across the world. These developments have evoked significant policy response in developing countries where the quality of health care is poor, resources are scarce and demands have to be immediately met. Telemedicine is gradually coming up as a viable policy option for the Governments in developing countries. This chapter gives an account of the telemedicine initiatives taken in India, describes emerging regional cooperation and its contribution for Sustainable Development Goals.

BACKGROUND

India, with its huge population of more than 1 billion and diverse geography that includes inaccessible hilly regions, tribal areas, deserts, coasts and islands, has long been struggling to provide minimum required health care to the people. The existing healthcare infrastructure is largely urban based. About 75% of health infrastructure, medical man power and other health resources are concentrated in urban areas where 27% of the populations live (Patil et al 2002). Government supported three tier healthcare

DOI: 10.4018/978-1-5225-3926-1.ch069

delivery system with limited medical experts and resources, is unable to provide healthcare facilities to the rural population (constituting about 70% of India's population).Further, most of the specialists are located in the urban areas and are reluctant to serve in the rural areas due to lack of basic amenities.

Contagious, infectious and waterborne diseases such as *diarrhea, amoebiasis, typhoid, infectious hepatitis, worm infestations, measles, malaria, tuberculosis, whooping cough, respiratory infections, pneumonia and reproductive tract infections* dominate the morbidity pattern, especially in rural areas. However, non-communicable diseases such as *cancer, blindness, mental illness, hypertension, cardio vascular disorders, diabetes, HIV/AIDS, accidents and injuries* are also on the rise (Patil et al, 2002 ; MOHFW, 2016). There is no health insurance policy and the common people are unaware of basic healthcare problems such as sanitation, hygiene, malnutrition, family planning, prevention, and preventive health. As India is struggling with these basic issues, new challenges of chronic diseases mostly cardiovascular illnesses and diabetes are creeping in due to changing life styles. There is growing threat of epidemic of HIV/AIDS, Malaria, Japanese Encephalitis, Chicken guinea etc. Providing healthcare and disease prevention to India's growing population is a challenge in the face of limited resources (MOHFW, 2016).Poor health care systems have adversely affected India's pursuit for Sustainable Development Goals (SDGs) and has significantly lowered important developmental indicators like life expectancy (63 years), infant mortality rate (80/1000 live births), maternal mortality rate (438/100 000 live births).

Why E-Health?

The India's performance on SDGs has to be taken seriously as one sixth of world's poor population lives in India (UN, 2016). Improved health care (SDG-3) for rural poor will directly or indirectly improve our performance on all the SDGs. However with the existing resources, infrastructure and expertise the demand cannot be met. There has to be paradigmatic changes in our policy concerns for the rural health. We have significant research base to conclude that e health is the only immediate solution available to meet the requirement. This is to be done in a holistic way, with a genuine effort to bring the poorest of the population to the centre of the fiscal policies. A paradigm shift from the current 'biomedical model' to a 'socio-cultural model', which should bridge the gaps and improve quality of rural life, is the current need (Patil et al 2002).The telemedicine coincides with worldwide developments of advancement in ICTs, need for continuing medical education, concerns for improved health care and its implications for poverty reduction. The following few developments have necessitated the practice of telemedicine in developing countries.

1. Increased Availability and Drop in cost of ICTs

Advances in Information and Communication Technologies (ICTs) have unfolded paradigmatically new ways of providing health care at affordable cost particularly for rural and underserved communities in developing countries which have long been confronting with lack of access to health care (World Bank, 2010). Such possibilities can help provide health care in critical situations, give rural practitioners access to specialist support and most importantly break the isolation of rural practice by upgrading their knowledge through tele-education or tele-CME. Developments have sparked interest in developing countries primarily due to increasing availability, utilization and drop in the cost of ICTs (World Bank, 2010).

2.   Increased Policy Level Sensitization

There has been an increased sensitization at national and international level that improved health care is required for sustainable livelihoods. Millennium Development Goals(UN 2000) and Sustainable Development Goals(UN 2015) of United Nations have laid emphasis on the improved health care for which all the major countries were signatory.

Such developments have given rise to a major policy thrust on ICT enabled health care services in resource starved developing countries to provide efficient and quality health services to its people (MOHFW, 2016). A revised National Health Policy addressing the prevailing inequalities, and working towards promoting a long-term perspective plan, mainly for rural health, is imperative. There is now a increasing realization among the decision making circles that the power of ICTs should be harnessed to connect the centres of excellences to remote areas. The low income countries and potential areas having limited health infrastructure are finding the options increasingly useful. Recent launch of National Rural Health Mission (NHRM) by the Ministry of Health & Family Welfare is a step in this direction.

3.   Heath Care for Vulnerable Communities and Heath Care Disaster Hit Areas

Developing countries suffer from huge disparities in the availability of quality health care primarily due to non availability of qualified health professionals and infrastructure in remote areas. Most of these remote locations inhabit socioeconomically most disadvantaged communities having poor access to conventional healthcare. Telemedicine has immense potential to enhance the reach of their health care services in remote and underserved areas at an affordable cost, improve quality of critical health care, improve administrative efficiency and improve tracking of chronic disease management. The health care in conflict and disaster hit areas becomes difficult due to high level of vulnerability of local population. Non availability of basic health care adversely affects their livelihoods. It has been observed that natural disasters make the rural poor more vulnerable for poverty .

4.   Need of Continuing Medical Education

The telemedicine is not just about extension of the health care to patients living in remote areas. It has a very strong purpose of providing continuing medical education to caregivers in such areas. Facilities for Continuing Medical Education are largely available in urban pockets which marginalize the health care givers posted in rural areas. Whereas the urban based professionals are able to update their expertise, their counterparts in rural interiors find it hard to catch up. It not only deincentivizes them to serve in rural areas but also adversely affects the quality of health care. Hence telemedicine services need to be promoted only for specialist care in rural interiors but also for capacity building of care givers. There is an immediate need for updating their knowledge and expertise which has to be responded by Universities and health care institutions through ICT enabled systems.

5.   Viability of Investments on Telemedicine Infrastructure

The use of telemedicine for the rural health care has been well discussed in existing research literature and outcomes have been described as favorable for developing countries and developed countries alike. Such projects have been observed to be highly beneficial for patient survival and recovery. However the equipments were expensive in the beginning and were also cumbersome. The technological advancements have brought down cost and also enhanced the usefulness of the equipments. Such developments have made telemedicine much more feasible to use in rural health care. settings

The telemedicine has also been observed to have accrued economic benefits to local community (Whitacre, 2011). Furthermore it leads to reduction in a number of other costs e.g. travel expenses for specialists and patient transfers which contributes for the economic viability of heath care access in a resource-constrained settings (Ecceles Nora, 2012). A recent study conducted by the Indian Institute of Public Opinion found that 89% of rural Indian patients have to travel about 8 km to access basic medical treatment, and the rest have to travel even farther. It amply justifies the policy level thrust on investments in telemedicine infrastructure in developing countries.

Making the E-Health Initiatives Work

The real challenge for the country is to reach 100% access to quality health care. It has been estimated by Kalam & Singh (2012) that poorest 20% of Indian population captures only 10% of total net public subsidy. The study also brings out the fact that top 20% receives more than thrice the subsidy received by the bottom 20%. Such disparities question the existing policies of health care and demand a paradigmatically new approach to address the health care requirements in rural and underserved areas. There have been several such best practices which can be customized in different socio economic contexts for different types of continuing educational requirements (Kalam and Singh, 2012).The content design, choice of media, scheduling etc need careful planning which should be planned in consultation with end users. Hence designing of entire delivery of the telemedicine services is crucial issue which needs to be taken in to consideration. Moreover such E-Health initiatives should converge with other developmental initiatives in the villages which will enhance utilization of electronic infrastructure and will reduce the cost of operation. Loni Providing Urban Amenities in Rural Areas (PURA) E-Health centre in Maharashtra presents a classic example for such initiative. This successful E health initiative has integrated the telemedicine initiatives with agriculture extension facilities, mobile clinics, capacity building of healthcare givers and a range of other developmental initiatives at village level.

How Does It Help?

Recent developments in technology mediated communication systems have made the telemedicine a viable opportunity for developing world. There is a interesting possibility to network different locations and pass on videos and pictures instantly. Such networked communication is helpful not only in rural areas but also in urban areas in conflict or disaster situations. Since the health care has to be immediately given at the site of disaster we need such technology mediated systems for immediate health care. However in most of the situations the telemedicine is required to overcome the constraints of distance. However in some of the cases the patients don't feel comfortable with in doctor's office, suffer from white coat syndrome or might need medical support without revealing their identity.

Telemedicine can additionally help in remote patient monitoring, reduce outpatient visits, enable remote prescription verification and drug administration oversight, potentially significantly reducing the overall cost of medical care. Most importantly it has created the interesting opportunity for grassroot level health caregivers to regularly interact with super specialists in urban based centers of excellences. It exposes them to advancements in their profession and share best practices more easily. The different types of telemedicine services and their relevance in the context of developing world are given below:

Table 1.

The Type of Telemedicine	Technological Application	The Use for Developing Countries
Tele-Neuropsychology	Patients with known or suspected cognitive disorders are evaluated using standard neuropsychological assessment procedures administered via video teleconference (VTC) technology.	The number of such neuropsychological cases are on rise, however experts are not available in sufficient numbers. Hence patients from remote areas need care at their doorsteps
Tele-Nursing	Use of telecommunications and information technology in order to provide nursing services in health care	Tele-nursing may help solve increasing shortages of nurses; to reduce distances and save travel time, and to keep patients out of hospital. A greater degree of job satisfaction has been registered among tele-nurses.
Tele-Pharmacy	Delivery of pharmaceutical care via telecommunications to patients in locations where they may not have direct contact with a pharmacist. Also refers to the use of videoconferencing in pharmacy for other purposes, such as providing education, training, and management services to pharmacists and pharmacy staff remotely.	It can be beneficial for patients far away from pharmaceutical care as they will not have to travel long distances
Tele-Rehabilitation (or *e-rehabilitation*)	Delivery of rehabilitation services over telecommunication networks and the Internet with commonly used mediums like webcams, videoconferencing, phone lines, videophones and WebPages containing rich internet applications	It can be beneficial to patients living in isolated communities and remote regions, who can receive care from doctors or specialists far away without the patient having to travel to visit them.
Tele-Trauma Care	Interaction with personnel on the scene of a mass casualty or disaster situation, via the internet using mobile devices and camera (pan, tilt and zoom) to determine the severity of injuries, to provide clinical assessments and determine whether those injured must be evacuated for necessary care.It may also includes delivering trauma education lectures to hospitals and health care providers worldwide using video conferencing technology.	Instant care can be given in those locations where the transport and communication networks are poor .
Remote Surgery	Performance of surgical procedures from remote locations using a robotic tele-operator system controlled by the surgeon. The remote operator may give tactile feedback to the user with the help of robotics and high-speed data connections.	Can prove to be extremely useful to overcome the lack of qualified surgeons in geographically isolated areas.
Specialist Care Delivery	Specialty care delivered by primary care physicians	It will be of tremendous help for a non specialist in remote locations
Tele-Cardiology	ECGs, or electrocardiographs, can be transmitted using smartphones with high internet connectivity.	Indigenous and customized solutions for tele transmission of ECG are being tried in several Asian countries which have proved useful
Tele-Psychiatry	Utilizes videoconferencing to offers wide range of services to the patients and providers, such as consultation between the psychiatrists, educational clinical programs, diagnosis and assessment, medication therapy management, and routine follow-up meetings.	Growing number of HIPAA compliant technologies are now available
Tele-Radiology	To send radiographic images (x-rays, CT, MR, PET/CT, SPECT/ CT, MG, US) from one location to another. For this process to be implemented, three essential components are required, an image sending station, a transmission network, and a receiving-image review station. The most typical implementation are two computers connected via the Internet. The computer at the receiving end will need to have a high-quality display screen that has been tested and cleared for clinical purposes. Sometimes the receiving computer will have a printer so that images can be printed for convenience.	Teleradiology is the most popular use for telemedicine and accounts for at least 50% of all telemedicine usage.
Tele-Pathology	Uses telecommunications technology to facilitate the transfer of image-rich pathology data between distant locations for the purposes of diagnosis, education, and research . Although digital pathology imaging is the major mode in developed countries, analog telepathology imaging is still prevalent for patient services in some developing countries.	Can be used for many applications including the rendering histopathology tissue diagnoses, at a distance, for education, and for research. Can eliminate the possible transmission of infectious diseases or parasites between patients and medical staff.
Tele-dermatology	Telecommunication technologies are used to exchange medical information (concerning skin conditions and tumours of the skin) over a distance using audio, visual and data communication	Health care management such as diagnoses, consultation and treatment as well as (continuing medical) education for teledermatologic service in a rural area underserved by dermatologists.
Tele-Dentistry	Information technology and telecommunications for dental care, consultation, education, and public awareness	Dentistry related problems are more and more prevalent in remote and rural areas
Tele-Ophthalmology	Eye care through digital medical equipment and telecommunications technology	It may help to reduce disparities by providing remote, low-cost screening tests such as diabetic retinopathy screening to low-income and uninsured patients.

Legal, Ethical and Socio-Economic Issues

Legal Issues in the Tele-Consultation in India

Telemedicine has provided a better platform for the better access of the healthcare services with efficiency and effectiveness. Millions of peoples are availing healthcare services through this platform. There are many legal issues related to utilization of telemedicine services which can be managed through better policy and guidelines.

Government sponsored telemedicine program in India has provided guidelines for the practice of teleconsultation between two medical practitioner. Here telemedicine practitioners bears the onus of any risk involved during the whole process of medical consultation. This is the reason why medical practitioners are not willing to practice the telemedicine even though there is strong need of such services in India (Mishra, 2013).

Health is the state matter in India which is major legal hurdle in the tele-consultation and the state governments are expected develop legal guidelines for telemedicine. However, even after so many years of telemedicine practices in India none of the Indian states has formulated any specific guideline, laws, advisory for the telemedicine practices. Indian Task Force on Telemedicine was constituted by the Ministry of Health & Family Welfare which has identified Legal, Ethical and Socio-economic aspects of Telemedicine as one of its "Terms of Reference". Taskforce has recommended many legal provisions but these recommendations are yet waiting to be framed as policies and laws (Task force on Telemedicine 2003).

Telemedicine network is expanding very fast in India and many public and private stakeholders are jumping into this filed which will increase the risk of malpractice and legal concerns in future . So there is strong need of a policy framework for Indian telemedicine program to avoid the serious consequences.

Medical Council of India, which is supreme body at central level need to frame guidelines and policies for its medical practitioners so that they can practice telemedicine without and fear of adverse legal consequences. Telemedicine is continuously getting acceptance in the population as well as in among the medical practitioners in India and taking the tele health services to the door steps of the patients . Lack of any legal framework at central and state level will hamper the growth of telemedicine program.

Tele consultation practices involve many sensitive data related to patients which need to be secured . There should be legal framework to secure the patient health information and medical records to prevent its misuse.

Ethical Issues in the Tele-Consultation in India

Telemedicine has brought tremendous improvement and convenience in the lives of millions throughout the world. It has brought patient and doctors very close. Lots of trust and intimacy issues are involved in tele-consultation. Application of technology in healthcare has shown cost effectiveness and benefitted millions. Patients and providers both are extremely satisfied with the tele consultation. Even though there is lots of benefits of tele consultation but it involves many ethical issues as we transmit patients personal information from one place to another. Taking pictures, making videos, recording health information and transmitting other personal details during the process of medical consultation needs to maintain the privacy and confidentiality.

Ethical issues should be well taken care of to ensure the faith and trust of patients in the tele-consultation and unfortunately there is no any specific guideline or laws at central and state level in India which force stakeholders to maintain the privacy and confidentiality into patients personal health records.

There is also issues of informed consent during the teleconsultation processes from distance which involves many individuals, in that case it become difficult to maintain the privacy and confidentiality of patients health information and we need to ensure that patient is aware about all the settings and consultation team and well informed and informed consent has been taken before the start of tele-consultation process.

In India where literacy is still big problem, understanding the technological process is not easy and need to deal with care while dealing with illiterate patients through tele consultation.

In India, where multiple languages are used, we need special attention while dealing with patients who are not aware the languages used by the healthcare providers and their teams to avoid the ethical concerns.

Socio Economic Issues in the Tele-Consultation in India

Although telemedicine has reached up to all level of healthcare delivery system still community is not fully aware about this technology and not prepared to accept the healthcare and medical services through distant. There is strong need to sensitize the community and make them ready to accept telemedicine services.

The socio-cultural aspects of relationship between doctor and patient cannot be ignored. This relationship has a cultural grounding on a personalized interaction and trust. The technological mediation between them could impinge on this relationship. With the technological advancement, the doctor and patient relationship has moved one step further. There is serious impact of losing touch on trust and the healing relationship nowadays. To maintain the strength of doctor patient relationship more personal attention needed to maintain the social bond between doctor and patient.

Telemedicine services are economical and brings cost efficiency in overburdened healthcare delivery system. It minimizes the travel of patients as well as physicians from one place to another and helped to fight the against the shortage of technical healthcare professionals.

There is also need to increase the standard of care through tele consultation to improve the quality of care so that patient feel comfortable and confident using telemedicine services.

Health insurance and payment reimbursement system should be strengthen to make telemedicine viable and successful.

Cost effective tools and technology which is acceptable by the community and society should be promoted for the tele consultations

Impediments in the Field of Telemedicine

Telemedicine plays an vital role in providing medical information and health services across space and time via telecommunication technologies ranging from the telephone to robotics (Sood et al., 2007) Telemedicine is mainly used to enhance the delivery of health care to geographically disadvantaged and medically underserved populations and it also provide a cost effective, quality healthcare (Akerman et al., 2010).

Telemedicine has shown its presence almost all corners of our lives. Telemedicine could be important in achieving care coordination and improvements in health disparity while avoiding duplication and wasting important resources (Rashid et al., 2013). Success of Telemedicine depends when it become an integral part of health care services and not as a stand-alone project. It is time for Telemedicine to move from experimental level to operational level and needed to be integrated with mainstream health services (LeRouge, et al., 2013).

Although telemedicine has achieved so much growth and success but still need to move further to achieve its main goals to become the routine part of the healthcare. Despite of so much development and work in field of telemedicine it has yet to become integral part of Indian healthcare system. Many technical, financial legal and cultural barriers has been observed in the development of telemedicine.

Technical Barriers

To run any system properly technical manpower is crucial. There is lack of champions in the field of telemedicine in India especially in the field of healthcare and only voluntary champions here and there are visible in the field of telemedicine. Most of doctors are not aware about the latest information technology and find difficulty to used modern IT gadgets. There is lack of telemedicine experts in healthcare sectors. There is need to include few chapters related to telemedicine in Medical education curriculum to sensitise and orient budding doctors to learn the technical part of this discipline. There should be separate telemedicine education secretariat and directorate in Ministry Medical Education like in Ministry of Health care which will promote the development of telemedicine. Because health is a state matter so state government should frame policies, program, guidelines and regulations regarding telemedicine practices and also allocate sufficient financial resources for telemedicine development. Policy level telemedicine exists but impediments appears at execution level so there is need to prepare the execution team for implementation and promotion of Telemedicine in India.

There is example of failure of successfully implemented telemedicine program in Madhya Pradesh, India by ISRO (Indian Satellite and Space Organization). Program failed only due to lack of interest of doctors in the telemedicine and lack of technical expertise in this field (Bali et al., 2016).

Other Technical barriers related to Information technology usability, reliability on machines, internet connectivity, remote data access, support for new technology, complexity in use, documentation and billing etc. are important barriers in the growth of telemedicine in India.

Financial Barriers

Cost incurred to install and maintain selected telemedicine services (telemedicine and communication equipment) is very high and do not give proper return on investment (ROI) so there is less economic benefits to the practitioners which leads to the bankruptcy and closure of many health facilities in rural communities and also prevents further telemedicine expansion to communities needing specialized services (Alverson et all 2004). Insurance companies do not reimbursed the tele consultation bills and payments which further force the practitioners to stop the telemedicine services.

Regulatory Barriers

Lack of definite guidelines, regulations and licensing policies prevents practitioners to practice teleconsultation due to fear of malpractice related legal issues. Malpractice liability is an important barriers in the practice of telemedicine services. There is certification and credential barriers which de-motivate practitioners. There are weak regulatory framework related to reimbursement in government as well as in private sectors against the teleconsultation services. End users are having privacy, confidentiality and security issues regarding their health information.

Lack of national and state level regulatory bodies are barriers in the development of telemedicine. Recently Government of India has constituted a National E Health Authority(NeHA) portal to remove this barrier in India. Implementation of telemedicine projects and programs without any specific framework is another barrier. There is no standardization in the telemedicine policy, program, implementation and practice.

Legal Barriers

Legal barriers are one of the most important obstacle in the growth of telemedicine in India. There is no legal framework of e-prescription or digital prescription or mobile based SMS prescription. Digital prescriptions are not approved and accepted by Medical Council of India(MCI). Most of doctors are afraid of Consumer Protection Act due to malpractice related issues. There is no standardised legal framework to protects practitioners as well as users. There is lack of specific standard operating procedure (SOPs) /guidelines for the telemedicine practice.

Service Provider Related Barriers

Most of the doctors still prefer to consult patients in traditional ways. They feel comfortable when they consult patients face to face and find difficulty in clinical examination. Another set of doctors have fear of losing job if something happens wrong. Because everything is on record so any error made by doctors can be easily caught so they try to bypass the digital consultation. Old doctors are not techno savvy and not aware of new information technology so find difficult to use telemedicine services. Even young doctors have hesitation to use telemedicine routinely because of lack of expertise in the subject.

User Related Barriers

Many patients are not aware of newer telemedicine technology and even if aware not feel comfortable to utilize it. There are many apprehensions about the treatment success rate and risk related to treatment through distant technology. Illiteracy is one of the major hindrance in acceptance of telemedicine services. Poor patient thinks it is not for them and avoid to visit the telemedicine centres. There is also apprehensions related to possibility of medical care through machine and through remote locations.

Cultural Barriers

There are lots of cultural barriers in the development of telemedicine in Indian healthcare sectors. Somewhere patients do not like to avail these services and somewhere healthcare professional do not like to provide services through telemedicine network due to various reasons. Few communities avoid to adopt the newer technology.

Administrative Barriers

It has been observed that even many policy makers are suspicious about the success of telemedicine in healthcare. In many healthcare institution health administrators are not supportive and do not like to set up telemedicine solution. Many health and nursing administrators are not convinced with telemedicine and do not support the implementation and day to day operations of telemedicine program.

The Impact So Far

Despite of so many barriers, telemedicine program is spreading in big way. Lots of successful projects has been launched and currently operational and benefiting population. Throughout the past sixty years, telemedicine has grown from its infancy to a noticeable and growing force in today's health landscape (Raoin, K. Datamonitor, 2007).

In India, telemedicine programs are actively supported by Department of Information Technology (DIT), Indian Space Research Organization (ISRO), North Eastern Space Applications Centre (NESAC), Apollo Hospitals, Asia Heart Foundation and other State governments (Dasgupta A et al 2008).

As pilot project basis, in year 2001, ISRO established about 60 telemedicine facilities in 60 remote hospitals, which were further connected to 20 super-specialty city hospitals (ISRO 2004).

Later on telemedicine system was started at the School of Tropical Medicine (STM), Kolkata and later connected with two remote District Hospitals of West Bengal namely Coronary Care Unit at Siliguri District Hospital, Siliguri, and Bankura Sammilani Hospital, Bankura in year 2001 (Dasgupta A et al 2008).

School of Telemedicine and Bioinformatics started in year 2003 and completed in year 2009 and since then providing telemedicine services to general population (STMI 2009).

In Madhya Pradesh India, telemedicine services were implemented in year 2008 through 16 telemedicine nodes. Most of the nodes are non-functional today (Bali et al 2016).

Telemedicine centre was established in AIIMS Bhopal in year 2013 with the help of Madhya Pradesh Government and ISRO. Many innovative projects were successfully launched and currently running at Telemedicine Centre, All India Institute of Medical Sciences(AIIMS)Bhopal, Madhya Pradesh.

Telemedicine Call Centre was inaugurated by on the occasion of Gandhi Jayanti 2, October, 2013 since then more than 60,000 patients have been consulted through the toll free (104) telephonic call centre. Call centre provides telephonic consultation services to the population.

Madhya Pradesh Government has also launched EHC(Electronic Healthcare Centres) pilot project in five districts in year 2015 with the support of Hewlett Packard. There is a single studio at the State head quarter (main telemedicine studio) and five remote district level studios. Both studios were connected through high bandwidth internet services. Patients come to the district level studio (which is build in a temporary shelter) and get examined by paramedical staff and patient also has opportunity to see and talk to doctor at main studio. Teleconsultation occurs through video conferencing and prescription is written at Main studio which can be printed at district level studio and patients can get all medicine free of cost at the local district pharmacy.

In year 2016, Telemedicine centre Bhopal launched ATM(Any Time Medicine) project at four primary health Centres(PHCs) in Betul District. Program was in pilot mode and was very successful. A telemedicine Unit (Monitor, Drug dispensing machine, and telephone) was kept at remote locations and were connected to the Call centre of AIIMS Bhopal over mobile phone. Patients from remote locations visited to the telemedicine unit for the consultation. Patients health information were sent from the remote centre on the mobile of physician posted at call centre, AIIMS Bhopal then doctor talked to patient to make diagnosis and later on sent command to drug vending machine to dispense required medicine through remote command. This telemedicine has investigation facility too. This was very simple project which did not need internet and worked on mobile connectivity and Voice and SMS based services. Consultation, laboratory investigations and medicine were available a single point. Patient were very satisfied with this pilot program as they received all their medical needs in very less time without spending any money.

Tele medicine Centre AIIMS Bhopal also has Video conferencing services connected with high band width National Knowledge Network (NKN). This telemedicine facility is used for continued medical education(CMEs), Clinical case discussions, expert consultations and seminar purposes.

Despite of all barriers, telemedicine network is expanding day by day and benefiting patients through removing the barriers in traditional health care seeking.

Regional Cooperation Through Telemedicine

Indian telemedicine program is well connected with other SAARC countries and India is helping to expand this network in neighboring countries. Collaboration of SAARC countries came in form of SACODiL(SAARC Consortium on Open and Distance Learning) to strengthen cooperation in the joint development of educational programmes, credit transfers, and promotion of equal opportunities and access to knowledge. Telemedicine has revealed many possibilities for regional cooperation in developing world. The Ministry Of External Affairs (MEA) Has Undertaken A Global Telemedicine Initiative In Africa And South Asia To Extend Its Telemedicine-Enabled Healthcare And Educational Services Under A South Asian Association For Regional Cooperation (Saarc) And Pan-African E-Network Project. Following the success of PAN African e learning project, Ministry of External Affairs (MEA) in India initiated an ambitious project called India Africa virtual university in 2011(MEA, 2011).(SAARC 2009)

SAARC Telemedicine Network

This platform provide the information related to telemedicine networking among SAARC countries. India as a leader in the field of telemedicine provide specialist healthcare facilities and treatments to all the members of SAARC countries. India also share medical experience and knowledge among doctors of SAARC countries. During the 14th SAARC summit at Delhi in year 2007, it was planned to connect one or two hospitals in each of the SAARC country with the super speciality hospitals in India like PGI Chandigath, AIIMS New DElhi, SGPGI Lucknow etc. (SAARC Telemedicine Forum 2009).

The SAARC e Network Telemedicine project is very popular and successful at SGPGI Lucknow, UP. This centre is providing proving telemedicine specialist services to the members of SAARC countries since year 2008 with the help of Telecommunications Consultants of India Limited(TCIL).

Statewide Telemedicine Network Implemented in Various States of India

If we look into the Indian healthcare scenario, there is lots of inequality and disparity in healthcare access across the urban and rural regions among different. Telemedicine is being used to fill the gap between urban and rural areas. All the stakeholders whether government or private actively participating in telemedicine program to ensure the quality and affordable healthcare(Mishra SK et el 2012)

Many states like Maharashtra, Orissa, Tamil Nadu, Madhya Pradesh are making strides in the field of telemedicine. These states running different types of telemedicine program to deliver better healthcare to the rural population where there is crises of health professionals and other paramedical staff. ISRO has spread its telemedicine network in these states and these network are being used for the purpose of education and healthcare delivery.

Orissa Trust of Technical Education and Training (OTTET) is working in close collaboration with Orissa government and has established modern ICT platform and network through Public Private Partnership (PPP). This platform is successfully providing promotive & preventive healthcare delivery to villagers in 51,000 villages of the state (OTTET 2011).

Punjab government has also established telemedicine network under a special Telemedicine Project at Government Medical College and Hospital to link the five polyclinics set up in the state.

In Himachal Pradesh 19 health centers at district, block and tehsil headquarters connected with Indira Gandhi Medical College, Shimla and Postgraduate Institute of Medical Education & Research Chandigarh through ISDN link (Mishra SK et al 2012).

Tamil Nadu and Maharashtra has connected its primary and secondary healthcare centre through telemedicine network.

Pan-African E-Network

The Ministry of External Affairs for the Government of India has implemented this project through Telecommunications Consultants India Ltd. (TCIL) to establish a VSAT-based telemedicine and tele-

Figure 1.
(Source: Indian Space Research Organization ISRO, Ahmadabad)

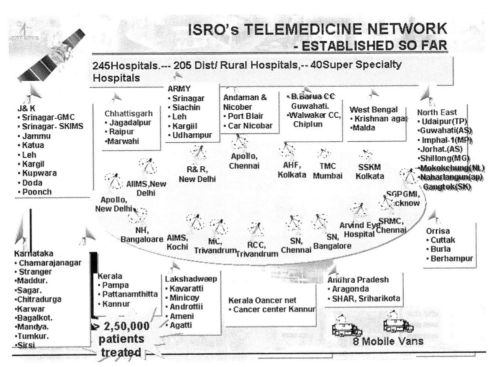

education infrastructure for African countries in 53 nations of the African Union. This has been successfully accomplished via a satellite and fiber-optic network that would provide effective tele-education, telemedicine, Internet, videoconferencing and VoIP services and also support e-governance, e-commerce, infotainment, resource mapping and meteorological services. Twelve super-specialty hospitals in India have been identified to provide tele-health services to 53 remote African hospitals. (SK Mishra et al 2012).

These remote hospitals are equipped with the medical equipments such as Electro-Cardio-Gram (ECG), Ultra Sound, and pathology and X-Ray at each location and each remote unit is equipped with Tele-Medicine hardware, camera and software. These hardware are integrated with telemedicine software for the patient management and day to day operations. and the complete system is HLA 7 compliant. The Super Specialty Hospitals in India are providing telemedicine services to Member States of the African Union AU with the 8 hours of consultation.(PAENP 2012).

CONCLUSION

The telemedicine holds a great promise for developing countries primarily due to huge population not being able to access the conventional health care facilities. It is not possible for the Governments to expand the conventional healthcare systems in such areas primarily due to resource crunch. The specialist medical experts are hesitant to work in such areas which is a major hassle in the expansion of health care systems. Moreover the areas where the targeted population lives are geographically isolated, poorly connected by transport and communication network and lack the civic amenities. It is also worth mentioning that the target areas are sparsely distributed in terms of population which makes the conventional health care systems economically non viable.

Many successful stories has been demonstrated using telemedicine technologies to enhance the community outreach of healthcare services (Bali et al 2005). Telemedicine has brought revolution in the field of healthcare. Barriers in healthcare seeking like distance, waiting time, monitory crisis, escort issues,

Figure 2.

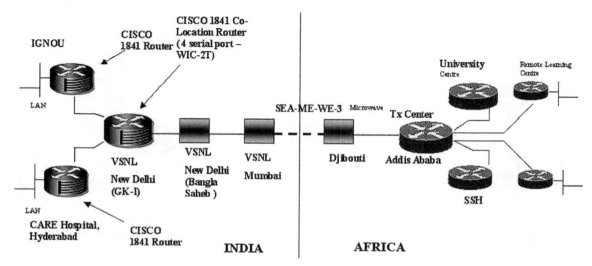

poverty, illiteracy etc. can be easily overcome using information technology in providing healthcare. Using satellite and terrestrial communications, information technologies more and more difficult areas can be covered and served.

There are certain constraints in the full development and utilization of telemedicine network which can be solved in due course of time through newer innovations and technologies.

Utilization of telemedicine technology will increase with the growth and development of television, telephone, and computer technologies. In future connectivity will increase which further help the technology to grow . Sooner or later sophisticated interactive multimedia programs, linked through television and computer capabilities will be common and can be used by doctors to enhance their outreach. (Zundel KM)

There are many barriers in the development of telemedicine in India like technological barriers, legal barriers, cultural barriers, social barriers and economic barriers etc. These can be removed easily in future and telemedicine can be used for the common person irrespective of cost, creed religion, distance, poverty and educational status.

Many pilot projects related to telemedicine have been successfully launched and demonstrated in last 50 years. These projects, programs were very successful at village, district, state, national and international level. India has shown its presence in the field of telemedicine at all level and now competing with the other developed countries.

Despite of its great promise to scale up health care in developing countries, telemedicine has varying levels of success across the developing world (World Bank, 2010).Though there have been sustainable pilot projects at several places such initiatives have not been mainstreamed. Reasons are largely a complex of human and cultural factors which prevent the mainstreaming of such initiatives. There has been a psychological rhythm which prevents change in conventional health care practices. The lack of ICT literacy, language barriers and cultural gaps between the service providers and patients are also the major factors which prevent change in conventional practices.

In future telemedicine will minimized the gap between urban rural, poor rich, literate and illiterate and also made access of quality healthcare services to remote and difficult terrain.

REFERENCES

Ackerman, M.J., Filart, R., Burgess, L.P., Lee, I., & Poropatich, R.K. (2010). Developing next-generation telehealth tools and technologies: Patients, systems, and data perspectives. *Telemed. e-Health, 16*, 93–95.

Alverson, D.C., Shannon, S., Sullivan, E., Prill, A., Effertz, G., Helitzer, D., Beffort, S., & Preston, A. (2004). Telehealth in the trenches: Reporting back from the frontlines in Rural America. *Telemed. e-Health, 10*, S-95–S-109.

Bali, S., Gupta, A., Khan, A., & Pakhare, A. (2016, April). Evaluation of telemedicine centres in Madhya Pradesh, Central India. *Journal of Telemedicine and Telecare, 22*(3), 183–188. doi:10.1177/1357633X15593450 PMID:26156940

Bali, S., & Singh, A. J. (2006). Enhancing the outreach of community medicine field team through mobile phones: A pilot study. *Indian Journal of Community Medicine, 31*(2), 80.

Bashshur. (2013). Compelling issues in telemedicine. *Telemed. e-Health, 19*, 330–332.

Dasgupta, A., & Deb, S. (2008). Telemedicine: A New Horizon in Public Health in India. *Indian Journal of Community Medicine: Official Publication of Indian Association of Preventive & Social Medicine, 33*(1), 3–8. doi:10.4103/0970-0218.39234 PMID:19966987

LeRouge, C., & Garfield, M. J. (2013). Crossing the Telemedicine Chasm: Have the U.S. Barriers to Widespread Adoption of Telemedicine Been Significantly Reduced? *International Journal of Environmental Research and Public Health, 10*(12), 6472–6484. doi:10.3390/ijerph10126472 PMID:24287864

Mishra, S. K. (2013). *Round-up of Snapshots of Tele-medicine/Tele-care/ Tele-rehabilitation and Their Economical and Legal Challenges: Telemedicine Scenario in India with special reference to legal, ethical and socio-economic issues.* Retrieved from https://www.jstage.jst.go.jp/article/jsmbe/51/Supplement/51_M-110/_pdf

Mishra, S. K., Singh, I. P., & Chand, R. D. (2012*). Current Status of Telemedicine Network in India and Future Perspective.* Retrieved from http://journals.sfu.ca/apan/index.php/apan/article/viewFile/54/pdf_54

Nora, E. (2012). Telemedicine in developing countries Challenges and Successes. *Harvard College Global Health Review.* Retrieved from https://www.hcs.harvard.edu/hghr/print/spring-2011/telemedicine-developing/

Orissa Trust of Technical Education and Training (OTTET). (n.d.). Retrieved from http://www.ottet.in/

Pan African e Network Project. (2012). Retrieved from http://www.panafricanenetwork.com/Portal/ProjectDetails.jsp?projectidhide=10&projectnamehide=Tele%20Medicine

Patil, A. V., Somasundaram, K. V., & Goyal, R. C. (2002). *Current health scenario in rural India.* Retrieved from https://www.ncbi.nlm.nih.gov/pubmed/12047509

Raoin, K. (2007). *Homecare Telehealth Expected to Grow Despite Current Barriers to Adoption.* Available online: http://it.tmcnet.com/news/2007/08/30/2897900.htm

Report of the Technical Working Group on Telemedicine Standardization. (2003). *Ministry of Communication and Information Technology (MCIT).* Recommended Guidelines & Standards for Practice of Telemedicine in India.

SAARC Consortium on Open and Distance Learning. (n.d.). Retrieved from http://saarc-sec.org/areaofcooperation/detail.php?activity_id=15

SAARC Telemedicine Forum. (n.d.). Retrieved from http://www.saarctf.org/

Sood, S., Mbarika, V., Jugoo, S., Dookhy, R., Doarn, C.R., Prakash, N., & Merrell, R.C. (2007). What is telemedicine? A collection of 104 peer-reviewed perspectives and theoretical underpinnings. *Telemed. e-Health, 13*, 573–590.

Whitacre, B. E. (2011). *Estimating the economic impact of telemedicine in a rural community.* Retrieved from http://ageconsearch.umn.edu/bitstream/117770/2/ARER%2040-2%20pp%20172-183%20Whitacre.pdf

WHO. (2010). *Telemedicine*. Opportunities and Development in Member States. WHO.

Zundel, K. M. (n.d.). *Telemedicine: history, applications, and impact on librarianship*. Retrieved from http://docplayer.net/15724378-Telemedicine-history-applications-and-impact-on-librarianship.html

This research was previously published in Open and Distance Learning Initiatives for Sustainable Development edited by Umesh Chandra Pandey and Verlaxmi Indrakanti, pages 339-354, copyright year 2018 by Information Science Reference (an imprint of IGI Global).

Chapter 70
Mobile Health Literacy to Improve Health Outcomes in Low–Middle Income Countries

Nafisa Fatima Maria Vaz
Goa Institute of Management, India

ABSTRACT

Despite improvements in health indicators over time, such as decreased mortality and morbidity, significant challenges remain with regard to the quality in the delivery of healthcare in low and middle-income countries (LMIC's), especially in rural and remote regions of developing countries. In the effort to find feasible solutions to these issues, a lot of importance is given to the information and communication technologies (ICTs) The author reviews the evidence of the role mobile phones facilitating health literacy to contribute to improved health outcomes in the LMIC's. This was done by exploring the results of ten projects. The author examines the extent to which the use of mobile phones could help improve health outcomes in two specific ways: in improving health literacy and promoting health and well-being, thus increasing life expectancy in LMIC's. Analysis of the papers indicates that there is important evidence of mobile phones boosting increased access, promoting education and increased health literacy leads to the better health status of the population.

INTRODUCTION

The world is developing at a very fast pace in the 21st century. The face of healthcare is changing! Digital technologies are changing the way in which the healthcare industry approaches the provision of care. By redefining the way services are provided and combining the use of technology and data analytics it has become possible to manage the health of patients and populations proactively (Bolton, Hausman, & Keisling, 2011). We can now get patients to help themselves by actually looking after their health and conditions. We have often heard the phrase "Prevention is better than Cure" and now with the growth of the Mobile health industry, this could be a reality if made use of judiciously.

DOI: 10.4018/978-1-5225-3926-1.ch070

In this paper, the author explores the scope of mobile health educational programs in improving the health and wellness status thus raising the life expectancy of its population in Lower and middle income countries (LMIC's). That can be achieved through predesigned health tips shared by practitioners or experts in the area, thus aiming at improving the lifestyles of the people within the given location. The aim was to design a mobile health pilot program from the inputs given.

The health care sector in many LMICs is constrained by the high financial and human resource costs, as well as lengthy implementation times, of expanding health facilities and training workforces based on accepted WHO standards (Schweitzer, 2010). With the coming in of Mobile health, healthcare has been taken to a different level where one can even warn the physician that they are likely to have an MI (myocardial infarct). Call centers that will continuously evaluate the data and interpret them and give valuable information to the patients have been running in several countries. Smart algorithm and feedback systems are changing the face of healthcare services (Kay, 2011).

The World Health Organization defines mobile health as "the spread of mobile technologies as well as advancements in their innovative application to address health priorities." (Kay, 2011). The National Institute of Health, on the other hand, defines mobile health as "the use of mobile and wireless devices to improve health outcomes, healthcare services, and health research." ("Mobile Health (M-Health) information and resources - Fogarty International Center @ NIH," n.d.)

Mobile Health is a rapidly developing field and has over 160,000 health apps that are currently available in the global market (Research2Guidance, 2015). Mobile health contributes to the empowerment of patients so that they are able to manage their health more actively, live independently focusing on self-assessment or remote monitoring solutions. Mobile health is an emerging part of e-health, where Information & Communication Technologies (ICT) are used to improve health products, services, and processes (Kay, 2011). It is a promising area to supplement the traditional delivery of healthcare and complements rather than replaces it. We can help the public attend to the social determinants of health-care in building a safer, healthier environment in order to lead a healthier lifestyle. We could help run the best healthcare system in the world. Mobile health can be used wisely to help people live a long healthy and happy life. We can try giving every person instant round the clock access to high-quality health care, at very affordable costs and access to the advice of highly skilled physicians across the country. Instead of making them travel to hospitals, we can take the hospital to them! What we can do is promote proactive preventive healthcare rather than reactive, when treating patients. That will go a long way in keeping patients out of the hospital. Ah doesn't this all sound divine in a world where health is still unaffordable to many.

Several studies, have shown us that mobile health has indeed worked wonders for patients adhering to medication intake, in patients suffering from cardiovascular disease and improvements in mother and child care etc. (Gandapur et al., 2016). When the success of the same has been proved, we need to move a step ahead in utilising this resource in the most positive way possible. These findings can be utilized in LMIC's where the doctors are scarce to cater to the population, and we wish to achieve the maximum we can to fill this gap.

More than 100 countries are now exploring the use of mobile phones to achieve better health (Report, Innovation, & Fund, 2015). Mobile health can be used to enhance health education and compliance to medication. One problem commonly faced is the shortage of medical practitioners in the country, especially in rural areas. That is a huge obstacle that comes in the way of delivery of health care services. This brings up a scope of opportunities to these countries, like organising support groups or communities for people with similar illnesses, access to reliable health care information, apps that remind patients of their medicine schedule, doctors' appointments, vaccinations, applications to monitor one's Blood pressure, heart rate and the list goes on.

A number of improvements are expected to come in healthcare with the large scale utilisation of M-health, the aid that this will provide will be huge considering that it would help increasing accessibility of health services, decrease the cost of healthcare, support chronic disease life care, provide suitable tools for timely management of healthcare in case of emergencies. Proper utilization of Mobile health will help by removing the restraint of time and location while increasing the coverage and the Quality of care (Adams, 2010). The health status of the public will improve which in turn would reduce the burden on the current health system.

This research aims to study the use of Mobile health in the reduction of mortality/morbidity rate amongst infants, maternal mortality and adult mortality at the same time increasing the life expectancy at birth. Mobile health, in this case, would be used to promote healthier lifestyles keeping each of the Cause of Death in mind. The main tool that this focuses on is Mobile health as a tool for increasing health literacy.

BACKGROUND AND MOTIVATION

The need to expand the mobile health evidence-base in LMICs was presented in a report in 2011 by the World Health Organization. The report featured that over 50% of low income and low-middle income countries that were surveyed, display a lack of knowledge of the possible mobile health applications and their public health outcomes which pose as a major barrier to mobile health implementation, substantiating the need for evaluation studies (Kay, 2011). There are several studies on mobile health feasibility in developed countries, all of which may not be replicable in LMIC's. Thus, we needed to build upon the studies in developing countries in order to provide satisfactory evidence to the policy makers.

The Role of Communication in Saving Lives

There are numerous, complex reasons why a large number of global deaths of pregnant women, infants and children under the age of five occurs in the developing world. Of course, poverty is one of the many reasons, besides this is significantly an insufficient number of skilled health workers, the lack of access to essential medicines and equipment, substandard living conditions and poor nutrition are issues to name a few. Health-related behaviors and social norms, beliefs, traditions, superstitions and local customs around delivering babies at home without access to skilled birth attendants or doctors also play a role (United Nations Children's Fund, 2013). The extent to which communication can help save lives depends inevitably on the complex interplay of these multiple factors. Nevertheless, decades of research and practice have established a strong evidence base that communication has a major role to play in improving health (Macpherson & Chamberlain, 2013). As Caroline Anstey, Managing Director of the World Bank Group, put it: "I firmly believe in the power of information to change lives." Media and communication can help to achieve health outcomes by improving knowledge, shifting attitudes and social norms and increasing people's confidence and motivation to act in the interests of their health.

They can also facilitate and stimulate public and interpersonal discussion, which in turn can support the adoption of healthier behaviors and greater accountability around health service provision and policy making. Researchers have identified verbal and non-verbal activities that are associated with patients changing behavior, increased health education being a major factor (Beck et al., 2002).

Methodology

In light of the theories as to how mobile health could help solve problems related to health education access and facilitate healthier citizens, the author sought to examine the existing evidence so as to confirm or refute the purported benefits advanced by the literature. Systematic literature searches were performed by searching Medline, Google scholar, academic publications and conference proceedings. A search strategy for gray literature was included to retrieve information from relevant sources, like the WHO and the World Bank, reference lists of included studies, and consulting experts related to the topic. In addition, generic and academic Internet searches and meta-searches were performed. The projects were selected according to the following criteria:

1. Studies that substantiate that health literacy increases life expectancy and reduces morbidity;
2. Mobile health Projects in the low-middle income countries are showing the impact on health outcomes;
3. Projects that show that healthier lifestyles can be led through health education;
4. Studies that clearly document the results and have evidence such that distinct conclusions can be drawn regarding the impact of mobile phones on the health outcomes of lowering morbidity and increasing the life expectancy via increased access to education.

RESULTS

There were ten studies that were suitable and are displayed in Table 1 with a brief summary of the findings. The search resulted in 64 studies in developing countries. The studies that did not match the criteria were excluded. Most mobile health related projects have been implemented in the developed countries of North America, and Asia-Pacific. Mobile health projects in the developing countries have been few and have a vast scope for research.

It was found that there is tremendous potential for M-Health to bring about considerable changes in the health status of the population in rural areas of developing nations. The studies chosen show a clear relationship with mobile phones being used fairly in rural areas of developing countries and a positive education outcome through M-education. M-Health intervention through health education results in behavior change which in turn leads to better health outcomes and lowered morbidity.

This assessment relies on relevant scientific literature and data. Literature evaluated included articles published in science and engineering journals, federal and state government reports, a nongovernmental organization (NGO) reports and industry publications. The research topic areas and projects described in the Study Plan were designed to meet the data and information needs of this assessment and were developed with substantial expert and public input.

Table 1. Summary of the studies referred

Study (Year)	Country	Intervention	Result
Mobile health Interventions in LMIC's.(2016)	Asia, Africa, Uganda & America	Mobile health education and behavior change initiatives.	Evidence exists for the efficacy of M-Health interventions in LMICs, especially in improving treatment adherence, appointment compliance, data gathering, and developing support networks for health workers (Hurt, Walker, Campbell, & Egede, 2016)
Education outcomes being improved by mobile phones in LMIC.(2010)	Countries in Asia	Reviewed the evidence of the role of mobile phone that facilitated M-Learning in contributing to improved educational outcomes in the developing countries	It was found that M-learning results in increased access, enables learner-centred education. Huge benefit for people who cannot avail traditional education (Valk, Rashid, & Elder, 2010)
Communications being the key to behavior change towards healthier lifestyles (2010)	-	Good communication, collaboration, and goal-setting in order to influence behavior change	Long-term behavior change needs to be promoted by health professionals (Davies, 2010)
Usage of mobile phones in LMIC (2015)	World data bank, LMIC	Lower prices of mobile phones have helped lower the digital divide. There is still a higher gap when it comes to smartphones.	There is a lowered digital divide, amongst LMIC. The penetration of smartphones not high enough in LMIC (Pew, n. d.)
The Impact of Mobile Health Interventions on Chronic Disease Outcomes in Developing Countries (2014)	LMIC (India, Malasia, Croatia, Uruguay, etc.)	Patient education, reminders, daily monitoring, diet tips and general health tips	Mobile health positively impacted on chronic disease outcomes, improving attendance rates, clinical outcomes, quality of life and was cost-effective (Beratarrechea et al., 2014)
Health literacy increases health outcomes leading to better life expectancy and reduced morbidity. (2007)	USA	Patient education by medics, reminders for medicine adherence, Education at a level understood	Self-management of health resulting in an improved health status (National Council on Patient Information and Education, 2007)
M-Health technology could impact greater health-care access to larger segments of rural populations and increased ability to meet the demand in developing countries. (2014)	India	A systematic review of studies in literature published for the last 10 years.	From 23 articles it was found that lack of suitable governmental regulation and oversight from health authorities had an impact on the results in terms of costs, benefits and utility of M-Health applications (Davey & Davey, 2014)
Evaluating feasibility, reach and potential impact of a text message family planning information service. (2012)	Tanzania and Kenya	Qualitative interview in family planning clinics	During the pilot period, 2870 unique users accessed m4RH in Tanzania, resulting in 4813 queries about specific contraceptive methods. A variety of changes in family planning use were mentioned after using the said programme, with reported changes consistent with where users are in their reproductive life cycle (L'Engle & Vahdat,2012))
Perspective on SMS mode for education on HIV prevention (2011).	Uganda	Survey of 1523 students	Data provides evidence that text messaging-based health programs, may be acceptable to secondary school students in Uganda (Mitchell, Bull, Kiwanuka, & Ybarra, 2011)
Evaluating the impact of mobile phone based 'health help line' service in rural Bangladesh	Bangladesh	Qualitative interviews	The field studies uncover enthusiasm from the rural people towards availing health help line services and the intervention's contribution to improved health-seeking behavior (Svensson, 2010)

Use of Mobile Phones in Education

In theory, M-learning increases access to education to those who are keen to learn but have limited or no access to education due to various constraints which could be either due to economic reasons associated with the high cost of education or the other constraints such as society, jobs, household activities or some other reason (OECD, 2007). The advantage of M-learning is that, if there is willingness to learn, M-education would remove all the barriers to education. It is useful in situations where the cost comes in the way or if situated in remote or rural areas or if proper education facilities are not available etc.

Health Literacy

Health literacy and literacy are closely related but are not the same. Literacy is defined as the ability of reading, writing, basic math, speech, and comprehension skills. If one visits remote rural areas in LMIC's, they would get a unique viewpoint about the country's public health system and would feel the urge to make health literacy the country's topmost priority. This health literacy cannot be imparted by just anyone, but authorized medical practitioners would need to develop clear communications and recommendations formulated, and it would be preferable if this team of medical practitioners belonged to the highest medical body in the country (Schillinger et al., 2002). For example, in India, it would be the Medical Council of India that could be given charge of creating the information to be imparted. Sustainable measures should be made to address the problem of health literacy in our keeping the goal of improving the health status within and across the populations in rural as well as urban areas. Past research has shown that individuals with low levels of health literacy are more likely to be hospitalized and have worse disease outcomes (Berkman et al., 2011). Health literacy is a fundamentally different concept compared to educational attainment. There is much research showing a strong relationship between poor literacy skills and health. This interest has led to the emergence of the concept of health literacy. That has taken a significant role in the healthcare world and has its focus in clinical care as well as in public health.

Low levels of health literacy are very common among patients who have low educational attainment and among the labourers, immigrants, geriatric patients and racial and ethnic minorities. A study of Medicare managed care enrollees showed that more than one-third of the enrollees had poor health literacy. The research also showed that poor health literacy is common among patients with chronic medical conditions like type 2 diabetes, cardiac related issues, asthma, AIDS (acquired immunodeficiency syndrome), and hypertension.

Research has shown that patients with poor health literacy have greater difficulties remembering their medications and adhering to medicines prescribed (Lin, Sklar, Oh, & Li, 2008). A project in South Africa called Project Masiluleke used to send over 1 million SMS messages every day to subscribers of a local telecommunications operator to promote HIV/AIDS testing (Kay, 2011). That was to encourage a behavior change amongst the people. These types of interventions have proven to be effective in propagating information; there are few studies that provide evidence of the impact of such programs on behavior change. There was also a study that showed the change in the behavior of the people when the communication by the doctors or nurses was higher, stressing on the fact that health literacy needs to be coming from healthcare sources. There is evidence that improved knowledge of one's condition may improve patient adherence to lifestyle changes and medication (Singleton & Krause, 2009).

The positive point to be noted is that 84% of women in LMIC's want better health care-related information while 39% of women express an interest in receiving health information through their mobile phones. (Deshmukh, Madhu & Mechael, 2013). Another interesting study showed that 73% of their population were interested in joining Mobile health programs in the future (Khatun et al., 2015).

The CDC has come out with the National Health Education Standards (NHES) which were developed to establish, promote and support health-enhancing behaviours for young students in all the classes at school. These students once have learned these health-enhancing behaviours are expected to promote further to family and community health (Waters, 2006).

The American Medical Association is promoting healthier lifestyles by implementing education and research projects all rooted in health literacy, to encourage wellness in rural disadvantaged communities worldwide.

Disease Burden

Chronic disease or non-communicable disease is a leading cause of morbidity worldwide. By 2030, it has been estimated that 23 million people will die annually from cardiovascular disease, with approximately 85% happening in LMIC. In addition, chronic health conditions have become a reason of the increasing health inequalities in LMIC, highlighting the urgent need to implement more cost-effective and quality interventions. Morbidity due to chronic diseases are largely preventable through counseling and medication adherence, but the implementation of these interventions is difficult in a resource-limited setting, which is the situation in most developing countries (Mechael et al., 2010). These interventions would work best if they are sponsored by the government and promoted in collaboration with the primary healthcare settings. They would need to be customized to the needs of the LMIC for them to be suitable in the sense of comprehension and usability especially for the disadvantaged groups. That can only be made possible by the involvement of the local healthcare practitioners in the primary healthcare settings.

Unfortunately, in fact, LMIC's face a dual burden of communicable and non-communicable diseases (Islam et al., 2014). See Figure 1 for a graph showing risk factors causing death based on income levels.

Figure 1. Ranking of 10 leading risk factors causing death, based on the income levels. Source: Risks, n. d. *Countries are grouped by gross national per capita income; low-income means (US$ 825 or less).

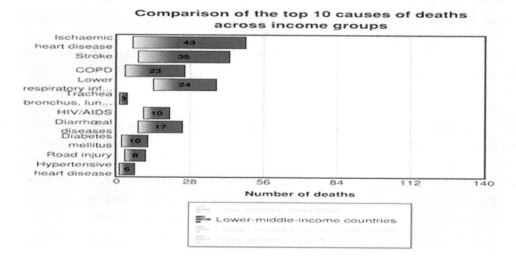

Mobile and Smartphone Usage

The Pew Research found that rates of Internet and smartphone usage are quickly rising in developing economies. As for smartphone ownership, the spike was even more dramatic, jumping from 21% in 2013 to 37% in 2015.

The Pew findings also highlighted strong correlations between income level, age and Internet connectivity. Across the globe, those that belonged to the age group of 18-34years were more likely to be connected to the Internet than other demographics. Research shows that there is great potential to convert those currently without Internet access into devoted Internet users. In a survey of 21 developing nations, 54% of adults reported using the Internet constituting a marked rise of 9% since 2013 (Poushter, 2016).

The statistics from growing economies reveals the extreme surge of smartphone and Internet usage in the recent years and the immense potential for app developers to capitalize on this trend. The increased explosion in the use of smartphones is due to their relatively lower prices, in some countries; a basic phone can be purchased for as little as US$30. Mobile apps are already beginning to proliferate in the developing world, resulting in a massive increase in the size of the app market. The use of the education apps has had a life-changing impact on those who use them. The potential of mobile health and e-health for resource-constrained environments becomes obvious when considering the following facts:

1. The global e-health market is estimated at $96 billion and growing, with many innovations coming from LMICs (Schweitzer, 2010);
2. 70% of all mobile phone users are in emerging markets, which are also the fastest growing markets (Africa, 2014);
3. Almost 90% of the world's population lives in areas with mobile phone coverage, providing a technology platform for mobile health applications (Kay, 2011).

From Figures 2 and 3 we can see that since major portions of developing countries are still not using smartphones, but a good number use mobile phones, our main focus should be directed to the health deprived population via mobile phones.

Thus, we can state the success of mobile health can be increased with:

- The involvement of healthcare professionals in setting it up;
- The focus on mobile phones more than or equal to smartphones;
- Constant dialogue with patient organizations;
- Ensuring the mode of delivery is patient friendly (Language);
- Initial and ongoing training of healthcare staff in the use of mobile technologies and incentives to encourage them to do so;
- Most importantly gaining the government support in launching this app and making it a success.

A MOBILE HEALTH MODEL FOR LMIC

In Lower and middle income countries the budget allocated for healthcare is on the lower side and is rarely sufficient to cover the populations healthcare needs. Here mobile health can come in very handy

Figure 2. Global divide on smartphone ownership. Source: Spring 2015Global Attitudes survey (Poushter, 2016).

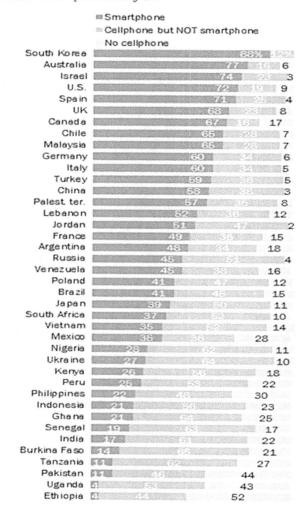

Global divide on smartphone ownership
Adults who report owning a ...

Note: Percentages based on total sample.

Source: Spring 2015 Global Attitudes survey. Q71 & Q72.

PEW RESEARCH CENTER

in reducing this burden and is a promising area to supplement the traditional delivery of healthcare rather than replacing it (see Figure 4).

This paper suggests a model that could be adopted by primary health center. The main idea of this should be to promote preventive healthcare.

Figure 3. Smartphone usage across the globe. Source: Spring 2015 Global Attitudes survey (Poushter, 2016).

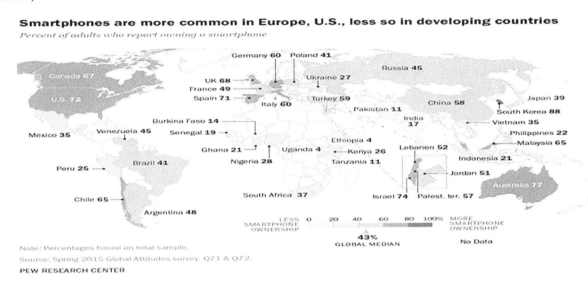

Figure 4. Mobile health model

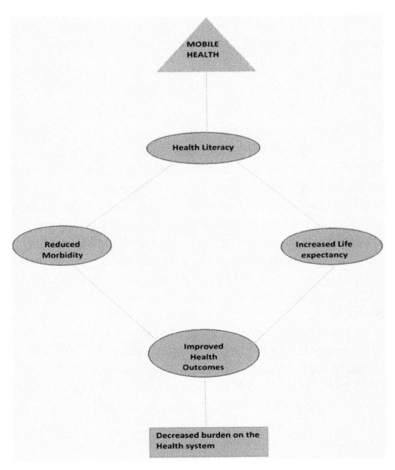

At this point, with low penetration of smartphones in LMIC's, it would be recommended to work with mobile phones. The cell phone usage in LMIC's has moved up the last few years from 89 per 100 in the year 2010 to 105 per 100 in year 2015. (Pews, 2016) This number is estimated to move up farther, and the trend is gradually shifting towards smartphones.

The App should be centrally managed for the entire country and region specific data should be provided which should be locally managed and tracked by the local clinics for a particular region.

The Mobile Phone Model should be focused on:

1. Communication with the health workers in case of emergency;
2. Health tips with a focus on the common illnesses faced by the population;
3. Warnings etc. in case of a breakout;
4. Information in case of availability of important vaccines, medicines or health camps;
5. Reminders for appointments.

Most importantly, one should ensure this App is created under the guidance of a team of specialist, approved by the Medical Council and available in the regional language.

Outcome Targeted

- Helps people take responsibility for their health and reduce hospital visits;
- Lowered burden on the current health system due to remote management;
- Healthier society, enhanced health and well-being, better health expectancy or lowered morbidity.

CONCLUSION

Analysis of the findings indicates that there is a strong evidence of mobile phones impacting education outcomes. On the other hand, we have seen substantial evidence that health literacy results in better health outcomes like lowered morbidity and increased life expectancy. With technology moving at a fast pace, research has shown that the people in LMIC's are also ready to adopt mobile health education, provided they be provided with the training to do so. This model of M-Health is created to benefit the inhabitants of rural areas in low and middle-income countries thus helping them to manage their health by getting health literate. That will have a positive impact resulting inefficiency of the healthcare delivery. Mobile health will work as an effective learning tool to promote health literacy, improve the health status amongst the rural population and thus lower the burden on the current health system of the developing countries. Considering the financial status of the target population, this model would need to be funded by the government.

The assessment of the cost-effectiveness of mobile health applications still needs to be done. It is a critical step as it will promote adoption by the government. Future research can be focused on exploratory/developmental research applications to study the adaptation and cost effectiveness of an innovative mobile health technology which is specifically designed for LMIC's. Future research could also focus on the health outcomes associated with the implementation of the new technology.

REFERENCES

Adams, R. J. (2010). Improving health outcomes with better patient understanding and education. *Risk Management and Healthcare Policy*, *3*, 61–72. doi:10.2147/RMHP.S7500 PMID:22312219

Africa, S. (2014). Consumer Emerging Markets.

Beratarrechea, A., Lee, A. G., Willner, J. M., Jahangir, E., Ciapponi, A., & Rubinstein, A. (2014). The impact of mobile health interventions on chronic disease outcomes in developing countries: A systematic review. *Telemedicine Journal and E-Health : The Official Journal of the American Telemedicine Association*, *20*(1), 75–82. doi:10.1089/tmj.2012.0328 PMID:24205809

Berkman, N. D., Sheridan, S. L., Donahue, K. E., Halpern, D. J., Viera, A., Crotty, K., & Viswanathan, M. et al. (2011). Health literacy interventions and outcomes: An updated systematic review. *Evidence Report/technology Assessment*, (199): 1–941. doi:10.1059/0003-4819-155-2-201107190-00005 PMID:23126607

Bolton, P., Hausman, V., & Keisling, K. (2011). Building Partnerships that Work: Practical Learning on Partnering in M-Health.

Davey, S., & Davey, A. (2014). Mobile-health technology: Can it Strengthen and improve public health systems of other developing countries as per Indian strategies? A systematic review of the literature. *Int. J. Medicine & Health*, *4*(1), 40–45. doi:10.4103/2230-8598.127121

Davies, N. (2010). Healthier lifestyles: Behaviour change. *Nursing Times*, *107*(23), 20–23. PMID:21834301

Deshmukh, M., & Mechael, P. (2013). Addressing Gender and Women's Empowerment In M-Health for MNCH An Analytical Framework.

Gandapur, Y., Kianoush, S., Kelli, H. M., Misra, S., Urrea, B., Blaha, M. J., ... Martin, S.S. (2016). The Role of M-Health for Improving Medication Adherence in Patients with Cardiovascular Disease: A Systematic Review. *European Heart Journal - Quality of Care and Clinical Outcomes*. Doi:10.1093/ehjqcco/qcw018

Health, M. (M-Health) information and resources - Fogarty International Center @ NIH. (n. d.). Retrieved from http://www.fic.nih.gov/RESEARCHTOPICS/Pages/MobileHealth.aspx

Hurt, K., Walker, R. J., Campbell, J. A., & Egede, L. E. (2016). M-Health Interventions in Low and Middle-Income Countries: A Systematic Review. *Global Journal of Health Science*, *8*(9), 183. doi:10.5539/gjhs.v8n9p183 PMID:27157176

Islam, S. M., Purnat, T. D., Phuong, N. T. A., Mwingira, U., Schacht, K., & Froschl, G. (2014). Non-Communicable Diseases in developing countries : A symposium report. *Globalization and Health*, *10*(1), 81. doi:10.1186/s12992-014-0081-9 PMID:25498459

Kay, M. (2011). M-Health: New Horizons for Health through Mobile Technologies. *World Health Organization*, *3*, 66–71. Doi:10.4258/hir.2012.18.3.231

Khatun, F., Heywood, A. E., Ray, P. K., Hanifi, S. M. A., Bhuiya, A., & Liaw, S. T. (2015). Determinants of readiness to adopt M-Health in a rural community of Bangladesh. *International Journal of Medical Informatics*, *84*(10), 847–856. doi:10.1016/j.ijmedinf.2015.06.008 PMID:26194141

Lin, J., Sklar, G. E., Sen Oh, V. M., & Li, S. C. (2008). Factors affecting therapeutic compliance: A review from the patient's perspective. *Therapeutics and Clinical Risk Management, 4*(1), 269–286. doi:10.2147/TCRM.S1458

Macpherson, Y., & Chamberlain, S. (2013). Can mobile phones save lives? *BBC Policy Briefing, 7*(February).

Mechael, P., Batavia, H., Kaonga, N., Searle, S., Kwan, A., & Goldberger, A. ... Ossman, J. (2010). Barriers and gaps affecting M-Health in low and middle income countries (Policy white paper).

Mitchell, K. J., Bull, S., Kiwanuka, J., & Ybarra, M. L. (2011). Cell phone usage among adolescents in Uganda: Acceptability for relaying health information. *Health Education Research, 26*(5), 770–781. doi:10.1093/her/cyr022 PMID:21536715

National Council on Patient Information and Education. (2007). Enhancing Prescription Medicine Adherence: A National Action Plan. *Education*, (August), 1–36.

OECD. (2007). Growth Building Jobs and Prosperity in Developing. *Why Growth Should Be at the Heart of Development Policy*.

Pew Research Center. (n. d.). Communications Technology in Emerging and Developing Nations.

Poushter, J. (2016). Smartphone Ownership and Internet Usage Continues to Climb in Emerging Economies. *Pew Research Center*. Retrieved from http://www.pewglobal.org/2016/02/22/smartphone-ownership-and-Internet-usage-continues-to-climb-in-emerging-economies/

Research2Guidance. (2015). M-Health App Development Economic 2015. *Research2Guidance, 5*(November), 35. Retrieved from http://research2guidance.com/r2g/r2g-M-Health-App-Developer-Economics-2015.pdf

Risks, G. H. (n. d.). 2 Results 2.1, 9–27.

Schillinger, D., Grumbach, K., Piette, J., Wang, F., Osmond, D., Daher, C., & Bindman, A. B. et al. (2002). With Diabetes Outcomes. *Primary Care, 288*(4), 475–482. PMID:12132978

Schweitzer, J. (2010). *The Economics of eHealth One of a series of discussion papers published by the M-Health Alliance The Economics of eHealth*. Health San Francisco.

Singleton, K., & Krause, E. M. S. (2009). Understanding cultural and linguistic barriers to health literacy. *The Online Journal of Issues in Nursing*. Retrieved from http://www.nursingworld.org/MainMenuCategories/ANAMarketplace/ANAPeriodicals/OJIN/TableofContents/Vol142009/No3Sept09/Cultural-and-Linguistic-Barriers-.htm

Svensson, J. (2010). *M4D 2010 M4D 2010. Development*.

United Nations Children's Fund. (2013). *Improving child nutrition. The achievable imperative for global progress*. doi:978-92-806-4686-3

Valk, J., Rashid, A. T., & Elder, L. (2010). March – 2010 Using Mobile Phones to Improve Educational Outcomes: An Analysis of Evidence from Asia. *The International Review of Research in Open and Distributed Learning*, *1*(1), 1–11.

Waters, M. (2006). National Health Education Standards.

This research was previously published in the International Journal of Reliable and Quality E-Healthcare (IJRQEH), 6(4); edited by Anastasius Moumtzoglou, pages 4-16, copyright year 2017 by IGI Publishing (an imprint of IGI Global).

Chapter 71

What E–Mental Health Can Offer to Saudi Arabia Using an Example of Australian E–Mental Health

Yamam Abuzinadah
Ministry of Education, Saudi Arabia & RMIT University, Australia

Bader Binhadyan
Ministry of Education, Saudi Arabia & RMIT University, Australia

Nilmini Wickramasinghe
Epworth HealthCare, Australia & Deakin University, Australia

ABSTRACT

Mental health have become a very influential topic around the world due to the increase of mental health issues that have been reported through national research and surveys. Many studies have been done along the years around the barriers in regards to seeking help in deferent countries and communities. This research aims to look closely into these barriers targeting issues and potential solutions, specifically for Saudi Arabia. Recently, the use of e-mental health services have proven to be an effective method to improve is barriers to mental health treatment. However, this chapter addresses the application and suitably of e-mental health programs for Saudi Arabia mental health services. To do so, a case study of Australian e-mental health services was selected to assist with the investigations.

INTRODUCTION

E-mental health is defined as providing treatment and/or support to people with different mental disorders through sensible technologies (Anthony et al., 2010; Christensen and Petrie, 2013b; Whittaker et al., 2012; e-Mental Health Alliance, 2014). E-mental health services have the ability to improve accessibility, reduce cost, provide flexibility, and better consumer interactivity and engagement (Lal and Adair, 2014). A number of the sensible technologies that are used in the delivery of e-mental health are

DOI: 10.4018/978-1-5225-3926-1.ch071

as follow: Short Message Service (SMS); Email; Website/apps; Shat or instant messaging (IM) tools; Social Media; Video/Audio via the Internet; Or Smart phones.

E-mental health services have the ability to overcome issues in the current mental health sector. These services have the ability to improve lack of access due to location, time or financial difficulties or poor mental health literacy (Booth et al., 2004). It also can reduce the load on mental health clinics which will improve the therapists' time efficacy and allow the service to be available for people who need higher level of medical attentions (Jorm et al., 2013; Jorm et al., 2007). However, there are a number of concerns found in the literature. These include lack of quality control; limited only for people with low to moderate mental illnesses; limited to people who are familiar with using technology (Lal & Adair, 2014)

The capability of e-mental can assist developed and developing countries to successfully deal with challenges that are currently exist in their mental health services. This by enabling early intervention and treatment, better promotion methods for various of people with different mental issues (Reavy, Hobbs, Hereford, & Crosby, 2012).

E-mental health is a useful tool to get information, treatments and support anonymously in most programs, which might help people avoiding the feelings of stigma. E-mental health also will help people who live in low population or rural areas, where access to mental health providers may be limited (Christensen & Hickie, 2010).

There is recognition globally that there are challenges to the current accessibility of mental health services. This includes stigma, location, service availability and geographic location (Lal and Adair, 2014; e-Mental Health Alliance, 2014; Gulliver et al., 2010). Besides these challenges, the Saudi Arabia has other challenges, which also found in some Muslim countries, that impact its mental health services accessibility, such as, religious healing (Koenig & Al Shohaib, 2014), gender versions (Al-Saggaf, 2004; Al-Shahri, 2002) and women's legal and social aspects (Saleh, 2014). These aspects are some of the factors that have been found that may impact mental health services delivery in a different way from the case (Australia) (Al-Saggaf, 2004; Koenig et al., 2014; Al-Shahri, 2002; Koenig and Al Shohaib, 2014; Saleh, 2014).

This study is investigating the capability of e-mental health services to facilitate the current mental health sector of Saudi Arabia. This will be by pointing out the potential of e-mental health to deal with challenges that affect the mental health services in Saudi Arabia. To do so, a case study of Australian e-mental health services was selected to assist with the investigations. Due to some of the main issues facing Saudi consumers such as: Mental health service provision, policies and legislations in Saudi Arabia, cultural barriers, stigma and religious healing and gender variation impact and women's legal and social aspects, e-mental health programs will be a productive solution for the mental health sector in Saudi Arabia. E-mental health services indicate significant outcomes to improve the barriers that affect traditional mental health services, as what will be discussed through examples of Australian e-mental health program.

BACKGROUND

Mental Health Service Provision, Policies, and Legislations in Saudi Arabia

Recently, the mental health sector has started to gain attention from Saudi authorities (Binhadyan, Troshani, & Wickramasinghe, 2014). In 2006, the national mental health policy was developed and special mental health programmers in the general medical system were established. The following year the Saudi Arabian Mental and Social Health Atlas was introduced, which aimed to establish a well-developed plan that would improve the quality of mental health services, mental health promotion/education and improve the mental literacy (Al-Habeeb and Qureshi, 2010). Almalki et al. (2011) argue that the aims of the current of mental health act include:

- Improving accessibility,
- Improving the accreditation of professionals and facilities,
- Ensuring better mental health policy and procedure enforcement,
- Protecting patients and their family member's rights,
- 48.93% of the total number of visitors to mental health clinics were women,
- 53.19% were between the age of 15-40,
- Depression 35%,
- Anxiety 36%.

Most statistics of mental illness cases in Saudi Arabia are based on the number of people who actually accessed the services. Between 2006 and 2012, the Ministry of Health (MoH) reported that the total number of outpatients seeking mental health services at public hospitals increased by 59.4% (from 310,848 to 495,484 cases), and the total number of inpatients increased by 12.9% (Moh, 2011; Moh, 2012). Moh (2012) used the International Classification of Diseases (ICD-10) to identify disease groups and reported the following in 2012:

… e-mental health has the potential to provide a better public health intervention on a mass scale through online surveys and data collection, in which will help to reach more audience with more accurate data.

The Saudi community is going through rapid social changes in all areas, and social problems are increasing with the developments and changes in the different aspects of Saudi life, which has become the dominant feature of life as a result of the complexity of social life and the cultural attitudes that go along with the structure and composition of Saudi society. Exposure of individuals to some psychological problems and difficulties has come to be expected under these circumstances; therefore, health care professionals have found that they must assist and guide members of the community who face social and psychological problems resulting from these changes through the creation of reliable channels to guide them to potential solutions to their problems.

According to Al-Krenawi (2005), recent studies have found an increase in cultural acceptance of community psychiatric care services in countries like Saudi Arabia. Nevertheless, counselling is a modern concept in Saudi society that has emerged in social and psychological studies, especially after the society underwent rapid and significant changes in a number of systems and social infrastructure. On the Ministry of Social affairs' (MoSA) official web-site, which is the governing body for social services, the MoSA defines psychological counselling as "a service that aims to help individuals through a professional relationship between mentors and guides, and this relationship is governed by the principles of professional ethics". The MoSA has sought to establish social and preventive guidance units to provide professional counselling for the problems faced by some members of Saudi society and to provide appropriate guidance to them through the many services that are offered (MoSA, 2016). However, one noticeable aspect is the "serious deficiency and lack" of mental health care services in Arab countries

(Al-Krenawi, 2005). The number of professionals working in mental health services still falls far below the demand for such services. Many workers in psychiatric facilities hold minimal training in mental health and social work (Al-Krenawi, 2005). Moreover, mental health related policy and legislation is almost "non-existent" in many Arab countries (Al-Krenawi, 2005).

Cultural Barriers, Stigma, and Religious Healing

A study shows that most religions have ways to practices religious healing and it is not limited to Islam (Koenig and Al Shohaib, 2014; Greenberg, 1997). Religious healing is widely used among Muslims (Koenig et al., 2014). Koenig and Al Shohaib (2014) argue an individual seeks such practice because it increases his/her wellbeing and improves his/her hope and self-esteem and provide a sense of belonging. In Islam, the religious healing is referred to as 'Ruqya' which applied for the healing through reading of the specific verses of the Quran (Rahman, 2014).

Despite the strong belief in the efficacy of religious healing in Islamic treatment, this practice can delay diagnoses and treatment for mental illness, and can increase the stigma (Koenig and Al Shohaib, 2014). In Saudi Arabia more than 50% of people first sought the advice of a religious healer for different mental illness (Al-Habeeb, 2002; Alosaimi et al., 2014). A pervious study shows that the majority of people who consult religious healers were suffering from depression and anxiety (Alosaimi et al., 2014). The knowledge of mental illness and stigma associated by religious healers is directly related to their educational level according to Al-Habeeb (2002). He also argues that religious healers do not refer their patients to a mental health clinic or express interested in working with mental health professionals due to many religious and social factors.

Gender Variation Impact and Women's Legal and Social Aspects

Due to many differences between males and females in roles and responsibilities in Saudi Arabia, it is noted in many published papers (Al-Krenawi & Graham, 2000) that this will have a major impact on women's mental heal and wellbeing. Gender is "a critical determinant of health, including mental health. It influences the power and control men and women have over the determinants of their mental health, including their socioeconomic position, roles, rank and social status, access to resources and treatment in society" (Astbury, 2001). In regard to seeking help in such a society, studies have shown that women will have a more positive attitude than men in regard to seeking professional help e.g counseling. Hence, men and women have different attitudes to seeking help (Haj-Yahia, 2002). Some studies have suggested that traditional gender roles may impact a person's decision in regard to seeking professional help which may affect their attitude as a women or a man about seeking help. In general, men are more affected by gender roles which may identify them as being "independent and in control" (Daoud et al., 2014).

Globally, most healthcare facilities allocate patients to shared rooms based on genders. However, The Saudi Health Services follow stricter sex-segregation. This is because Islam requires that men are prohibited to mix with unrelated women and this applies to the work environment, education, hospitals (Al-Saggaf, 2004). This means male patients are examined by male mental health professional, and female patients are seen by female mental health professional. To meet these requirements is a challenge that mental health services delivery in Saudi currently faces. Quite often, men demand a female doctor to examine their female relatives, or a female will be refused to be seen by a male doctor (Al-Shahri, 2002). This power relationship between men and women might influence access to mental treatment.

According to Haj-Yahia (2005), the occupational structure of patriarchal societies leaves women with very few alternatives. However, the availability and perceived status of occupations and jobs open to women are inferior to those available to men, which will affect women's incomes and their dependence on their family members or "guardians" (Haj-Yahia, M. 2005). This effect may lead to emotional and mental disorders such as anxiety and by default this will affect their children's lives. He gives an example of Palestinian society in Israel which is a Middle Eastern society that shares many concepts with Saudi Arabian society. For this and other reasons, in many cases Palestinian women earn less than men who are employed in the same jobs. Without having access to good jobs, women will continue to be economically dependent on their spouses or partners (Haj-Yahia, 2005). Economic dependence is one of the factors that force battered women to continue living with a violent spouse. For them, divorce or separation means poverty (Haj-Yahia, 2005).

Depression is the most diagnosed mental illness globally and it is found in women more than men (Piccinelli & Wilkinson, 2000). In Saudi Arabia, 50.19% of visitors to psychiatric clinics were women (Moh, 2011). Many other social issues affect women more than men in Saudi Arabia. Divorce is one major example which might have a direct impact on Saudi women's mental health wellbeing. Unfortunately, Saudi Arabia has the highest divorce rate among the Gulf Cooperation Council countries at 35% and are also above the world average rate of 22% (Saleh, 2014). Another example is women limitation in moving freely out and about due to insufficient public transport and the public cultural ban on women against driving their own vehicles (Alghamdi & Beloff, 2014). Due to that, the access for mental health services for women might become a challenge.

The negative impacts of the factors mentioned earlier are some of the barriers to mental health access and treatment in Saudi Arabia. As mentioned, the number of people seeking mental health attention is increasing, which can be a challenge mental health providers may face in the future. Therefore, the need for e-solutions that will make more productive mental health sector is needed. E-mental health services indicate significant outcomes to improve the barriers that affect traditional mental health services.

METHODOLOGY

This study was conducted as a document review for the purpose of understanding the current Australian literature on e-mental health and it relevance to applying the knowledge in Saudi Arabia. E-mental health in Saudi Arabia has not been previously explored and it lacks defined characteristics. As such, an exploratory qualitative research method is the most suitable method and a single case study will be used (Yin, 2008). At this stage of the research, the answer to the research question of "How are e-mental health services implemented to facilitate the current mental health in Saudi Arabia?" will be examined and explored.

Case Study: Australian E-Mental Health Development

The Australian government is investing heavily in e-mental health services because of technology can assist in overcome issues that are preventing young people from seeing mental health services and providers and creating barriers to treatment. Problems include; lack of access of mental health services due to location, time or perhaps financial matters (Booth et al., 2004); stigma incurred by seeing a therapist (Burns, Davenport, Durkin, Luscombe, & Hickie, 2010; Christensen & Hickie, 2010) and therapist time and efficacy (Jorm, Wright, & Morgan, 2007). Reynolds, Griffiths, and Christensen (2011) argue that there are two types of e-mental health programs in Australia:

According to the e-mental health alliance (2014), there are five main types of e-mental health programs, they have summaries it in:

1. Health promotion, wellness promotion and psycho-education such as Byondblue.
2. Prevention and early intervention support and assessment such as MoodGym.
3. Crisis intervention and suicide prevention diagnostics tools and screening methods such as LIFELINE.
4. Treatment these programs are designed to treat or manage specific mental illness such as depression and anxiety such as myCompass.
5. Recovery and mutual peer support Blueboard.

The Australian Government has invested $70.4 million to date in developing and funding e-mental health services and telephone crisis assistance, also the Australian Government will invest a further $110.4 million in the next four years targeting young adults (Australian Govermment, 2012). In addition, an estimate conducted between 2012 - 2013 showed that 96.5% of 15- to 24-year olds use the Internet in Australia (Australian Bureau of Statistics, 2014). This commitment to adoption of technology in Australia makes the country a potentially rich site in which to consider possibilities.

Finding and Discussion

To be able to the service provision will help identify the need for e-mental health programs. There is a difference between the types of mental health service provider in Saudi Arabia compared to Australia.

In Australia, Mental health patience and or the consumers of such services will be able to access more mental health providers and will have a variety of workers, doctors and/or nurses to help (WHO,2012). According to the mental health atlas created by WHO. Table 1 summarizes the type of mental health service providers with some example in comparison between Saudi Arabia and Australia.

Table 1.

Type of Service Providers	Saudi Arabia	Australia
Psychiatrics	Available mostly to prescribe medicines, First point of contact	Available to give some therapy and prescribe medicine if needed
Psychologists	Limited, due to insufficient training programs	Available to give therapy, diagnose and refer to other services
Counsellors	Not available	Available to support, give therapy and refer as needed
Social workers	limited due to insufficient training programs	Available to provide support with other issues patency may face, therapy, referral and education
Mental health nurses	Available to practice in psychiatric units in hospitals only	Available to provide support, therapy, medicine instrumenting in and out of the hospital
Allied health (Other therapy and lifestyle intervention)	unknown	Available to provide therapy, other support service "meditation, e.g." mental health education, referral to services

In Table 1, it is noted that mental health provider maybe limited in access and resources, and many of the service provider may find it challenging to service people with mental health issues and their families due many factor such as: insufficient training, limited resources, gender role, local availability, and ease of access.

In regards to e-mental health, a new intuitive by the name "Qareeboon" which is an Arabic word referrer to "close" or being close is recently offered through the National Committee for the promotion of mental health (NCPMH) in Saudi Arabia. It was launched September 2013 as an online application. This application works on all smart devices. NCPMH climes on their website, that it is managed by consultants and specialists in the Saudi mental health field. Their websites suggest that the application is the first of its kind in the Middle East on smart devices. The application makes it possible to write a psychological consulting requests (free of charge), which are answered by consultants, psychologists and specialists in this field.

The application contains: Mental health educational materials (like: sings symptoms, issues) techniques to deal with emotional distress through visual content. Such as images and info-graphics, daily updated information, specialist educational text Variety content suitable for both genders and all age groups. Moreover, a link to communicate with suitable mental health providers.

The application however dose not state reliable references and the resource of the data and content available for consumers, and there is no evidence for any research conducted to come up with the content, or any recent scientific reference available on their website whatsoever. Furthermore, when targeting the Saudi consumer, such applications need to cautious with the presenter of the video material and content as it is a male, some consumers might feel it is only targeting male audience due to the cultural sensitivity with gender role in Saudi Arabia (Al-Krenawi, 2014). Moreover, the application does not direct people to further knowledge such as other websites, books, and/or any other useful resources. Also, it is not integrated to any other e-mental health services if exist. However, the application might be improved and enhanced and it will be a stepping stone for e-mental health in Saudi Arabia, as it has good potential.

FUTURE RESEARCH DIRECTIONS

E-mental health is an emerging new field of research and there is limited literature was conducted on the use of E-mental health in Saudi Arabia (Binhadyan, Peszynski, & Wickramasinghe, 2016; Binhadyan et al., 2014). Further research in e-mental health application and benefits will contribute to further understanding the Saudi consumers' concepts, beliefs, perspectives and attitudes toward mental health issues and service access. It will also help to understand some of the obstacles and difficulties they face to access/use available social and welfare services and how e-mental health could be the answer. The program reviewed earlier "Qareeboon" will be a good start, with further enhancement it will have good grounds to further the potential of e-mental health in Saudi Arabia. Also, due to some of the implications on e-mental health, such as internet access and literacy, further studies need to examine the challenges that might encounter Saudi consumers when using e-mental health programs.

CONCLUSION

The service provision, policies and legislations in Saudi Arabia, the stigma of mental illness, Gender variation and all the issues that is facing the Saudi consumer in Saudi Arabia plays a major role in affecting people's attitudes toward mental health in general and its considered a key factor in mental health literacy (Jorm,2013). In terms of literacy, there is a need for accurate information about psychotherapy to help reduce public stigma in Saudi Arabia. Education efforts can be applied through e-mental health programs similar to the Australian version of *Beyondblue* reach out and the *Black Dog Institute*. Even brief intervention programs have been shown to have short-term effects on people's attitudes (Pinfold et al., 2003 E-mental health programs can enhances the awareness and the intervention of the evidenced-based medical, psychological and alternative treatments available such as online therapy, scientific knowledge based information about mental health issues, there symptoms and treatments. As a result, people will be more aware of such problems which may be a good tool to decrease stigma and help people with other berries they may face.

REFERENCES

Al-Habeeb, A., & Qureshi, N. (2010). Mental and Social Health Atlas I in Saudi Arabia. *EMHJ, 16*(5).

Al-Krenawi, A. (2014). *Context and Change: The Structure of Arab Society Psychosocial Impact of Polygamy in the Middle East* (pp. 25–50). Springer. doi:10.1007/978-1-4614-9375-4_2

Al-Krenawi, A., & Graham, J. R. (2000). Culturally sensitive social work practice with Arab clients in mental health settings. *Health & Social Work, 25*(1), 9–22. doi:10.1093/hsw/25.1.9 PMID:10689599

Al-Saggaf, Y. (2004). The effect of online community on offline community in Saudi Arabia. *The Electronic Journal of Information Systems in Developing Countries, 16*(2), 1–16.

al-Shahri, M. Z. (2002). Culturally sensitive caring for Saudi patients. *Journal of Transcultural Nursing, 13*(2), 133–138. doi:10.1177/104365960201300206 PMID:11951716

Alghamdi, S., & Beloff, N. (2014). Towards a comprehensive model for e-Government adoption and utilisation analysis: The case of Saudi Arabia. *Paper presented at the 2014 Federated Conference on Computer Science and Information Systems (FedCSIS).* doi:10.15439/2014F146

Almalki, M., Fitzgerald, G., & Clark, M. (2011). Health care system in Saudi Arabia: An overview. *Eastern Mediterranean Health Journal, 17*(10). PMID:22256414

Alosaimi, F. D., Alshehri, Y., Alfraih, I., Alghamdi, A., Aldahash, S., Alkhuzayem, H., & Albeeeshi, H. (2014). The prevalence of psychiatric disorders among visitors to faith healers in Saudi Arabia. *Pakistan Journal of Medical Sciences, 30*(5), 1077. PMID:25225530

Astbury, J. (2001). Gender disparities in mental health. *Paper presented at the 54th World Health Assemble on Mental health Ministerial Round Tables.* Who, Geneva, Switzerland. Retrieved from http://vuir.vu.edu.au/1656/

Australian Bureau of Statistics. (2014). Personal internet use. *8146.0 - Household Use of Information Technology, Australia, 2012-13*. Retrieved from http://www.abs.gov.au/ausstats/abs@.nsf/Lookup/8146.0Chapter32012-13

Australian Government. (2012). *E-mental health strategy for Australia*. Retrieved from http://www.health.gov.au/internet/main/publishing.nsf/Content/7C7B0BFEB985D0EBCA257BF0001BB0A6/$File/emstrat.pdf

Binhadyan, B., Peszynski, K., & Wickramasinghe, N. (2016). Using e-Mental Health Services for the Benefit of Consumers in Saudi Arabia. In N. Wickramasinghe, I. Troshani, & J. Tan (Eds.), *Contemporary Consumer Health Informatics* (pp. 367–377). Cham: Springer International Publishing.

Binhadyan, B., Troshani, I., & Wickramasinghe, N. (2014). Improving the treatment outcomes for ADHD patients with IS/IT: An actor-network theory perspective. [IJANTTI]. *International Journal of Actor-Network Theory and Technological Innovation*, *6*(4), 38–55.

Booth, M. L., Bernard, D., Quine, S., Kang, M. S., Usherwood, T., Alperstein, G., & Bennett, D. L. (2004). Access to health care among Australian adolescents young people's perspectives and their sociodemographic distribution. *The Journal of Adolescent Health*, *34*(1), 97–103. doi:10.1016/S1054-139X(03)00304-5 PMID:14706412

Burns, J. M., Davenport, T. A., Durkin, L. A., Luscombe, G. M., & Hickie, I. B. (2010). The internet as a setting for mental health service utilisation by young people. *The Medical Journal of Australia*, *192*(11), S22. PMID:20528703

Christensen, H., & Hickie, I. B. (2010). E-mental health: A new era in delivery of mental health services. *The Medical Journal of Australia*, *192*(11), S2. PMID:20528702

Gulliver, A., Griffiths, K. M., & Christensen, H. (2010). Perceived barriers and facilitators to mental health help-seeking in young people: A systematic review. *BMC Psychiatry*, *10*(1), 113. doi:10.1186/1471-244X-10-113 PMID:21192795

Haj-Yahia, M. M. (2002). Attitudes of Arab women toward different patterns of coping with wife abuse. *Journal of Interpersonal Violence*, *17*(7), 721–745. doi:10.1177/0886260502017007002

Jorm, A. F., Wright, A., & Morgan, A. J. (2007). Where to seek help for a mental disorder? *The Medical Journal of Australia*, *187*(10), 556–560. PMID:18021042

Koenig, H. G., & Al Shohaib, S. (2014). *Understanding How Islam Influences Health and Well-Being in Islamic Societies*. Springer. doi:10.1007/978-3-319-05873-3_12

Lal, S., & Adair, C. E. (2014). E-Mental Health: A Rapid Review of the Literature. *Psychiatric Services (Washington, D.C.)*, *65*(1), 24–32. doi:10.1176/appi.ps.201300009 PMID:24081188

MOH. (2011). *Statistical Book for the Year 1432*. Retrieved from http://www.moh.gov.sa/en/Ministry/Statistics/book/Documents/1431.rar

NCMH. (2013). Qareeboon. Retrieved from http://ncmh.org.sa/index.php/pages/view/90/15

Piccinelli, M., & Wilkinson, G. (2000). Gender differences in depression Critical review. *The British Journal of Psychiatry*, *177*(6), 486–492. doi:10.1192/bjp.177.6.486 PMID:11102321

Rahman, F. N. (2014). Spiritual Healing and Sufi Practices. *Nova*, *2*(1), 1–9.

Reavy, K., Hobbs, J., Hereford, M., & Crosby, K. (2012). A new clinic model for refugee health care: Adaptation of cultural safety. *Rural and Remote Health*, *12*(1). PMID:22263874

Reynolds, J., Griffiths, K., & Christensen, H. (2011). Anxiety and depression-online resources and management tools. *Australian Family Physician*, *40*(6), 382. PMID:21655483

Saleh, R. H. (2014). *The Supporting Role of Online Social Networks for Divorced Saudi Women. (Masters)*. University of Ottawa.

The National Committee for the promotion of mental health. (2016). Qareeboon. Retrieved from http://ncmh.org.sa/index.php/pages/view/90/15

Wickramasinghe, N., & Binhadyan, B. (2016). *An Investigation of the Role of Using IS/IT in the Delivery of Treatments for ADHD in University Students.*

Yin, R. K. (2008). *Case study research: Design and methods* (4th ed.). Thousand Oaks, Ca: Sage.

This research was previously published in the Handbook of Research on Healthcare Administration and Management edited by Nilmini Wickramasinghe, pages 178-187, copyright year 2017 by Medical Information Science Reference (an imprint of IGI Global).

Chapter 72
Equipping Advanced Practice Nurses With Real-World Skills

Patricia Eckardt
Stony Brook University, USA

Brenda Janotha
Stony Brook University, USA

Marie Ann Marino
Stony Brook University, USA

David P. Erlanger
Stony Brook University, USA

Dolores Cannella
Stony Brook University, USA

ABSTRACT

Nursing professionals need to assume responsibility and take initiative in ongoing personal and professional development. Qualities required of nursing graduates must include the ability to, "translate, integrate, and apply knowledge that leads to improvements in patient outcomes," in an environment in which "[k]nowledge is increasingly complex and evolving rapidly" (American Association of Colleges of Nursing, 2008, p. 33). The ability to identify personal learning needs, set goals, apply learning strategies, pursue resources, and evaluate outcomes are essential. Nursing professionals must be self-directed learners to meet these expectations. Team-based learning (TBL) is a multiphase pedagogical approach requiring active student participation and collaboration. Team-based learning entails three stages: (1) individual preparation, (2) learning assurance assessment, and (3) team application activity.

National health care has undergone a dramatic restructuring where inter-professional teams comprised of nurses, physicians, dentists, social workers, dieticians, pharmacists, and ancillary paraprofessionals deliver healthcare to the US population. This transformation in the health care delivery system has included a call to educate thousands of nurses as advanced care (graduate education completed) providers,

DOI: 10.4018/978-1-5225-3926-1.ch072

and hundreds of thousands as entry-level (undergraduate education completed) providers, to organize and lead these healthcare teams, while delivering direct patient care and conducting outcomes effectiveness research. This is a daunting task, as nurses enter the practice of professional registered nursing from diverse trajectories. As the entry into practice differs, so does the educational pathways through nursing undergraduate and graduate studies differ, with many traditional professional nursing educational programs lacking the resources to provide students with the skills required for inter-professional success. Nursing programs also need to meet the challenges of educating nurses who live and practice in communities that historically do not have access to academic medical center care and education. In this chapter, we outline how programs of nursing studies within universities and colleges can meet these challenges, by incorporating innovative methods for curricula delivery and learning evaluation. Computer-based education is a critical component for successfully educating nurses- particularly when these nurses are located throughout the world serving in the armed forces or with a humanitarian mission. This chapter provides exemplars of how to prepare nurses with the real-life skills needed to practice in and lead inter-professional care delivery and research teams across their communities. These three case studies illustrate the effectiveness of three distinct computer-based innovative approaches to curricula and evaluation: a social cognitive constructivist approach to graduate nursing computer- based statistics education, a team-based learning approach to undergraduate nursing computer-based statistics education, and a hybrid (face to face and computer-based sessions) team science approach to advanced practice nursing education. The incorporation of these approaches within advanced and entry level practice nursing programs can provide the essentials for the clinical real world- patient practice skills needed to deliver quality patient care to complex patient populations.

BACKGROUND

Current State of Health Care Delivery System and Nursing Curriculum Response

The national healthcare delivery model has changed drastically over the past few years and further changes are underway. These changes include who provides primary healthcare, where the healthcare is delivered, guidelines for health management of populations, and reimbursement and accountability for healthcare services payment (Dykema Sprayberry, 2014; Forbes, 2014; Scott, Matthews, & Kirwan, 2014; Spetz, 2014). The nursing workforce in the United States is approximately 3.5 million and is expected to increase over the next ten years (U.S. Department of Health and Human Services HRSA, 2014). Nurses are being called to increase their leadership skills, scientific knowledge and practice competencies, educational preparation and to practice to the fullest extent of their education (IOM, 2011).

As the educational and competency requirements increase and role definitions for practice models expand, nursing curriculum content and delivery methods have changed in response (AACN Essentials for Education, 2010, 20111, 2012). However, faculty is insufficient to provide the expertise required to deliver the curriculum and evaluate student learning. Faculty are insufficient in number and often in training to meet the suggested curriculum essentials (IOM, 2011). Faculty lack of preparation in research and statistical knowledge are cited across programs as a roadblock to preparing our students to meet the new educational and practice environment demands (Hyat, Eckardt, Higgins, Kim, & Schmeige, 2013).

Nursing student populations are more diverse than ever. Many students are now entering nursing programs after attaining undergraduate and graduate degrees in other disciplines, and some specific student populations, such as males and minorities, are increasing as compared to the trajectories of the past twenty years (Banister, Bowen-Brady, & Winfrey, 2014). To increase the number of nurses educated to practice, and meet the new guidelines, nursing programs now offer many different pathways to the entry and advanced levels of practice (AACN, 2012). For example, some schools admit students from high school for programs that lead to doctoral degrees, while in contrast, others admit only master's prepared nurses to doctoral programs of study (Starr, 2010).

In addition to the changes within the healthcare system in the US, and the nursing professional and educational environments, the way that information is shared on an individual, local, and global level has been revolutionized by the computer and the internet. Like much of the world's citizens, nursing students and faculty rely on the internet and computers for personal, social, and educational needs. The reliance on the internet and computer usage for daily information has a significant impact on the needs and learning patterns of students and educators and should be considered when structuring curriculum delivery and evaluation (Costa, Cuzzocrea, & Nuzacci, 2014).

Nursing educators have been incorporating elements of computer –based learning into nursing curriculum for both students and practitioners for over thirty five years (Johnson-Hofer, & Karasic, 1988; Love, 1974). However, the incorporation has not been uniformly implemented or evaluated across the discipline. Reasons for lack of continuity in implementation are resource availability, attitudes and beliefs towards technology adoption, and organizational constraints (Chow, Herold, Choo, & Chan, 2012). Regardless of reasons for lack of continuity across the discipline in using computer-based learning to deliver curriculum, the need for nursing students to have access to the most current state of nursing science education persists and must be addressed.

Varied approaches to implementing computer-based learning that will successfully meet this need and prepare nurses for practice are currently in practice. Successful adoption of computer-based delivery of curriculum requires evidence of its effectiveness in real-world settings. Due to the resources required for this type of research, investigator-initiated adoption of the various approaches to implementing computer-based learning is feasible only with a pilot or case study design. Funding mechanisms are available for implementation and evaluation of nursing education programmatic redesign in response to the changes in the external environment (Stevens & Ovretveit, 2013). These funding opportunities are from private and governmental sources that are stakeholders in the future of the delivery of health care services (Blum, 2014; Thompson & Darbyshire, 2013). However, these funding sources remain very competitive and most require some evidence of an intervention on a pilot or case study level before consideration for funding support of research of a larger scale. Our faculty have been implementing and evaluating small investigator-initiated studies to lay the foundation for programmatic research initiatives centered on computer- based or computer-supported curriculum delivery. This chapter outlines three investigator-initiated pilot case studies on computer-based curriculum delivery: a social cognitive constructivist approach, a team-based learning approach, and an interprofessional approach to computer-based learning. Each approach provides evidence that supports further investigation on a larger scale.

THREE CHOSEN CASE STUDIES FOR COMPUTER-BASED DELIVERY OF INSTRUCTION

Background for Case Study 1: A Social Cognitive Constructivist Approach to Graduate Nursing Computer-Based Statistics Education

Graduate nursing educators are called to prepare nurse leaders who can engage in higher level practice by deriving and translating evidence from population level outcomes into practice through innovative care models (AACN, 2011). To meet these graduate education essential outcomes requires a sound undergraduate foundational level knowledge of statistics. As a fixed estimate of prior statistical learning is not appropriate given the variability of the population of students, an initial assumption of no prior knowledge at the outset of each learning module is wise. To teach from an initial assumption of no prior knowledge requires an individualized instruction strategy that incorporates a later adjustment in teaching to account for individual students' prior knowledge bases, assumptions around learning, and learning styles. Individualized instruction strategy is an application of social cognitive constructivist learning theory that also provides tools for educators and learners to enhance knowledge retention and knowledge development (Luciano & Ontario Institute for Studies in Education, 2001).

Learning can be framed by four principles:

1. Social and formal education is critical for learning development to occur.
2. Learning is motivated by needs of the learner.
3. Instruction should be scientifically based.
4. Instruction should consider individual differences (Schunk, 2004).

One approach to instruction is one that is: learner-centered, based on knowledge of the skills and processes employed by experts/successful learners (e.g., what does the successful quantitative researcher know), and seeks to help students develop the cognitive processes that are used by "skilled practitioners" (Schunk, Pintrich, & Meece, 2008). This approach fits well for professional nurses who must be skilled in academics of their science as well as their clinical practice.

A grand theory of learning that incorporates other learning theories, such as constructivist, attribute and goal theory, is Bandura's Social Cognitive Theory (Zimmerman & Schunk, 2003). Social cognitive theory stresses the idea that much of learning occurs in a social environment by observing others, and that the individual learner constructs his own knowledge based on prior learning and new information. According to social cognitive theorists, this knowledge construction is a function of triadic reciprocity. Triadic reciprocity is the interaction of the learner's personal factors, behaviors, and environmental factors. Learner personal factors include age, learning style, and personal theory of intelligence. Behavioral factors to consider are self- regulatory behaviors and self-evaluator mechanisms. Lastly, environmental factors may include social setting of instruction, tools used by instructor, and mode of delivery of curriculum (Zimmerman & Schunk, 2001). Computer-based instruction provides the opportunity for manipulation of each of the elements of the triadic reciprocity functions (students' personal factors, behaviors, and environmental factors), and is well-suited for applied statistics content when a constructivist approach is used.

In applied statistics learning, there are two distinct lines of inquiry, computation and conceptualization. Computation involves learning the use of rules, procedures, algorithms, while conceptualization is the learning to use problem solving strategies. Graduate nursing statistical knowledge requirements should focus on conceptualization, with minimal requirements in basic computational skills. With computational skill development, students' errors reflect their knowledge construction and arise from exposure to new problem types or poor knowledge of facts. A key goal of computation instruction is for the learner to use the most efficient strategy to solve a problem. Computational skill is first represented as declarative knowledge, facts about steps are memorized through mental rehearsal and overt practice; after more practice, representation becomes "domain-specific procedural representation" and eventually full automaticity is achieved. In conceptualization, problem solving involves problem translation, and problem categorization. Here, students must accurately identify the problem type through relevant information, then select appropriate strategy. Problem categorization requires student to attend to problem type rather than content resulting in deep instead of surface structure learning (Schunk, 2004). Conceptualization allows for a generalization of knowledge to a different problem, and can incorporate elements of computational skill. Computer-based podcast and video cast libraries that are linked by problem type and also by content augment this process. Generalization is an example of authentic learning (Zimmerman & Schunck, 2003). Authentic learning is a deep understanding of learned material that can be demonstrated by the application of knowledge gained in one setting to another setting or situation. Nurses are very familiar with authentic learning in their clinical practices as generalization needs to occur when treating multiple patients and various patient subpopulations.

A social cognitive constructivist approach to instruction allows the teacher to provide authentic learning in the virtual classroom through learning that is vicarious, peer learning, and active learning. Vicarious instruction is when the student learns through observing expert solution to a problem. Peer learning and active learning is such that a student accommodates or assimilates knowledge through scaffolded direction. Through a consideration and manipulation of the elements of triadic reciprocity, a constructivist approach to education promotes and demonstrates outcomes of deep authentic learning. Computer-based learning tools, such as interactive synchronous lesson reviews, podcast libraries of specific problem steps and solutions that can be reviewed as often as needed, and computer-simulated distribution construction can be integral to vicarious, and peer and active learning for graduate nursing students.

Vygotsky's sociocultural perspective of learning provides a constructivist theory of learning within a social cognitive framework for statistical learning (Henson, 2003). This perspective of learning emphasizes the importance of society and cultural environment of learning for promoting cognitive growth and knowledge development. Social interactions during the learning process are critical, as knowledge is co-constructed between two people, such as the teacher-student dyad or the student-student dyad. In the computer-assisted learning environment the instructor can continually engage students in meaningful and challenging activities, and help them perform those activities successfully even when in an asynchronous format. The social setting of the graduate online computer-based classroom is ideal for the formation of multiple dyadic learning experiences, as well as reciprocal experiences that involve more than two persons through active and vicarious learning. Both active and vicarious learning involve self-regulation of learning.

Self-regulation is an important component of learning in constructivist learning theory, and is developed through internalization (developing an internal representation) of actions and mental operations that occur in social learning interactions. Learning development occurs through the cultural transmission of tools, such as language and symbols. Language is the most critical tool as it aids in learning for self-regulation by internalizing others' speech (professor or peers) to develop private speech to guide learning and steps of problem solving, that eventually becomes covert speech (or inner speech) to guide and direct problem solving and learning. An example of this is the mouthing of words as you read a manuscript with new language, such as this one. You have mastered reading, now you are mastering the application of Vygotsky's learning theory components with private speech in an online nursing curriculum. The development of inner speech is nurtured by accessible and repeatable on-line lecture libraries of course lessons that students can view and play and practice as often as needed individually. Inner speech is further honed as a skillset in the asynchronous and synchronous discussion threads available to students throughout the semester. Participation is neither graded nor mandatory, but rather gentle redirection and discussion points and worked examples are inserted into the discussions by the professor. These discussion formats are not available in traditional classroom settings.

The use of the tool of language for learning occurs within each student's individual zone of proximal development (ZPD). The ZPD is the difference between what statistics students can do on their own in constructing new knowledge, and what they can do with interaction. Interactions with peers and professors (competent others) in the ZPD promote cognitive development. Obuchenie is a term used by Vygotsky that represents the interaction between teaching and learning and occurs within the ZPD through scaffolding. Scaffolding of students is the guided instruction of students into new knowledge development that is outside of their current domain. Scaffolding provides continual feedback and clarification as students incorporate new learning of the language and tools of statistics into their existing framework, also known as schema (Niess, 2005). The new knowledge development and its association to existing schema generalize the knowledge and result in increased authentic learning. Scaffolding and teaching within the ZPD can be achieved with an online computer-based approach to teaching graduate statistics. Using the resources available to them such as an online stats knowledge portfolio, instructor created podcast lesson library, virtual office "minutes"- as often as needed increases the opportunity for each student to have an educational experience that is tailored to their unique learning needs.

Situated learning is a familiar model in nursing clinical practicum educational settings, and can also be applied to a cognitive constructivist approach to teaching graduate statistics. The learner begins by studying a model of an expert's approach to the problem. Experts' approaches tend to focus on deeper aspects of problem rather than its surface features. The learner engages in vicarious knowledge acquisition by observing the expert with a worked example. An example of this is the observation of graduate students as the expert provides coaching for statistical approach and analysis to "real world-real time" questions brought by other students and faculty to the virtual classroom setting. This use of "real world-real time" worked examples for statistical learning involves the use of situated cognition by the expert and the novices.

Although instructional design approaches, such as the novice to expert, typically begin with analysis of skills entailed by performance of expert, this task analysis of expert performance does not capture the expert's capacity to respond to the variability in the real work situation, whereas the situated learning worked examples does. Here the talk- alouds of the expert are genuine and demonstrate the responsiveness of the expert's decisions for design and analysis to the incremental information elicited from and then provided by the novice practitioner engaged in the situated learning dyad. Though these exchanges require expertise and comfort in full exposition of thought by the teacher, they also provide a cross-sectional view into the machinations of decision-making and refining of decisions during statistical problem solving of real issues. Situated learning examples are incorporated into a graduate statistics course with invited expert nurses bringing their research proposal or project to the virtual classroom for a statistical consult within the classroom setting by the expert faculty. This is an introduction to application of statistics within a practice setting for students who are being prepared to lead healthcare delivery reform in their current practices.

Using a social cognitive constructivist approach to the design and delivery of graduate nursing online computer-based statistics education allows the teacher to employ multiple modalities of instruction, and teaching aids and add-ons while also individualizing student mentoring and resources to meet each student at their ZPD. The following Case Study A describes and evaluates the effectiveness of this approach over one semester of instruction.

Application Case Study 1: The Effect of a Social Cognitive Constructivist Teaching and Evaluation Approach on Graduate Student's Statistical Efficacy and Knowledge

The aim of this case study was to explore the effect of approaching online graduate nursing course in statistics from a social cognitive constructivist approach for one semester (Spring 2011). The course had been developed in an online computer-based format and delivered in a static mode (read a posted presentation, answer test exam questions, receive a grade) for the previous four semesters. A secondary goal of the case study was to provide data from the student and professor perspective that supported a paradigm shift for delivery of all quantitative method curriculum in the social cognitive constructivist framework within the School of Nursing graduate nursing program.

Methods

This was a retrospective observational mixed methods case study. A grounded theory approach to the analysis of the qualitative data was used and descriptive data for the analysis of quantitative data.

Sample

The convenience sample (n=36) consisted of graduate nursing students from one school of nursing and three graduate nursing programs from one semester. The students represented the larger nursing school graduate student population in regard to demographics (age, gender, and race), entry level into programs, program of study, and placement in course progression.

Setting

The school of nursing graduate program is a part of a large suburban academic medical center health sciences center in the Northeastern United States. Students within the graduate program have applied and been accepted into a program that was delivered completely on-line except for clinical practicums that additionally required on-site intensive curriculum. Students are in their second to third semester of their programs, on average, when they take this course. This is the only graduate statistics course in the curriculum for all students in the graduate nursing program. A prerequisite of an undergraduate statistics course within ten years prior to admission to the program is required. This course is a 15 week 3 credit statistics course with a state approved course outline and syllabus.

Intervention

The state-approved curriculum was unchanged for the case study. The delivery of the material and the supporting resources presented on-line and via add-ons such as Skype and FaceTime and google chat were additions to mode of delivery and support. A self- assessment of statistical knowledge was completed by students before coursework commenced. The self-assessment included twenty basic statistical knowledge questions and definitions and a 0-10 Likert scale to rank their statistical knowledge and competence. After self-assessments were completed, a library of podcasts and interactive skill-building applications were made available to students on the course webpage. To support all learning styles and encourage vicarious and peer learning, students were given the choice to work individually or in teams of up to four members for all assignments. Students were given the chance to submit assignments as many times as needed to meet the course objectives. Each iteration of the assignment that was submitted was graded and given individual feedback from instructor using a shared computer screen of the submission and a voice-over and highlighter marking points to discuss and revisit. A worked-example, or exemplar, of each assignment was available to students for comparison and contrast to their own assignments to increase knowledge building. Discussions with students and student groups were available by appointment through non-traditional office "minutes" via phone, shared computer screen, and through various applications such as: Skype, google chat, FaceTime, GoToMeeting, and join.me. The seven course assignments all built upon each previous assignment and culminated in a final project where the goal was to incorporate all prior summative evaluations and resubmit their previous summative work product. The final also included a narrative section for students to describe their experience with the course delivery and their beliefs about their statistical efficacy after taking the course.

Results and Discussion

A total of 35 students (97%) who began the case study course completed it. The one student who dropped the course did so after one week as they left the program all together for health reasons. The students were majority white women (70%) enrolled in the neonatal nursing program (60%), with an average age of 35 years. Most students chose to work in teams (77%) while some students chose to work independently (23%). All students resubmitted at least one assignment, and the majority of students resubmitted over half of the assignments (82%). Students self –efficacy pre-course assessment for statistics was an average of 3.34 (SD 2.07). The qualitative data after the course ended was analyzed using a grounded theory framework. Two researchers read the responses and coded independently and grouped into themes independently then met to compare common themes identified. Themes that emerged were: feeling better about statistics; importance of statistics applied to practice; pride with own ability; high satisfaction with course structure; high satisfaction with professor availability and feedback. Saturation was reached on each theme that emerged after 14 narratives analyzed. Feedback from students at their program exit evaluation (twelve months and eighteen months after course completion) continued to demonstrate authentic learning and self-efficacious belief with statistical application to practice and studies. Students reported using the knowledge acquired in the statistics course within their practice settings to appraise research reports for application to patient care, and also reported using the skills obtained in other course assignments (e.g. Research and advanced pharmacology courses). One student reported at the end of the program that the "statistics course took the distant out of distance learning". Though anecdotal this comment provided additional support for this approach to graduate statistics education.

The results are limited due to the non-experimental nature of the course and lack of randomization, a control group, and a pre and post- test of the same measure. The results however do provide support for a social cognitive constructivist approach to graduate statistics course delivery. However, as this framework and approach to teaching and evaluation requires faculty resources of time and comfort with technology, the availability of such faculty can be a limitation. An effective constructivist approach to teaching entails competence in three areas: *content knowledge, pedagogical content knowledge, pedagogical knowledge* (Shulman, 1987). This requires faculty preparation in each area. There are varied approaches to attaining these faculty competencies. Some involve the use of experts in each area to co-teach or scaffold educators through identified areas of lack of expertise, while others suggest additional education of professors or interdisciplinary approaches to statistics education (Garfield, Pantula, Pearl, & Utts, (2009).

Implementing the constructive approach requires a shift in thinking and a willingness to be open to change for nurse educators. It likely that instructors' of statistics learned statistics under the traditional problem solving model of instruction, in a lecture based classroom setting and with a focus on computations and methods. Utilizing technology, recent findings from statistics education research, and planning active learning activities and exercises may initially involve substantial effort and time investment. The potential reward of such efforts may include transforming student attitudes and mindsets towards the topic of statistics into one of fun, excitement, enthusiasm, and deeper understanding of its relevance and practical use.

Conclusion

There are no known standardized competency guidelines or curriculum standards for teaching statistics to nursing students. The AACN essentials publications only vaguely refer to a need for students to learn something about statistics. This is especially problematic for nurse faculty developing curricula for graduate nursing students. For example, the PhD Essentials publication (AACN, 2010) only includes a single mention of statistics on page 5, citing the phrase "Advanced research design and statistical methods" in the section on Expected Outcomes and Curricular Elements. This brief mention is not informative or useful in developing course objectives, deciding on course content, pedagogy, or depth of material. Statistics is a stand-alone discipline and is composed of many areas, specialties, and sub-disciplines. For example, the meaning and content of "basic applied statistics" may be interpreted quite differently by different statistics educators. There is a great need for tailored degree-specific standardized competency guidelines for teaching statistics to graduate nursing students.

The approach presented here may be useful and effective in addressing many challenges that naturally arise with teaching statistics to graduate nursing students. Some of these challenges may include the diversity in student background and preparation for statistics coursework, the anxiety and fear of the topic, and the daunting task of balancing didactic and clinical coursework in an already full nursing curriculum. The case study described here provide a computer-based approach to meeting the challenges of educating nurses in statistics within a social cognitive constructivist framework. The timeliness of this approach to instruction is well aligned with the focus on patient centered care and personalized medicine and will serve to address the need for graduate nursing students to learn and understand statistics.

Background for Case Study 2: A Team-Based Learning Total Computer-Based Undergraduate Nursing Statistics Course

The TBL strategy was conceived by Larry Michaelsen in the late 1970's to allow for the benefit of small group learning in large classes (Parmelee, Michaelsen, Cook, & Hudes, 2012). According to Michaelsen, at that time he was a professor of Business at the University of Oklahoma and he developed TBL as a solution to better know what students were thinking during his lecturing, and to provide them with opportunities for engaging in real-world problems they would face after graduation (Parmelee et al.). In 2001, the US Department of Education Find for the Improvement of Postsecondary Education funded TBL promotion for faculty development workshops, symposiums, and the scholarship of teaching and learning (Parmelee et al.). At present, TBL is used in more than 60 US and international health science professional schools at several levels of education: undergraduate, graduate, and continuing education (Parmelee et al.).

According to the literature, there are four reasons use of TBL in higher education is rapidly being adopted. One reason is the increased need for active engagement of students in larger classes while maintaining positive student learning outcomes, and TBL provides this opportunity (Parmelee, Michaelsen, Cook, & Hudes, 2012). Another reason is that many higher education accrediting agencies are requiring that schools document student active learning and using the established TBL pedagogical approach makes this possible (Liaison Committee on Medical Education, 2011). Additionally, students must be equipped with real-world skills needed to work with interprofessional teams, which TBL enforces (Interprofessional Education Collaborative Expert Panel, 2011). Lastly, faculty are increasingly frustrated with poor attendance at lectures, and using TBL requires students to actively participate in their educations (Parmelee et al.).

What Is Team-Based Learning?

Team-based learning is a pedagogical approach designed to scaffold learning through high performing team interactions and provide opportunities for significant learning by engaging the teams (Michaelsen, Knight, & Fink, 2002). It allows students opportunities to learn and apply course materials, develop skills needed for working on teams, and foster appreciation for the team approach to solving intellectual tasks (Millis & Cottell, 1998). Team building follows a trajectory of collaboration that includes four stages: forming, storming, norming, and performing (Michaelsen, 2008). These stages allow the team to become an effective unit.

The TBL approach, designed to encourage team collaboration and impact team outcomes, shifts the passivity of learning to a more active and constructive process (Grady, 2011). Promoting active participation in learning is valued as it has far reaching potential and provides students with skills that impact life-long learning (Li, An, & Li, 2010). The TBL approach design was developed for use in on-site classrooms but the concepts can be adapted to the meet the demands of distance education.

Team-based learning is an established and structured collaborative team approach to education. There is significant evidence to support the benefits of collaborative learning in all disciplines (Parmalee, 2010). Collaborative-problem solving is necessary to ensure 21st century higher education graduates' success. Use of TBL provides collaborative learning opportunities by way of individual and team discovery (Cheng, Liou, Tsai, & Chang, 2014).

In all three stages of TBL, students actively contribute and participate in individual and team learning. Research shows that this type of learning consistently improves student performance (Beatty, Kelley, Metzger, Bellebaum, & McAuley, 2009; Cheng, Liou, Tsai, & Chang, 2014; Chung, Rhee, & Baik, 2009; Grady, 2011; Marz, Plass, Weiner, 2008). Data demonstrates that weaker students have the greatest overall performance improvement with TBL (Koles, Stolfi, Borges, Nelson, & Parmelee, 2010). The literature supports TBL use, in courses using the TBL strategy student overall performance is significantly improved (Carmichael, 2009; Cheng, Liou, Tsai, & Chang, 2014; Letassy, Fugate, Medina, Stroup, & Britton, 2008; Persky & Pollack, 2011; Pogge, 2013, Tan et al., 2011; Thomas & Bowen, 2011; Zgheib, Simaan, & Sabra, 2010; Zingone et al., 2010). The TBL pedagogy allows for all learners a potential for improved outcomes (Fujikura et al., 2013).

Team-Based Learning Design

Teams

Teams are central to the design of the TBL experience. In TBL design, teams are distinctly different than groups. While both teams and groups have more than two members that interact on a common activity, teams are characterized by high levels of individual commitment to, and trust, for the members (Michaelsen, 1999; Sweet & Michaelsen, 2012). The teams of TBL are purposely formed and managed by the instructor. According to TBL theorists, team membership should be diverse, cohesive, and permanent for the term of the course (Michaelsen & Black, 1994; Michaelsen, Black & Fink, 1996). To facilitate diversification of the team, assignments should be made considering student ethnicity, gender, and academic abilities (Michaelsen, Fink, & Knight, 1997). Diversification should promote cohesiveness as it reduces the chance of subgroups based on background factors. Instructors should also consider and avoid including members with previously established relationships when assigning teams (Michaelsen, 1999). Instructor organization of teams is an essential first step in the implementation of TBL design.

The development of the team is essential to the success of TBL. Distance education team development poses challenges, but may be fostered by applying some essential concepts. Evaluating student accountability is a key strategy to encourage team-building. Michaelsen (2008) recommends encouraging team-building within teams by having students conduct peer assessments of team-mates for predetermined percentages of the course grade. The peer-evaluation process reinforces this accountability, and should be used to provide constructive feedback. Team-based learning theorists also recommend public posting of *team learning assurance assessment* scores to encourage competition between teams (Michaelsen, 2008).

The underlying premise with TBL design is that no member of a team outperforms the team as a whole (Michaelsen & Black, 1999). The TBL strategy targets learners at different levels of knowledge and understanding (Fujikura et al., 2013). The TBL design is a multiphase approach that requires students to be active participants in learning (Michaelsen, 1999). The motivation for student participation in the TBL teaching and learning strategy is encouraged by a grading policy that allocates significant and student selected percentages to *learning assurance assessments, peer evaluations,* and *team application activities* (Michaelsen, 1999).

Stages of TBL

There are three stages that makeup the TBL instructional activity sequence (Figure 1). The stages include *(1) individual preparation, (2) readiness assurance assessments, and (3) course concept team applica-*

Figure 1. TBL instructional activity sequence

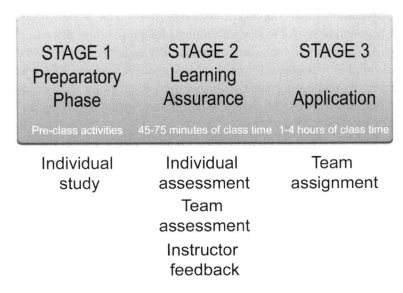

STAGE 1 Preparatory Phase	STAGE 2 Learning Assurance	STAGE 3 Application
Pre-class activities	45-75 minutes of class time	1-4 hours of class time
Individual study	Individual assessment Team assessment Instructor feedback	Team assignment

tion activities (Michaelsen, Sweet, & Parmalee, 2009). When using TBL design, it is recommended the course be divided into approximately five to seven major instructional units over the course of a semester (Michaelsen, 1993). The three stages of TBL are then repeated for each unit.

Stage one of the TBL sequence begins with faculty developing and assigning *individual preparation* to students. This is an individual student activity and completion is required prior to participating in the instructional unit (Michaelsen, Sweet, & Parmalee, 2009). Examples of *individual preparation* include: completion of required readings, viewing of podcasts, reviewing presentations prior to the instructional unit, or gathering data/ evidence on a given topic. Students are accountable for completing this stage and are evaluated on their preparation in stage two.

Stage two in the TBL sequence is *readiness assurance assessments*. These are performed by the students individually and again as a team. According to Michaelsen, Parmalee, McMahon, and Levine (2008), the instructor diagnoses student understanding and provides immediate and frequent feedback during stage two. Diagnosing student understanding is done using the results of the *readiness assurance assessment* (Sweet & Michaelsen, 2012). Since TBL was developed for onsite instruction, *readiness assurance assessments* are recommended to be provided in-class. The *readiness assurance assessment* process was adapted for computer-based learning. Individual *readiness assurance assessments* were provided asynchronously, students were provided a schedule for submission. The *team readiness assurance assessment* is the same examination provided to each individual student, but is now provided to the teams. The team *readiness assurance assessment* for distance education requires team collaboration. The team must complete the team *readiness assurance assessment* synchronously, so the team must establish a time to work collaboratively within the established schedule. The teams are provided immediate feedback through the distance education learning management system. Team *readiness assurance assessment* grades are determined by the number of tries the team requires to choose the correct response. Using the learning management system, these attempts can be tracked. If the team chooses the correct answer on the first attempt, the team earns full credit. If the team takes several attempts to correctly answer the question, the grade earned reflects the number of attempts.

The *readiness assurance assessments* are dependent on the individual student and the student as a team member's participation in stage one, *individual preparation*. The process of assurance assessment promotes individual accountability for materials required for preparation prior to class. Results of the *readiness assurance assessments* are then used by the faculty to focus the review of course content for the major instructional unit (Michaelsen, Parmalee, McMahon, & Levine, 2008). This is possible with computer-based learning by adding rationale with specific resources for each *readiness assurance assessment* topic/ question. According to Michaelsen, Sweet and Parmalee (2009), the entire second stage should take up approximately 45-75 minutes.

Stage three of the TBL sequence involves application of course concepts through in class *team application activities*. The *team application activities* should account for most of the time allotted for the course, upwards of one to four hours per major instructional unit (Sweet & Michaelsen, 2012). The *team application activities* require the team effectively interact and collaborate (Michaelsen, Watson & Black, 1989). *Team application activities* require team collaborative problem-solving, and possibly even more so when computer-based curriculum is delivered.

Ideal *team application activities* of stage three are designed to assess student teams' mastery of subject matter (Michaelsen & Sweet, 2008). *Team application activities* foster accountability within and between teams (Sweet & Michaelsen, 2012). Strong *team application activities* adhere to the "4S's" which denotes that each assignment: be significant to the student, be the same assignment for all teams, require specific choice to be made, and have all teams simultaneously report (Michaelsen, 2008). A significant problem should be an authentic representation of a situation the students would encounter in the professional realm. Answers for the significant problem should be complex and require discussion within the team (Parmelee, Michaelsen, Cook & Hudes, 2012). Every team should be working on the same problem at the same-time, ideally the different teams will each provide alternative answers for the same assignment. The assignment should allow the teams to provide a specific choice for easy distribution to all teams and not lengthy documentation (Parmelee et al.). All teams should distribute their specific choices for the same significant problem at the same-time. This poses somewhat of a challenge with distance education and requires creative use of assignments.

Appeals Process

The TBL design provides opportunity for students to appeal the *team readiness assurance* if they choose to challenge an answer. The appeals process requires the team provide a re-written question or rationale with references supporting the appeal. Only teams that take the steps to write the appeal should be eligible for credit if this is supported (Parmelee, Michaelsen, Cook, & Hudes, 2012).

Peer Evaluation/ Grading Percentages

Student to student peer evaluation is also part of the TBL process and encourages accountability. It is recommended that the students, not the faculty, establish the percentages of the final course grade for the individual and team *readiness assurance assessments*, *team application activities,* and *peer evaluations* (Michaelsen, 1993). This can be done by conducting an anonymous poll with several options for the students to choose percentages.

Peer evaluation ensures student accountability (Sweet & Michaelsen, 2012). This type of evaluation is easily implemented in computer-based learning. Michaelsen (2008), offers standardized evaluation forms that can easily be adapted for distance education, as individual accountability does not change based on curriculum delivery method. It is recommended that peer evaluation be done anonymously, however students should be encouraged to speak directly to their team members providing feedback. There are several models for conducting peer evaluation outlined later in the "Getting Started" section.

Getting Started with Team-Based Learning

An initial and integral part of developing a TBL computer-based learning course includes team formation. There are four principles that should be applied to the team formation process: students are not permitted to self-select, identify determinants of a successful team member, ensure there is representative diversity in each team including success determinants, and make the team assignment process transparent to all students (Parmelee, Michaelsen, Cook, & Hudes, 2012).

Students need to be oriented to the process of TBL. Most higher education students are not accustomed to preparing prior to class as is required with TBL and thus this must be explained to them prior to their participation. Orientation can be accomplished using a module that is a sample session.

As mentioned previously, peer evaluation is an integral part of the TBL process. There are several methods recommended for peer evaluation. Peer evaluations can be quantitative or qualitative. There are guidelines and tools developed by experts for the evaluation of team members that can be utilized. A percentage of the TBL course grade is devoted to peer evaluation and this may be assigned by a team member to a team member or by the faculty. One method is by allowing the team members to assign grades for their teammates based on their interpretation of peer contribution. Another method is for faculty to assign a grade to the team member who is submitting an evaluation of a teammate on the thoroughness and objectivity of the evaluation.

Overall course grade percentages are also integral the TBL design. There is a significant amount of time students devote to preparation and this must be reflected in the overall course grade. Additionally, each component of the TBL process should carry some weight as each is essential: the *individual* and *team assurance assessments*, the *team application activities*, and *peer evaluation*. The grading percentage breakdown can be predetermined by the educator and administration or it can be determined by the students.

Educators must develop TBL modules using backward design (Wiggins & McTighe, 1998). The process of backward design includes three steps in the following order: establish learning goals, develop feedback and assessment activities, and create teaching and learning activities. First the educator must write clear, specific, and meaningful learning goals using Bloom's taxonomy of expertise and mastery. Once these goals are established the educator needs to create or find an authentic interprofessional scenario for the *team application activity* applying the 4 S's. Finally, the educator prepares the *readiness assurance assessment*.

TBL requires faculty development. A formal program for faculty TBL development and support throughout the process should be established prior to implementation. Workshops should be provided to faculty and administration, either by supporting attendance at local and national TBL conferences or by inviting consultants to campus. Creating a TBL community on campus, possibly an interprofessional faculty community is important. Student orientation, as mentioned early is essential for students. Also, collection and review of constructive student feedback is important to the ongoing evaluation of TBL.

Lastly, physical space and environment is important to consider when implementing TBL. The TBL design has been implemented in large lecture halls with fixed seating and some universities have developed classrooms to accommodate TBL teams specifically. Ideally, TBL can be implemented in any setting if the educator has the ability to circulate the space and if all the students are able to speak and be heard by all.

Why Team-Based Learning?

There is significant data supporting the use of collaborative problem-solving in higher education. The TBL process is versatile: it can be adapted for large classes or small classes, it can be used for entire courses or to cover certain topics blending with lectures, it can be applied to onsite and computer-based learning. The team formation of TBL strengthens the team members' abilities to work in teams which is essential especially in the health professions. The advance preparation required with TBL will assist students in developing skills to guide their own learning.

Team-based learning is a structured step-wise approach that allows for collaborative problem-solving for students in a 21st century technology-rich environment. The use of TBL for computer-based learning is a unique opportunity for educators to develop real-world skills in student graduates. There is increasing evidence to support the use of TBL and the academic effectiveness of this collaborative teaching and learning strategy.

Case Study 2: The Effect of a Team-Based Learning Approach on Students' Experiences in an Undergraduate Online Statistics Course

The aim of this case study was to examine the effects of a Team-based learning approach on students' experiences in an undergraduate on-line statistics course to inform further curriculum development with team-based learning design.

Methods

This was a retrospective observational qualitative design. Grounded theory approach to the analysis of the qualitative data was used to identify themes.

Sample and Setting

The sample (n=38) consisted of the students in an on-line undergraduate statistics course. All undergraduate nursing students are required to take a statistics course. Students self-selected into on-line or traditional face- to- face delivery of instruction. Students within the on-line course were comparable to the face-to-face courses in demographic composition. The course was delivered completely online over a fifteen week semester.

Intervention

A systematic approach was utilized to adapt the undergraduate nursing statistics course to a distance education TBL design course. An expert panel was convened that included faculty with nursing education experience, educators with statistical degrees, and TBL design consultants. The process applied to the development and implementation of TBL pedagogy in the distance education undergraduate nursing statistics course for Registered Nurse to baccalaureate students is outlined in the following section.

Before adapting the undergraduate nursing statistics course to a TBL designed computer-based learning course from the traditional distance education the expert panel asked the course faculty to divide the course into five to seven distinct modules. Each module had a theme and specific content outlined. These modules became the foundation for the course design.

Then the expert panel, with the assistance of the course faculty and administration, determined the success determinants for this undergraduate statistics course. The success determinants that were agreed upon included: previous formal statistics courses, and degrees in statistics or related fields. Teams were also comprised of males and females to insure heterogeneity of students in teams.

A formal orientation module was designed for this specific course and to be used in all future courses adapted to include TBL pedagogy. The module required all students log in to the course for this mandatory orientation, the time of the mandatory online orientation was provided prior to registration for the undergraduate nursing statistics course. Once students were officially registered they received an email with an article attached and instructions to read the article prior to the orientation. The article used is available at: http://www.teambasedlearning.org/Resources/Documents/TBL+Handout+Aug+16-print+ready+no+branding.pdf

The orientation module followed the TBL process. The module was delivered using an online video conferencing software. Immediately students were asked to complete an *individual readiness assurance assessment* in the learning management system, this was a timed 10 multiple choice question quiz based on the article assigned. All students were then informed of their groups, which were randomly selected for this activity. They were provided 20 minutes to complete the same *readiness assurance assessment* now as a team. They could see their scores on the *team readiness assurance assessment* with immediate feed-back as the system provided them with a correct or incorrect indicator with each submission. They were provided the opportunity to continue until they chose the correct answer. This was followed by a *team application activity*. The *team application activity* was an assignment that required the students to discuss the merits of TBL and design a grading percentage structure using guidelines provided to them which provided ranges for each of the TBL graded components.

Using all of the grading percentage submissions developed by the teams during the orientation *team application activity* a student poll was anonymously distributed. The students were then permitted to select a grading percentage scale from the submissions. The grading percentage was determined by majority vote.

The process of adapting the asynchronous undergraduate statistics course curriculum began using the backward design. The course was offered in the past as an 8 module course over a 15 week semester to undergraduate nursing students earning a baccalaureate degree in nursing. The expert panel reviewed the former course objectives and adapted them to include language that incorporated the collaborative problem-solving focus of the new curriculum.

The second step with backward design is the development of *team application activities* incorporating the 4 S's. This was accomplished through the efforts of the expert panel using real-world scenarios and creating activities that had significance to the nursing profession with specific choices to conclude. A calendar with dates to allow students a small time-frame to meet virtually was drafted, taking into consideration each students' hectic scheduling. This time-frame and an online forum shared by all students registered for this course allowed for simultaneous submission.

The third and final step with developing a TBL course applying the backward design is composing *readiness assurance assessments.* The course faculty, most familiar with the content and requirements of the undergraduate nursing statistics course, was charged with formulating 10 multiple choice questions for each module. These questions were then loaded into the learning management system for students to take both as individuals and then as virtual teams.

Materials

Distance Education Course Adaptation Checklist

1. Review course objectives.
2. Determine measurable course outcomes.
3. Divide course content into five to seven major instructional units.
4. Establish semester schedule with dates for all TBL modules and activities.
5. Develop all *individual preparation* assignments.
6. Create *learning assurance assessments* using course objectives and measurable outcomes.
7. Adapt *team application activities* to meet measurable outcomes.
8. Apply standardized TBL peer evaluation tools.
9. Implement evaluation protocol for student learning.
10. Use evaluation data to modify as needed.

Procedure

Expert Panel Recommendations for Distance Education Course Sequencing

The expert panel for TBL design implementation in distance education established recommendations for replication. These recommendations are presented as sequencing for course events, with specifics on how these recommendations were operationalized for the nursing statistics course (Table 1).

The nursing statistics distance education course design followed the checklist and recommendations for sequencing. The course was modified over a semester prior to implementation. Students were aware they were enrolled in a TBL designed course as it was described in the course description. Faculty members teaching the course were familiar with the TBL design, and had experience teaching TBL design on-site. The course followed the sequencing, and no unforeseen problems were encountered.

Results and Discussion

The majority of students (74%) completed the course evaluation and narrative responses asked to describe their overall impression of the course, the course structure, and team-based learning. The theories that emerged from the qualitative narratives were: overall satisfaction with team-based learning; enjoyment of the interaction with peers; high perceptions of own ability in the course. As is common with any curriculum delivery design change, there are lessons to be learned. Student buy-in is necessary; therefore, it is important to include the following: (1) background of TBL design to students, (2) the benefits to them as learners, and (3) the expectations required in a TBL course. The peer evaluation process provided some student distress, as students verbalized they did not feel their evaluations should be reflected in a

Table 1. Recommendations for distance education course sequencing

Sequence Recommendation	Implementation Action in Undergraduate Nursing Statistics Course
At the beginning of the course, all students are invited to participate in an anonymous online poll to determine the percentage of the course final grade allotted to each graded TBL segment (*learning assurance assessments, peer evaluations*, and *team application activities*).	Link to anonymous online poll with three (3) options for students to choose from determining the percentage of the course final grade allotted to *learning assurance assessments, peer evaluations,* and *team application activities.* *Option one: learning assurance assessments- 2.5 points Individual/ 2.5 points Team, peer evaluations- 2.5 points,* and *team application activities- 2.5 points* *Option two: learning assurance assessments- 1 point Individual/ 4 points Team, peer evaluations- 2.5 points,* and *team application activities- 2.5 points* *Option three: learning assurance assessments- 4 points Individual/ 1 point Team, peer evaluations- 1 point,* and *team application activities- 4 points*
The course content is divided into five to seven major instructional units.	The course content was divided into the following seven major instructional units: descriptive statistics, inferential statistics, hypothesis testing, correlational techniques, research methods, statistics in epidemiology, and statistics in medical decision making.
Individual preparation assignments should incorporate multiple delivery modalities to engage all learner preferences.	*Individual preparation* assignments include required text readings, podcasts, and power point presentations with animation.
Asynchronous individual *learning assurance assessments* are provided with schedules for submission.	Individual *learning assurance assessments* are provided with a schedule for asynchronous submission.
Synchronous team *learning assurance assessments,* the same examination provided to each individual student, are provided to the teams based on the schedule the team determined.	Team *learning assurance assessments* are provided for synchronous team determined submission.
The teams are provided immediate feedback on team *learning assurance assessments* through the distance education learning management system. Immediate and frequent instructor feedback is provided in the form of rationale and resources. This feedback is provided immediately following final submission of each question on the team *learning assurance assessment.*	The teams are provided immediate feedback on team *learning assurance assessments* through the distance education learning management system. The immediate and frequent instructor feedback is provided in the form of rationale and resources for the topic/ content on the assessment. Feedback is provided immediately following final submission of each question on the team *learning assurance assessment.*
Team *learning assurance assessments* are graded in learning management system based on number of attempts required for correct response. The team grade incrementally decreases with every wrong choice as indicated by the system.	Team *learning assurance assessments* are set up to be graded in learning management system based on number of attempts required for correct, students earn 100% for a correct response first attempt, 75% for a correct response second attempt, 50% for a correct response third attempt, and 0% for a correct response fourth attempt.
Team application activities are course worksheets required for submission.	Seven *team application activities* or course worksheets are required for submission.
Team participation should be enforced by having each student's contribution being acknowledged.	Team participation should be enforced by having each student use a different color ink.
The *peer evaluation* process requires each team member comment on participation of peers. Use of a standardized TBL *peer evaluation* form or development of a new tool.	The *peer evaluation* process had students use a standardized TBL evaluation form available from Michaelsen & Sweet (2008).

classmates final course grade. A solution to this would be to allow students to develop the peer evaluation tool as a group providing faculty guidance and suggestions. As is consistent in the literature, faculty workload with TBL design implementation is increased. Provision of faculty resources and support to assist with the increased work load associated with this change.

Background for Case Study 3: An Interprofessional Approach to a Nursing and Dental Graduate Student Hybrid Course on Team Science Delivery of Community Care

The delivery of care to at-risk and traditionally underserved communities continues to be an issue of unmet access needs for many in the New York area. This care is not limited to medical care, it also includes nursing, dental, and behavioral health care. Of particular issue are the lack of access of at-risk populations to screening and monitoring of health issues to prevent chronic disease and hospitalization. The populations we serve are comprised of multiple at-risk populations: undocumented immigrants and migrant workers, working poor families, and poverty-level elderly (Gaines & Kaimer, 1994; U.S. Census Bureau, 2011). Unmet oral and primary health care needs are more prevalent in individuals whose access to health care services is compromised by a shortage of qualified health providers and/or lack of resources and/or access to multiple healthcare specialties (Allukian, 2008).

Additionally, the provision of quality health care requires a complex response from a team of health professionals. These teams are often called interprofessional healthcare delivery teams. Although interdisciplinarity has become a favored model of care delivery, the assumption that interdisciplinary work is intuitive and can be performed without training is short-sighted (Larson, Cohen Gebbie, Clark, & Saiman, 2001). Interprofessional education requires education in both the machinations of the interprofessional care delivery model and the competency cross-training of care delivery to be successful (Charles & Alexander, 2014). Interprofessional education has instituted in academic medical centers across the United States over the past ten years and is increasing in popularity in response to the health care reformation of the past five years (Bowser, Sivahop, & Glicken, 2013).

The success of the educational initiatives have been evaluated with measures of clinical competencies, interdisciplinary respect and valuing collegiality and practice expertise (Delunas & Rouse, 2014; Larson, et al. 2001). Interprofessional education has been demonstrated to be more effective in clinical competency development and practice expertise with the use of simulated patient experiences with computer-assisted programs. Authentic learning has been demonstrated and participation in activities increased with the addition of on-line self-directed computer-based curriculum to enhance the in-classroom meetings (Clouder, 2008). This mode of curriculum delivery is often called a hybrid model. Interprofessional health care teams educated within a hybrid interprofessional education model will develop cross- disciplinary competencies and mutual respect that supports better health outcomes for at-risk patient populations.

Case Study 3: The Effect of a Hybrid Interprofessional Course on Advance Practice Nurses' and Dental Students' Competencies and Confidence with Health Screenings and Interprofessional Education

Aim: Educators from the Stony Brook University School of Nursing (SON) and School of Dental Medicine (SDM) implemented an interprofessional education (IPE) model that expanded opportunities to engage and educate advanced practice registered nursing (APRN) and dental students to work in interprofessional teams, improve oral-systemic health outcomes and meet professional education standards.

Methods

This was a prospective observational mixed methods study. A phenomenological approach to the analysis of the lived experience of graduate nursing and dental students in a hybrid interprofessional education course was used to interpret the qualitative findings. Simple descriptives analysis was used to examine quantitative data.

Sample and Setting

The sample (n=44) consisted of APRN and dental students enrolled in their first year of studies in the nursing and dental school professional programs. Participants were representative of the populations sampled as enrollment was not optional, but rather was a required course in both programs. The participants were mostly young adult women (68%). The average age was 35 years with a majority of white participants (80%). The nursing and dental students differed in demographics with nursing students comprised of more women, on average older than dental students, and more white participants.

Intervention

The model was designed to enhance confidence and credible familiarity with established screening tools for oral systemic disease. Learning outcomes for the APRN students included becoming conversant and skilled in performing oral cancer screening exams, salivary analysis, denture prostheses evaluation, and caries/periodontal risk assessment. Learning outcomes for the dental students included clinical fluency in the screening and monitoring of hypertension, type 2 diabetes mellitus, and nutritional/hydration status, as well as implementation of a smoking cessation protocol. By targeting the vulnerable elderly community, this initiative was designed to strengthen the utilization of medical and dental screening tools and early referral while expanding the healthcare community's engagement in oral-systemic health issues.

Prior to implementation of the IPE model, APRN and dental students completed assessments regarding their perceived readiness and ability to participate in interprofessional team-based care, and had the opportunity to state their expectations about IPE and provide input regarding IPE activities. To obtain foundational knowledge related to oral health and health promotion, APRN and dental students completed on-line self-directed learning modules which were embedded within each student's program curricula.

Oral health content was delivered through the Smiles for Life program; a free, online, comprehensive oral health curriculum designed specifically for primary care clinicians (Clark, et al, 2010). Students completed the following modules: *The Relationship of Oral and Systemic Health, Adult Oral Health Promotion and Disease Prevention, The Oral Exam*, and *Geriatric Oral Health*. Online modules related to Smoking Cessation and Motivational Interviewing were completed via the Tobacco Recovery Resource Exchange (Professional Development Program, et al., n.d.). Presentations focusing on health promotion and prevention were developed specifically for this program and included instruction on management of diabetic and hypertensive patients, medication reconciliation, and the use of the *Fagerstrom Nicotine Dependence Test* (Heatherton, et al, 1991) and the *Mini Nutritional Assessment* (Vellas, et al., 2006) in clinical practice.

Following the self-study modules, APRN and dental students were brought together to facilitate the development of competencies in interprofessional collaborative practice, including interprofessional teamwork; interprofessional communication; roles and responsibilities; and, values and ethics for interprofessional collaborative practice (IPEC, 2011). The five-hour session began by using interactive strategies to assign students to interprofessional practice teams and team-based learning exercises that include individual and group assessments to evaluate understanding of online self-study materials and discussion of the application of interprofessional principles in clinical practice. Students then engaged in a series of simulated exercises, including faculty-facilitated skills stations and encounters with standardized patients. During these exercises, students applied their knowledge and skills as they engaged in team-based activities related to oral health (e.g., caries and periodontal risk assessment; salivary analysis; head and neck exams), general health (e.g., mini nutritional assessment, tobacco and alcohol assessment, management of diabetes and hypertension), and attainment of interprofessional competencies.

Following these simulated experiences, students once again completed self-assessments regarding their perceived readiness and ability to participate in interprofessional team-based care.

Utilizing the knowledge and skills gained during earlier components of the model, the APRN and dental students were again placed in interprofessional practice teams and engaged in collaborative practice at a state veterans home (SVH). The SDM had a well-established clinical rotation program for dental students at the SVH and the SON established a similar clinical rotation for APRN students to create opportunities for interprofessional collaboration. During their rotations, APRN students had opportunities to join the dental team and participate in the provision of oral health services and dental students had opportunities to participate in medical rounds and interprofessional care planning meetings for SVH residents. Students were evaluated by their respective program faculty and assessed on their ability to work collaboratively as part of an interprofessional team.

The team-based model culminated in an interprofessional oral cancer screening and health promotion community health fair. Student teams provided health care services and health promotion education to veterans, caregivers, and their families living in the community served by the SVH.

Results and Discussion

To evaluate the success of this program, at the conclusion of their experience APRN and dental students evaluated their ability to learn about each other, from each other, and with each other and provided feedback about their ability to work effectively in interprofessional care teams. Several themes emerged:

- Recognition that both APRN's and dentists are primary care providers;
- By working together, APRN and dental students can enhance their knowledge, strategies and approaches to patient care; and
- Interprofessional teams ensure care of the whole patient which lead to improved patient outcomes.

Evaluation data related to specific aspects of the model are helpful to faculty for revising and refining the model. Student evaluation data are especially useful when assisting faculty to plan professional development activities related to teamwork and collaborative practice and for the continuous quality improvement of courses and teaching methods.

Evaluation of the students by faculty of both programs described competence from providers in all areas of clinical and IPE performance. Themes that emerged from the evaluation of the care provided to the community and veteran's home residents and staff were comfort level increase with the provision of care by teams over independent providers and increase in self-care knowledge was also reported. Data regarding the quality of the clinical practice site and experience can inform the development of additional clinical practice environments that facilitate team-based competencies and a culture of collaborative practice.

The resources required to provide this level of IPE and interprofessional health care delivery are significant when compared to traditional delivery model of curriculum resources. The results of this pilot study support further development of further research studies around the effect of IPE and interprofessional health care teams on the student and community health outcomes.

CONCLUSION

Health care reform continues to be a subject of national debate and concern. As the political agenda and representation change over the next few years, constraints around health care delivery models are also expected to change. However, the needs of patient populations and the nurses and the inter-professional teams that deliver their care will not change. Access to quality care for health maintenance and treatment by well-prepared practitioners will always remain a constant. Incorporating advances in technology and computer-based instruction provides nursing educators with the tools needed to meet the increasing demand to educate more nurses while maintaining quality. The model for nursing educational interventions will continue to change and adapt to the world around it in order to meet its populations needs.

Moving forward, the next steps in our research plan include the development and incorporation of psychometrically sound tools to measure the effectiveness of the computer-based models of curriculum delivery within our nursing student populations. Though many tools do exist measuring efficacy of nursing students with computer-based educational interventions, measures of effectiveness of the intervention on learning outcomes are not as convincing. There are many diverse subpopulations of nursing students in graduate and undergraduate courses of study. These populations each need to be assessed for effectiveness of the curricula delivery interventions on a pilot scale before any large scale deployment. The three approaches outlined in the case studies in this chapter are all scientifically and theoretically supported approaches to teaching in other student populations. The daunting task here will be to assure validness and reliability in the effectiveness of these interventions within and between our student subpopulations. We hypothesize this will require adjustment of interventions to be effective for each student phenotype identified. Though this will require multiple iterations of testing and tool development and redesign of interventions, we expect a more robust intervention will be the end product for increased effectiveness of curriculum delivery for our students.

ACKNOWLEDGMENT

The authors would like to thank Ms. Sarah A. Eckardt, MS, and Ms. Amanda Tischler for their continuing assistance and contributions to this chapter.

REFERENCES

Allukian, M. Jr. (2008). The Neglected Epidemic and the Surgeon General's Report: A Call to Action for Better Oral Health. *American Journal of Public Health*, 98(Suppl 1), S82–S85. doi:10.2105/AJPH.98. Supplement_1.S82 PMID:18687628

American Association of Colleges of Nursing. (2008). *The essentials of baccalaureate education for professional nursing practice*. Washington, DC: American Association of Colleges of Nursing.

American Association of Colleges of Nursing. (2010). *The Research-Focused Doctoral Program in Nursing: Pathways to Excellence*. Washington, DC: American Association of Colleges of Nursing.

American Association of Colleges of Nursing. (2011). *The Essentials of Master's Education for Advanced Practice Nursing*. Retrieved August 15, 2015, from http://www.aacn.nche.edu/educationresources/MastersEssentials11.pdf

American Association of Colleges of Nursing. (2012). *New AACN Data Show an Enrollment Surge in Baccalaureate and Graduate Programs amid Calls for More Highly Educated Nurses*. Retrieved August 15, 2015, from http://www.aacn.nche.edu/news/articles/2012/enrollment-data

Banister, G., Bowen-Brady, H. M., & Winfrey, M. E. (2014). Using Career Nurse Mentors to Support Minority Nursing Students and Facilitate their Transition to Practice. *Journal of Professional Nursing*, 30(4), 317–325. doi:10.1016/j.profnurs.2013.11.001 PMID:25150417

Beatty, S. J., Kelley, K. A., Metzger, A. H., Bellebaum, K. L., & McAuley, J. W. (2009). Team based learning in therapeutics workshop sessions. *American Journal of Pharmaceutical Education*, 73(6), 100. doi:10.5688/aj7306100 PMID:19885069

Blum, C. A. (2014). Evaluating Preceptor Perception of Support Using Educational Podcasts. *International Journal of Nursing Education Scholarship*, 11(1), 1–8. doi:10.1515/ijnes-2013-0037 PMID:24615492

Bowser, J., Sivahop, J., & Glicken, A. (2013). Advancing Oral Health in Physician Assistant Education: Evaluation of an Innovative Interprofessional Oral Health Curriculum. *Journal of Physician Assistant Education*, 24(3), 27–30. doi:10.1097/01367895-201324030-00005 PMID:24261168

Carmichael, J. (2009). Team based learning enhances performance in introductory biology. *Journal of College Science Teaching*, 38(4), 54–61.

Charles, G., & Alexander, C. (2014). An Introduction to Interprofessional Concepts in Social and Health Care Settings. *Relational Child & Youth Care Practice*, 27(3), 51–55.

Cheng, C., Liou, S., Tsai, H., & Chang, C. (2014). The effects of team-based learning on learning behaviors in the maternal-child nursing course. *Nurse Education Today*, 34(1), 25–30. doi:10.1016/j.nedt.2013.03.013 PMID:23618848

Chow, M., Herold, D. K., Choo, T., & Chan, K. (2012). Extending the technology acceptance model to explore the intention to use Second Life for enhancing healthcare education. *Computers & Education*, 59(4), 1136–1144. doi:10.1016/j.compedu.2012.05.011

Chung, E., Rhee, J., Baik, Y., & A, O.-S. (2009). The effect of team-based learning in medical ethics education. *Medical Teacher*, *31*(11), 1013–1017. doi:10.3109/01421590802590553 PMID:19909042

Clark, M. B., Douglass, A. B., Maier, R., Deutchman, M., Douglass, J. M., Gonsalves, W., … Bowser, J. (2010). Smiles for Life: A National Oral Health Curriculum. 3rd Edition. *Society of Teachers of Family Medicine*. Retrieved August 15, 2015, from http://www.smilesforlifeoralhealth.com

Clouder, D. L. (2008). Technology-enhanced learning: Conquering barriers to interprofessional education. *The Clinical Teacher*, *5*(4), 198–202. doi:10.1111/j.1743-498X.2008.00243.x

Costa, S., Cuzzocrea, F., & Nuzacci, A. (2014). Uses of the Internet in Educative Informal Contexts. Implication for Formal Education. *Comunicar*, *22*(43), 163–171. doi:10.3916/C43-2014-16

Delunas, L. R., & Rouse, S. (2014). Nursing and Medical Student Attitudes about Communication and Collaboration Before and After an Interprofessional Education Experience. *Nursing Education Perspectives*, *35*(2), 100–105. doi:10.5480/11-716.1 PMID:24783725

Forbes, T. H. III. (2014). Making the Case for the Nurse as the Leader of Care Coordination. *Nursing Forum*, *49*(3), 167–170. doi:10.1111/nuf.12064 PMID:24393064

Fujikura, T., Takeshita, T., Homma, H., Adachi, K., Miyake, K., Kudo, M., & Hirakawa, K. et al. (2013). Team-based learning using an audience response system: A possible new strategy for interactive medical education. *Journal of Nippon Medical School*, *80*(1), 63–69. doi:10.1272/jnms.80.63 PMID:23470808

Gaines, L., & Kamer, P. M. (1994). The incidence of economic stress in affluent areas: Devising more accurate measures. *American Journal of Economics and Sociology*, *53*(2), 175–185. doi:10.1111/j.1536-7150.1994.tb02584.x

Grady, S. E. (2011). Team-Based Learning in Pharmacotherapeutics. *American Journal of Pharmaceutical Education*, *75*(7), 136. doi:10.5688/ajpe757136 PMID:21969722

Hayat, M. J., Eckardt, P., Higgins, M., Kim, M., & Schmiege, S. (2013). Teaching Statistics to Nursing Students: An Expert Panel Consensus. *The Journal of Nursing Education*, *52*(6), 330–334. doi:10.3928/01484834-20130430-01 PMID:23621121

Heatherton, T. F., Kozlowski, L. T., Frecker, R. C., & Fagerstrom, K. (1991). The Fagerstrom Test for Nicotine Dependence: A revision of the Fagerstrom Tolerance Questionnaire. *British Journal of Addiction*, *86*(9), 1119–1127. doi:10.1111/j.1360-0443.1991.tb01879.x PMID:1932883

Interprofessional Education Collaborative Expert Panel (IPEC). (2011). *Core competencies for interprofessional collaborative practice. Report of an expert panel*. Washington, DC: Interprofessional Education Collaborative.

IOM (Institute of Medicine). (2011). *The Future of Nursing: Leading Change, Advancing Health*. Washington, DC: The National Academies Press.

Johnson-Hofer, P., & Karasic, S. (1988). Learning about Computers. *Nursing Outlook*, *36*(6), 293–294. PMID:3186471

Jones, R., Higgs, R., DeAngelis, C., & Prideaux, D. (2001). Changing face of medical curriculum. *Lancet, 357*(9257), 699–703. doi:10.1016/S0140-6736(00)04134-9 PMID:11247568

Koles, P. G., Stolfi, A., Borges, N. J., Nelson, S., & Parmelee, D. X. (2010). The impact of team based learning on medical students' academic performance. *Academic Medicine, 85*(11), 1739–1745. doi:10.1097/ACM.0b013e3181f52bed PMID:20881827

Larson, E. L., Cohen, B., Gebbie, K., Clock, S., & Saiman, L. (2011). Interdisciplinary research training in a school of nursing. *Nursing Outlook, 59*(1), 29–36. doi:10.1016/j.outlook.2010.11.002 PMID:21256360

Letassy, N. A., Fugate, S. E., Medina, M. S., Stroup, J. S., & Britton, M. L. (2008). Using team-based learning in an endocrine module taught across two campuses. *American Journal of Pharmaceutical Education, 72*(5), 103. doi:10.5688/aj7205103 PMID:19214257

Li, L., An, L., & Li, W. (2010). Nursing students self-directed learning. *Chinese General Nursing, 8*(5), 1205–1206.

Liaison Committee on Medical Education. (2011). *Accreditation standards.* Retrieved August 15, 2015, from www.lcme.org/standard.htm

Love, R. L. (1974). Continuing Education Garnished with Computer Assisted Instruction. *Journal of Allied Health, 3*, 86–93.

MacDonald, C. J., Archibald, D., Trumpower, D., Cragg, B., Casimiro, L., & Jelley, W. (2010). Quality standards for interprofessional healthcare education: Designing a toolkit of bilingual assessment instruments. *Journal of Research in Interprofessional Practice and Education, 1*(3), 1–13.

Michaelsen, L. K. (1983). Team learning in large classes. In C. Bouton & R. Y. Garth (Eds.), *Learning in Groups. New Directions for Teaching and Learning Series* (Vol. 14). San Francisco: Jossey-Bass.

Michaelsen, L. K. (1998). Three keys to using learning groups effectively. *Teaching Excellence: Toward the Best in the Academy, 9*(5), 1997-1998.

Michaelsen, L. K. (1999). Myths and methods in successful small group work. *National Teaching & Learning Forum, 8*(6), 1–4.

Michaelsen, L. K., Bauman-Knight, A., & Fink, D. (2003). *Team-based learning: A transformative use of small groups in college teaching.* Sterling, VA: Stylus Publishing.

Michaelsen, L. K., & Black, R. H. (1994). Building learning teams: The key to harnessing the power of small groups in higher education. In S. Kadel & J. Keehner (Eds.), *Collaborative learning: A sourcebook for higher education* (Vol. 2). State College, PA: National Center for Teaching, Learning and Assessment.

Michaelsen, L. K., Black, R. H., & Fink, L. D. (1996). What every faculty developer needs to know about learning groups. In L. Richlin (Ed.), *To improve the academy: Resources for faculty, instructional and organizational development* (Vol. 15). Stillwater, Oklahoma: New Forums Press.

Michaelsen, L. K., Fink, L. D., & Knight, A. (1997). Designing effective group activities: Lessons for classroom teaching and faculty development. In D. DeZure (Ed.), *To improve the academy: Resources for faculty, instructional and organizational development* (Vol. 17). Stillwater, OK: New Forums Press.

Michaelsen, L. K., Knight, A. B., & Fink, L. D. (2002). *Team-based learning: A transformative use of small groups.* Westport, CT: Greenwood Publishing Group.

Michaelsen, L. K., Parmalee, D., McMahon, K., & Levine, R. (Eds.). (2008). *Team-based learning for health professions education: A guide to using small groups for improving learning.* Sterling, VA: Stylus Publishing.

Michaelsen, L. K., & Sweet, M. (2008). Teamwork works. *NEA Advocate, 25*(6), 1–8.

Michaelsen, L. K., Sweet, M., & Parmalee, D. (2009). Team-based learning: Small group learning's next big step. *New Directions for Teaching and Learning, 116,* 7–27.

Michaelsen, L. K., Watson, W. E., & Black, R. H. (1989). A realistic test of individual versus group consensus decision making. *The Journal of Applied Psychology, 74*(5), 834–839. doi:10.1037/0021-9010.74.5.834

Millis, B. J., & Cottell, P. G. Jr. (1998). *Cooperative learning for higher education faculty.* Phoenix, AZ: Oryx Press.

Persky, A. M., & Pollack, G. M. (2011). A modified team-based learning physiology course. *American Journal of Pharmaceutical Education, 75*(10), 204. doi:10.5688/ajpe7510204 PMID:22345723

Pogge, E. (2013). A team-based learning course on nutrition and lifestyle modification. *American Journal of Pharmaceutical Education, 77*(5), 103. doi:10.5688/ajpe775103 PMID:23788814

Professional Development Program, Rockefeller College, University at Albany, State University of New York. (n.d.). *Tobacco Recovery Resource Exchange.* Retrieved August 15, 2015, from http://www.tobaccorecovery.org/

Schunk, D. (2012). *Learning Theories: An Educational Perspective* (6th ed.). Boston: Pearson.

Scott, P. A., Matthews, A., & Kirwan, M. (2014). What is nursing in the 21st century and what does the 21st century health system require of nursing? *Nursing Philosophy, 15*(1), 23–34. doi:10.1111/nup.12032 PMID:24320979

Spetz, J. (2014). How Will Health Reform Affect Demand for RNs? *Nursing Economics, 32*(1), 42–44. PMID:24689158

Sprayberry, L. D. (2014). Transformation of America's Health Care System: Implications for Professional Direct-Care Nurses. *Medsurg Nursing, 23*(1), 61–66. PMID:24707672

Starr, S. S. (2010). Associate degree nursing: Entry into practice -- link to the future. *Teaching and Learning in Nursing, 5*(3), 129–134. doi:10.1016/j.teln.2009.03.002

Stevens, K. R., & Ovretveit, J. (2013). Improvement research priorities: USA survey and expert consensus. *Nursing Research and Practice, 2013,* 1–8. doi:10.1155/2013/695729 PMID:24024029

Sweet, M. S., & Michaelsen, L. K. (2012). *Team-based learning in the social sciences and humanities: Group work that works to generate critical thinking and engagement.* Sterling, VA: Stylus Publishing.

Tan, N. C., Kandiah, N., Chan, Y. H., Umapathi, T., Lee, S. H., & Tan, K. (2011). A controlled study of team-based learning for undergraduate clinical neurology education. *BMC Medical Education, 11*(1), 91. doi:10.1186/1472-6920-11-91 PMID:22035246

Thomas, P. A., & Bowen, C. W. (2011). A controlled trial of team-based learning in an ambulatory medicine clerkship for medical students. *Teaching and Learning in Medicine, 23*(1), 31–36. doi:10.10 80/10401334.2011.536888 PMID:21240780

Thompson, D. R., & Darbyshire, P. (2013). Reply... Thompson D.R. & Darbyshire P. (2013) Is academic nursing being sabotaged by its own killer elite? Journal of Advanced Nursing 69(1), 1–3. *Journal of Advanced Nursing, 69*(5), 1216–1219. doi:10.1111/jan.12123 PMID:23521594

U. S. Census Bureau. (2011). *Profile of selected social characteristics: Suffolk County, N.Y. Author.*

U.S. Department of Health and Human Services, Health Resources and Services Administration, National Center for Health Workforce Analysis. (2014). The Future of the Nursing Workforce: National- and State-Level Projections, 2012-2025. Rockville, MD: Author.

Vellas, B., Villars, H., Abellan, G., Soto, M. E., Rolland, Y., Guigoz, Y., & Garry, P. et al. (2006). Overview of the mini nutritional assessment: Its history and challenges. *The Journal of Nutrition, Health & Aging, 10*(6), 456–465. PMID:17183418

Wiener, H., Plass, H., & Marz, R. (2009). Team-based learning in intensive course format for first-year medical students. *Croatian Medical Journal, 50*(1), 69–76. doi:10.3325/cmj.2009.50.69 PMID:19260147

Wiggins, G., & McTighe, J. (1998). *Understanding by design.* AlexandrIa, VA: ASCD.

Zgheib, N. K., Simaan, J. A., & Sabra, R. (2010). Using team-based learning to teach pharmacology to second year medical students improves student performance. *Medical Teacher, 32*(2), 130–135. doi:10.3109/01421590903548521 PMID:20163228

Zingone, M. M., Franks, A. S., Guirguis, A. B., George, C. M., Howard-Thompson, A., & Heidel, R. E. (2010). Comparing team based and mixed active learning methods in an ambulatory care elective course. *American Journal of Pharmaceutical Education, 74*(9), 160. doi:10.5688/aj7409160 PMID:21301594

ADDITIONAL READING

American Association of Colleges of Nursing. (2011). *The Essentials of Master's Education for Advanced Practice Nursing.* Retrieved August 15, 2015, from http://www.aacn.nche.edu/educationresources/MastersEssentials11.pdf

American Association of Colleges of Nursing. (2012). *New AACN Data Show an Enrollment Surge in Baccalaureate and Graduate Programs amid Calls for More Highly Educated Nurses.* Retrieved August 15, 2015, from http://www.aacn.nche.edu/news/articles/2012/enrollment-data

Hayat, M. J., Eckardt, P., Higgins, M., Kim, M., & Schmiege, S. (2013). Teaching Statistics to Nursing Students: An Expert Panel Consensus. *The Journal of Nursing Education, 52*(6), 330–334. doi:10.3928/01484834-20130430-01

Interprofessional Education Collaborative Expert Panel (IPEC). (2011). *Core competencies for interprofessional collaborative practice. Report of an expert panel.* Washington, DC: Interprofessional Education Collaborative.

IOM (Institute of Medicine). (2011). *The Future of Nursing: Leading Change, Advancing Health.* Washington, DC: The National Academies Press.

Jones, R., Higgs, R., DeAngelis, C., & Prideaux, D. (2001). Changing face of medical curriculum. *Lancet, 357*(9257), 699–703.

MacDonald, C. J., Archibald, D., Trumpower, D., Cragg, B., Casimiro, L., & Jelley, W. (2010). Quality standards for interprofessional healthcare education: Designing a toolkit of bilingual assessment instruments. *Journal of Research in Interprofessional Practice and Education, 1*(3), 1–13.

Michaelsen, L. K. (1983). Team learning in large classes. In C. Bouton & R. Y. Garth (Eds.), *Learning in Groups. New Directions for Teaching and Learning Series* (Vol. 14). San Francisco: Jossey-Bass.

Michaelsen, L. K. (1999). Myths and methods in successful small group work. *National Teaching & Learning Forum, 8*(6), 1–4.

Michaelsen, L. K., Knight, A. B., & Fink, L. D. (2002). *Team-based learning: A transformative use of small groups.* Westport, CT: Greenwood Publishing Group.

Schunk, D. (2012). *Learning Theories: An Educational Perspective* (6th ed.). Boston: Pearson.

Scott, P. A., Matthews, A., & Kirwan, M. (2014). What is nursing in the 21st century and what does the 21st century health system require of nursing? *Nursing Philosophy, 15*(1), 23–34. doi:10.1111/nup.12032

Tan, N. C., Kandiah, N., Chan, Y. H., Umapathi, T., Lee, S. H., & Tan, K. (2011). A controlled study of team-based learning for undergraduate clinical neurology education. *BMC Medical Education, 11*, 91.

Wiener, H., Plass, H., & Marz, R. (2009). Team-based learning in intensive course format for first-year medical students. *Croatian Medical Journal, 50*(1), 69–76.

This research was previously published in the Handbook of Research on Technology Tools for Real-World Skill Development edited by Yigal Rosen, Steve Ferrara, and Maryam Mosharraf, pages 163-189, copyright year 2016 by Information Science Reference (an imprint of IGI Global).

Chapter 73
Big Data and Healthcare:
Implications for Medical and Health Care in Low Resource Countries

Kgomotso H. Moahi
University of Botswana, Botswana

ABSTRACT

Big data and its application to healthcare has captured the world's imagination because of the ability of data analysts to combine huge disparate datasets and be able to produce trends, patterns and predictions. This ability lends itself to the quest to improve healthcare in terms of quality as well as cost. This chapter explores what big data is and how it can be applied to health care and medicine. To do this, the first sections address the question of what big data and data analytics are and what they encompass. An exploration of the potential benefits of big data is provided, with examples of applications, most of which are from the more developed nations of the United States and Europe. The chapter then considers what might be possible from implementing big data in low resource countries, with some examples of what already pertains. It looks at the challenges of implementing big data in health care in both developed and low resource countries.

INTRODUCTION

The data explosion that is being experienced in these times was long foretold by Vannevar Bush in his seminal paper of 1945. In that paper, he proposed an information storage and retrieval tool called the "Memex" which could function as a library for scientists and enable them to access information in a non-linear manner. To many people, his ideas must have seemed far-fetched, but time has proven him to be prescient. Digitization of many aspects of our lives has resulted in treasure troves of data waiting to be analyzed and used for business and other functions (Luna et al., 2014; Mayer-Schoenberger & Cukier, 2014; Manyika et al., 2011). Sectors such as banking and retail are realizing the value of big data to their businesses. Data from retail store loyalty cards is being analyzed for purchasing trends and patterns in order to determine marketing and delivery preference information. As various digital tools and applications are being used, "data exhaust" or "digital trail" is being generated, which lends

DOI: 10.4018/978-1-5225-3926-1.ch073

itself to a myriad of uses for innovation, productivity and competition (Manyika et al., 2011; Mayer-Schoenberger & Cukier, 2014), but also other less benevolent purposes. This data trail has immense potential in both private businesses as well as in the sphere of social services. The data is known as big data and its manipulation and use as big data analytics. Big data and its analysis have been touted as a means to generate information and knowledge in aid of decision making in various areas and domains. Healthcare is one of the domains typically covered in the literature (Asokan & Asokan, 2014; Austin & Kusumoto, 2016; Bellazi, 2014). Indeed public health in the USA has been cited as a beneficiary of big data analytics through Google Flu trends (Mayer-Schoenberger & Cukier, 2014).

Healthcare in general is information intensive and is characterized by immense data or record keeping (Raghupathi & Raghupathi, 2013). Information is critical for all aspects of healthcare such as patient care; public health, disease surveillance, decision support, and evidence based medicine. The use of computers in healthcare has a long history going back to the 1960s. Early applications of technology advanced as technology capabilities also developed. Much of the information used in health is digitized, for example electronic health records and clinical laboratory tests. Digitization of health data is not restricted only to developed economies (high income economies), but also to low and middle income economies where nascent e-health systems are being implemented. Furthermore, the move by many jurisdictions towards e-government means that even more information about their populations is coming on stream, and adding to the already burgeoning data trails and digital information.

Data produced in healthcare is characterized by high volumes, variety and velocity which are characteristics shared with big data (Belle et al., 2015). Big data is composed not only of structured data obtained from health information application, but also other data (unstructured) gleaned from various activities people engage in, in technology enabled services and applications – such as social media, location specific data enabled by sensors in mobile devices, searches on the Internet, and the content created on various applications. This type of data collection has been facilitated by rapid developments in technology, but has until recently not been harnessed and used effectively to improve health outcomes for a number of reasons. The reasons include the distributed and unrelated nature of the data, and the inability of traditional operations to manipulate the data (Belle at al., 2015). However, developments in cloud computing and data processing software such as Google's MapReduce and Apache Hadoop mean that more can be done with such data (Mayer-Schoenberger & Cukier, 2014).

Clinical data can now be combined with unstructured non-clinical data such as people's location and movement, lifestyles and behavior patterns to provide a composite image of the individual, and give healthcare providers the potential to influence lifestyle and behavior towards improved health outcomes. The use of big data analytics provides opportunity for data to be used to make predictions, to inform interventions, discern trends, and to ensure that the costs of health care do not escalate needlessly by addressing problems before they develop (Belle et al., 2015).

This chapter explores potential and actual uses of big data in healthcare and medicine. The literature is reviewed to define big data, big data analytics, and to describe some big data applications in healthcare. The review focuses on the benefits and the challenges of implementing big data in healthcare. The chapter also explores how healthcare and medicine in developing (low and middle income countries) might benefit from big data analytics and what the impediments to implementation are and how these may be addressed.

BACKGROUND

What Is Big Data?

There does not seem to be a standard definition of big data in the literature, other than the fact that big data is data sets so large and varied that current hardware and software cannot handle (Mayer-Schoenberger & Cukier, 2014). De Souza & Smith (2014) describe big data as the growing amounts of available data as well as increasing abilities to create and use value from it. However, what is not clearly defined, and some say, may be difficult to do is to put a figure to the amount of data or threshold that would qualify to be called big data (Gandomi and Haider, 2015). Big data is typically defined as data that is of high volume, variety and velocity that standard data management and analysis technologies and tools cannot handle. Many other authors agree with this definition (Gupta et al. 2016; Luna et al. 2014; Kim & Park 2016). Using the 3 V's (Volume, variety and velocity) has been a *common framework to describe big data* (Gandomi and Haider, 2015:138). The emphasis seems to be on the size and different formats that data takes, as well as the speed with which it is amassed; this also includes new methods and tools of storing, managing, analyzing, and most significantly, using such data (Raghupathi & Raghupathi, 2013). Big data is also described as systems that are able to efficiently process distributed data, thus leveraging on the volume, variety and velocity of available data (Asokan and Asokan, 2015; IDS Policy Briefing, 2015). The 3 V's are generally used to characterize big data and also to indicate the challenges that the management, analysis and use of big data presents. But Boyd and Crawford (2011) maintain that what is critical about big data is not its big size, but that data from disparate sources can be put together and analyzed for patterns, trends, and predictions. It is the ability of making connections between various data items. The remainder of this section discusses the characteristics of big data.

Volume – as indicated earlier, e-health applications around the world have generated significant amounts of data as a result of using technology to harness information required to deliver quality and efficient healthcare. In addition, data that is amassed from the use of social media, mobile and wireless devices is said to be moving into Exabytes (10006 bytes) (Kim & Park, 2016). This volume refers to the amount of data that is generated every time individuals use their computing and communication devices, the Internet for searching, social media, purchasing, blogging, etc. The data is located in many disparate and distributed sources, making integration for management and analysis a challenge (Belle et al., 2015).

Variety refers to the structural heterogeneity of a dataset (Gandomi and Haider, 2015:138). Essentially meaning that big data contains data that is both structured (which standard databases can handle) and unstructured (such as text, images, sound, and video) which need special tools to handle and analyze. It can also be said that big data is also characterized by collection of vast amounts of unstructured data from activities that have not been previously quantifiable (Stevens et al, 2015). Mayer-Schoenberger & Cukier (2014) refer to this phenomenon as "datafication" - the possibility to extract data from information hitherto not considered worth much as a source of data. What makes the variety of data remarkable today is the advance in technology that has given rise to new methods of managing and analyzing such data.

Velocity refers to the rate and speed with which data is generated and should be analyzed to derive value from it. It is now possible for real-time analysis to be carried out in aid of quick turnaround in decision-making, planning, intervention and marketing. Big data technologies are able to handle large amounts of data instantaneously.

According to IDS Policy Briefing (2015), 90% of the world's data was created in the last 2 years (from 2013 to 2015) – a truly exponential rise. Big data is further defined "as the ability to generate, analyze, manipulate and synthesize data to create or even destroy value" (IDS Policy Briefing, 2015:1). According to the IDS Policy Briefing, big data has both positive and negative potential, and that it will be up to governments and civil society to ensure that big data is used in such a way that it benefits government, corporations, but in particular the ordinary person or citizen in the areas of economic, human development, and rights. Data has been growing exponentially since 2010, and it is estimated that annual data is expected to grow from 1.2 zettabytes in 2010 to 35 zettabytes in 2020 (Kim & Park, 2016). Healthcare generates approximately 10 Gigabytes of structured data per day, but much higher volumes of unstructured data are collected (Gupta et al. (2016). Digital data sources in health care include electronic health records, genomics data, medical images, and medical sensor data.

Big Data Analytics

In spite of the fact that data gathering has been with us for many years, it is only in recent years that it has become a topical issue. The reason behind this is the remarkable advances in technology that make it possible for disparate data items to be aggregated, managed, and analyzed to produce trends, patterns, and predictions that can guide decision making. As indicated, data comes in many varieties and in structured and unstructured formats. Developments in storage (becoming cheaper and more sophisticated), in management (developments of software that enable aggregation and organization of data for various purposes), and in analysis (algorithms developed to be able to sort and make correlations amongst data), have driven the value of data up. Much of the data that is being generated ends up being used for purposes other than those it was collected for – in a word, data can be used as required by those who know what they want with it and what to do with it. To be able to make sense of data, data analytics must be applied. Data Analytics are fast becoming a skill that is in high demand, and yet is not in steady supply. Gandomi and Haider (2015) describe some of the data analytics techniques for structured and unstructured data. Text analysis, text summarization, question answering, and sentiment analysis are typically used to analyze unstructured data. They further identified audio analysis, video analysis, and social media analysis. Predictive analysis, which uses future and historic data to make predictions of what may happen in the future, is used to analyze structured data. Predictive analysis largely employs statistical techniques to make correlations. Big data analytics enable correlations as opposed to establishing causation (Mayer-Schoenberger & Cukier, 2014). Correlations do not necessarily tell the why of a situation, but they make it possible to identify trends and patterns to be able to make predictions. It has become less of an effort to determine or measure correlations between millions of data items and variable.

Statement of the Problem

Most people in developing countries reside in rural areas and are the most underserved in respect of social services, including healthcare. Kai and Ahmed (2013) divide this challenge into two: insufficient healthcare facilities and unavailability of health care experts. In addition, other challenges include low patient to doctor ratios, lack of trained clinical personnel in various specialties, limited resources in terms of equipment and even drugs, the high cost of healthcare, exacerbated by increased occurrence of non communicable diseases from changed lifestyles.

These aforementioned make primary healthcare/preventive care all the more crucial in such settings. Because of the need to emphasize preventive over curative care, the ability to conduct health surveys so as to detect problems early becomes critical. It is also critical that populations are educated on lifestyle and behavior change to prevent/postpone the onset of avoidable diseases and conditions. Thus the potential of big data is especially high in such environments. The availability of mobile phones and smart phones has provided a glimmer of hope in terms of providing healthcare and collecting data to inform timely intervention. The 2016 International Telecommunications Union (ITU) report on measuring the information society indicates that mobile telephony uptake in developing countries continues its rise and truly demonstrates the ideas of leapfrogging technology.

Developing countries located in the African continent have the greatest challenges to contend with in the provision of health and medical care to citizens. One of these is the high rate of HIV and AIDS requiring large spending on the provision of anti retroviral drugs (ARVs). Malaria is also a big threat, as are other highly infectious diseases such as Ebola. The health systems in these countries are barely able to cope without assistance from international donors and organizations. Jee and Kim (2013) identified the healthcare problems faced by developing countries as health finance reforms and effective analysis of healthcare related information. Health financial reforms are an issue because most of these countries are challenged to deliver optimally through their public healthcare systems. Health related information is required to facilitate better planning and delivery, and yet, is not readily available.

A great deal of hope is placed on big data and its analytics for health care. This study establishes the possibility of big data as part of the solution to some of the problems of providing healthcare in developing countries. This is done through a review of the literature on the use of big data for health care in both developed and developing countries. The researcher is however aware that many other developments or implementations of technology in health care have been touted as possible solutions to the problems in developing countries, but that the promise has not been delivered. The view taken in this paper is that for as long as the identified challenges of implementing big data for health care are not addressed, then big data will be one of those 'fads' that end up not accounting for any improvement in the situation.

BIG DATA IN MEDICAL AND HEALTHCARE

Since the 1960s health systems particularly in the US have experimented with electronic health records to capture patient demographics, medical history, medical episodes, clinical tests and treatment. However, it was not until 2009 that an Act was passed in the US for health care providers to adopt the electronic health record. On the other hand, in developing countries, a study conducted in 2011 found that 15 countries in Africa documented use of patient record systems, mostly using open source systems (Akanbi et al., 2012).

Baro et al., (2015) conducted a systematic review of papers on big data in healthcare in a bid to determine a literature driven definition of big data in healthcare. This definition seems to tally with other definitions in that it determined that big data was data of such volume, variety, and velocity as to defeat the traditional means of organizing, analyzing and managing such data. Data in healthcare is voluminous as it can be obtained from clinical data, medical imaging, doctor's and nurses notes, prescriptions, genomics, medical sensors data, clinical trials, etc. It may also be derived from other non-clinical data such as data on the searches conducted by individuals, their Facebook posts, tweets, blogs, e-mails, purchases both online and in store, movements, location, and activities. This last category of data may be used to make predictions concerning a variety of health related issues using big data analytics. The rate that healthcare data is generated is also very high and would demand the use of modern techniques to analyze and understand its implications for healthcare. Veracity is another critical issue in healthcare, signaling the need to consider how such data may be validated to ensure that its analysis does not have life threating impact.

Literature and policy reports have indicated positive potential for big data application to ensure effective and efficient public health systems, identification of appropriate treatments for patients, monitoring and enhancement of the safety of healthcare systems, and ensure well-run health systems in general (Jee and Kim, 2013).

Patient and Lifestyle Records

The combination of patient records and lifestyle behavior related data has provided significant amounts of data that can be analyzed to provide information that would help improve healthcare quality and efficiency (Luna et al., 2014). These are identified as:

1. Generating new knowledge about the patients in relation to their lifestyle that would not otherwise be available or divulged by the patient.
2. Disseminating knowledge in the form of decision support systems for practitioners – the information obtained on lifestyle and other behavioral indicators could provide information for decision-making.
3. Aiding development of personalized medicine – an in-depth understanding of the patient, their genetic makeup, lifestyle, etc. could lend itself to this type of health care.
4. Empowering patients through provision of information regarding their health, lifestyles, likely risks, etc.
5. Improving epidemiological surveillance through location data provided by mobile devices.

Big data can facilitate personalized health care based on analysis of patient characteristics. Personalized medicine is also known as Precision Medicine (Estape et al. (2016). Personalized healthcare is made possible by the availability of genetic, environmental and behavior based information on individual patients. *The objective is to more effectively target their physiological and pharmacological responses to a specific treatment. Personalized medicine enables physicians and other care providers to treat individuals as unique, using observations from the individual patient as well as harnessing the power of aggregated data drawn from millions of other patients' data* (Estape et al., 2016:10). Such data is obtainable from the patient medical record (which contains demographic, medical history, medical tests, previous diagnosis and treatments, etc.). Other sources of information available, especially in developed countries include patients' genetic information. The cost and time for genetic sequencing has fallen to make it an option for some patient to opt for treatment to be tailored to themselves. Mayer-Schonberger & Cukier (2014) recount the story of Steve Job's fight with cancer and how his doctors were able to use his genetic information to find treatment that would likely work for him. Personalized healthcare can therefore lead to targeted and better quality health care - perhaps at a fraction of the cost it would take to try out different courses of treatment, until the right one is found. The abundance of data lends itself to being mined and analyzed to inform better clinical and treatment decision-making (Estape et al., 2016). Insurance providers are likely to benefit from personalized healthcare since diseases will be identified and treated earlier and to specification (Austin & Kusumoto, 2016).

Risk Factors, Disease Prevention and Interventions

Although scientists are still grappling with how to use big data in healthcare, its applicability has been demonstrated in 3 areas: disease prevention; identification of modifiable risk factors for disease prevention, and the design of interventions for health behavior change (Hansen et al., 2014). Big data analytics provide the possibility of deriving insights, trends, and patterns that may lend themselves to information and knowledge leading to better and improved health care, provided at a lower cost both in terms of the health of populations (especially in developing countries where there is a shortage of medical care such that people's conditions may have deteriorated by the time they receive the medical care), as well as in the resources that would be expended on patients once conditions are predicted before they develop or are caught fairly early in the stages. Big data holds the promise of making many systems in healthcare more effective than they were when limited amounts of data were used. Big data affords the synthesis of disparate data sets to 'map' health problems (IDS Policy, 2015).

Identification of patients or people at risk of particular conditions from a combination of data from electronic health records, data on people's location and movement, lifestyle data obtained from wearable or mobile applications that track people's activity (movement, what and when they eat, how much they sleep, how active they are), data gleaned from store reward cards that provide data on the food bought, and products used both in homes and for personal care. This kind of data could also provide information for patient profiling, to enable personalized or targeted healthcare.

Public health services have benefited in that some countries are now able to generate geographic health maps, and the possibility for population risk stratification using electronic health records integrated with other sources of information, such as environmental information. Public health is a domain that is heavily dependent on timely data and information in order to facilitate planning that is required for a number of activities. These activities include identification of disease patterns to inform the resources and planning required to address such situations; the tracking of disease outbreaks to inform speedy responses; knowing ahead of time the patterns of disease outbreaks, such as flu strains so that targeted vaccinations and treatments can be availed.

Disease Surveillance and Population Health Management

Big data promises to support healthcare functions such as disease surveillance and population health management (Raghupathi & Raghupathi, 2014:1). The literature has highlighted a number of areas.

Asokan and Asokan (2015) discuss the potential of big data to enhance the performance of one health – a system based on collaborative approach to human and animal health. They describe how big data contributes in the fight to control disease outbreak caused by zoonoses through use of data to detect disease trends, outbreaks, pathogens and causes of outbreaks (Asokan & Asokan, 2015:312). The ability to put together and analyze data from a variety of sources that track human and animal movements, climactic conditions, etc., can provide the much needed information to identify potential problems and enhance the speed and magnitude of interventions required to address the impending problems.

Stevens et al (2015) discuss how the mining of big data can have the potential to detect disease occurrence from first evidence and help to control a full scale outbreak using for example, postings on Twitter which is real-time and provides the immediacy required to detect first occurrences of cases. Big data can lead to better population health outcomes by enabling the provision and sharing of information and knowledge for better planning of interventions, services, and resources as required.

Biomedical Research

Biomedical research will benefit from big data and its analysis, contributing new models of healthcare delivery. There are a number of areas that should and could benefit from big data implementations, and these include molecular biology and molecular medicine; literature analysis and analysis of biomedical knowledge bases (Bellazzi, 2014). Big data analysis also has the potential to advance real-time research (Asokan & Asokan, 2015) leading to enhanced responsiveness and health interventions before situations escalate.

Better clinical trials are a possibility because big data enables research using large data sets as opposed to carefully selected samples whose results are then extrapolated to the research population. Although big data is "messy" due to its sheer volume and variety, the sheer volume and variety of the data outweighs its messiness and provides greater predictive power that according to Hansen et al., (2014) can produce hypotheses that can then be tested by scientists on carefully selected data. Big data also enables variations in the subjects to be taken into account. If one can imagine a drug trial administered to a larger number of patients rather than to a carefully selected number. The analytic tools would then be used to show the correlations between any number of data items about the patients with the outcome of the trial so as to be able to state clearly that the drug may work with patients whose characteristics it can enumerate.

Connecting Stakeholders

Health stakeholders such as clinical staff, patients and populations, administrators and policy makers, public health specialists, insurance companies, etc. can benefit from the analysis of a variety of data pertaining to patients. In fact, Grove et al. (2013) indicated that many applications have been built around big data analytics in the US that would be of benefit to a number and variety of healthcare stakeholders. For example, it is possible through mining insurance claims data for healthcare insurance companies to identify any instances of claim fraud.

Enhanced Clinical Decision Support

Clinicians around the world have embraced the concept of using the best scientific evidence available to inform their clinical decisions (Grover et al., 2013). Big data provides a platform for evidence-based medicine, as practitioners would have the ability to establish from the data how conditions were identified and treated, and what the outcomes were. The possibilities for rare conditions are particularly significant, as a practitioner would be able to find information on any similar cases and what worked or did not work so as to inform their course of action. Big data analytics can lead to better clinical decision support, as the practitioner will be able to form a complete picture of the patient when they have all data available and when associations are made between the different types of data. For example data about the patient's characteristics, previous conditions, tests, diagnosis, genomics, lifestyle, may enable the practitioner to quickly determine a diagnosis, possible tests that are targeted and more cost effective due to the information gleaned from the data, and also be in a position to make prescriptions that are likely to make a difference given the patient's data. Big data gleaned from sensors on patients such as premature babies, can be used to monitor the babies and intervene before problems escalate (Mayer-Schoenberger & Cukier, 2014).

When big data is synthesized and analyzed—and those aforementioned associations, patterns and trends revealed—healthcare providers and other stakeholders in the healthcare delivery system can develop more thorough and insightful diagnoses and treatments, resulting, one would expect, in higher quality care at lower costs and in better outcomes overall. (Raghupathi & Raghupathi, 2013:2)

Reduced Healthcare Costs

Overall, big data can lead to reduced healthcare costs as associations that are made between patient characteristics, healthcare records, and available interventions can inform decisions on most cost effective and sustainable responses (Raghupathi & Raghupathi, 2013). The availability of national registries, genetic information etc., can help healthcare providers minimize costs by taking preemptive steps. Further, data can be mined to identify the most effective treatments for particular conditions. In hospitals, existing admissions data combined with other patient specific data can be mined to identify patterns of hospital readmissions and factors associated with it.

Consumers/patients could be provided with better information to make informed decisions and manage their own conditions, based on the data gathered through wearable devices, social media activities, and their health profiles. This would enable reduced costs as they could be empowered to recognize instances that do or do not warrant hospital visits.

Genomic analysis has been identified by Raghupathi & Raghupathi (2014) who indicate that genetic sequencing can be executed more efficiently and cost effectively than in the past, and can become part of the data considered in determining treatments and interventions.

The management of healthcare facilities can benefit from use of large amounts of data that are collected and include clinical data, financial data, patient data, supply chain data, human resource data, to better plan and manage facilities.

SOME EXAMPLES OF BIG DATA AND HEALTHCARE IMPLEMENTATIONS

Implementation of big data for healthcare has not been as straightforward as those writing about its applications might have made it sound. Chang & Choi (2016:154) state that *a seamless integration of big data into our healthcare systems may seem to lie in still in the distant future.* Writing in 2014, De Souza & Smith determined that big data analytics were not used as extensively in the area of social services as in the more technical and business areas. However, they went on to describe some applications of big data in health care. These examples included the use of big data analytics by Merck the pharmaceutical company to identify areas where pollen allergens are at their highest in order to target the market with adverts of the allergy medication Claratin. Other applications included the use of mobile phone generated data to study the migration patterns of people after a disaster and use this to study and predict the potential spread of infectious diseases.

Research institutions in the US (Department of Health and Human Services Agency for Healthcare Research) and the UK (Health and Social Care Information Center) have collected electronic health records into data sets that can be used in conjunction with other data sets for research and for providing health care (Simpao et al (2015). The authors further describe how anesthesia data sets can be analyzed with visual analytics tools to enable easier identification of trends and patterns. The 100,000 Genome

Project in the UK is one of the largest whole genome sequencing initiatives and its aim is to integrate genomic sequencing of patients with rare diseases and their families, as well as patients with common cancers into routine healthcare in the UK's National Health Service (NHS) (Chang & Choi, 2016: Genomics England). Another project is the National Institute of Health (NIH) Big Data to Knowledge and Precision Medicine Initiatives in the US that is aimed at ensuring that available biomedical data is accessible and discoverable for healthcare providers to harness and use for providing precision or personalized healthcare (Chang & Choi, 2016; Big Data to Knowledge Initiative).

According to McCormack (2013) a number of companies in the US are already providing big data solutions for healthcare. These include Explorys which provides tools for clinical decision support, at risk patient population management, and cost of care measurement. Propeller Health uses data obtained from sensors attached to asthma inhalers to provide data that could be used in asthma management. NextBio is another company that provides genomic data at individual levels using clinical information and evaluating genome data. IBM Watson Health has integrated big data and machine learning for healthcare, by collecting vast amounts of data from medical records, clinical trials, data from wearable devices, health insurance information, and medical research into its Watson Health Cloud. They are thus able to provide health and medical care solutions to patients, health providers, and insurance administrators (Cheng & Choi, 2016).

Hospital systems too are tapping into the potential of big data. The University of Pittsburg Medical Center (UPMC) also uses a combination of genomic, clinical, financial and administrative data to experiment on breast cancer treatments, and also provide personalized healthcare. Nambiar et al (2013) provide more examples where the Center for Disease Control (CDC) is reportedly using big data analytics to combat influenza in the US. This is done by collecting data on flu episodes in its FluView application. Raghupathi & Ragupathi (2014) report real time data analytics use at North York Hospital in Toronto Canada to improve health outcomes and provide insight into healthcare delivery costs; data analytics are also reportedly used to develop healthcare protocols and case pathways using the IBM cloud datasets.

THE POSSIBILITIES OF BIG DATA FOR HEALTHCARE IN LOW RESOURCE COUNTRIES

Big data in healthcare has not made any significant inroads in developing or low and middle income countries. The 3rd global survey of eHealth conducted by the WHO Global Observatory for eHealth in 2015 shows few countries having sound eHealth foundations in terms of national policies and strategies; It also shows there is still significant work that needs to be done to develop the legal framework for eHealth; a significant number of countries, especially in low resource environments do not have national electronic patient records, they use mHealth and social media in a limited manner, and they do not report having big data policies or strategies. However, the path towards big data application is being forged through a number of applications and technology use in the healthcare sector, as well as in other areas such as data gathering in retail, some use of social media, and the high adoption of mobile technology in general and some applications for healthcare in these countries. Some jurisdictions are piloting and using electronic health information systems, and developing e-health strategies that include e-health records, telemedicine, medical image processing, mobile devices for mHealth (Chigona et al, 2013).

The Promise of Cloud Computing

Purkayastha & Braa (2013) present a case for the use of cloud computing for big data analytics application in developing countries – as it involves provision of infrastructure, platform, software and analytics as services. Taking advantage of this could free healthcare organizations to focus on improving healthcare without worrying about purchase, maintenance and management of infrastructure, platforms, securing expertise for running software and for carrying out analytics required to inform healthcare.

Evidence of Potential for Low Resource Settings

Research conducted in developed countries holds promise for implementation in developing countries. Young (2015) reports research carried out to use data gleaned from mobile phones, social media and other mobile applications to determine HIV related risk behavior that could inform prevention strategies. The report specifically mentioned analysis of Twitter messages to identify posts that could shed light on behaviors that are linked to high HIV risk and found a correlation between the location of these tweets and areas identified by the Centre for Disease Control (CDC) to be high risk areas. Such use of big data could lead to possibilities for HIV remote monitoring and surveillance, as well as HIV prevention efforts (Young, 2015).

Stevens et al. (2015) shed some light on how early warning systems could be effected through data mining Twitter posts and filtering Tweets by specific keywords. They also recount the use of search term surveillance on Google in Africa that enabled the analysis of Ebola outbreaks in Guinea, Liberia and Sierra Leone. This means that Internet based surveillance systems have the potential to provide early warning in developing countries too. Having volunteers submit information on their symptoms which can then be aggregated and analyzed for patterns is also a tool that could be looked into for areas that are prone to periodic outbreaks. Kshetri (2014) gives an example of how the UN used an analysis of social media posts (tweets) to establish how well its Every Woman Every Child (EWEC) project accomplished its goal of delivering health messages. The UN further used an analysis of social media posts made by parents of children to determine and track their attitudes towards immunization. Using the 2014 Ebola outbreak, Amankwah-Amoah (2016) demonstrates how big data, specifically digital surveillance can be used to report and control the spread of diseases. In this case call data records were used to identify areas where the disease was and to determine where to set up treatment centers. The analysis of Twitter updates assisted in the tracking of the spread of cholera in Haiti during the 2010 earthquake (Ragipathi & Ragupathi, 2014).

The use of mobile phones is one way of collecting data and a number of applications have been identified in the literature. The significant growth and uptake of mobile telephony has been noted in developing countries. In 2010 more than 5 billion mobile phones were in use, more than 80 percent of them in developing countries. The percentage of people owning mobile phones in Sub-Saharan Africa increased from 32.1 percent in 2008 to 57.1 percent in 2012, and it is expected to rise to 75.4 percent by 2016. (De Souza & Smith, 2014). This growth has offered people in developing countries better opportunities to improve their quality of life. For example, Cell Life, a South African organization, created a mass messaging mobile service called Communicate, which reminds patients to take their medications, links patients to clinics, and offers peer-to-peer support services such as counseling and monitoring. Cell Life also developed Capture, a service that makes it possible for health care workers in the field to collect and save information in digital form using their mobile phones (De Souza & Smith, 2014). In Kenya, mobile phone records were used to provide travel and human movement information to understand the spread of malaria (Hilbert, 2016).

However, Chigona et al. (2013) report mHealth applications in developing countries are focused mostly on health promotion and promotion of positive health behavior through the use of text messaging. They report applications that combine the use of mobile phones and sensoring equipment. Examples include eCompliance in India to encourage treatment adherence for TB patients by using a combination of biometric and mobile technologies (Chigona et al, 2013:4). They also discuss a remote patient monitoring system application called Autocare in Bangladesh used to monitor breast cancer patients through mobiles and wearable sensor applications. Wyber et al (2015) outline the challenges faced by low and medium income countries in collecting, reporting and analyzing routine health data from their public health systems. The challenge has been the vertical program reporting and its impact on the collection of quality data that can be used for localized decision-making. They conclude that the use of computers, mobile phones and tablets to collect data will go a long way to mitigate the challenge and generate data for immediate and future analysis to enable timely intervention when disease outbreaks strike.

Challenges of Implementing Big Data Analytics in Both Resource Rich and Poor Environments

De Souza & Smith (2014) identified a number of issues that make use of big data difficult in the social services arena: these include the fact most data is buried in administrative systems, making the logistics for its extraction somewhat cumbersome; lack of data governance standards to guide on how data is structured, stored, and curated; recognition that not all data is reliable; the unintended consequences of using data for purposes other than that it was collected for. Wyber et al (2015) reiterated that the challenges besetting big data application can be classified as logistical, technical and governance related.

The complexity of healthcare data in terms of the volumes and variety, as well as its time frames affects the implementation of big data for healthcare and is the source of a myriad of challenges of implementation (Jee & Kim, 2013). The distributed nature of healthcare data presents a challenge to effective use (Austin & Kusumoto, 2016; Costa, 2014) as healthcare data is generated and used by many stakeholders (individual health care providers, health insurance companies, laboratory services, hospitals, etc.). Consumers/patients could be provided with better information to make informed decisions and manage their own conditions, based on the data gathered through wearable devices, social media activities, and their health profiles. This would enable reduced costs as they could be empowered to recognize instances that do or do not warrant hospital visits. Most healthcare data is largely unstructured (Austin & Kumumoto, 2016), making it imperative for advanced analytics to analyze this unstructured data. The tools for managing and analyzing the data also present a challenge for implementation. The architectural framework required has 4 components: the data sources themselves; how they are aggregated, transformed and managed; the tools/software used for the analysis; and the types of analytics implementation (Raghupathi & Raghupathi, 2014).

According to the authors the sources of big data themselves are complex and require specific handling. Data can come from internal sources which include electronic health records; from external sources which may include laboratory data, government, pharmacies; the data may come in multiple formats given the multiple sources, and may be structured and unstructured; It also resides in multiple locations – internally, externally, etc., using different types of formats that must be accommodated. The data has to be organized and maintained so that when it is required it is available despite its format and location, etc. It has to be aggregated, transformed and managed to facilitate use when required. For this purpose there are a number of options that may include data warehousing. Decisions have to be made regarding the platforms to use for big data analytics which include, Hadoop which is an open source distributed data processing platform (Raghupathi & Raghupathi, 2014).

Further, the growth and rate of big data generation presents problems/challenges associated with the storage and security of the data (Luna, 2014; Costa, 2014; Gupta et al. 2016). The structured and unstructured nature of healthcare data presents problems of storage and retrieval, and is compounded by the fact that even with the falling price of storage, using a cloud storage with 10 TB would cost up to 20 Thousand USD per month without factoring in maintenance costs (Gupta et al., 2016). It might be less expensive to generate data than to store, secure and analyze it, especially healthcare data (Costa, 2014).

Governance issues such as data security, ownership, privacy are yet other areas that have been identified in the literature (Austin & Kusumoto, 2016; Raghupathi & Raghupathi, 2014). As health data becomes more available and analysis of disparate data sets becomes a reality, there will be issues of keeping data secure to ensure its integrity; of protecting the privacy of individuals; and of providing policies and regulations on data ownership and what it may or may not be used for. According to Kostkova (2016), using big data to conduct research for improved decision-making and healthcare raises issues of ownership of the data. Such data includes the integration of data from electronic health records, real-time geo-located data from wearable and tracking devices, and from use of various social media platforms (Facebook, Twitter) and the World Wide Web search engines such as Google. Much as use of this data can generate knowledge that could be instrumental to a variety of applications as outlined in this chapter, questions of the privacy of the individual open up the issue of personal data ownership. Who does this data belong to? To what extent should the privacy of individuals be subjugated for the greater good? What needs to be done to ensure that data cannot be traceable to individuals? According to Luna et al (2014:39), unlike traditional database software, big data software does not have the "granular security policies that protect data at various levels". This means that personal data might be at a risk of being accessed and used, and even possibly altered without proper authorization and permission. Authors such as Vayena et al (2015) have considered the ethical challenges arising from using big data for Digital Disease Detection (DDD). DDD involves the use of data sources such as the Internet, mobile devices, online shopping platforms and enables digital surveillance. Members of the population do not necessarily have to visit health facilities for such surveillance to happen in today's digital world. Luna et al (2014) suggest the need for policies and strategies to safeguard the security of data, the protection of personal, private information, and disclosure on how data is to be used. Developing countries could take a leaf from the US that enacted the Health Insurance Portability and Accountability Act (HIPAA) on rules to govern how personal information should be protected. There is need for appropriate legal and regulatory frameworks.

In a study conducted in the Republic of Korea, Kim and Park (2016) established the critical success factors for the implementation and use of big data in health care. They conducted a literature review and surveyed experts in the field in Korea to determine what factors were prioritized as critical for promoting big data in health care. They found that:

1.   Data exerted high influence in the implementation of big data in healthcare. Issues such as data quality, data privacy and security were critical. Also important were data integration and sharing (open data).

2. Investments in the analytics and application capabilities of healthcare organizations were also slated as important players in implementing big data in healthcare.
3. There was need for appropriate laws, regulations and policies.
4. Having the appropriate technology to handle big data. Although the technology might not be much of an issue since cloud computing and software such as Hadoop are available.

Challenges in Developing Countries

Big data in developing countries may not be in the same magnitude as that generated in developed countries in terms of volumes, variety, and velocity due to disparities in technology availability, adoption and use (Kshetri, 2014). Speaking specifically about developing countries Wyber et al (2015: 204) had this to say: *the big data approach inherently demands more technical skills, specialized equipment, interoperability standards, coherent data collection and analysis systems and regulatory oversight. Beyond the technical aspects, an organizational culture of quality is one of the key drivers of an effective health information system. Health care providers and system administrators in most countries have not been trained on data science.* These issues are at the heart of the challenges facing both resource rich and resource poor environments, but especially more so for resource poor environments found in most developing countries.

Developing countries are said to be afflicted by a multi-level digital divide the goes beyond the issue of lack of access to technology. Instead the countries face a 3 level divide: inequality of Access to ICTs; inequality of capability or capacity to make use of ICT; and finally, inequality of outcomes resulting from the use of the ICTs (such as productivity) (Purkayastha & Braa, 2013). Limited access to big data creates new digital divides (Boyd & Crawford, 2011). For developing countries, the lack of money to purchase data from those who own it (like Facebook or Google) is very real, and the issue of the computational skills required is magnified. For developing countries the debate in using technology has always been centered on prioritization – where does one put priority, should it be in improving medical facilities or information systems that hopefully will lead to improved services as an outcome? Given the third level of inequality of outcomes in developing countries, this question is very real and presents itself as a chicken and egg question. But the lack of access to technology is also a major player. IDS Policy Briefs (2015) indicate the need for reliable Internet connections for healthcare organizations to be able to utilize cloud computing and big data analysis software.

Luna et al (2014) point out that key to any big data project is the availability of robust infrastructure (hardware and communications) to handle the distributed nature of big data. But many developing countries lack the infrastructure required to take advantage of big data. They lack communications infrastructure required to access as well as effectively synthesize data for healthcare purposes; they have issues with power production and provision. However cloud computing applications described by Purkayastha & Braa (2013) may offer solutions to these challenges, and availability of open source analytics software such as Hadoop mitigate the cost of purchasing or licensing software.

Big data management and analysis require skills that are not as yet widely available. For example, according to Raghupathi and Raghupathi (2014), to install and use Hadoop is complex and requires skills that are not yet in abundance. These skills include advanced computing skills, mathematical and statistical skills, with a healthcare related background. According to Luna et al, (2014:38), "these resources are not only scarce in developing countries: it is estimated that the US will have a shortage of 160, 000 professionals with these skills by 2018. Most of these scientists are recruited by major technology companies in the core countries, with the consequence that countries with fewer resources will suffer this deficit even more".

Big data generally utilizes data of a variety of formats from a variety of sources. For such data to be usable, it has to be integrated and that integration can only be achieved if there is an agreement regarding standards of metadata used to make data and systems interoperable. The agreement on metadata is at the crux of interoperability and involves discussion and collaboration towards a common purpose. The fact that many countries are moving towards e-government and pushing the e-health agenda means that some headway will be made in ensuring use of common standards.

Although the problems of adopting big data are largely economic, covering infrastructural, access, as well as skills, one of the challenges is the understanding and attitudes of those in authority of the potential of big data and more than that, the significance of data as an organizational asset that must be managed and put to good use. Until an understanding is reached as to how data management and analysis can contribute to organizational effectiveness and efficiency, the promise of big data will be just that a promise, and no more.

CONCLUSION

This chapter has defined big data, big data analytics, and applications in healthcare. A discussion of the potential of big data analytics for developing or low resource setting countries has been provided. The challenges and pitfalls of big data implementation in general and for developing countries have been identified. Overall, the chapter is optimistic about the role of big data analytics in addressing some of the issues faced by developing countries. Resource poor environments cannot afford to deal with disease outbreaks and would therefore benefit from analysis of data that would indicate the likelihood of problems before they occur. The hope for such countries is in having robust public health systems that generate timely and accurate data that can be used for planning interventions such as information and education, as well as other preventive measures. Analyzing environmental data, climactic conditions, people's movements and lifestyles, animal movements, and disease prone areas to form correlations would yield data and information to contain situations, and thus bring down the cost of dealing with problems when they have escalated. The literature has revealed that big data analysis can help improve healthcare quality and efficiency by generating new knowledge that can be used to prevent problems; by disseminating knowledge in the form of decision support systems for practitioners – this is particularly significant in low resource environments where practitioners experience a dearth of information and knowledge; empowering patients by providing them with information regarding health, lifestyles and likely risks; and improving epidemiological surveillance (Luna et al., 2014).

REFERENCES

Akanbi, O. M., Ocheke, N., Amaka, A. A., Daniyam, P. A., Emmanuel, C. A. I., Okeke, N. E., & Ukoli, O. C. (2012). Use of electronic health records in sub Saharan Africa: Progress and challenges. *Journal of Medical Tropics*, *14*(1), 1–6. PMID:25243111

Amankwah-Amoah, J. C. (2016, September). Emerging economies, emerging challenges: Mobilizing and capturing value from big data. *Technological Forecasting and Social Change, 110*, 167–174. doi:10.1016/j.techfore.2015.10.022

Asokan, G.V., & Asokan, V. (2014). Leveraging "big data" to enhance the effectiveness of "One Health" in an era of health informatics. *Journal of Epidemiology & Global Health, 5*, 311-314.

Austin, C., & Kusumoto, F. (2016). The application of big data in medicine: current implication and future directions. *Journal of Interv Cardiovascular Electrophysiology*.

Baro, E., Degoul, S., Beucart, R., & Chazard, E. (2015). Towards a literature driven definition of big data in healthcare. *BioMed Research International*, 1–9. doi:10.1155/2015/639021

Bellazzi, R. (2014). Big data and biomedical informatics: A challenging opportunity. IMIA. *Yearbook of Medical Informatics, 9*(1), 8–13. doi:10.15265/IY-2014-0024 PMID:24853034

Belle, A., Tiagarajan, R., Soroushmehr, S. M. R., Navidi, F., Beard, A. D., & Najarian, K. (2015). Big Analytics in Healthcare. *Biomedical Research, 2015*, 1–16. doi:10.1155/2015/370194 PMID:26229957

Big data to knowledge initiative. (n.d.). National Institutes of Health. Accessed 28 November 2016 from: https://datascience.nih.gov/bd2k/about

Boyd, D., & Crawford, K. (2011). *Six Provocations for Big Data*. Presented at Oxford Internet Institute's "A decade in Internet time: Symposium on the dynamics of the internet society".

Chen, M., Ma, Y., Song, J., Lai, C., & Hu, B. (2016, October). Smart clothing connecting human with clouds and big data for sustainable health monitoring. *Mobile Networks and Applications, 21*(5), 825–845. doi:10.1007/s11036-016-0745-1

Cheng H. & Choi M. (2016). Big data and healthcare: building an augmented world. *Healthcare Informatics Research, 22*(3), 153-155.

Chigona, W., Nyemba-Mudenda, M., & Metlula, S. A. (2013). A review in mHealth research in developing countries. *The Journal of Community Informatics, 9*(2).

Costa, F. F. (2014, April). Big data in biomedicine. *Drug Discovery Today, 19*(4), 433–440. doi:10.1016/j.drudis.2013.10.012 PMID:24183925

De Souza K. & Smith L. K. (2014, Summer). Big data for social innovation. *Stanford Social Innovation Review*, 39-43.

Estape, S. E., Mays, H. M., & Sternke, A. E. (2016, January). Translation in data mining to advance personalized medicine for health equity. *Intelligent Information Management, 8*(1), 9–16. doi:10.4236/iim.2016.81002 PMID:27195185

Gandomi, A., & Haider, M. (2015). Beyond the hype: Big data concepts, methods and analytics. *International Journal of Information Management, 35*(2), 137–144. doi:10.1016/j.ijinfomgt.2014.10.007

Genomics England (Internet). (n.d.). London: Department of Health. Accessed 28 November 2016 from: https://www.genomicsengland.co.uk/the-100000-genomes-project/

Groves, P., Kayyali, B., Knott, D., & Van Huiken, S. (2013). *The 'big data' revolution in healthcare: accelerating value of innovation.* McKinsey & Co.

Gupta, G. V., Bora, S. G., & Mavuduru, S. R. (2016). Big data in third world countries. so the means justify the end? letter to editor of. *Technology and Health Care, 1*, 1–2.

Hansen, M. M., Miron-Shatz, T., Lau, A. Y. S., & Paton, C. (2014). Big data in science and healthcare: A review of recent literature and perspectives. *IMIA Yearbook of Medical Informatics, 2014*(1), 21–26. doi:10.15265/IY-2014-0004 PMID:25123717

Hilbert, M. (2016). Big data for development: A review of promises and challenges. *Development Policy Review, 34*(1), 135–175. doi:10.1111/dpr.12142

Hussain, S., Bang, H. J., Han, M., Ahmed, I. M., Amin, B. M., Lee, S., & Parr, G. et al. (2014). Behaviour life style analysis for mobile sensory data in cloud computing through MapReduce. *Sensors (Basel, Switzerland), 14*(11), 22001–22020. doi:10.3390/s141122001 PMID:25420151

IDS Policy Briefing. (2015). Ensuring Developing countries benefit from Big Data. Author.

ITU. (2016). *Measuring the information society report.* Accessed 25 November 2016 from: http://www.itu.int/ITU-D/Statistics/Documents/publications/mirr2016/MISR2016-w4.pdf

Jee, K., & Kim, G-H. (2013). Potentiality of big data in the medical sector: focus on how to reshape the healthcare system. *Healthcare Information Research, 19*(2), 79-85.

Kai, E., & Ahmed, A. (2013). Technical challenges in providing remote health consulting services for the unreached Communities. *International Conference on Advanced Information Networking and Application workshop.* IEEE Computer Society.

Kim, M., & Park, J. (2016). *Identifying and prioritizing critical factors for promoting the implementation and usage of big data in healthcare.* Information Development. doi:10.1177/02666669

Kostkova, P., Brewer de, L., Fattelli, G. B., Hart, G., Koczan, P., Knight, P., ... Tooke, J. (2016). Who own the data? Open data for healthcare. *Frontiers in Public Health February, 4*(7) 1-6.

Kshetri N. (2014, July). The emerging role of big data in key development issues: opportunities, challenges, and concerns. *Big Data and Society,* 1-20.

Luna, D. R., Mayan, J. C., Garcia, M. J., Almerares, A. A., & Hauseh, M. (2014). Challenges and potential solutions for big data implementation in developing countries. *IMIA Yearbook of Medical Informatics, 2014*(1), 36–40. doi:10.15265/IY-2014-0012

Manyika, J., Chui, M., Brown, B., Bughin, J., Dobbs, R., Roxburgh, C., & Byers, H. A. (2011). *Big data: The next frontier for innovation, competition, and productivity.* McKinsey Global Institute.

Mayer-Schoenberger, V., & Cukier, K. (2014). *Big data a revolution that will transform how we live, work and think.* Boston: Houghton Mifflin, Harcourt.

McCormack, N. (2013). *What is big data in healthcare and who's already doing it?* Accessed 25 November 2016 from: http://profitable-practice.softwareadvice.com/what-is-big-data-in-healthcare-0813

Nambiar, R., Bhardwaj, R., Sethi, A., & Vargheese, R. (2014). A look at challenges and opportunities of big data analytics in healthcare. *2013 IEEE International Conference on Big Data*, 17-22.

Purkayastha, S., & Braa, J. (2013). Big data analytics for developing countries – using cloud for operational BI in Health. *Electronic Journal of Information Systems for Developing Countries*. Accessed: 27 July 2016 from: http://ejisdc.org/ojs2/index.php/ejidsc/article/view/1220

Raghupathi, W., & Raghupathi, V. (2014). Big data analytics in healthcare: promise and potential. *Health Information Science and Systems, 2,* 1-10. Accessed 27 July 2016 from: http://www.hissjournal.com/content/2/1/3

Simpao, A. F., Ahumada, L. M., & Rehman, M. A. (2015). Big data and visual analytics in anesthesia and healthcare. *British Journal of Anaesthesia*. Accessed 25th November from: http://bija.oxfordjournals.org

Stevens, B. K., & Pfeiffer, U. D. (2015). Sources of spatial animal and human health data: Casting the net wide to deal more effectively with increasing complex disease problems. *Spatial and Spatio-temporal Epidemiology, 13,* 15–29. doi:10.1016/j.sste.2015.04.003 PMID:26046634

Vayena, E., Salathé, M., Madoff, L. C., & Brownstein, J. S. (2015). Ethical challenges of big data in public health. *PLoS Computational Biology, 11*(2), e1003904. doi:10.1371/journal.pcbi.1003904 PMID:25664461

World Health Organization. (2016). *Atlas of eHealth country profiles: the use of eHealth in support of universal health coverage: based on the findings of the third global survey on eHealth 2015.* Accessed 27 July 2016 from: www.who.int/goe/publications/atlas_2015/en/

Wyber, R., Vaillancourt, S., Perry, W., Mannava, P., Folaranmi, T., & Celi, L. A. (2015). Big data in global health: Improving health in low and middle income countries. *Bulletin of the World Health Organization, 93*(3), 203–208. doi:10.2471/BLT.14.139022 PMID:25767300

Young, D. S. (2015). A big data approach to HIV epidemiology and prevention. *Preventive Medicine, 70,* 17–18. doi:10.1016/j.ypmed.2014.11.002 PMID:25449693

ADDITIONAL READING

Mittelstadt, B. D., & Floridi, L. (2016). The ethics of big data: Current and foreseeable issues in biomedical contexts. *Science and Engineering Ethics, 22*(2), 303–341. doi:10.1007/s11948-015-9652-2 PMID:26002496

Murdoch, B. T., & Detsky, A. K. (2013). The inevitable application of big data to health care. *Journal of the American Medical Association, 309*(13), 1351–1352. doi:10.1001/jama.2013.393 PMID:23549579

Shultz, T. (2013). Turning healthcare challenges into big data opportunities: A use case review across the pharmaceutical development life cycle. *Bulletin of the American Society for Information Science and Technology, 39*(5), 2–53.

Wu, J., Li, H., Cheng, S., & Lin, Z. (2016, December). The promising future of healthcare services: When big data analytics meets wearable technology. *Information & Management, 53*(8), 1020–1033. doi:10.1016/j.im.2016.07.003

KEY TERMS AND DEFINITIONS

Big Data: Data sets so large and varied that current hardware and software cannot handle.

Big Data Analytics: The analysis of large set s of data to reveal patters, trends and to make predictions.

Cloud Computing: The use of large networks of remote servers to store data and to conduct various analysis of such data.

Precision Medicine: Personalized medical care based on analysis of genomic and other data for a given individual.

This research was previously published in Health Information Systems and the Advancement of Medical Practice in Developing Countries edited by Kgomotso H. Moahi, Kelvin Joseph Bwalya, and Peter Mazebe II Sebina, pages 14-32, copyright year 2017 by Medical Information Science Reference (an imprint of IGI Global).

Chapter 74
Patient Privacy and Security in E-Health

Güney Gürsel
Gülhane Military Medical Academy (GATA), Turkey

ABSTRACT

In the digital era, undoubtedly, e-health is a major contributor for decision support, education, research and management activities in healthcare. It provides tremendous benefits by easy store and access to data. This easiness brings a big problem together with the benefits. Users have easy access to vast amount of sensitive health data about patients. This may give way to misuse and abuse. That is why the concepts of privacy and security becomes very popular and point of major concern. This chapter is a descriptive study aimed to give principles of these concepts and invoke awareness about.

INTRODUCTION

Electronic health, E-Health, is in the intersection of medical informatics, public health and business, can be defined as the use of information and communication technologies to improve health care (Eysenbach, 2001). E-Health has grown and developed rapidly. From primary care institutions to big healthcare centers, every healthcare organization uses an information system and records every piece of patient data electronically. As the amount of data increases, using it helps improve not only the quality of services given in healthcare, but also healthcare education, research etc. Easy access to huge amounts of healthcare data brings some problems and dangers together with the benefits. One of the biggest dangers is the violation of Patient Privacy and Security. Patient Privacy and Security is becoming a popular issue as the e-health continues to improve. With the electronic storage and access of patient health data, staff has the opportunity to access huge amounts of data that they would never have when they are in paper forms. The electronic patient data also lures many organizations, who are big actors in healthcare business such as drug companies, medical device companies, insurance companies etc. Many people are in a competition to use this huge amount of patient data for legal or illegal purposes with legal and illegal access.

Patient Privacy and Security is a challenge for every e-health application and healthcare organization using e-health technologies. E-health has many advantages and benefits to both patients and caregivers,

DOI: 10.4018/978-1-5225-3926-1.ch074

healthcare managements take advantage of these benefits, but the possibility of misuse and abuse of patient health data emerges.

This chapter is a descriptive study that examines the concepts and issues related to Patient Privacy and Security and techniques used to protect it. The purpose of the study is to take attention to the importance of the Patient Privacy and Security and invoke awareness of the students, academics, researches having studies and works related to healthcare and patient data.

The chapter is organized as follows: In Background section, the definition and description of patient Privacy and Security will be given. The main part is in the heading of "Patient Privacy and Security" comprising the seriousness of the situation, Patients' Rights and Healthcare Providers' Responsibilities, Privacy and security trends that affect healthcare, Laws and Regulations on Patient Privacy and Security, Security and Privacy Auditing in E-health. In the end are the future research directions and conclusion parts interpreting the chapter.

BACKGROUND

Health data is the most private data of a person. It is so sensitive that it can make a person ashamed and upset. There may be some details even the person himself wants to forget. Because of these assets of patient health data, the notion of Patient Privacy and Security has arisen.

Although privacy and security are two different things, they are used together as a repetition for patient data. In healthcare, these two terms are used together as a concept, in which one refers to what is going to be protected, privacy, and the other refers to how it will be protected, security. In this section, to avoid misusage and confusion, brief descriptions about what is intended with patient privacy and security, will be examined. Exact description of health information is going to be given to clarify what to protect.

Health Insurance Portability and Accountability Act (HIPAA, 1996) defines health information as "whether oral or recorded in any form or medium, that

- Is created or received by a health care provider, health plan, public health authority, employer, life insurer, school or university, or health care clearinghouse; and
- Relates to the past, present, or future physical or mental health or condition of any individual, the provision of health care to an individual, or the past, present, or future payment for the provision of health care to an individual."

HIPAA (1996) defines *individually identifiable health information as* "a subset of health information, including demographic information collected from an individual, and:

- Is created or received by a health care provider, health plan, employer, or health care clearinghouse; and
- Relates to the past, present, or future physical or mental health or condition of an individual; the provision of health care to an individual; or the past, present, or future payment for the provision of health care to an individual; and
  - That identifies the individual; or
  - With respect to which there is a reasonable basis to believe the information can be used to identify the individual."

HIPAA (1996) defines *Protected Health Information* (PHI) as "individually identifiable health information that is:

- Transmitted by electronic media;
- Maintained in electronic media; or
- Transmitted or maintained in any other form or medium."

PHI that is electronically collected, stored, used and sent is called as Electronically Protected Health Information (EPHI).

In this chapter, the scope is limited to privacy and security of EPHI.

Patient privacy deals with any medical data (medical condition, test result, payment info etc.) at any from (paper, electronic etc.) that belongs to a patient, meaning what is protected and who will be permitted to use this information (Upstate Medical University, 2011). It is the term used for notion of the confidentiality and access restrictions of patients' PHI, which contains sensitive and personal information (Sun, Zhu, Zhang, & Fang, 2012).

Security means protecting the valuable resources against malicious attempts. Patient Security is safeguarding the patient privacy, in another words, states how the information will be protected (Upstate Medical University, 2011).

Privacy and security concerns of EPHI fall into two general categories (Electronic Health Record Vendors Association (EHRVA), 2008):

- Inappropriate release from authorized users of provider organizations, or from non-authorized users who intrude into an organization's information system with malicious intent.
- The flow of PHI between providers, payers and secondary users, with consent or with "implied consent" to conduct treatment, payment and healthcare operations.

PATIENT PRIVACY AND SECURITY

How Serious?

The numbers in the report of Health Research Institute at PricewaterhouseCoopers (PwC) in 2011 are striking and frightening, which can support the seriousness of these concepts. PwC report is composed of survey of 600 executives from U.S. hospitals and physician organizations, health insurers and pharmaceutical and life sciences companies. Findings can be summarized as (Clinical Innovation + Technology, 2011);

- Sixty-six percent of the reported health data breaches over the past two years up to 2011 are theft. Also, medical identity theft is rising. Thirty-six percent of healthcare provider organizations stated that they had patients seeking services, using somebody else's name and identification.
- Fifty-five percent of health organizations do not have privacy and security policies associated with the use of mobile devices.
- Fifty-four percent of health organizations have at least one issue with information privacy and security over the past two years.

- Improper use of PHI by an internal party is the most reported privacy and security violation. Over the past two years up to 2011, 40 percent of providers reported an incident of improper internal use of PHI. Because of the lack of awareness or training, breaches can occur with greater probability from mishandling of paper documents, people talking in the elevator, or comments made via social media.
- Among health insurers and pharmaceutical and life science companies, the most frequently reported issue was the improper transfer of PHI to unauthorized parties. Over the past two years up to 2011, 21 percent pharmaceutical and life sciences companies and 25 percent of health insurers improperly transferred files containing protected health information.
- Healthcare organizations; more than half allow access to social media while at work; less than half have a policy for the use of social media outside of work.
- Thirty-seven percent of the health organizations have the issue of use of mobile devices and social media, in their company privacy training.
- Forty-one percent of health insurers and 58 percent of providers include the appropriate use of EHRs as in their employee privacy training.

Patients' Rights and Healthcare Providers' Responsibilities

Patients have a right to (Cooper & Collman, 2005):

- Disclosure of how PHI is used and protected from providers and health plans,
- Given copies of their healthcare records,
- Request justification of their healthcare records,
- An explanation of disclosures made for purposes other than treatment, payment and healthcare operations.

Additionally, patients can (Xiong, 2012);

- Request restriction of the usage and disclosure of his PHI
- File a complaint if he believes privacy rights were violated
- Request notification of privacy practices used in the organization such as:
  - How medical information is used and disclosed,
  - How to access and obtain a copy of their medical record,
  - How to file a complaint.

Health care organizations should devise policies for PHI access such as (Oracle, 2011):

- Need-to-know and context. Is the access essential to perform the user's job related activities? As an example a receptionist or database administrator has no need to see PHI. A lab technician may need a part of medical information to perform his task.
- Privilege/authorization. Right to copy and/or modify PHI, or simply read.
- What applications have access to PHI?
- Who requires access to those applications? In what context and what functions/capabilities of the application the user is authorized to use?

Healthcare organizations can also (Australian Department of Health, 2013):

- Ensure that they comply with all security and technical requirements defined by the laws.
- Ensure their policies and procedures are up to date and the staff are well informed of.
- Ensure they have mechanisms to audit the System Operator individuals who have accessed or uploaded information.
- Ensure the information system infrastructure is clean of viruses and appropriately protected.
- Ensure the staff are well informed and educated about the Healthcare information system (HCIS), especially in privacy and security features.
- The staff's awareness is increased by reinforcing the importance of protecting and not sharing access credentials.

Privacy and Security Trends that Affect Healthcare

Experts of idexperts, a service provider for data breach care, forecast 12 top trends in data breach, privacy and security. In this section, the forecasts of idexperts about the trends that affect healthcare are going to be given. The trends that may affect healthcare are (idexperts, 2013):

- **Global Criminals:** Criminals became globally connected and they are part of organized crime. They are in an attempt to intrude into databases and capture PHI illegally.
- **Advanced Persistent Threat (APT):** APT is a huge threat to every type of organization, hackers gain access to the system somehow and standby for a long period of time to capture the PHI and they cannot be detected for a long time.
- **Malicious Attackers:** Intruders of the systems. They may have commercial purposes such as capturing and selling the data, or can hack the system to damage the reputation of the organization.
- **Data Breaches:** Breaches affect all kinds of organizations and give way to intruders.
- **Infinitely Distribution Possibility of Electronic Data:** PHI can be stolen from anywhere in the world, distributed to infinite number of locations for an infinite period of time and can cause limitless damage.
- **Increased Enforcement Risk:** Regulators increasingly aggressive in investigating security breaches and obtaining substantial monetary settlements or penalties from responsible organizations.
- **Identity Theft:** Authentication mechanisms employ identity verification to do many things in the systems. Theft of identity is a big risk, because the capturing person causes big damages by pretending to be the person of the stolen identity.
- **Ubiquity of Digital and Mobile Devices:** The systems use a wide range of digital and mobile devices, and they are increasing in number as the technology improves, to collect and digitize PHI. This both provides more opportunities for governments to resell consumer data, forcing consumers to demand better privacy protections and read/approve/decline company privacy statements, and give a road to malicious intruders.
- **Long-Term Monitoring:** Data captured by hacking, theft or unauthorized access, can't be used immediately always. Organizations should develop plans for persistent, long-term monitoring, for the possibility of lag time that may occur between the time of the breach and the fraudulent use of consumer information.

- **Mistaken Dependency on Technology:** Organizations believe that data security and cyber privacy is an outsourced product that can be purchased. It is for sure, but it is not enough by itself, it's the humans using this product (in the case of most breaches, it is not). Organizations should focus on training the staff and invoke awareness of them about the valuable data.

LAWS AND REGULATIONS ON PATIENT PRIVACY AND SECURITY

There are many non-governmental organizations releases standards and measures to provide Patient Privacy and Security beside the governmental organizations that arrange this issue by means of laws. Health Insurance Portability and Accountability Act (HIPPA), Healthcare Information Systems Management Society (HIMSS), Healthcare Information Technology Standards Panel (HITSP) are some examples. In this section HIPAA Privacy Rule and Security Rule, Health Information Technology for Economic and Clinical Health (HITECH) Act, Healthcare Information Systems Management Society (HIMSS) privacy and security toolkit, and European Regulations on Privacy and Security is going to be examined.

HIPAA Privacy Rule and Security Rule

The Office for Civil Rights department of the United States in Department of Health and Human Services (HHS) enacted the Health Insurance Portability and Accountability Act (HIPAA) in 1996 and it is updated regularly. The last update is made in 2013. It has four basic rules:

- Privacy rule,
- Security rule,
- Breach Notification rule,
- Enforcement Rule.

This chapter will examine the privacy and security rule of HIPAA. HIPAA privacy rule applies to all forms of patients' PHI, whether electronic, written, or oral whereas HIPAA security rule is applied to EPHI only (Center of Medicare & Medicaid Services, 2007).

There are three safeguards for security in HIPAA security rule (Webb-Morgan, 2013):

- **Administrative Safeguards**: Comprehensive staff training, limited access to electronic health records, contingency plans in case of emergencies.
- **Physical Safeguards:** Computer monitor privacy filters, locks to prevent equipment theft, limited access to areas that host data.
- **Technical Safeguards:** Limited access to EPHI:
  - Access Controls,
  - Audit Controls,
  - Integrity,
  - Person or Entity Authentication,
  - Transmission Security:
    - Integrity Controls,
    - Encryption.

Healthcare administrations should take cautions to comply with both security and privacy of health data. The security rule assigns duties in the heading of "Administrative safeguards" to the healthcare managements. Especially invoking awareness of the healthcare staff is an important issue that healthcare managements deal with. Most of the staff either is not aware of privacy and security issues or they do not take even simple precautions because of negligence. Employee negligence is a major source of data breach in the healthcare institutions (Wallace, 2015).

Health Information Technology for Economic and Clinical Health Act (HITECH)

Health Information Technology for Economic and Clinical Health (HITECH) Act is the part of the American Recovery and Reinvestment Act of 2009. It has four basic goals (Blumenthal, 2010):

- Define meaningful use,
- Encourage and support the attainment of meaningful use through incentives and grant programs,
- Bolster public trust in electronic information systems by ensuring their privacy and security, and
- Foster continued Healthcare Information Technologies (HIT) innovation.

HITECH strengthened HIPAA's privacy and security guidelines by imposing new privacy obligations, expanding and clarifying business associates requirements; adding provisions related to EHR, health information exchange (HIE), and personal health records (PHR), increasing enforcement and monetary civil penalties (Hiller, McMullen, Chumney, & Baumer, 2011).

HITECH extends HIPAA's Privacy and Security Rules, by addressing the privacy and security issues related to the electronic transmission of PHI (Kobus, 2012).

HITECH, enforces the healthcare organizations to report immediately breaches that affect 500 or more people mandatorily, to both HHS Secretary and the media and notify affected individuals, breaches affecting less than 500 individuals are supposed to be reported to the HHS Secretary on an annual basis (HHS, 2009).

Managing Information Privacy and Security in Healthcare by HIMSS

Healthcare Information Systems Management Society (HIMSS) defines itself as "...a global, cause-based, not-for-profit organization focused on better health through information technology (IT). HIMSS leads efforts to optimize health engagements and care outcomes using information technology" (HIMSS, 2014). HIMSS has a toolkit for privacy and security, which is the improved and moved to a dashboard format version of "CPRI Security Toolkit", created by Computer based Patient Record Institute's (CPRI) charter Work Group on Confidentiality, Privacy, and Security, in response to HIPAA (Collman & Demster 2013).

HIMSS privacy and security toolkit is a free resource to educate the healthcare industry on privacy and security, the dashboard includes 11 major categories (Collman & Demster 2013):

- **Introduction/Concepts:** Basic Foundation Knowledge,
- **Laws/Regulations:** Local, state, federal, and international,
- **Best Practices:** Industry produced guidelines,
- **Case Studies, Use Cases, Forms and Formats:** Real world experiences,
- **Personal Health Records:** P&S issues unique to PHR,

- **Policies and Procedures:** Requirements and Samples,
- **Privacy:** All privacy related content,
- **Executive Information:** C-Suite considerations,
- **Security:** All security related content,
- **Business Associates and Health Information Exchanges:** Issues unique to BAs and HIEs,
- **Specialty Segments:** LTC, HHA, Physician Practices, Medical Devices among others.

European Regulations on Privacy and Security of PHI

The Organization for Economic Cooperation and Development (OECD) declared Guidelines on the Protection of Privacy and Transborder Flows of Personal Data (OECD Privacy Guidelines) in 1980 which contain (Hiller, McMullen, Chumney, & Baumer, 2011),

- Limitation of data collected,
- Maintenance of data quality,
- Specification of the collection purpose,
- Limitation of data use to that specified purpose,
- Adequate security,
- Transparency,
- Individual access to and control of data collected, and
- Accountability.

These guidelines are updated when required.

In addition to OECD guidelines, there are two directives that privacy and security is based on: 1995 directive (95/46/EC), from which Article 29 Board is created, related to the protection of individuals with regard to the processing of personal data, and 2002 directive (2002/58/EC), related to the processing of personal data and the protection of privacy in the electronic communications sector (Hiller, McMullen, Chumney, & Baumer, 2011).

1995 directive is designed to protect the privacy and security of all personal data (not only health data) collected for or about EU citizens (Mirkovic, Skipenes, Christiansen, & Bryhni, 2015).

2002 directive, on privacy and electronic communication complements, regulates the protection of privacy when processing personal data using new telecommunication technologies (Mirkovic, Skipenes, Christiansen, & Bryhni, 2015).

Article 29 Board declared the "Working Document on the Processing of Personal Data Relating to Health in Electronic Health Records" in 2007, which provides an interpretation of the application of privacy principles to electronic health records, and recommends adoption of eleven specific legal protections to protect individual health privacy (Hiller, McMullen, Chumney, & Baumer, 2011). The requisites of the report can be summarized as (Hiller, McMullen, Chumney, & Baumer, 2011);

- **Explicit Consent:** An entity may collect and process PHI only if the owner of the PHI (patient) grants explicit consent. This consent must be given as specific, voluntary, informed, and not forced in any way.

- **Vital Interests:** The consent can be given on behalf of patient when he is "physically or legally incapable of giving his consent". This exception can only be applied to a "small number of cases."
- **Health Professionals:** For health professionals to process PHI, the requisites are:
  ○ Processing must be required for the purpose of "preventive medicine, medical diagnosis"
  ○ For the "provision of care or treatment or the management of health-care services," and
  ○ The health professional processing the PHI have to comply with the professional secrecy.
- **Public Interest:** PHI can be used for Public interest purposes if the requisites below are met;
  ○ There must be a special legal basis for the need,
  ○ PHI processed under the system must be necessary and proportional to the need, and
  ○ Specific and suitable safeguards for fundamental privacy have to be employed.

The latest regulation in EU about the patient privacy and security was performed in Prague, on the 19th of October, 2009, by the attendance of European Union Health Ministers to the conference, "eHealth for Individuals, Society and Economy" (Hiller, McMullen, Chumney, & Baumer, 2011). In this conference the official "Prague Declaration" was announced. The declaration stated paying close attention to legal and ethical issues including data protection and privacy issues (Hiller, McMullen, Chumney, & Baumer, 2011).

SECURITY AND PRIVACY AUDITING IN E-HEALTH

Audit mechanisms are employed by all sectors in information systems. The purpose is to trail the electronic records accessed and store the issues committed in these accesses. The information in the audit logs should contain the data accessed, the user who accessed that data, time of access, type of access, type of action done (read, update, delete, print), the hardware information of the access (the computer name or IP, the printer if a print is done etc.).

Recording all the audit data is not enough of course. They must be analyzed and the violations have to be spotted in time. To be capable of doing this, normal and abnormal access conditions should be clearly defined. Data mining mechanisms can be employed to detect the anomalies and outliers.

Instead of recording every action in the HCIS, some events can be selected to store in audit trails. The recommendations of the NEMA/COCIR/JIRA Security and Privacy Committee (SPC) (2001) are;

- PHI-Related Events:
  ○ Create Events:
    ▪ Creation of records that contain PHI,
    ▪ Import of records that contain PHI.
  ○ Modify Events:
    ▪ Editing of data (e.g. appending, merging, modifying),
    ▪ Re-association of data,
    ▪ De-identifying of PHI.
  ○ View Events:
    ▪ Access to PHI by any user,
    ▪ Export of PHI to digital media or network,
    ▪ Print or FAX of PHI.

- ◦ Delete Events:
  - ▪ User command to delete PHI,
  - ▪ User command to delete PHI before the correct transmission of PHI was confirmed by the receiver,
  - ▪ Automated command to delete PHI.
- • Non-PHI Events:
  - ◦ General:
    - ▪ Machine startup and shutdown,
    - ▪ Successful login and logout of users,
    - ▪ Changes to user accounts (creation, modification, deletion),
    - ▪ Automatic logout of a user after exceeding a locally-defined time of inactivity,
    - ▪ Switching to another user's access or privileges after logging in with one's own identification,
    - ▪ Software or hardware modification,
    - ▪ Update of virus signatures.
  - ◦ Operational Events:
    - ▪ Login attempts with failed identification or authentication, also known as failed login attempts,
    - ▪ Changes of the time or date of the system,
    - ▪ Emergency mode operation,
    - ▪ Detection of a virus,
    - ▪ Detectable hardware errors,
    - ▪ Changes to log files (creation, deletion, configuration)
  - ◦ Communication Events:
    - ▪ Network link failures,
    - ▪ Device connection failure due to device identification or authentication failure (also known as a failed connection attempt),
    - ▪ Network and device connections dropped,
    - ▪ Data integrity verification failure for information transmitted over a network,
    - ▪ Message authentication failure for information transmitted over a network,
    - ▪ Evocation of a network abnormality alarm,
    - ▪ IP addresses of successful and unsuccessful connections,
    - ▪ Changes to network security configuration (e.g., firewalls if part of a medical IT system).

SOLUTIONS AND RECOMMENDATIONS

Patient privacy and security is a very important issue. There can be great and unbearable outcomes when violated. To avoid violations and assure protection of patient rights, the institutions dealing with patient data should be beware of threats first. They have to know and inform their staff that there are many people and organizations chasing after the patient data, and motivated to capture it legally or illegally. Second, they have to know there are regulations to abide by. These regulations should be studied and related measures have to be taken.

Staff training is an important issue. With very simple measures, most of the breach risks can be eliminated. There are institutions giving this training.

The last but not the least, patients have to be well informed about their rights. In most of the cases, the patients do not know the rights. They either do not give importance to that issue, or exaggerate their rights and request more than they deserve. In this case, this is the duty of public authorities to inform the patients by drawing attention. The healthcare institutions also may employ patient's rights departments to both handle the disputes and inform the patients. Staff training is also a solution to avoid disputes, by enabling the staff to inform the patient first about their rights and then start giving healthcare.

FUTURE RESEARCH DIRECTIONS

As seen, privacy and security of the EPHI is very critical, violations have both legal and moral consequences. Protection of patient privacy and security is major concern for every healthcare organization and bodies that deal with PHI.

Securing technologies will be the major future work item, in both technical and managerial concern, for both electronic and manual ways. Security is the challenge of all information technologies not only in healthcare but in all sectors. It is improving in an ongoing way. E-health will take advantage of the general improvements, as well as the healthcare specific works and researches.

Literature tells, most of the breaches occur as a result of insider related activities, mostly by negligence of the users. Security professionals think the risks posed by negligent insiders (65%) is the biggest security concern (SANS, 2013). Intruders and malicious attacks have less shares in the security breaches than the insider negligence. Employee negligence is a major source of data breach in the healthcare institutions (Wallace, 2015). Development of strategies for invoking the awareness of the staff and ensuring that they take the tiny measures for protecting the patient privacy is another future work candidate. It is not possible to secure the EPHI, without being sure that the staff does not take part in the violations whether intentionally or mistakenly.

Protection of patient privacy and security in mobility is another future work item. Mobility is the miracle of the era. There is a large number of mobile applications in healthcare and they are growing in a tremendous way. The ubiquity of the mobile devices whets the application developers and health investors' appetite. As a result of this appetite, mobility becomes a huge application area. There should be great concern and work about the patient privacy and security in mobility. Especially unexperienced users about mobile device security can give breaches to malicious people and applications, by not employing necessary security measures.

CONCLUSION

The privacy and security of patient data is a research and application area in e-health and healthcare. There are conferences dedicated to this subject, certification programs are available.

It has been found that electronic data breaches occur three times as many as paper based breaches and affect 25 times more people (Torrieri, 2011). E-health has many advantages, there is no need to mention or list them here again. What we should know and be aware is, it has challenges and problems together with the benefits.

Most electronic breaches are caused by are insider theft or human errors other than hacking. Especially when the subject is healthcare, because of the dynamics of it, security and privacy will be its weakness. The staff does not like the security issues and sees it as an obstacle to doing his work properly. This issue must be gently and seriously handled by the managements.

I want to end the chapter with the saying of Peter Harries, principal and co-leader, Health Information Privacy and Security Practice, PwC. "To protect patient trust and their own brand reputation, organizations need to go beyond minimum regulatory requirements and adopt an integrated approach that combines privacy, security and compliance within a culture where all employees see themselves as champions of confidentiality and where privacy is part of the patient experience" (Techtw, 2011).

ACKNOWLEDGMENT

Part of this work was presented in The International Journal of Arts & Sciences' (IJAS) International Conference for Technology and Science on 30 June – 03 July 2015 in Brussels.

REFERENCES

Act, H. I. P. A. A. (1996). Health insurance portability and accountability act of 1996. *Public Law*, *104*, 191.

Australian Department of Health. (2013). *What can you do? Learning center, E-health*. Retrieved from http://www.ehealth.gov.au/internet/ehealth/publishing.nsf/content/elearning

Blumenthal, D. (2010). Launching HIteCH. *The New England Journal of Medicine*, *362*(5), 382–385. doi:10.1056/NEJMp0912825 PMID:20042745

Center of Medicare & Medicaid Services. (2007). *Security 101 for Covered Entities* (Vol. 2). Retrieved from http://www.hhs.gov/ocr/privacy/hipaa/administrative/securityrule/security101.pdf

Clinical Innovation + Technology. (2011). *PwC: Healthcare is underprepared to protect patient info*. Retrieved from http://www.clinical-innovation.com/topics/ehr-emr/pwc-healthcare-underprepared-protect-patient-info

Collman, J., & Demster, B. (2013). *HIMSS Privacy and Security Toolkit Executive Summary*. Retrieved from http://www.himss.org/files/HIMSSorg/Content/files/CPRIToolkit/version6/v7/D01_Executive_Summary.pdf

Cooper, T., & Collman, J. (2005). Managing information security and privacy in healthcare data mining. In H. Chen, S. Fuller, C. Freidman, & W. Hersh (Eds.), *Medical Informatics* (pp. 95-137). Springer US. Department of Health and Human Services (HHS) (2009). *HITECH Breach Notification Interim Final Rule*. Retrieved from http://www.hhs.gov/ocr/privacy/hipaa/understanding/coveredentities/breachnotificationifr.html

Electronic Health Record Vendors Association (EHRVA). (2008). *Privacy and Security Whitepaper*. Retrieved from http://www.himssehra.org/docs/20080506PS_Whitepaper.pdf

Eysenbach, G. (2001). What is e-health? *Journal of Medical Internet Research, 3*(2), e20. doi:10.2196/jmir.3.2.e20 PMID:11720962

Healthcare Information Systems Management Society (HIMSS). (2014). Retrieved from http://www.himss.org/

Hiller, J., McMullen, M. S., Chumney, W. M., & Baumer, D. L. (2011). Privacy and security in the implementation of health information technology (electronic health records): US and EU compared. *BUJ Sci. & Tech. L, 17*, 1.

idExperts, (2013). *12 Trends in Privacy and Security.* Retrieved from http://www2.idexpertscorp.com/press/12-trends-in-privacy-and-security-infographic-available-a-decade-of-data-br/

Kobus, T. J. III. (2012). The A to Z of healthcare data breaches. *Journal of Healthcare Risk Management, 32*(1), 24–28. doi:10.1002/jhrm.21088 PMID:22833327

Mirkovic, J., Skipenes, E., Christiansen, E. K., & Bryhni, H. (2015, April). Security and privacy legislation guidelines for developing personal health records. *Proceedings of Second International Conference on eDemocracy & eGovernment (ICEDEG)* (pp. 77-84). IEEE.

NEMA/COCIR/JIRA Security and Privacy Committee (SPC). (2001). Security and Privacy Auditing in Health Care Information Technology. Retrieved from http://www.medicalimaging.org/wp-content/uploads/2011/02/Security_and_Privacy_Auditing_In_Health_Care_Information_Technology-November_2001.pdf

Oracle, (2011). *HITECH's Challenge to the Health Care Industry.* Retrieved from http://www.oracle.com/technetwork/database/security/owp-security-hipaa-hitech-522515.pdf

SANS Institute. (2013). *Inaugural Health Care Survey.* Retrieved from http://www.sans.org/reading-room/analysts-program/2013-healthcare-survey

Security Week. (2011). *Health Industry Under-Prepared to Protect Patient Privacy, Says PwC Report.* Retrieved from http://www.securityweek.com/health-industry-under-prepared-protect-patient-privacy-says-pwc-report

Sun, J., Zhu, X., Zhang, C., & Fang, Y. (2012). Security and Privacy for Mobile Health-Care (m-Health) Systems. In S. K. Das, K. Kant, & N. Zhang (Eds.), *Handbook on Securing Cyber-Physical Critical Infrastructure* (pp. 677–704). USA: Elsevier. doi:10.1016/B978-0-12-415815-3.00027-3

Techtw. (2011). *Health Industry Under-Prepared to Protect Patient Privacy: PwC (Posted by Geek Girl).* Retrieved from https://techtw.wordpress.com/category/analyst-reports/

Torrieri, M. (2011). *Mobile Technology and the Rise of Healthcare Data Breaches.* Retrieved from http://www.physicianspractice.com/blog/mobile-technology-and-rise-healthcare-data-breaches

Upstate Medical University. (2011). *Protecting Patient Confidentiality and Security.* Retrieved from www.upstate.edu/forms/documents/F84037.pdf

Wallace, I. M. (2015). Is Patient Confidentiality Compromised With the Electronic Health Record?: A Position Paper. *Computers, Informatics, Nursing*, *33*(2), 58–62. doi:10.1097/CIN.0000000000000126 PMID:25532832

Webb-Morgan, M. (2013, June 12). *How to safeguard patient info in the digital age*. Retrieved from http://www.healthcarecommunication.com

Xiong, L. (2012). *CS573 Data Privacy and Security Lecture notes*. Retrieved from http://www.mathcs. emory.edu/~lxiong/cs573_s12/share/slides/0320_healthcare.pdf

KEY TERMS AND DEFINITIONS

Data Breach: An incident in which sensitive, protected or confidential data has been viewed, stolen or used by an unauthorized body.

E-Health: E-health is the use of information and communication technologies to improve health care.

HIMSS: HIMSS is a global, cause-based, non-profit organization, focused on better health through information technology.

HIPAA: HIPAA is the federal Health Insurance Portability and Accountability Act of 1996.

HITECH: The HITECH Act is an incentive program that urges healthcare organizations to use a certified Healthcare Information System for everyday practice and use.

Privacy: The state of being free from being observed or disturbed by other people.

Protected Health Information (PHI): PHI is the individually identifiable health information of a patient.

Section 6
Critical Issues and Challenges

Chapter 75
The Administrative Policy Quandary in Canada's Health Service Organizations

Grace I. Paterson
Dalhousie University, Canada

Jacqueline M. MacDonald
Annapolis Valley Health, South Shore Health and South West Health, Canada

Naomi Nonnekes Mensink
Dalhousie University, Canada

ABSTRACT

This chapter examines the process for administrative health service policy development with respect to information sharing and decision-making as well as the relationship of policy to decision making. The challenges experienced by health service managers are identified. The administrative health policy experience in Nova Scotia is described. There is a need for integrated policy at multiple levels (public, clinical, and administrative). The quandary is that while working to share health information systems, most Canadian health service organizations continue to individually develop administrative health policy, expending more resources on policy writing than on translation/education, monitoring, or evaluation. By exploring the importance and nature of administrative policy as a foundation for quality improvement in healthcare delivery, a case is made for greater use of health informatics tools and processes.

INTRODUCTION

In its simplest form, a policy tells people what to do and a procedure tells how to do it. (Cryderman, 1999, p. 17)

Policies provide structure to decisions. They allow consistent, informed decisions to be made about situations that have previously been encountered in health organizations, allowing clinicians, patients, users, and employees at any level to respond to a situation. Policies, based on the mission or purpose

DOI: 10.4018/978-1-5225-3926-1.ch075

Copyright © 2018, IGI Global. Copying or distributing in print or electronic forms without written permission of IGI Global is prohibited.

of the organization, provide the framework of objectives and measures that will allow decisions to be made and actions to be taken (Althaus, Bridgman, & Davis, 2007). Administrative policy is policy that: identifies the governing principle that enables or constrains decisions and action, is institution or group-wide, supports compliance with applicable law, and is mandated by the highest authority within the institution or group of institutions (University of Arizona, 2011).

According to the Canada Health Act, the primary objective of Canadian health care policy is "to protect, promote, and restore the physical and mental well-being of residents of Canada and to facilitate reasonable access to health services without financial or other barriers" (Nova Scotia Department of Health and Wellness, 2012, p. 9).

In this chapter, we explore the nature and purposes of administrative policy. We discuss the relationship of policy to decision making at both the administrative and clinical levels and the importance of well-developed policy for healthcare practice, as that relates to health information systems. We explore the importance and nature of administrative policy as a foundation for quality improvement in healthcare delivery through health informatics tools and processes such as electronic health records and health decision support systems; and for analysis for policy that focuses on the needs of policymakers.

We address the quandary that, while working to share health information systems, most Canadian health service organizations continue to individually develop administrative health policy, expending more resources on policy writing than on translation/education, monitoring or evaluation. Although policy can be most effective in bringing about improved health outcomes and organizational efficiencies, it is often difficult to see a relationship between health policy and health information systems. There is an absence of good policy-oriented data on which to base decisions. As an example, researchers found that Canada's wait-list information and management systems were inadequate and did not track outcomes to allow for continuous refinement of the criteria and weights used to prioritize patients in the wait-list policy (Lewis, Barer, Sanmartin, Sheps, Shortt, & McDonald, 2000). A systematic approach using health informatics skills and knowledge can empower policymakers to use data to develop policy, use information technologies to strategically communicate policy, and use outcomes data to monitor adherence to and effectiveness of policy.

Most research literature on health policy is concerned with public policy and clinical policy. There is a research-practice gap surrounding many aspects of administrative health policy (MacDonald, Bath, & Booth, 2008). The literature review for this chapter includes research on the relationship between policy and health informatics, and on health service managers' decision making at the administrative policy level. It focuses on what health service managers actually do rather than what they should do. We identify several challenges experienced by policymakers that provide opportunities for health informatics leadership and research. We also draw on experiences of OP3 (One Province, One Process, One Policy), a group working to share policies at the District Health Authority (DHA) level in Nova Scotia.

THE NATURE OF POLICY

With its many layers, health policy is more complex than "what to do" and "how to do it" (Cryderman, 1999, p. 17). The highest and most authoritative level is law or legislation. In Canada, the most general principles reside in the Canada Health Act where requirements for provincial and territorial government health service delivery are outlined. Each province or territory has legislation, such as the Nova Scotia Health Services and Insurance Act, that describes the "what". The regulations contained in the legislation describe the "how" with the attendant penalties listed. The process of passing Bills into laws is one of the main tasks of provincial legislative assemblies. A Bill becomes an Act, and thus provincial law, when it receives Royal Assent by the Lieutenant Governor. Acts are then translated into multi-organization policies for the levels of authority that apply the legislation to healthcare delivery in each geographic area or for specific patient groupings. The purpose of any policy is to guide corporate and individual decision-making at each level.

There is a complex set of historical, cultural, and socio-political forces that shape the policy environment (Bell, 2010). A fundamental policy assertion is that government should not solve a problem until it understands the problem. Being able to perceive the explicit, implicit and pragmatic dimensions of the policy problem is key to understanding the barriers and challenges associated with a particular policy goal and context.

Two frameworks for examining multi-layered health policy have been identified. Caldwell and Mays (2012) use macro-meso-micro frame analysis to study the transition of a policy from high-level idea to program in action where macro is national policy, meso is national programme and micro is local context. The Canadian Health Services Research Foundation (2000) identified three types of health policy decisions: public policy decisions that deal with determining what health services will be provided; administrative policy decisions that are concerned with operations including where specific health services will be located and how they will be offered; and clinical policy decisions that include determining criteria to identify who qualifies for specific services and how these services are to be managed. The informational uncertainty of clinicians is resolved more readily by research than is the informational uncertainty faced by government and managers (Canadian Health Services Research Foundation, 2000).

Provincial and federal governments, health researchers, and leaders of professional associations are more likely to be concerned with public policy and clinical policy than they are with administrative policy. Administrative and operating policies are more likely to be concerns at local levels, such as in hospitals and DHAs where, despite expected similarities, each health service organization has traditionally developed its own policy and procedure documents.

There has been little discussion in the literature of the differences between the above policy decision types and how they are integrated. There is a lack of understanding of their relationship with each other and with legislation and professional standards; and of whether the different types of health policy are best developed together or separately. It is not clear whether and how these policy decision types might relate to strategic, consequential, and far-reaching decisions; tactical, medium-range and moderate decisions that support strategic decisions; and operational decisions—the everyday decisions that support tactical decisions (Heller, Drenth, Koopman, & Rus, 1988).

RELATIONSHIP BETWEEN POLICY AND HEALTH INFORMATICS

As it pertains to curricula, the concept of "Health Informatics Policy" is usually considered to encompass topics such as leadership and ethics; information security; health communication; social implications of computing; and, negotiation and conflict resolution (Martz, Zhang, & Ozanich, 2007).

The form and characteristics of the system, the information exchange it enables, the permitted access and the permitted sharing are all based on policies within the organization or from multiple organizations that place enablers and constraints on the system since each participating organization has its own purposes. For example: who can enter prescriptions in a drug information system and whether the system is available near the bedside in a hospital (both policy based) often affects the quality of ordering and measurement of effectiveness. The policies, in turn, are based on the purpose and values of the organization. If improvement of patient health/condition is the over-riding purpose, health information systems have different characteristics and sharing procedures than if the over-riding purpose is risk management. Policies governing health information flow and use in one part of an organization may be different from those in another part of an organization based on unique purposes and constraints.

The concept of "Health Policy Informatics" as a subdiscipline of health informatics is emerging. It would tackle the challenges and problems arising from the multidimensional nature of information that is used for policy creation, dissemination, implementation, and evaluation; and would also address the challenges experienced by health service managers.

CHALLENGES EXPERIENCED BY HEALTH SERVICE MANAGERS

Knowledge Management

An organization's approach to knowledge management should be reflected in its culture, commitment to knowledge services, skills and use of information technology (Walton & Booth, 2004). The challenge is to ensure that information systems are designed to enable clinical knowledge management—supporting clinicians (of any kind) with information about, critical analysis of, and learning-oriented dissemination of health related information about individuals and groups (Booth & Brice, 2004). A feedback loop that uses data from health records along with research evidence from clinical literature provides knowledge about what works in the local context (Zitner, Paterson, & Fay, 1998).

A study that examined health services managers' information behaviour found that managers rarely referenced external research-based information for their decision making. They were more often influenced by explicit organizational knowledge such as policies and guidelines (MacDonald, Bath, & Booth, 2008).

Multiple Communities of Practice

Policymakers need to address the multidimensional aspects of knowledge-making for policy (Bell, 2010). There are perspectival differences in how knowledge is acquired and understood by the multiple communities that are impacted by policy as described in the CHAMP (Clinicians, Health Informaticians, Administrators, Medical Educators, Patients) framework (Paterson, 2008). Communities of practice have vested interests in both the process and the outcomes. An assessment of needs should consider the advantage to be gained or lost in the planning process (Mensink, 2004). The authors' experience is that multiple communities of practice rarely work collaboratively to influence policy and legislation that affects all of them.

Researchers need to pay attention to the gaps in policy as these tell their own story. In Keshavjee et al.'s policy framework analysis for Electronic Medical Records (EMR), they acknowledge that policy at the macro (public policy) level lags client needs significantly (Keshavjee, Manji, Singh, & Pairaudeau, 2009). That framework focused on policies such as incentives for uptake of EMRs, engagement of key stakeholders from affected communities of practice, creation of suitable Information and Communication Technology (ICT) infrastructure, implementation of interoperability standards, and engagement of patients and their advocacy groups. To achieve interoperability with external systems in hospitals, laboratories and other health care provider communities, strong health information technology policies are required at the macro level.

Organizational Inertia

There are multiple and disparate processes for policy approval. A policy on the same topic, e.g., handheld devices, may come from multiple departments. In the experience of the authors, such policies may be identified as "universal" policy without reference to any approval process.

Embedding Policy in Information Systems

Whether or not to embed policy in information systems is a challenge, since an information system has a level of inertia inherent, such that it may continue to reflect outdated policy if no decision is made to systematically update it. This could lead to ignoring explicit policy because the current policy is not integrated with information systems and clinical workflow. This may result in workarounds by staff that are costly and a challenge to quality (Mensink & Paterson, 2010).

According to Grant et al., the health informatics research agenda should be dominated by the requirements for usable, useful and used systems (Grant, Moshyk, Kushniruk, & Moehr, 2003). If the effort needed to access policy resources at the clinician level is high, its usefulness will be diminished (Smith, 1996). A theoretical framework, the Normalisation Process Model, aims to identify factors that promote and inhibit the implementation of decision support technologies in routine practice (Elwyn, Légaré, van der Weijden, Edwards, & May, 2008).

There are programming challenges that may be difficult to overcome, including vendor agreements and information systems that do not fully fit with the purpose for which they were acquired. Collaboration is needed in the development and management of information resources to better ensure recognition of the differences in information structure and information needs based on varying philosophies of care and service as well as sites of care (Mohaghan & Cooke, 2004).

Protection of Health Information and Interprofessional Practice

A seamless integrated circle of care requires sharing of information across the settings of care, supported by legislation and policies at the local level. The regulatory and medico-legal barriers to interprofessional practice were identified (Lahey & Currie, 2005). Through collaboration between academics and policymakers the Regulated Health Professions Network Act was introduced (Lahey, 2012). Once passed, this legislation will enable interdisciplinary care and collaboration, and improve processes that may involve the different health professions involved in a patient's care (such as the investigation of a patient complaint for an adverse event, the sharing of competencies among the scopes of practice and the appeals process) (Wedlake, 2012). Policies that will be implemented need to be monitored to measure the impact of this Act.

At the macro level in Nova Scotia, the Personal Health Information Act, proclaimed on December 4, 2012 and effective June 1, 2013, "governs the collection, use, disclosure, retention, disposal and destruction of personal health information" (Nova Scotia Department of Health and Wellness, 2012). This act recognizes and supports the circle of care.

COACH, Canada's Health Informatics Association, publishes guidelines for the protection of health information. They state, "Health organizations must develop policies and procedures to protect the privacy, confidentiality, and security of personal health information under their control, to help mitigate the risk of unauthorized access, use or disclosure of such information, and to prevent against its loss or unnecessary destruction" (COACH, 2001). COACH publications are being continuously updated to align with changing legislation and new ways of delivering health information to patients and their caregivers.

Common Health Language

Policy committees need a standardized health glossary to achieve common policies and reduce the resource-intensive nature of administrative policy formulation. While there are medical dictionaries and online glossaries we are not aware of one that is specifically for health care professionals that melds written and spoken words and uses standardized health nomenclature that is grounded in a reference terminology. Access to a common language will support communication between professions, departments and health districts and help new health services staff. Use of a standardized health vocabulary is fundamental to both communications and information technology. It also enables semantic interoperability in ICT infrastructure (Paterson, 2008).

Generalization and Scaling Up of Policy

We need to pay systematic attention to how the benefits achieved in successful pilot or experimental projects can be expanded to serve more people more quickly and more equitably (Simmons & Shiffman, 2007). Policy is the articulation of a government program. Program development requires an interactive, iterative, and process-oriented approach to be sustainable.

High-level policy may be overly detailed and rigid, creating challenges for those who are tasked with implementing those policies locally. Such policies may require elements or processes that may not be available locally. However, these high level policies do have the advantage of authority and support. "In contrast, decentralized approaches allow local initiative, autonomy, spontaneity, mutual learning and problem-solving. Their obvious disadvantage is that they do not have the reach of central authorities, and often do not command sufficient influence or resources to ensure appropriate policy reform" (Simmons & Shiffman, 2007, p. 15).

Since electronic information sharing has such a broad reach, central principles concerning this have to be clear and universally applied. This is especially true of information that is used for overall program quality management where policies and practices have to be consistent across different settings.

Creating/Developing a Learning Organization

A learning organization is one that creates and uses administrative policy to best manage changing conditions, and is not rigidly bound by rules that emphasize standardization (Simmons & Shiffman, 2007). Administrators of health information systems are responsible for enabling clinical care. They need to ensure that clinical knowledge management systems are available for clinicians and their patients where and when needed.

Despite lots of education and public discussion about the concept of a multi-disciplinary team involvement in care, formal hospital-based medical records that are used as a basis for sharing information with other clinicians may contain only information that has been approved by a central administrative committee that is primarily responsible for the legal status of the health record (Capital Health, 2011). Because of this approval process, there may be little information retained on the shared record from members of the team who are not hospital-based health practitioners. Examples include external (to the hospital) physiotherapists, family counselors, family caregivers and service staff who may have made important observations about the patient or been the most frequent confidant of the patient's wishes when in hospital. This affects not only the total care provided but also the richness of information available to researchers and others for quality improvement.

Shared Administrative Health Policy Development, Implementation, and Evaluation

There is an opportunity for efficiency if multiple organizations share policies. There must be a policy development framework with capacity, authority, and resourcing to achieve province-wide policy development, approval and distribution. In addition, policy readers need to be queried about their policy documentation needs and uses, and the barriers and challenges they encounter in finding and using institutional level policies.

Results arising from an evaluation of the effectiveness of program may identify policy issues. An independent evaluation of the Summary Care Records and HealthSpace programs in the UK (Greenhalgh, Hinder, Stramer, Bratan, & Russell, 2010) led to the closing of HealthSpace—a free, secure online health organizer—on December 14, 2012 and the destruction of all data in compliance with the Data Protection Act (NHS Connecting for Health, 2012). The findings raised questions about how this eHealth program in England was developed and approved at the policy level. The evaluation revealed that the benefits anticipated by policy makers were not achieved.

HEALTH SERVICE MANAGERS, ADMINISTRATIVE POLICY, AND DECISION MAKING

Health services have been described as the most complex of organizations to manage (Glouberman & Mintzberg, 2001). Elsewhere they are referred to as "high velocity" environments "in which there is rapid and discontinuous change … such that information is often inaccurate, unavailable, or obsolete" (Stephanovich & Uhrig, 1999, p. 198). Within this environment, health service managers are accountable for health service quality, resource use, employee effectiveness and wellbeing, and workplace safety and productivity.

Little research directly related to administrative health policy development has been identified. A mixed-methods study of 116 Australian health administrators' policy-related decision making practices used interviews and surveys to explore resource allocation decision situations (Baghbanian, Hughes, Kebriaei, & Khavarpour, 2012). Conclusions included that policy makers were "enlightened by" research that reached them indirectly. Managers made policy decisions by involving others with knowledge of the situation rather than by following formal procedures and reading primary research or systematic reviews. Decisions were characterized by ambiguity and complexity, short deadlines, incomplete information and significant unknowns. A UK study that used 21 interviews, document analysis and embedded research to assess understanding about national (macro level) policy translated to programs (meso level) and implemented locally (micro level) attributed differences to local contexts and different approaches to knowledge translation and concluded that a common understanding of purpose and objectives contributed to success (Caldwell & Mays, 2012).

Research on what health service managers actually do includes ten workplace studies of their information and decision making behavior. Five studies of health service managers and their workplace information access and use, each conducted in a different country and with a slightly different focus, found similar challenges related to information access and use (Head, 1996; Kovner & Rundall, 2006; Mbananga & Sekokotla, 2002; Moahi, 2000; Niedźwiedzka, 2003) despite difference in the wealth of the country (G8 or not), degree of computerization (desktop access to databases and the Internet, or not), single hospital or multi-site health service, and health service funding (whether public or private). These studies observed the importance of internal or local information to healthcare services. An additional five other studies of health service managers in their workplaces shared the finding that much of their work time was spent in meetings (Arman, Dellve, Wikström, & Törnström, 2009; Baghbanian, Hughes, Kebriaei, & Khavarpour, 2012; MacDonald, 2011; Moss, 2000; Tengelin, Arman, Wikström, & Delive, 2011).

The remaining literature on health service managers has tended to focus either on what they should do (Gray, 2009; Innvaer, Vist, Trommald, & Oxman, 2002; Innvær, 2009) or why they do not do what they should do (Kadane, 2005; Willis, Mitton, Gordon, & Best, 2012).

We do not know the cost to a health service organization of developing a single administrative policy or the potential return on investment of shared administrative policy development. OP3 members individually estimated the number of employees involved and the time needed to complete each task in the policy process model used by OP3. When tasks were totaled, the cost of developing a policy ranged from $10,000 to $200,000 with legal advice a factor contributing to higher policy development costs.

No research has been identified that explores how administrative policy decisions are made, how administrative policies are used or who uses them, whether policy development practices might be improved, or what the costs and benefits of shared policies are. Further research is needed to know whether problems solved and decisions made at health service managers meetings are shared within the organization and how they are shared, whether informally (either orally or through email) or formally (as administrative policy to support structured decision making).

ADMINISTRATIVE HEALTH POLICY IN CANADA

Through the 1980s and 1990s, Canadian hospitals were guided through policy and procedure manual development by Paula Cryderman (Cryderman, 1987). By the end of the 1990s, Cryderman recommended an overhaul to hospital policy manuals, citing forces of change that rendered manuals obsolete (Cryderman, 1999).

The Canadian Policy and Procedure Network (CPPN) has served since 2004 as "an informal forum for health care professionals to share and discuss policy and procedure topics for the improvement of health care" (Canadian Policy and Procedure Network, 2010). The CPPN is a moderated Yahoo Group with over 200 members. Members post an average 2,500 policy questions and requests for examples of policy and procedure documents per year.

The Canadian Association for Health Services and Policy Research (CAHSPR) is Canada's largest health services and policy research association. CAHSPR holds an annual conference and uses social media tools, such as Twitter, to build a community working towards evidence-based health care and health policy. "CAHSPR's mission is to improve health and health care by advancing the quality, relevance and application of research on health services and health policy" (Canadian Association for Health Services and Policy Research, 2012). Annual conferences feature policy forums and panel discussions which encourage true dialogue and debate. Citizen participation is important to a democracy and to the development of health policies that reflect the type of society that citizens want.

Accreditations Canada has performance indicators to measure the degree to which a health care facility delivers health care services according to criteria. Personnel in charge of administrative health policy are often the ones who participate in the assessment, which makes visible to the reviewers how well a facility abides by its health policies. As part of the dissemination of knowledge, Accreditations Canada developed a searchable Leading Practices Database to recognize innovative solutions to improving the quality of healthcare services delivery (Accreditations Canada, 2012).

ADMINISTRATIVE HEALTH POLICY EXPERIENCE IN NOVA SCOTIA, 2007-2012

In 2005, recognizing the resource-intensive complexity of policy development within their DHAs, Chief Executive Officers (CEOs) of Nova Scotia's nine DHAs and the Izaak Walton Killam Health Centre (IWK, pediatric and obstetric health centre for the Maritime Provinces) commissioned a feasibility study of shared policy development. The study identified fifteen opportunities for efficiencies with shared policies (Table 1).

In response to the study, the DHA/IWK CEOs established a working group in 2007, initially with one representative from each organization. The group expanded to include representatives from the Nova Scotia Department of Health and Wellness Policy and Planning Branch, and from the Health Association of Nova Scotia Policy, Planning and Decision Support Unit. All members of this group, known as OP3, have full time responsibilities in their own organization. Two guides, Policy Development, Implementation and Evaluation (Capital Health, 2012) and Style Guide, provide standard approaches to writing and formatting policy documents (OP3: One Province, One Process, One Policy, 2011).

Table 1. Opportunities for efficiency for NS DHAs/IWK in shared policy development

Coordinated Policy Processes	Coordinated Policy Structures	Coordinated Policy Skills and Competencies	Coordinated Policy Technology/ Enablers
1. Coordinated issue identification. 2. Centralized research support. 3. Centralized policy development. 4. Centralized communication and education content development. 5. Coordinated archiving and storage. 6. Coordinated compliance monitoring. 7. Provincial coordination of practice guidelines and procedures.	8. Formalize the policy 'community of interest' or network. 9. Leverage existing provincial committees. 10. Create new policy development committees.	11. Provincial Policy researcher/ coordinator.	12. Common policy templates and formats. 13. Collaboration tools. 14. Document management tools. 15. Access to Common templates.

By the fall of 2012, the group accomplished five of the fifteen opportunities for efficiency (numbers 5, 8. 12, 13, and 14 in Table 1) including coordinated archiving and storage in the form of a Web-based platform for shared policy management (http://policy.nshealth.ca/). In 2012, although policy manuals for most DHAs remain incomplete, an average of 500 policies per DHA is available on the site. Some DHAs have over 1,000 policies on the OP3 site.

In 2011, to inform strategic planning, OP3 members began considering evaluation of both group and policy process. A review of meeting minutes identified 45 tasks in the policy process that might be evaluated (Appendix A). To help explain the administrative policy development process to a DHA Policy Committee willing to develop a pilot evaluation survey, these 45 tasks were grouped under 15 main headings, and arranged graphically as cogs in a policy process cycle (Figure 1).

In an effort to build a business case for a single office in Nova Scotia, OP3 members are considering how to best estimate or track the cost of developing a single policy in one DHA. Research is required to accurately calculate this cost. A suggested approach is to ask OP3 members to consider an estimated cost for a sample of policies in each DHA. By considering each of the 45 tasks listed in Appendix A, OP3 members could estimate or track: 1) whether the task is routine in a DHA, 1a) if it is not routine, whether the member believes the task should be routine or 1b) if the task is routine, the number of employees typically engaged in the task, and 2) the average length of time required of a single employee engaged in the task.

Figure 1. Administrative policy process: graphic representation of steps in the OP3 shared policy development process (©South Shore Health Authority and used with permission)

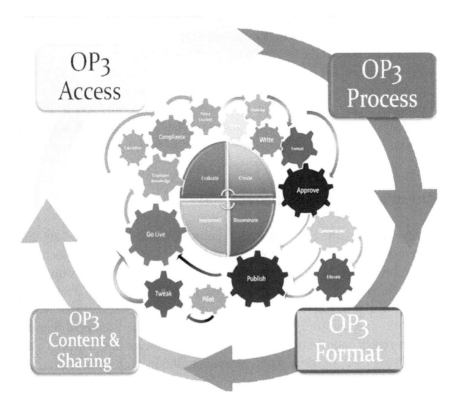

DISCUSSION

Using the experience of one author with the OP3 working group process described above, we identified four particularly challenging areas that could benefit from an increased role of health informatics in health policy and management. We also discuss two additional areas where there is a relationship between health informatics research and administrative policy development at the health services level.

The Research Practice Gap

Managers need research to provide solutions to their problems rather than explanations of why things happen or instruction telling them what not to do. This "relevance gap" where either the research subjects or focus are not relevant to managers' needs has been suggested as the reason why managers make little use of research (Davies, 2006). Labadie uses the metaphor of a burning house to show how different the cultures are: "Decision makers put out fires, and researchers want to let the fire burn to understand how it spreads" (Labadie, 2005).

The research practice gap with respect to health policy generally, and in health informatics research specifically, can be expressed by the lack of administrative health policy research in several areas that impede OP3 working group progress.

A Variety of Sources for Rules

The relationship between provincial and federal legislation related to health, public health policy, clinical health policy, administrative health policy, professional standards, clinical competencies and practice guidelines is not clear. Typically various document types exist to address a subject, each created independently without reference to the others, each with their own sets of definitions and references. Administrative policy, intended to give clear policy guidance to practicing health professionals within a particular setting, must address local context while taking into consideration the full array of other influencing policies, practice guidelines and practice standards. This can leave health professionals and administrators confused so that they must rely on their own best judgment and hope that it is consistent with the purposes of the organization, congruent with current research and compliant with legislation and other rules.

Policy Contributor and Policy Approver

In the experience of the authors, the difference between the roles of these two stakeholder groups is not always clear and there is no system to support effective management of contributions and approvals. Historically, in single site health service organizations, tracking contributions during policy development has been accomplished through a printed one page tracking sheet. This documentation is handled separately from the approval process, with approvals managed through signatures on the original copies of printed policies. Multi-site, multi-organizational shared policy development requires an automated system or mechanism to track contributions from various sites and groups. There is a need to clarify for each policy the level of approval necessary for implementation in each organization and track whether that approval has been granted.

Shared Health Policy Language

A review of the 400 publicly available policies available on the OP3 policy site in April 2011 identified >1,000 terms defined within the policies. Some of these terms had as many as 18 different definitions created independently by the policy writer with inconsistencies between and within departments and DHAs. A study by a graduate student completed in 2012 identified terms defined as clinical, technical, administrative and general (Phinney, MacDonald, & Spiteri, 2012). The study concluded that of 26 potential policy languages examined, the best source of definitions for the variety of administrative health policy terms in Nova Scotia administrative health policies on the OP3 site was the Unified Medical Language System (U.S. National Library of Medicine, 2012). The best way to introduce and implement a standard language has not been identified.

A Critical Conflict Inherent in Health Informatics Policy: Privacy of Health Information

Health informatics policy implicitly affects two core values within healthcare delivery. One is the practice of patient-centered, collaborative healthcare through all parts and among all providers within the healthcare system. The other is protecting the privacy of patient information. Health informatics provides the tools, mechanisms and processes to share critical patient and patient-care information among the full range of healthcare providers and others critical to care and well-being of the patient. It also provides ready access to clinical research for evidence-based practice. Ideally, this information is also shared with the patient (or patient proxy) so that the patient is the driver of his/her own health care. Appropriately applied, health informatics methods reduce the risk of "private" information becoming known to others outside of the care network.

Risk management is an important consideration. The risk of unwanted publicity or legal action against care providers and health organizations on the basis of information available must be managed through health informatics processes based on health informatics policy.

The Role of Administrative Health Policy in Education and Innovation

Another core value inherent in health care is that of innovation: continuous exploration into the best ways to deliver healthcare through complex systems of organizations and professionals. A sound health informatics policy encourages exploration and innovation by providing a statement of principles/values that encourages both exploration and its careful management. Such a policy also includes guidance and processes on introduction and integration of innovations, in care and professional practice, into the work of the organization and its associated care providers. Current areas of administrative innovation in this area are the use and dissemination of electronic health records, both within the organization and among related community healthcare providers.

Along with innovation (the introduction of new concepts and practices) comes the need for continuous learning among those who must change their practice and processes. Sound administrative policy related to health informatics and health information systems provides the framework and guidelines for what needs to be learned. Part of the administrative practice would then be to collaboratively learn new or varying practice principles and patterns. By learning together, administrative and clinical professionals discover the areas of potential challenge. By working through those challenges together in a continuous learning environment, the result is improved practice and health outcomes. Health services will be enabled by health information systems based on policy at all three levels: public, clinical and administrative.

CONCLUSION

The introduction and use of health information systems throughout health organizations and among members of multi-site organizations is still considered innovative. Health service organizations experience continuing change in practice and administration. Organization-wide innovations often require lengthy periods of time and iterative processes to accomplish (Rogers, 1983). Cost-effective shared administrative policy development to provide clear overall guidance for health services and for health informatics solutions designed to support health services is essential.

ACKNOWLEDGMENT

We acknowledge the assistance of Angela Clifton, South Shore Health Authority, for work on the administrative policy development cycle and task list. The work of the 2012 OP3 Working Group members is also acknowledged.

REFERENCES

Accreditations Canada. (2012). *Leading practice: Recognizing innovation and creativity in Canadian health care delivery*. Retrieved 12 16, 2012, from http://www.accreditation.ca/news-and-publications/publications/leading-practices/

Althaus, C., Bridgman, P., & Davis, G. (2007). *The Australian policy handbook* (4th ed.). Sydney, Australia: Allen & Unwin.

Arman, R., Dellve, L., Wikström, E., & Törnström, L. (2009). What health care managers do: Applying Mintzberg's structured observation method. *Journal of Nursing Management, 17*(6), 718–729. doi:10.1111/j.1365-2834.2009.01016.x PMID:19694915

Baghbanian, A., Hughes, I., Kebriaei, A., & Khavarpour, F. A. (2012). Adaptive decision-making: How Australian healthcare managers decide. *Australian Health Review, 36*(1), 49–56. doi:10.1071/AH10971 PMID:22513020

Bell, E. (2010). *Research for health policy*. Oxford, UK: Oxford University Press.

Booth, A., & Brice, A. (2004). Knowledge management. In G. Walton & B. Andrew (Eds.), *Exploiting knowledge in health services*. London, UK: Facet Publishing.

Caldwell, S. E., & Mays, N. (2012). Studying policy implementation using a macro, meso and micro frame analysis: The case of the collaboration for leadership in applied health research & care (CLAHRC) programme nationally and in North West London. *Health Research Policy and Systems*, *10*(1), 32. doi:10.1186/1478-4505-10-32 PMID:23067208

Canadian Association for Health Services and Policy Research. (2012). *About CAHSPR*. Retrieved 12, 16, 2012, from https://cahspr.ca/en/about

Canadian Health Services Research Foundation. (2000). *Health services research and evidence-based decision-making*. Ottawa, Canada: Canadian Health Services Research Foundation.

Canadian Policy and Procedure Network. (2010). *Canadian policy & procedure network*. Retrieved 12, 16, 2012, from http://ca.groups.yahoo.com/group/cppn/

Capital Health. (2011). *Health record forms management*. Retrieved from http://policy.nshealth.ca/Site_Published/DHA9/document_render.aspx?documentRender.IdType=6&documentRender.GenericField=&documentRender.Id=34962

Capital Health. (2012). *Policy development, implementation and evaluation*. Retrieved 12 16, 2012, from http://policy.nshealth.ca/Site_Published/DHA9/document_render.aspx?documentRender.IdType=6&documentRender.GenericField=&documentRender.Id=17121

COACH. (2001). *Guidelines for the protection of health information*. Edmonton, Canada: COACH - Canada's Health Informatics Association.

Cryderman, P. (1987). *Developing policy and procedure manuals*. Ottawa, Canada: Canadian Hospital Association.

Cryderman, P. (1999). *Customized manuals for changing times*. Ottawa, Canada: CHA Press.

Davies, H. (2006). Improving the relevance of management research: Evidence-based management: Design, science or both? *Business Leadership Review*, *3*(3), 1–6.

Elwyn, G., Légaré, F., van der Weijden, T., Edwards, A., & May, C. (2008). Arduous implementation: Does the normalisation process model explain why it's so difficult to embed decision support technologies for patients in routine clinical practice. *Implementation Science; IS*, *3*(1), 57. doi:10.1186/1748-5908-3-57 PMID:19117509

Glouberman, S., & Mintzberg, H. (2001). Managing the care of health and the cure of disease-Part II: Integration. *Health Care Management Review*, *26*(1), 70–84. doi:10.1097/00004010-200101000-00007 PMID:11233356

Grant, A. M., Moshyk, A. M., Kushniruk, A., & Moehr, J. R. (2003). Reflections on an arranged marriage between bioinformatics and health informatics. *Methods of Information in Medicine*, *42*(2), 116–120. PMID:12743646

Gray, J. A. (2009). *Evidence-based healthcare and public health: How to make decisions about health services and public health*. London: Elsevier Health Sciences.

Greenhalgh, T., Hinder, S., Stramer, K., Bratan, T., & Russell, J. (2010). Adoption, non-adoption, and abandonment of a personal electronic health record: Case study of HealthSpace. *British Medical Journal*, *341*, c5814. doi:10.1136/bmj.c5814 PMID:21081595

Head, A. L. (1996). *An examination of the implications for NHS information providers of staff transferring from functional to managerial roles.* Aberystwyth, UK: University College of Wales.

Heller, F. P., Drenth, P., Koopman, P., & Rus, V. (1988). *Decisions in organizations: A three county comparative study.* London: Sage.

Innvær, S. (2009). The use of evidence in public governmental reports on health policy: An analysis of 17 Norwegian official reports (NOU). *BMC Health Services Research*, *9*(1), 177. doi:10.1186/1472-6963-9-177 PMID:19785760

Innvaer, S., Vist, G., Trommald, M., & Oxman, A. (2002). Health policy-makers' perceptions of their use of evidence: A systematic review. *Journal of Health Services Research & Policy*, *7*(4), 239–244. doi:10.1258/135581902320432778 PMID:12425783

Kadane, J. B. (2005). Bayesian methods for health-related decision making. *Statistics in Medicine*, *24*(4), 563–567. doi:10.1002/sim.2036 PMID:15678444

Keshavjee, K., Manji, A., Singh, B., & Pairaudeau, N. (2009). Failure of electronic medical records in Canada: A failure of policy or a failure of technology? In J. G. McDaniel (Ed.), *Advances in Information Technology and Communication in Health* (pp. 107–114). Amsterdam: IOS Press BV.

Kovner, A. R., & Rundall, T. G. (2006). Evidence-based management reconsidered. *Frontiers of Health Services Management*, *22*(3), 3–22. PMID:16604900

Labadie, J.-F. (2005). Inter-regional front-line services knowledge brokering alliance. In *Proceedings of the Fourth Annual National Knowledge Brokering Workhop* (p. 8). Retrieved from http://www.cfhi-fcass.ca/migrated/pdf/event_reports/National_Workshop_Report_2005_e.pdf

Lahey, W. (2012, November 29). Collaboration vital to better health care, improved regulation. *The Chronicle Herald*.

Lahey, W., & Currie, R. (2005). Regulatory and medico-legal barriers to interprofessional practice. *Journal of Interprofessional Care*, *19*(S1), 197–223. doi:10.1080/13561820500083188 PMID:16096156

Lewis, S., Barer, M. L., Sanmartin, C., Sheps, S., Shortt, S. E., & McDonald, P. W. (2000). Ending waiting-list mismanagement: Principles and practice. *Canadian Medical Association Journal*, *162*, 1297–1300. PMID:10813011

MacDonald, J., Bath, P., & Booth, A. (2008). Healthcare services managers: What information do they need and use? *Evidence Based Library and Information Practice*, *3*(3), 18–38.

MacDonald, J. M. (2011). *The information sharing behaviour of health service managers: A three-part study.* (Unpublished PhD Dissertation). Sheffield, UK: University of Sheffield Information School.

Martz, B., Zhang, X., & Ozanich, G. (2007). Information systems and healthcare XIV: Developing an integrative health informatics. *Communications of AIS, 19*.

Mbananga, N., & Sekokotla, D. (2002). *The utilisation of health management information in Mpumalanga Province*. Retrieved from http://www. hst. org. za/research

Mensink, N., & Paterson, G. (2010). The evolution and uptake of a drug information system: The case of a small Canadian province. *Studies in Health Technology and Informatics, 160*(Pt 1), 141–145. PMID:20841666

Mensink, N. M. (2004). *Facilitating the development of a graduate-level university program using processes and principles of adult education*. (Unpublished MAdEd thesis). St. Francis Xavier University, Antigonish, Canada.

Moahi, K. H. (2000). *A study of the information behavior of health care planners, managers and administrators in Botswana and implications for the design of a national health information system(NHIS)*. (Unpublished PhD dissertation). University of Pittsburgh, Pittsburgh, PA.

Mohaghan, V., & Cooke, J. (2004). The health and social care context. In G. Walton & B. Andrew (Eds.), *Exploiting knowledge in health services* (p. 16). London: Facet Publishing.

Moss, L. J. (2000). *Perceptions of meeting effectiveness in the capital health region*. (Unpublished MA thesis). Royal Roads University, Victoria, Canada.

NHS Connecting for Health. (2012). *HealthSpace*. Retrieved 12, 16, 2012, from http://www.connectingforhealth.nhs.uk/systemsandservices/healthspace

Niedźwiedzka, B. (2003). A proposed general model of information behaviour. *Information Research, 9*(1), Paper 164.

Nova Scotia Department of Health and Wellness. (2012,). *Overview and discussion paper, health services and insurance act*. Retrieved 12, 16, 2012, from http://www.gov.ns.ca/health/hsil/doc/OverviewDiscussionDocument.pdf

Nova Scotia Department of Health and Wellness. (2012). *Personal health information act*. Retrieved 12, 16, 2012, from https://www.gov.ns.ca/dhw/phia/

OP3: One Province, One Process, One Policy. (2011). *Style guide for writers and developers of NS DHA and IWK policy documents*. Retrieved 12 16, 2012, from http://policy.nshealth.ca/Site_Published/dha9/document_render.aspx?documentRender.IdType=5&documentRender.Id=29030

Paterson, G. I. (2008). *Boundary infostructures for chronic disease: Constructing infostructures to bridge communities of practice*. Saarbrücken, Germany: VDM Verlag Dr. Muller.

Phinney, J., MacDonald, J. M., & Spiteri, L. (2012). *A health policy language for Nova Scotia: A Dalhousie school of information management reading course project*. Paper presented at APLA 2012: Discovering Hidden Treasures. Wolfville, Canada.

Rogers, E. M. (1983). *Diffusion of innovations* (3rd ed.). New York: Free Press.

Simmons, R., & Shiffman, J. (2007). Scaling up health service inovations: A framework for action. In R. Simmons, P. Fajans, & L. Ghiron (Eds.), *Scaling up health services delivery from pilot innovations to policies and programmes* (pp. 1–30). Geneva, Switzerland: World Health Organization.

Smith, R. (1996). What clinical information do doctors need? *British Medical Journal, 313*(7064), 1062–1068. doi:10.1136/bmj.313.7064.1062 PMID:8898602

Stephanovich, P. L., & Uhrig, J. D. (1999). Decision making in high-velocity environments: Implications for healthcare. *Journal of Healthcare Management, 44*(3), 195–205.

Tengelin, E., Arman, R., Wikström, E., & Delive, L. (2011). Regulating time commitments in healthcare organizations: Managers' boundary approaches at work and in life. *Journal of Health Organization and Management, 25*(5), 578–599. PMID:22043654

University of Arizona. (2011). *Administrative policy formulation.* Retrieved 12, 16, 2012, from http://policy.arizona.edu/policy-formulation

U.S. National Library of Medicine. (2012). *Unified medical language system (UMLS®).* Retrieved 12, 16, 2012, from http://www.nlm.nih.gov/research/umls/

Walton, G., & Booth, A. (2004). *Exploiting knowledge in health services.* London: Facet Publishing.

Wedlake, S. (2012). *Law amendments bill 147 - An act respecting the Nova Scotia regulated health professions network.* Retrieved 12, 16, 2012, from http://nslegislature.ca/pdfs/committees/61_4_LAC-Submissions/20121129/20121129-147-03.pdf

Willis, C. D., Mitton, C., Gordon, J., & Best, A. (2012). System tools for system change. *BMJ Quality & Safety, 21*(3), 250–262. doi:10.1136/bmjqs-2011-000482 PMID:22129934

Zitner, D., Paterson, G. I., & Fay, D. F. (1998). Methods for identifying pertinent and superfluous activity. In J. Tan (Ed.), *Health Decision Support Systems* (pp. 177–197). New York: Aspen Publishers, Inc.

KEY TERMS AND DEFINITIONS

Data Quality Framework: Aggregation of data from individual patient records to fulfill data requirements for measuring patient and population health and health system performance.

eHealth: Health care practice which is supported by electronic information and communication systems.

Health Data Standards: Standards developed by international standards organizations and adopted or adapted by Canada's Standards Collaborative to determine how health data is classified or grouped, and how it is encoded in machine-readable representation for electronic manipulation.

Health Informatics Policies: Explicit statements directing how to address issues that arise with the introduction of information technology into the health system, including topics such as ethics; information security and privacy; interoperability; health communication; social implications of computing; and, quality, risk and patient safety.

Health Organization Models: Health organization models of care delivery vary based on the philosophies of care and service as well as sites of care and use of multi-disciplinary care teams.

Health Policy Informatics: A subdiscipline of health informatics that addresses challenges experienced by health service managers and other policymakers and problems that arise from the multidimensional nature of information used for policy creation, dissemination, implementation and evaluation.

Knowledge Management: Aims to leverage the intellectual capital held in the skills and expertise of personnel so that the knowledge that is critical to them is made available in the most effective manner to those people who need it so that it can add value as a normal part of work.

Policy Implementation: Policy management across the lifecycle including release, communication, translation, compliance monitoring, effects evaluation and revision.

Policy Monitoring: Feedback loop that allows you to monitor for policy effects.

Shared Health Policy Development: Inter-organizational policy development, ideally using a framework that addresses capacity, authority and resourcing to achieve policy development, approval and distribution at the meso and macro levels.

This research was previously published in Research Perspectives on the Role of Informatics in Health Policy and Management edited by Christo El Morr, pages 116-134, copyright year 2014 by Medical Information Science Reference (an imprint of IGI Global).

APPENDIX

Table 2. Tasks in the Administrative Policy Process identified by the OP3 Working Group

Quadrant	Policy Process (Cog)		Task	Definition
Create	Initiate	1.	Identify Issue	Recognize policy need
Create	Initiate	2.	Consult	Consult with several colleagues to see what they think of an issue
Create	Initiate	3.	Compare Situations	Compare 2-3 similar incidents and decide whether a policy is needed
Create	Initiate	4.	Respond	Respond to provincial policy or legislation with DHA policy
Create	Initiate	5.	Acknowledge	Recognize policy gap and decide to create a policy
Create	Initiate	6.	Set Policy Level	Decide where admin or other type of policy is needed
Create	Initiate	7.	Stakeholders	Identify stakeholders & contributors & approvers, including legal, ethics
Create	Initiate	8.	Plan For Education	Decide whether education will be required
Create	Initiate	9.	Plan For Monitoring	Decide whether monitoring will be required
Create	Initiate	10.	Plan For Evaluation	Decide whether evaluation will be required
Create	Initiate	11.	Plan Timing	Decide when policy should go live (ideally)
Create	Develop	12.	Literature Search	Search for current research evidence and best practice
Create	Develop	13.	Environmental Scan	See who is doing what in similar organizations
Create	Develop	14.	FEMA (Failure Mode Effect Analysis)	Consider effect of policy failures and design policy for maximum success
Create	Develop	15.	Appraise	Appraise, synthesize and integrate information gathered
Create	Develop	16.	Review Rules	Ensure congruency with legislation and provincial health policy
Create	Develop	17.	SBAR	Create SBAR to communicate policy need
Create	Write	18.	Draft	Create first draft
Create	Write	19.	Define	Define less familiar terms
Create	Write	20.	Revise	In plain language and appropriate writing style
Create	Write	21.	Reference	Support text with references and reference list
Create	Write	22.	Procedure	Identify and draft associated procedures
Create	Write	23.	Forms	Identify form requirements and locate or create forms
Create	Write	24.	Appendix	Create required appendices
Create	Format	25.	Algorithms	Create decision tree
Create	Format	26.	Template	Format in appropriate template
Create	Format	27.	Toc	Add table of contents
Create	Write	28.	Input	Seek stakeholder input
Create	Write	29.	Revise	Synthesize, appraise and integrate stakeholder format

continued on following page

Table 2. Continued

Quadrant	Policy Process (Cog)		Task	Definition
Create	Write	30.	Legal/ethical	Seek and integrate input from legal and ethical experts
Create	Write	31.	Review	Seek stakeholder input on revisions
Create	Write	32.	Director	Seek input & approval from org unit director
Create	Write	33.	Committee	Seek input and approval from DHA policy committee
Create	Approve	34.	Approve	Have DHA authority approve policy
Disseminate	Communicate	35.	Communicate	Design and implement communication plan
Disseminate	Educate	36.	Educate	Design and deliver education
Disseminate	Publish	37.	Publish	Make policy available on op3 site
Implement	Pilot	38.	Pilot	Test policy in limited setting for limited period
Implement	Tweak	39.	Tweak	Revise pilot following user experience
Implement	Go Live	40.	Go Live	Release policy effective DHA wide
Evaluate	Evaluate	41.	Evaluate Employee Knowledge	Test to determine employee awareness of policy
Evaluate	Evaluate	42.	Evaluate Policy Content	Survey to determine if content meets needs
Evaluate	Evaluate	43.	Evaluate Policy Education	Survey to determine if education was effective
Evaluate	Evaluate	44.	Evaluate Policy Compliance	Monitor to establish DHA complies with policy
Evaluate	Evaluate	45.	Evaluate Policy Outcomes	Determine whether policy meets need

Chapter 76
Exploring Physicians' Resistance to Using Mobile Devices:
A Hospital Case Study

Paola A. Gonzalez
Dalhousie University, Canada

Yolande E. Chan
Queen's University, Canada

ABSTRACT

Mobile communication technology is emerging as an area of major importance in healthcare. By enabling ubiquitous real-time access to patient information and state-of-the-art medical knowledge, this technology has the potential to support the integration of health records, the practice of evidence-based medicine, and to improve productivity among provider organizations. However, its adoption and implementation have faced many challenges; an important one has been users' resistance. For instance, many physicians are still reluctant to embed these technologies in their medical practices. This chapter, hence, explores factors that influence this resistance to using mobile devices, thereby hindering the potential benefits that these technologies can bring to healthcare. Specifically, the authors present the results of an empirical study conducted at a local hospital where two mobile technologies were examined. The findings highlight several important factors that, if not addressed in healthcare settings, can result in user resistance to the implementation of this technology.

INTRODUCTION

The healthcare industry constantly faces a number of challenges, including high costs, a growing incidence of medical errors, inadequate staffing, and lack of coverage in rural areas. Healthcare professionals at the same time are under pressure to provide high quality services to more people but using constrained financial and human resources. One proposed solution to this crisis is the adoption of mobile devices or MDs (Varshney, 2003).

DOI: 10.4018/978-1-5225-3926-1.ch076

MDs are important health information technology (IT) based solutions to support and streamline medical practice. Different from fixed computers or nursing workstations, the use of MDs aims to facilitate the access to patient and medical information at the bedside, thereby enhancing medical decisions and knowledge integration (Fontelo, Ackerman, Kim, & Locatis, 2003). These devices can help healthcare professionals cut down the time involved in searching for forms and knowledge at the bedside, and can reduce the risk of prescribing errors (Amarasingham, Plantinga, Diener-West, Gaskin, & Powe, 2009). By enabling ubiquitous real-time access to patient information and up-to-date medical knowledge, these technologies have the potential to support the integration of health records and the practice of evidence-based medicine[1] (Scott, Seidel, Bowen, & Gall, 2009). Mobile devices are thus perceived as a potential solution to not only improve quality of medical services but also reduce long-term costs.

As MDs become more pervasive in healthcare institutions, several challenges remain. One of them is persuading healthcare professionals, specially physicians, to use these devices. Physicians are aware of the importance of being able to access and input medical and patient information from anywhere, at any time in their medical practices (Davenport & Glaser, 2002). Health IT is also perceived as a solution to support and enhance team collaboration among physicians and across healthcare institutions. Despite these advantages, physicians are still often reluctant to embed these technologies in their medical practices. "Physicians enjoy high levels of autonomy; they are sufficiently powerful that the institutions they work for are reluctant to tinker with their work processes; and, perhaps most important, they do most of their work away from a computer screen" (Davenport & Glaser, 2002, p. 111).

A common pattern in the literature of physicians' resistance toward health IT lies in the perceived distraction and unintended consequences that these technologies bring to the medical practice. For instance, Freudenheim (2004) reported the case of the Sinai Medical Center at Los Angeles where physicians resisted the use of a newly implemented computerized physician order entry (CPOE) because they felt the system was disturbing their medical duties. Physicians forced its withdrawal after it was already online in two-thirds of the 870-bed hospital. Another study, conducted in a children's hospital, found that mortality among critically ill children increased after the installation of a popular commercial CPOE. This mortality rate was mainly attributed to changes in clinicians' workflow patterns after the installation (Han, Carcillo, & Venkataram, 2005). These findings suggest that due to the newness of, and unfamiliarity with, the technology, physicians spent excessive amounts of time at the computer screen when they would have previously been at their patients' bedsides. A similar pattern has been seen in the adoption of MDs in healthcare institutions. Although device portability has been perceived as an asset, some physicians have pointed out that excessive portabilty can be a deterrent to their use (e.g., too small key strokes, easy to lose) (Ammenwerth, Buchauer, Bludau, & Haux, 2000; Goldstein, Wilson, & VanDenkerkhof, 2007). Lack of users' acceptance and resistance have long been a barrier to successful IT adoption and implementation in healthcare.

Researchers and advocates call for more studies to help overcome the challenges faced when implementing these technologies, especially research that examines the functionality of healthcare technologies and factors leading to physicians' resistance to using them (Agarwal, Gao, DesRoches, & Jha, 2010; Varshney, 2003). Hence, the purpose of the research discussed in this chapter is to explore technological, psychological and environmental factors that inhibit or enable physicians' mobile device usage during their medical practice.

The rest of the chapter proceeds as follows. In the next section, we present key concepts and literature related to healthcare IT and the use of mobile devices in healthcare settings. Then we present a sociotechnical model that explores the inhibitors and enablers of mobile devices usage, and we discuss preliminary results from a survey and interviews conducted with physicians at a local hospital. We end the chapter by presenting our research conclusions and recommendations for practitioners.

LITERATURE REVIEW

Healthcare Information Technologies and Systems

Healthcare information technologies and systems (health IT/IS thereafter) refer to information and communication technologies to improve the quality, safety, and efficiency of healthcare (Juciute, 2009). Benefits of these technologies range from offering better access to integrated patient information in the form of information systems (or clinical systems) to patients' empowerment in healthcare practices (Hillestad et al., 2005). Medpac (2004) classifies health IT/IS applications in three main categories:

- Administrative and financial systems to support billing, accounting, and other administrative tasks;
- Clinical systems to support medical work. They facilitate or provide input into the care process; and
- Infrastructure that supports both the administrative and clinical applications.

In addition to supporting healthcare providers and enhancing patient care and satisfaction, health IT/IS are considered a solution for the fragmented healthcare delivery system (Medcap, 2004). The urgency of the care, and the constant moving of patients across locations, make coordination and integration of patient healthcare records very daunting tasks. Health IT/IS have formed a "virtual" or electronic integrated delivery system (e.g., electronic medical records (EMRs) or healthcare records (HERs) that offers solutions for this lack of integration and collaboration across healthcare professionals.

The Institute of Medicine (IOM) identified health IT/IS as a critical force that could radically improve health care quality and safety (IOM, 2001). A RAND[2] study reported that the health system could save $77 billion annually upon full implementation of a Health IT/IS system. "The Congressional Budget Office recently estimated that requiring physicians and hospitals to have Electronic Health Records (EHRs) as a condition of participation in Medicare would save the federal government $33 billion over 10 years, a number that does not include private sector savings" (Blumenthal, 2009, p.4). These results motivate governments to invest in the promotion and adoption of these technologies. For example, as part of the American Recovery and Reinvestment Act of 2009, the U.S. government included $19 billion to promote the adoption and implementation of health IT/IS by healthcare providers across the country (Blumenthal, 2009).

Health IT/IS is also perceived as a key tool to facilitate evidence-based medicine (Eysenbach & Jadad, 2001). For example, as healthcare professionals treat patients, they need access to information and they must collaborate with other colleagues to ensure that patients receive the right treatments at the right time (Hansen, Nohria, & Tierney, 1999). Healthcare professionals work together as a team, sharing evidence-based information in a timely manner to provide high quality care (Scott et al., 2009). Health IT/IS must be developed to support collaborative, clinical work and not increase the workloads of these rushed, professionals. Particularly, these technologies should be designed to support the mobile nature of healthcare delivery (Bardram, 2005).

Mobility is a central characteristic of healthcare delivery (Bardram, 2005). Healthcare professionals are always on 'the go' and constantly move between wards, outpatient clinics, diagnostic and therapeutic departments, and conference rooms. Thus, their many information and communication needs at various locations, and at different times, are difficult to satisfy. Clinical systems have only partly fulfilled these needs. While computer workstations allow easy storage, retrieval, and sharing of patient and medical information, they do not fully support the mobility aspect of healthcare delivery (Bardram, 2005; (Banitsas, Georgiadis, Tachakra, & Cavouras, 2004). Physicians have little time to spend with patients during rounds, and going back and forth to a fixed computer workstation only adds time to their practice (Goldstein, 2010). Traditional paper charts support this mobility, but are limited by inefficient and insufficient information accessibility and lack of simultaneous access by multiple users.

Mobile Devices in Healthcare

Mobile devices combine advantages of paper charts and computer workstations in their portability (Kuziemsky, Laul, & Leung, 2005) and support for information access needs at anytime, anywhere (Dahl, Svanes, & Nytro, 2006). These devices, including tablet computers and personal digital assistants (PDAs), are generally small, portable, lightweight computers connected to wireless networks. Since their introduction in the 1990s, their acceptance has steadily increased. A systematic review of PDA use by healthcare professionals indicated an adoption rate increase from 45% to 85% of those surveyed between 2000 and 2005, with hospital-based physicians classified as the most likely users (Garritty and El Emam, 2006). Initially, these devices were used mainly as organizing tools (e.g., contacts, calendar, appointments), but as they became more technologically powerful and more health IT/IS were developed, MDs were used for more administrative and clinical activities in healthcare settings. Today, the devices are used for: administrative support (e.g., billing and scheduling); professional activities (e.g., patient tracking, electronic prescribing, lab readings); documentation; decision support (e.g., clinical and drug reference); and education and research (Prgomet, Georgiou, & Westbrook, 2009).

Easy access to real-time information at anytime, anywhere brings undoubtedly many benefits to healthcare delivery. A systematic review identified three main benefits of handheld technology (i.e., mobile devices) in supporting hospital healthcare professionals' work and patient care: rapid response, medication error prevention, and data management and accessibility (Prgomet et al., 2009). In regard to rapid response, mobile devices allow physicians to expedite early diagnoses and treatments by permitting earlier notification, resource preparation and mobilization of staff. Respondents in these studies referred to the benefits of accessing up-to-date information (e.g., patient and drug interaction) at the point-of-need, which assisted them in making more informed treatment decisions, thereby improving patient care.

The review also showed that medication errors were prevented. Mobile devices could address issues related to drug order illegibility and errors in transcription. Direct input of medications into an information system tends to reduce errors in medication and transcribing documentation. Although these benefits also apply to fixed computers, physicians commented on the inconvenience of moving back and forth to a computer workstation, preventing them from using the direct input and instead using the traditional paper system (Grasso, Genest, Yung, & Arnold, 2002; Shannon, Feied, Smith, Handler, & Gillam, 2006). Nevertheless, when physicians were asked about their choice preferences of direct input, some physicians still opted for the fixed computer. They commented on the cumbersomeness of entering data into a handled device via a stylus (i.e., it is slower, more erroneous and less pleasant than using a QWERTY keyboard) (Haller, Haller, Courvoisier, & Lovis, 2009).

The use of mobile devices also improved data management and accessibility. Although, the studies did not indicate a significant difference between the use of mobile devices and paper processes in this area, a decrease in documentation discrepancies was noticeable. "As most patient information is obtained at the bedside providing physicians with devices that allow data entry at the point of care can promote more complete documentation and decrease the length of patient encounters" (Prgomet et al., 2009, p. 797). Having accurate information in a timely fashion is a critical requirement for making decisions under pressure, as is the case in healthcare environments. For that reason, mobile devices are perceived as a technology that can offer portable, complete, accurate and up-to-date patient- and medical-related information, thereby facilitating more accurate and timely patient management.

Other studies have counter argued these benefits and examined the extent to which these devices produced unintended consequences and became instead a distracting tool for healthcare professionals during their work. Technical characteristics of the device, poor wireless connectivity, and perceptual factors related to comfort with the technology are among the common barriers to using these mobiles. Issues related to the device included size, limited memory and battery life, and speed of data exchange (Fischer, Stewart, Mehta, Wax, & Lapinsky, 2003). Physicians who resisted the technology also commented on their physical constraints such as eyesight and comfort with the device. Others expressed their frustration with data entry, "it just takes too long and is too disruptive to the day" (McAlearney Schweikhart, & Medow, 2004, p. 3). For these non-users, the use of these devices was proned to cause medication and prescription errors as well as to shorten their time per patient during medical rounds and thus decrease their quality of care (McAlearney et al., 2004). Although, some research has examined physician's resistance toward health IT, little research has theoretically and empirically examined physicians' resistance to mobile technology usage.

THEORETICAL FOUNDATION

We recognize that resistance cannot be conceptualized as the opposite of acceptance (Laumer & Eckhardt, 2012) and that resistance takes many forms and occurs over time. However, we used both literatures because this exploratory study was part of a larger project that examines knowledge sharing behaviors through mobile technologies in healthcare settings (see Gonzalez, Chan & Goldstein, 2013). We initially focused on physicians' adoption of these technologies but quickly realized that the more interesting and challenging research issues concerned non-acceptance, non-adoption, and resistance. Hence, both acceptance and resistance are examined in this research, and the related literatures informed our understanding.

The use of mobile devices by physicians also involves two basic usage aspects: (1) the user's motivation to share information, and (2) the user's acceptance and adoption of the technology as an enabler of this process (Ba, Stallaert, & Whinston 2001). To analyze these components, we used the dual-factor model of IT usage proposed by Cenfetelli (2004) to explore the second aspect and the social exchange theory (SET) to explore the former.

Cenfetelli's (2004) theoretical model aims to bridge the gap between research on IT acceptance and IT resistance by identifying inhibiting and enabling factors that influence IT usage. His model supports the argument that "the barriers to the use of technology are in many cases qualitatively different from the extensively studied positive features" (Cenfetelli, 2004, p. 485). This model is based on the premise that beliefs about a system's design and functionality exist, and these beliefs act mainly to discourage, but not encourage. SET has been widely used in IS research as a theoretical lens to identify the motivators and barriers to share knowledge through IT (e.g., Kankanhalli, Tan, & Wei, 2005a; Wasko and Faraj, 2005). The next subsections describe these theories briefly and present a summary of key factors found in Kankanhalli et al.'s and Wasko and Faraj's studies.

Inhibitors and Enablers as Dual Factor Concepts in Technology Usage

Cenfetelli (2004) proposes a theoretical model of IT usage by examining the enabling and inhibiting factors that influence a user's general attitude, intentions, and behavior to either continue or stop using a system, similar to Lewin's (1947) notion of opposing forces. He defines enabling factors as "those external beliefs regarding the design and functionality of a system that either encourage or discourage usage" (Cenfetelli 2004, p. 475) (e.g., systems, that are perceived to be reliable are used whereas unreliable ones are not). On the other hand, inhibiting factors are "the perception held by a user about a system's attributes with consequent effects on a decision to use a system. They act solely to discourage use" (Cenfetelli 2004, p. 475), but do not necessarily favor usage when they are absent. Inhibitors are not necessarily the opposite of enablers, but are qualitatively different factors that are independent or may coexist with enablers. Cenfetelli (2004) also posits that inhibiting and enabling perceptions have different antecedents and consequent factors, and argues that usage inhibitors deserve an independent investigation.

To illustrate the influence of inhibitors, Cenfetelli (2004) describes the case of an online purchase as follows: "If an online purchase transaction is completed without incident, it is likely not noticed, let alone favorably perceived. Therefore, if a user were to not have an inhibitor perception, this absence of perception would play no role in enabling use. The existence of these "inhibitors" may explain why people fail to adopt, or worse, outright reject a system" (p. 475-76). Using this argument, Cenfetelli (2004) emphasizes that although the absence of inhibitors alone will not encourage use, inhibitors and enablers will respectively have negative and positive effects on use. He points out that rejection of technology – a separate decision from adoption – may be best predicted by inhibitors, whereas adoption may best be predicted by enablers.

Cenfetelli (2004) compares the influecing power of inhibitors and enablers, and argues that the presence of an inhibitor will lead to salient negative perceptions about the system, thereby increasing the resistance to using the system. This is due to the power of presence over absence of negative information and a user's attributions asymmetry regarding the source of negative versus positive perceptions. The perception of a negative atribute can act much more as a strong cue relative to a positive attribute (Skowronski and Carlston, 1987). Similarly, inhibitors may also bias perceptions and other beliefs about the system in ways that enablers will not (Cenfetelli 2004).

This theoretical model was motivated by examining the extent to which IT usage theories, such as the technology acceptance model (TAM) (Davis, Bagozzirp, & Warshawpr, 1989) and the unified theory of acceptance and use of technology (UTAUT) (Venkatesh, Morris, Davis, & Davis, 2003), have centered their core on users' positive (enabling) perceptions related to IT usage (e.g., perceived usefulness and ease of use), while disregarding negative (inhibiting) perceptions that may impede IT usage. An earlier empirical study supported Cenfetelli's argument of inhibitors as perceptions that may hinder IT usage. Speier and colleagues (Speier, Vesseyi, & Valachi, 2003) found that system interruptions, such as pop-up advertisements on a web site, 'you've got mail' announcements in an e-mail system, and animation characters offering help with word documents, can hinder IT usage and task performance, yet, the lack of such interruptions does not enhance IT usage. Also, "the independent nature of enablers and inhibitors in Cenfetelli's model is consistent with prior empirical findings that IT acceptance and resistance are driven by different motivators" (Bhattacherjee and Hikmet 2007, pp. 726). Therefore, Cenfetelli's (2004) model provides a theoretical bridge to link research on IT acceptance and IT resistance.

Social Exchange Theory

Social exchange theory has been used to explain non-contractual interactions among people (Chadwick-Jones, 1976) and to examine a variety of social exchanges including market relations, work relations, friendships and love (Blau, 1964), as well as knowledge sharing behaviors (Cummings, 2004). Social exchange proposes that social behavior is the result of an exchange process. An exchange indicates that one party provides something to another party. An implicit or explicit obligation is then created in the receiving party. The receiving party must provide some sort of benefit to the first in order to discharge this obligation. The returns may be either direct or indirect.

Social exchange critically differs from economic exchange in that social exchange generally entails unspecified obligations (Blau, 1964). In the context of information sharing, the process of social exchange involves the user's willingness to share or exchange information in an indirect reciprocal way, with the technology serving as the intermediary between knowledge contributors and seekers (Fulk, Flanagin, Kalman, Monge, & Ryan, 1996; Kankanhalli et al., 2005a).

Social exchange theorists have suggested that by increasing the benefits (or motivators) and reducing the costs (inhibitors) of information sharing, individuals can be encouraged to share information. Some of the costs and benefits are affected by the specifics of the technology used as a medium for the exchange. These authors suggest that the perceived usefulness and ease of use of the technology also impact information sharing. Table 1 summarizes the key factors identified in previous studies. [3]

We considered five of these factors in this study because they were found to be more relevant in the healthcare context. For instance, extant literature on physicians' motivation to share their information through IT has shown that physicians are less sensitive to organizational rewards when they do not perceive a link between knowledge sharing and quality of care (e.g., Doolan & Bates, 2002; Karimi & Chiang Choon Poo, 2009). This has been a critical part in promoting evidence-based medicine, and thus intrinsic rewards appear to be more useful incentives in this context (e.g., image, reciprocity). Also, for reasons of model parsimony, we needed to balance the social and technical factors influencing information sharing behaviors through a technology. That is, the research framework needed to include internal and external aspects such as those derived from the information seeker and/or contributor and those from the technical artifact.

RESEARCH MODEL

In this study, we define IT acceptance as the willingness to use IT (Saga & Zmud, 1994) and IT resistance as low levels of IT use (Martinko, Zmud, & Henry, 1996). In our research model, IT resistance is our dependent variable. We recognize that while some users develop an intention to accept mobile devices, others develop an intention to resist the technology, based on perceived technology-related qualities and threats (Lapointe & Rivard, 2005). The model is presented in Figure 1 and the research propositions – related to technological, psychological, and environmental factors – are discussed below.

Table 1. Inhibiting and enabling factors to information or knowledge exchange

Factor	Exchange	Relation	List of Sources
Loss of knowledge power	Knowledge is perceived as a source of power, and individuals may fear losing their power or value if others know what they know.	–	Davenport & Prusak (1998); Gray (2001) Kankanhalli et al. (2005)
Codification effort*	Time and cost associated with sharing knowledge.	–	Ba et al. (2001); Markus (2001); Kankanhalli et al. (2005)
Organizational rewards	Rewards such as increased pay, bonuses, job security or career advancement can encourage knowledge sharing.	+	Ba et al. (2001); Hall (2001); Kankanhalli et al. (2005)
Image*	The perception that knowledge sharing enhances one's reputation or image.	+	Hall (2001); Kankanhalli et al. (2005a); Wasko & Faraj (2005)
Reciprocity*	The belief that contributing knowledge would lead to future request for knowledge being met.	+	Davenport & Prusak (1998); Kankanhalli et al. (2005a); Wasko & Faraj (2005)
Knowledge self-efficacy	The confidence in one's ability to share knowledge that is valuable.	+	Constant et al. (1996); Kankanhalli et al. (2005a)
Enjoyment in helping	The pleasure received from helping others through knowledge contribution.	+	Kankanhalli et al. (2005a); Wasko & Faraj (2005)
Centrality	An individual's structural position (i.e., has a direct and strong ties with other members) in a network.	+	Wasko and Faraj (2005)
Commitment	Individuals who have a sense of belonging to a collective or organization.	+	Wasko & Faraj (2005)
Quality of output*	The perceived quality of the output provided by an information system in terms of relevance, reliability, and timeliness of knowledge.	+	Huang et al. (1998) Kankanhalli et al. (2005b)
Resource Availability*	The time and opportunities to access the technology.	+	Culnan (1984) Kankanhalli et al. (2005b)

Note. Factors marked with an asterisk were adopted in the study and are further explained in our discussion of the research framework.

Figure 1. Research model

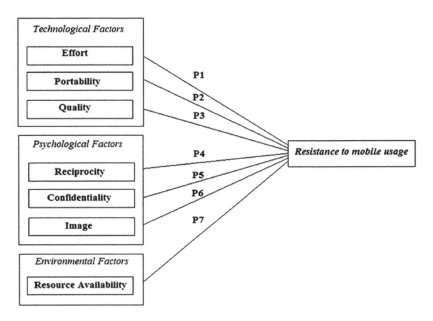

Effort

Effort relates to the degree of ease of use of a technology and the time devoted to share information (Ba et al., 2001; Markus 2001). Based on the social exchange theory, effort can be considered as a cost or a resource that individuals are willing to give away (Kankanhalli et al. 2005a). Effort or perceived ease of use has been deemed as an important predictor of technology acceptance (Venkatesh et al., 2003) and resistence (Cenfetelli, 2004). Users will avoid a system and develop resistance if their perceptions towards the system are negative. For instance, initial negative experiences related to the difficulty of learning to use a system may result in sustained negative perceptions and discourage the continued use of the system (Cenfetelli, 2004).

In a recent hospital case study, for example, data input and retrieval were perceived as major problems in the implementation of electronic medical records (Trimmer, Beachboard, Wiggins, & Woodhouse, 2008). The study revealed that the resistance to using the system was associated with the time required to codify the information and the complexity of the information system. Physicians are generally very busy with little discretionary time. They wish to focus their efforts on patient care and not on system usage. Previous research suggests that physicians may resist using IT because of the extra time required to learn how to use a new medical device or how to enter information in an electronic medical repository (Lu, Sears, & Jacko, 2005). Therefore, we expect that,

P1: The more effort required to use mobile devices, the more likely will physicians resist using these devices.

Portability

The appropriate degree of portability of an IT system has been related to the use and effectiveness of the technology (Garfield, 2005). In contexts with high levels of mobility of stakeholders and nomadic information, portability of information systems is crucial to support these needs. The healthcare environment is one example. Healthcare professionals are characterized by being constantly on the move and their offices are where they stand (Bardram, 2005). Thus, mobile devices are considered an important technology to support their work. Studies have shown that convenient access to medical information at the point of care increases the likelihood that clinicians will rely on these devices as part of their daily workflow (Kuziemsky, Lau, & Leung, 2005). Convenience facilitates the use of technology to access information within a healthcare system (Westbrook, Gosling, & Coiera, 2004). Sackett and colleagues (1998) reported that giving physicians easy access to evidence-based resources while making rounds increased the extent to which evidence was sought and incorporated into patient care decisions. Therefore, we expect that an object of resistance (Cenfetelli, 2004; Lapointe & Rivard 2005) may be fixed computer workstations. Without mobile technology, practitioners have to interrupt their patient care to go to these workstations. Yet, with mobile devices, they can access information whenever and wherever desired, even at the patient's bedside. Therefore, we expect that,

P2: Physicians who do not have mobile devices will be more likely to resist using healthcare IT/IS.

Quality

Quality is associated with higher levels of usefulness of a technology (Kankanhalli et al., 2005b). The performance expectancy of a technological device has been highlighted in the technology acceptance (Venkatesh & Davis, 2003) and resistance literatures (Cenfetelli, 2004). Important aspects of content quality such as the relevance, reliability, and timeliness of knowledge embedded in the IT device are perceived to be useful for job performance, and thus are enablers of technology use. An empirical study that investigated the usefulness of tablet PCs in patient care showed that the physicians who were given a poor information system showed higher resistance to using their devices than other physicians who used the same devices with a better system (Lottridge et al., 2007). Hence, when the quality of either output or content of the system embedded in the technology is poor, physicians are likely to harbor negative attitudes towards, and show reluctance to using, the mobile device to accomplish their patient care tasks. Therefore, we expect that,

P3: The lower the perceived quality of the content and output retrieved from mobile devices, the more likely will physicians resist using these devices.

Reciprocity

One of the intrinsic benefits of social networks is reciprocity (Kankanhalli et al., 2005a). Eckhardt and colleagues (Eckhardt, Laumer, & Weitzel, 2009) discuss the importance of social networks and conclude that the interaction with other users within the organization influences the adoption of IT. Reciprocity refers to the belief that future requests (e.g., for information) are likely to be met, when the healthcare professionals have met others' current requests. For example, physicians often rely on colleagues to gain new information, interpret the medical literature, and obtain specific advice about the care of their patients. Consequently, reciprocity has been shown to be a key factor in the formation of new networks among practicing physicians (Davenport and Glaser, 2002). These networks may also play an important role in the diffusion of new technologies (Coleman et al., 1966), "by shaping beliefs, attitudes, preferences and sharing of new information among members of the network" (Keating, Ayanian, Cleary, & Marsden, 200, p. 794).

Hew and Hara (2006) reported that reciprocity was a critical factor that encouraged critical care and advanced practice nurses to share their knowledge in a longstanding online community of practice. These healthcare professionals felt obligated to contribute their knowledge to the listserv as a result of reciprocity because they had received help at some point in the past from other community members. Therefore, we anticipate that if healthcare professionals perceive that their information requests have not been met satisfactorily through the use of the IT, they may be discouraged to use the technology. Thus, we expect that,

P4: The lower the perceived reciprocity when using mobile devices, the more likely will physicians resist using these devices.

Privacy Concerns

Privacy has been a major concern in healthcare applications. Health-related patient information is private in nature and, as such, it is considered a key governing principle of the patient-physician relationship (Hodge & Gostin, 2004) . Two most common threats of information privacy through IT recognized in the literature are: accidental disclosure and unauthorized intrusion (Rindfleisch, 1997). Accidental disclosure refers to the occasional unintentional behavior of healthcare professionals when using IT. For instance, these professionals can unintentionally disclose patient information to others (e.g., due to an e-mail message sent to wrong recipients, inadvertent web-posting of sensistive data, leaving the IT device unattended or not logging off the information system). Unauthorized intrusion can occur from inside or outside of the orgnization. From inside, disgruntled current employees can use data inapropriately (e.g., employees peek at data of celebreties in the hospital) and from outside, intruders can hack the hospital network to gain access to patient information or render the system inoperable (Appari & Johnson, 2010).

Wireless technology has increased these privacy concerns. As information becomes more ubiquitious, the greater is the risk of privacy breaches. Since wireless media is more vulnerable than wired media, attackers find it easier to intrude. Also, mobile devices permit healthcare professionals to share patient information away from the patient's bedside. A study of a wireless voice recognition technology in a hospital found that it was underused because users felt that they were divulging patient information in front of others when using the mobile device (Vandenkerkhof, Hall, Wilson, Gay, & Duhn, 2009). Therefore, we expect that,

P5: The higher the perceived likelihood of privacy breaches when using mobile devices, the more likely will physicians resist the use of these devices.

Image

SET suggests that individuals are discouraged from sharing or exchanging knowledge when they perceive that the resources given away surpass those received in return. That is, people normally behave in ways that maximize their benefits and minimize their costs (Molm, 1997). Reputation or image has been found to be a crucial factor in position and power (Markus, 2001). Previous research has found that the degree of use of an innovation or new IT system can impact both image and status (e.g., Kankanhalli et al., 2005a; Wasko & Faraj, 2005). The knowledge management literaure posits that individuals can receive intrinsic rewards (e.g., enhanced self-concept) and extrinsic rewards (e.g., monetary or recognition rewards) when contributing to electronic knowledge repositorios (Ba et al., 2001; Hall, 2001).

However, image can be an inhibitor of IT usage in healthcare environments. Health IT research has shown that some physicians feel that their image or status is negatively affected when using IT, a job that they associate with nurses and clerks (Ammenwerth et al., 2000). In these studies, some physicians expressed that writing medical reports in these systems was not part of their jobs. This perception may be due to the traditional relationship between nurses and physicians in which nurses are perceived as healthcare professionals restricted to carrying out the physicians' orders, including clerical work (Fagin et al., 1992). Therefore, we expect that,

P6: The lower the perceived image when using mobile devices, the more likely will physicians resist the use of these devices.

Resource Availability

In this research, resource availability refers to the time and opportunities healthcare professionals have to access mobile devices. Availability of resources makes the use of technology possible, although easy access does not ensure that the technology will actually be used. Previous studies have demonstrated that access to technology is positively related to the use of online information (Culnan, 1984). In exploring the factors that impact knowledge seeking from electronic knowledge repositories, Kankanhalli et al. (2005a) found that when individuals are provided with resources to access the repositories, they are more likely to do so. The resources can take the form of the availability of computers as well as time and opportunities to use these devices. Therefore, we expect that when healthcare profesionals' schedules are not adjusted to provide them with the time and opportunities needed to use mobile devices (i.e., devices are not available or devices are unfamiliar because of limited training which makes their use cumbersome), they will be less motivated to use these devices.

P7: The lower the availability of mobile device resources, the more likely will physicians resist using these devices.

RESEARCH METHODOLOGY AND SETTING

Given the exploratory nature of this research, and the context of the study (e.g., healthcare), an embedded case study was suitable (Yin, 2009). The research setting was a 456-bed acute-care facility providing health services to approximately 500,000 people in Southeastern Ontario, Canada. This facility is a teaching hospital affiliated with the local university. The units in which the study was conducted are the critical care and anesthesiology units because they had introduced mobile technologies. This research site became available because one of the project's researchers is an attending physician at the hospital and was the head of one of the mobile devices projects (i.e., the Tablet Personal Computer) and its specialized information system (e.g., the Acute Pain Management System). Two mobile devices: the Tablet Personal Computer (TPC) and Workstation On Wheels (WOW) permitted us to explore healthcare professionals' resistance to use mobile devices in this context (Gurteen 1998; Hansen et al. 1999).

Data collection included participant observation, field notes, and semi-structured interviews. A pilot study was first conducted to refine the field instruments (interview guides, etc.). Three healthcare professionals considered technology champions of the mobile devices and two academic experts in information systems reviewed and modified the initial constructs and questions. The semi-structured interviews were used to gather information on: a) the purposes and frequency with which the device was used, and the user's familiarity with mobile devices in general; b) interviewee perceptions of the influence of each of the factors identified in the research model; and c) other information offered by the interviewee that s/he considered relevant. Examples of questions are as follows:

- For what purposes do you use the mobile device (e.g., TPC, WOW)? (Please describe a situation in which you would use the device; please describe a situation where you could use the device but would not want to).
- What type of information do you enter and look for in the device (e.g., patient-related information, process-related information, medical information)?
- What type of information do you enter and retrieve from the device (e.g., patient-related information, medical-related information)?
- Is the mobile device easy to use (i.e., is it easy to enter/retrieve information)? Why or why not?
- Does the use of the mobile device enhance your practice at the hospital (i.e., does it take less time whit the device?)? Why or why not?
- Do you think that the information embedded in the mobile device is of high quality (i.e., it is well-documented, reliable, up-to-date)? Why or why not?
- Do you think that by using (i.e., entering and retrieving information) the mobile device, your future queries for information will be answered? Why or why not?
- Is it easy to have access to the device (i.e., are there many opportunities to use it)? Why or why not?
- Do you think that your prestige or professional status is enhanced by using the mobile device? Why or why not?
- Can you think of any other factor that may interfere with the use of the mobile device?

Our study incorporated a mixed-methods approach to data collection, using a survey and interviews. We derived most of the questionnaire items from Kankanhalli et al.'s (2005a, 2005b) studies, adapting them to a healthcare context when appropriate. We also developed questions (e.g., on mobility and privacy) that were assessed and revised by a panel of scholars in the medical field. Survey responses used a five-point Likert scale: 0 - not applicable, 1- never, 2 - rarely, 3 - once in a while, 4 - sometimes, 5 - almost every day. These scores measured the frequency of device usage. Lower scores indicated resistance. Data related to enabling/inhibiting factors were also scored on a five-point Likert scale: 0 - not applicable, 1 - strongly disagree, 2 - disagree, 3 - neutral, 4 - agree, 5 - strongly agree. The questions we used to measure the constructs in our model are presented in Table 2. To distribute the questionnaires, we followed Dillman's protocols (Dillman, 2000). We also conducted 6 interviews, lasting 30-45 minutes each, and distributed as follows: TPC - three attending physicians and a nurse practitioner, WOW - two attending physicians and a resident. Field notes and e-mail exchanges between the authors and study participants complemented the interview data collection.

DATA ANALYSIS AND RESULTS

The Tablet Personal Computer (TPC)

The TPC is used by attending physicians, residents and nurse practitioners in the Anesthesiology and Perioperative Department. The TPC is a portable personal computer equipped with a 12'' touchscreen. Healthcare professionals can enter or retrieve information from the device by using either the stylus pen on the screen keyboard or an external keyboard attached to the base body. The device is mainly used in the perioperative setting to assess patients' acute pain in pre- and post-operative phases through the

Table 2. Survey questions

Construct	Item ID	Question
Effort	EF1 EF2	It is laborious to enter/share information in the mobile device. It is laborious to look for information in the mobile device.
Image	IMG1 IMG2 IMG3	Using the mobile device enhances my professional status. Clinicians who use the mobile device have more prestige than those who do not. When I use the mobile device, the people I work with respect me.
Resource Availability	RA1 RA2 RA3	I have easy access to the mobile device. I have many opportunities to use the mobile device. I have the time to use the mobile device.
Reciprocity	REC1 REC2 REC3	When I use the mobile device, I expect others to respond when I need their information. When I use the mobile device to assist others, I believe that my own future queries for information will be answered. I use the mobile device because I expect others to respond to my work-related inquiries.
Mobility	MOB1 MOB2 MOB3	I use the mobile device because it is a portable device. I use the mobile device because I can enter information and knowledge whenever and wherever I need. I use the mobile device because I can look for information and knowledge whenever and wherever I need.
Quality	QUA1 QUA2 QUA3	I use the mobile device because the output is relevant for my work. I use the mobile device because the output is trustworthy. I use the mobile device because the output is up-to-date.
Confidentiality	CF1 CF2 CF3	Using the mobile device forces me to reveal personal information in front of others. Using the mobile device forces me to reveal patient information in front of others. Patient privacy is an issue when I use the mobile device.
Usage	USG1 USG2	I use the mobile device to access the APMs during the acute pain rounds. I use the mobile device to access the PCS during the acute pain rounds.

Acute Pain Management System (APMS). The APMS software provides the healthcare professional with a (1) checklist template for pain assessment, (2) information on side-effect therapy, (3) drug usage, (4) notable events, (5) consultations, (6) lab results, (7) pharmacy, (8) imaging, and (9) billing. APMS "consults" are entered into the APMS application, available via the hospital intranet, either through the TPC or a nursing workstation.

The APMS software was developed by a group of physicians and a nurse practitioner who received a research grant to start the project. The primary goal of the software development was to standardize and monitor the assessment of patients' acute pain. After developing the system, the intention was to make it available at the patient bedside. Thus, in 2001, personal digital assistants (PDAs) were given to these professionals. Several issues arose during this implementation. First, the wireless infrastructure of the hospital was not robust enough to properly support these devices, and users often lost connectivity when conducting their rounds. Second, users complained that the PDAs were too small, making it cumbersome to enter and retrieve information at the bedside. Aiming to solve these issues, TPCs were introduced a year later.

The field notes, direct observation and interviews revealed that, although the TPC provides effective medical decision support, usage of the device is very low. Arguably no more than 20 percent of healthcare professionals choose to use the TPC. Non-users bring their notes on a clipboard from their rounds and walk to the nearest nursing workstation at which they enter the information. Low TPC usage has affected the level of detailed information available for pain assessments in the perioperative setting, even via the system. A physician commented:

Sometimes, you click on the consultation assessment and you don't find a thorough assessment from the previous day. (active TPC user expressing frustration that non-TPC user information in the APMS is less complete. This statement emphasizes the important of reciprocity as an enabler of IT use).

Currently, there are three TPC devices available to be signed out by healthcare professionals completing acute pain rounds; however, their use has been limited. Only few healthcare professionals use the TPC. An user commented:

There is always a Tablet available when I need it. Only a few times, I have not used it because the system is down. (TPC user)

However, when asked about the resource availability of these devices, a non-user had a different perception and expressed the following:

It is a problem when your rounds are on the weekend because the Tablets are usually locked up in the department. (Non-user)

The APMS and patient care system can also be accessed from the nursing workstations; hence, physicians who resist using the TPCs can document their assessments using these workstations. The doctor who actively championed the use of TPCs argues that physicians who do not often use TPCs sometimes do not check lab results before seeing patients, which introduces risks when they prescribe medication for pain, for example. He maintains that physicians usually enter all patients' consultations in the nursing workstation after seeing an average of 25 patients per round. Therefore, the probability of recalling detailed information from each patient is very low. This practice, he claims, hinders detailed and comprehensive recording of patient consultations.

The main reasons reported for the lack of usage among the non-users were initial negative experiences with the device. Problems were being corrected as the technology was being implemented, and users started to feel discomfort with the APMS and TPC project in general. Some non-users referred to the system and device as "[doctor's name]'s project". There was little encouragement from the hospital management or other professionals to use the system. Some respondents also pointed out the limited number of available devices and described technical challenges (e.g., intermittent wireless connectivity) as important factors deterring their continued use.

The interviewed physicians did not perceive the use of the mobile devices as enhancing their professional status or image. However, a nurse practitioner who was highly involved in the project and is an active user had a different view and responded to the question related to image:

Physicians do not usually ask questions to nurses, but because I'm one of the most experienced [TPC] users, they have to call me when they face issues with the device.

Perception of portability was also an important factor among the active users. They perceived value in the portability attribute of the devices because they were strong believers of the need for patient and medical information at the bedside. One of the physicians commented: "The portability of the Tablet is the key issue for me because my office is where I stand."

Survey Results

The sample consisted of 54 physicians and one nurse pain practitioner. Of the 55 participants contacted, 26 (or 47%) replied. Evaluation of the questionnaires revealed that 11 of the 26 (42.3%) participants - 10 attending physicians and the nurse - were active users of the TPC, but the frequency of usage varied. The majority (57.7%) did not use, or resisted using, the technology. Users' and non-users' age and experience did not differ significantly. One-way analyses of variance were performed to test for differences between the two groups of users and non-users on the factors analyzed.

Unidimensionality was assessed using Cronbach's alpha and item-total correlations. The resulting alpha values, ranging from 0.74 to 0.95, were above the threshold of 0.70 suggested by Nunnally and Bernstein (1994). In order to test the propositions and appropriately handle the small sample size of 26 responses, we conducted separate linear regression analyses. This technique is usually conducted to identify antecedents of a phenomenon and test interaction effects between the independent and dependent variables (e.g., see Kankanhalli et al., 2005a, 2005b). Table 3 summarizes the results of the regressions.

The results show that required effort and confidentiality had no significant relationship with mobile device usage, and P1 and P5 were not supported. On the other hand, image, resource availability, reciprocity, mobility, and quality of output were significant antecedents to TPC usage in this hospital department, and P2, P3, P4, P6, and P7 were supported. The standardized coefficients indicated that image, reciprocity, quality of output and mobility had a comparable degree of importance in the model. Resource availability had the strongest impact on TPC usage by healthcare professionals in the Department of Anesthesiology and Perioperative Care.

The comparative results between users and non-users show that these two groups were significantly different in their perception of mobility. The mobility mean for users was 3.9 whereas the mean for non-users was 2.9; this difference was statistically significant, $F(1,11) = 6.20$, $p < 0.05$, and marginally different regarding the antecedents of required effort and resource availability. Clearly, the TPC usage by users was significantly higher in comparison to non-users. The usage mean for users was 3.2 whereas the mean for non-users was 1.37; this difference was statistically significant, $F(1,11) = 10.7$, $p < 0.01$. We also examined the impact of control variables on TPC usage. Age and work experience did not have a significant impact on TPC usage.

The Workstation On Wheels (WOW)

The Workstation On Wheels (WOW), also known as a computer on wheels, is basically a notebook placed on a mobile cart. The device used in the intensive care unit (ICU) is a StyleView® 19" LCD

Table 3. Regression results for the TPC case

Factors	β	R²	F
Effort	.243	.059	1.2
Image	.563*	.318	10.24
Resource Availability	.730**	.533	22.9
Reciprocity	.551*	.303	7.83
Mobility	.568***	.323	8.6
Quality of Output	.516*	.266	6.2
Privacy	.083	.007	.124

widescreen cart with a drawer. As a trial technology, the device was introduced in the ICU to facilitate storage and retrieval of patient-related information at the bedside. The WOW was perceived as a solution to eliminate frequent walking to, and logging in and out of the computer at, the nursing workstation. The technology could be transported alongside the healthcare professional who could stay logged in. Due to the early stage of the hospital's Electronic Medical Records (EMR) adoption model[4], the Patient Care Information System (PCS) did not provide data entry capability for healthcare professionals. Thus, they used the device simply to access test and lab results, x-rays, pharmacy information, and previous assessments. The device was also connected to the Internet; so some physicians sometimes used it to access medical research in an up-to-date electronic medical repository.

The WOW was primarily used during rounds. Two groups of physicians (i.e., a group consisted of an attending physician and residents) performed the rounds twice a day. The device was then accessible to one of the groups (i.e., there was a single device for the unit). Normally, at the start of each round, one of the residents logged onto the system and the WOW was then transported to each patient visit during the round. Physicians retrieved patient information and sometime accessed online medical resources (e.g., UpToDate®) for teaching and diagnoses purposes. Because the EMR was still in its early stages, current patient information was not always accessible electronically. This information was available but was sometimes on paper, in a queue to be scanned and entered in the system. It took usually 2-4 days for this information to be available in an electronic form. For this reason, physicians referred to the system as a "hybrid" (i.e., paper and electronic).

Physicians valued the portability attribute of the device and mentioned the efficiency gains when having the device during their rounds. One physician commented:

If I don't have the WOW, it is less likely that I look for a patient's past lab results. I can do it if I log into the PCS from the nursing workstation, but it will take me longer...I need to log in and out for every patient.

However, they stated that the device would have been more effective if information input was available. The major complaint was related to the 'hybrid system'. A physician commented:

I have to go back and forth from the [paper] chart to the WOW. For previous admissions, I go to the computer but for the current, I need the chart.

An interesting fact was a workaround observed during the onsite visits. One of the residents was also using his laptop to write patients' assessments. These assessments were printed out and placed in the paper charts at each patient's bed. Because of the limitations of the EMR and physicians' need to have updated and legible patient assessment at the bedside, the medical director of the unit and a group of residents were developing internal electronic documentation. The system had firewall protection and only a selected group was given access to it.

Additional complaints were related to technical issues resulting from the hospital's wireless infrastructure and device configurations. When the WOW was first introduced, the hospital did not have enough access points on the floor and users experienced difficulties when logging into the system. Poor wireless infrastructure and processing power of the device also made the system accessibility and browsing speeds very slow. Users also complained about the unfriendly interface of the PCS.

Survey Results

The sample consisted of 26 physicians and residents altogether. Of the 26 participants contacted, 14 (or 53%) replied. Nine were attending physicians and five were residents. More than 60% of the respondents had five or more years of experience at the hospital. All reported that they were active users of the WOW and eight participants reported that they used their personal laptops as a form of WOW (i.e., placing the laptop on a mobile cart during their rounds).

Not all survey questions applied to this case because the device allowed only retrieval of information. Questions related to effort focused on the effort associated with the retrieval of the information. Reciprocity did not apply in this case either. The dependent variable was restricted to the use of the device to retrieve patient and medical information. The resulting alpha values ranged from 0.61 to 0.96 with three factors marginally below the acceptable threshold of 0.70. The small sample size may have contributed to this slightly low score. As with the analyses of the TPC, separate linear regression analyses were performed to identify important antecedents to the resistance to use the device (Kankanhalli et al., 2005a, 2005b). Table 4 summarizes the results of the regressions.

The results show that effort, image, resource availability, and privacy had no significant relationships with mobile device usage. On the other hand mobility, and quality of output were significant antecedents to WOW usage in this hospital department. The standardized coefficients indicated that the two factors had a comparable degree of importance in the model. Moreover, quality of output had the stronger impact on WOW usage by physicians in the ICU.

DISCUSSION

Our study was exploratory and the findings we present are preliminary. They suggest that image, resource availability, reciprocity, mobility, and quality of output are factors that impact physicians' decisions to continue or stop using mobile devices in their medical practice. However, the extent to which the factors enable or hinder the use of these devices varies by the device; for example, image, resource availability and reciprocity influenced TPC usage but not WOW usage. One reason for the lack of influence of these factors on the WOW usage can be attributed to the restricted retrieval usage capabilities of the information system. As previously mentioned, the EMR allowed only patient information retrieval, but not information input.

The results from the TPC case suggest a significant positive relationship exists between image and mobile usage. Physicians may resist using these devices if they feel their professional status diminishes as a result of entering information in an electronic form and dealing with potential technical issues when

Table 4. Regression results for the WOW case

Factors	β	R²	F
Effort	.342	.087	1.6
Image	-.119	.014	.172
Resource Availability	-.016	.001	.003
Mobility	.454*	.240	3.1
Quality of Output	.654**	.427	8.21
Privacy	.148	.022	.27

using these technologies. A possible explanation relies on the traditional hierarchical relationship between nurses and physicians. Fagin and Garelick (2004) observe that nurses are seen as order-takers whereas doctors are order-givers. If physicians perceive the process of entering and retrieving information from a device to be a mere documentation activity, they may feel that this is not part of their practice, and therefore may resist using these devices.

Moreover, reciprocity significantly affected TPC usage by healthcare professionals. This relationship suggests that healthcare professionals are more willing to use a health IT/IS, if they think that their future requests for information will be met through these systems. Our results showed that low scores of reciprocity were associated with low scores of TPC usage, and greater resistance. An example of this resistance occured with using the free consultation option of the APMS. This option offered the opportunity to provide more details about patients' conditions in a free-text-entry format. In spite of the advantages of having complete and detailed patient assessments at the bedside, physicians rarely used this feature, in part because others were not doing so. There was a 'vicious cycle' of non-use and resistance because there was little likelihood of reciprocity. The physician who championed the initiative was frustrated by the lack of usage of the free-text-entry option.

Lack of resource availability was also a significant deterrent to use. Availability (i.e., easy access, opportunities to use and time to use the TPC) was a key enabler of mobile usage. The unit possessed only three TPCs. Differences in perceived resource availability appeared related to the ability to incorporate the technology into the work processes of the users – a nurse practitioner, attending physicians and residents. Time was a particularly important aspect of availability. Healthcare professionals who could not smoothly integrate the technology into their regular work practices seemed more aware of the time required to operate the device and more resistant to using the TPC. This was not the case for the WOW technology. Although, the unit possessed only one WOW, physicians who were part of the group developing the internal documentation system used their own laptops as WOWs. Therefore, they did not perceive this factor as an inhibitor.

Quality of the output was an important factor for both devices. The robustness of wireless infrastructures, the technical attributes of the devices, and the amount of training provided to users influenced the quality of the output and the required effort to use both devices (respondents indicated that limited training had been provided). Some users opted to use a fixed computer (or their personal laptop in the case of WOW) instead of the mobile devices because they did not find the devices reliable or satisfactory. A common complaint, related to the quality of the output, was the low screen resolution and limited ability of the devices to display sharp images (e.g., x-rays). This reduced the perceived value of the technology (McAfee, 2006).

Users also complained about the information systems accessed through these devices. While WOW users complained about the hybrid EMR (i.e., only allowed online 'information pull' and the 'information push' happened on paper) of the hospital and the unfriendliness of the PCS interface, the non-users of the TPC did not find the standarization of the APMS data reliable. For instance, a non-user commented on her discomfort with the scale used to assess pain. This suggested that the information transmitted and the device are interconnected. Frustration with one side (e.g., the information system) may spillover into frustration with the other side (e.g., the device), resulting in increased user resistance.

Quality of the output has been an important factor in the study of user satisfaction with IT. The user satisfaction paradigm (e.g., DeLone & McLean, 1992; DeLone, 2003) suggests that the beliefs about the technical quality of the system itself (e.g., reliability) or the semantic quality of the information provided by the system (e.g., up-to-dateness, timeliness, accessibility) can be important enablers but also inhibitors that decrease likelihood of IT use (e.g., Rai, Lang, & Welker, 2002; Teng & Calhoun, 1996; Wixom & Todd, 2005). That is, systems that are perceived to have high quality are used; others are not.

Mobility was also a critical factor for both devices. TPC users were less willing to share detailed evidence-based information when the technology was at a fixed location. Similarly, WOW users commented on the key aspect of portability. For these users, accessing the information at the bedside reduced the time spent per patient and enhanced their medical diagnoses. This finding is supported by previous research demonstrating that portability is a key factor for evidence-based medicine (e.g., Sackett & Straus, 1998; Westbrook et al., 2004). In healthcare settings, increasing device portability will likely reduce resistance to use.

Although, the degree of physical portability was an important factor, having to carry the device all the time could hamper its use. In this way, paradoxically, the high portability of the device, for instance, could hinder its adoption. Some TPC users reported that a practical solution would be to place the device on a mobile cart, thereby converting it to a WOW. Thus, although portability generally seemed positively related to use, different users desired different degrees of portability, and portability could also act as a deterrent if not designed appropriately to suit the task and users' needs and preferences.

The propositions that were not statistically supported involved required effort and privacy. Most of the respondents reported high usage of wireless devices for personal purposes and even at work (for example, they were used to using pagers). As a result, they were skilled at using the devices per say and did not see effort as a deterrent to their use. The healthcare professionals' resistance related more to reliability problems than to design issues. In addition, the respondents were not particularly concerned about breaching patients' confidentiality when using the devices. First, the information in the system was encrypted. Second, the information remained in an online database and not in the device. It could only be accessed with a username and password. For these reasons, the healthcare professionals were not concerned about the confidentiality of patient information accessed through the devices. Resistance to using the devices, in this hospital setting, was not linked with privacy concerns.

CONCLUSION

By combining insights from the IT resistance and social exchange theories, we identified potential factors influencing the use of mobile devices in healthcare environments. Specifically, we explored technical, psychological and environmental factors that inhibited or enabled physicians to use mobile devices in their medical practice. Our findings suggest that image, reciprocity, resource availability, quality of output, and portability are important factors to consider when designing and introducing mobile technologies in the healthcare industry. Some of these factors have been studied in the IT acceptance literature as antecedents or enablers of IT usage. However, in this study, we found that they can also act as inhibitors that discourage IT usage, specifically mobile usage.

In addition, the study revealed that user complaints about "poor Internet connectivity," and negative "initial experiences that turned them off" discouraged physicians to continue using the technology. These findings suggest and reaffirm the need to ensure that the complementary aspects of the technology (e.g., drivers, wireless robustness, software) are properly in place prior to technology adoption. Healthcare institutions should try to provide positive first experiences to users, especially to physicians who are often rushed and feel that they have very limited time.

These findings are preliminary and should be interpreted in the context of the study's limitations. The sample size was small and only simple statistical analyses could be conducted. Constraints such as the limited willingness of physicians to participate in non-clinical research, and their busyness, made it difficult to overcome this limitation. We recognize also that the data were gathered from physicians in a single hospital, and focused on the use of two specific mobile technologies (e.g., the TPC and WOW). It is possible that the results could vary for other hospital units and other technologies. We invite other researchers to replicate and extend our exploratory study.

REFERENCES

Amarasingham, R., Plantinga, L., Diener-West, M., Gaskin, D. J., & Powe, N. R. (2009). Clinical information technologies and inpatient outcomes: A multiple hospital study. *Archives of Internal Medicine*, *169*(2), 108. doi:10.1001/archinternmed.2008.520 PMID:19171805

Ammenwerth, E., Buchauer, A., Bludau, B., & Haux, R. (2000). Mobile information and communication tools in the hospital. *International Journal of Medical Informatics*, *57*(1), 21–40. doi:10.1016/S1386-5056(99)00056-8 PMID:10708253

Appari, A., & Johnson, M. E. (2010). Information security and privacy in healthcare: Current state of research. *International Journal of Internet and Enterprise Management*, *6*(4), 279–314. doi:10.1504/IJIEM.2010.035624

Ba, S., Stallaert, J., & Whinston, A. B. (2001). Research Commentary: Introducing a Third Dimension in Information Systems Design–The Case for Incentive Alignment. *Information Systems Research*, *12*(3), 225–239. doi:10.1287/isre.12.3.225.9712

Banitsas, K. A., Georgiadis, P., Tachakra, S., & Cavouras, D. (2004). Using handheld devices for real-time wireless teleconsultation. In *Proceedings of Engineering in Medicine and Biology Society,* (Vol. 2, pp. 3105–3108). IEEE. doi:10.1109/IEMBS.2004.1403877

Bardram, E. (2005). Activity-based computing: Support for mobility and collaboration in ubiquitous computing. *Personal and Ubiquitous Computing*, *9*(5), 312–322. doi:10.1007/s00779-004-0335-2

Bhattacherjee, A., & Hikmet, N. (2007). Physicians' resistance toward healthcare information technology: A theoretical model and empirical test. *European Journal of Information Systems*, *16*(6), 725–737. doi:10.1057/palgrave.ejis.3000717

Blau, P. M. (1964). *Exchange and power in social life*. Transaction Publishers.

Blumenthal, D. (2009). Stimulating the adoption of health information technology. *New England Journal of Project Management*, *24*(1), 1477–1479. doi:10.1056/NEJMp0901592 PMID:19321856

Cenfetelli, R. T. (2004). Inhibitors and enablers as dual factor concepts in technology usage. *Journal of the Association for Information Systems*, *5*(11), 3.

Chadwick-Jones, J. K. (1976). *Social exchange theory: Its structure and influence in social psychology*. Published in cooperation with European Association of Experimental Social Psychology by Academic Press.

Constant, D., Sproull, L., & Kiesler, S. (1996). The kindness of strangers: The usefulness of electronic weak ties for technical advice. *Organization Science, 7*(2), 119–135. doi:10.1287/orsc.7.2.119

Culnan, M. J. (1984). The dimensions of accessibility to online information: Implications for implementing office information systems. *ACM Transactions on Information Systems, 2*(2), 141–150. doi:10.1145/521.523

Cummings, J. N. (2004). Work groups, structural diversity, and knowledge sharing in a global organization. *Management Science, 50*(3), 352–364. doi:10.1287/mnsc.1030.0134

Dahl, Y., Svanes, D., & Nytro, O. (2006). Designing pervasive computing for hospitals: learning from the media affordances of paper-based medication charts. In Pervasive Health Conference and Workshops, 2006 (pp. 1–10). doi:10.1109/PCTHEALTH.2006.361673

Davenport, T. H., & Glaser, J. (2002). Just-in-time delivery comes to knowledge management. *Harvard Business Review, 80*(7), 107–111. PMID:12140850

Davenport, T. H., & Prusak, L. (2000). *Working knowledge: How organizations manage what they know.* Harvard Business Press.

Davis, F. D., Bagozzi, R. P., & Warshawpr, P. R. (1989). User acceptance of computer technology: A comparison of two theoretical models. *Management Science, 35*(8), 982–1003. doi:10.1287/mnsc.35.8.982

Delone, W. H. (2003). The DeLone and McLean model of information systems success: A ten-year update. *Journal of Management Information Systems, 19*(4), 9–30.

DeLone, W. H., & McLean, E. R. (1992). Information systems success: The quest for the dependent variable. *Information Systems Research, 3*(1), 60–95. doi:10.1287/isre.3.1.60

Dillman, D. A. (2007). *Mail and internet surveys: The tailored design method.* John Wiley & Sons Inc.

Doolan, D. F., & Bates, D. W. (2002). Computerized physician order entry systems in hospitals: Mandates and incentives. *Health Affairs, 21*(4), 180–188. doi:10.1377/hlthaff.21.4.180 PMID:12117128

Eckhardt, A., Laumer, S., & Weitzel, T. (2009). Who influences whom? Analyzing workplace referents' social influence on IT adoption and non-adoption. *Journal of Information Technology, 24*(1), 11–24. doi:10.1057/jit.2008.31

Eysenbach, G., & Jadad, A. (2003). Evidence-based Patient Choice and Consumer health informatics in the Internet age. *Journal of Medical Internet Research, 3*(2), e19. doi:10.2196/jmir.3.2.e19 PMID:11720961

Fagin, C. M. et al. (1992). Collaboration between nurses and physicians: No longer a choice. *Academic Medicine: Journal of the Association of American Medical Colleges, 67*(5), 295–303. doi:10.1097/00001888-199205000-00002 PMID:1575859

Fischer, S., Stewart, T. E., Mehta, S., Wax, R., & Lapinsky, S. E. (2003). Handheld computing in medicine. *Journal of the American Medical Informatics Association, 10*(2), 139–149. doi:10.1197/jamia. M1180 PMID:12595403

Fontelo, P., Ackerman, M., Kim, G., & Locatis, C. (2003). The PDA as a portal to knowledge sources in a wireless setting. *Telemedicine Journal and e-Health, 9*(2), 141–147. doi:10.1089/153056203766437480 PMID:12855037

Freudenheim, M. (2004). Many hospitals resist computerized patient care. *New York Times,* p. 6. Retrieved from http://www.contrib.andrew.cmu.edu/usr/rk2x/mmmjune05/ithealth.pdf

Fulk, J., Flanagin, A. J., Kalman, M. E., Monge, P. R., & Ryan, T. (1996). Connective and communal public goods in interactive communication systems. *Communication Theory, 6*(1), 60–87. doi:10.1111/j.1468-2885.1996.tb00120.x

Garfield, M. J. (2005). Acceptance of ubiquitous computing. *Information Systems Management, 22*(4), 24–31. doi:10.1201/1078.10580530/45520.22.4.20050901/90027.3

Goldstein, D., Wilson, R., & VanDenkerkhof, E. (2007). Electronic monitoring in an acute pain management service. *Pain Medicine, 8*(3), 94–100. doi:10.1111/j.1526-4637.2007.00373.x

Gonzalez, P., Chan, Y., & Goldstein, D. (2013). Exploring the use of mobile devices for knowledge sharing in healthcare: A hospital case study. In *Proceedings of the 9th Americas Conference on Information Systems*. Chicago, IL: Academic Press. Retrieved from http://aisel.aisnet.org.proxy.queensu.ca/amcis2013/HealthInformation/GeneralPresentations/6

Grasso, B. C., Genest, R., Yung, K., & Arnold, C. (2002). Reducing errors in discharge medication lists by using personal digital assistants. *Psychiatric Services (Washington, D.C.), 53*(10), 1325–1326. doi:10.1176/appi.ps.53.10.1325 PMID:12364687

Gray, P. H. (2001). The impact of knowledge repositories on power and control in the workplace. *Information Technology & People, 14*(4), 368–384. doi:10.1108/09593840110411167

Gurteen, D. (1998). Knowledge, creativity and innovation. *Journal of Knowledge Management, 2*(1), 5–13. doi:10.1108/13673279810800744

Hall, H. (2001). Social exchange for knowledge exchange. In *Proceedings of International Conference on Managing Knowledge*. Leicester, UK: University of Leicester.

Haller, G., Haller, D. M., Courvoisier, D. S., & Lovis, C. (2009). Handheld vs. laptop computers for electronic data collection in clinical research: A crossover randomized trial. *Journal of the American Medical Informatics Association, 16*(5), 651–659. doi:10.1197/jamia.M3041 PMID:19567799

Han, Y., Carcillo, J., & Venkataram, S. (2005). Unexpected increased mortality after implementation of a commercially sold computerized physician order entry system. *Pediatrics, 116*(6), 1506–1512. doi:10.1542/peds.2005-1287 PMID:16322178

Hansen, M. T., Nohria, N., & Tierney, T. (1999). What's your strategy for managing knowledge? *Knowledge Management: Critical Perspectives on Business and Management, 322.*

Hew, K. F., & Hara, N. (2006). Identifying factors that encourage and hinder knowledge sharing in a longstanding online community of practice. *Journal of Interactive Online Learning, 5*(3), 297–316.

Hillestad, R., Bigelow, J., Bower, A., Girosi, F., Meili, R., Scoville, R., & Taylor, R. (2005). Can electronic medical record systems transform health care? Potential health benefits, savings, and costs. *Health Affairs, 24*(5), 1103–1117. doi:10.1377/hlthaff.24.5.1103 PMID:16162551

Hodge, J. G., & Gostin, L. O. (2004). Challenging themes in American health information privacy and the public's health: Historical and modern assessments. *The Journal of Law, Medicine & Ethics, 32*(4), 670–679. doi:10.1111/j.1748-720X.2004.tb01972.x PMID:15807355

Huang, K. T., Lee, Y. W., & Wang, R. Y. (1998). *Quality information and knowledge.* Prentice Hall PTR.

Juciute, R. (2009). ICT implementation in the health-care sector: Effective stakeholder's engagement as the main precondition of change sustainability. *AI & Society, 23*(1), 131–137. doi:10.1007/s00146-007-0168-4

Kankanhalli, A., Tan, B. C., & Wei, K. K. (2005a). Contributing knowledge to electronic knowledge repositories: An empirical investigation. *Management Information Systems Quarterly*, 113–143.

Kankanhalli, A., Tan, B. C. Y., & Wei, K. K. (2005b). Understanding seeking from electronic knowledge repositories: An empirical study. *Journal of the American Society for Information Science and Technology, 56*(11), 1156–1166. doi:10.1002/asi.20219

Karimi, F., & Chiang Choon Poo, D. (2009). Personal and external determinants of medical bloggers' knowledge sharing behavior. *Proceedings of the American Society for Information Science and Technology, 46*(1), 1–23. doi:10.1002/meet.2009.1450460242

Keating, N. L., Ayanian, J. Z., Cleary, P. D., & Marsden, P. V. (2007). Factors affecting influential discussions among physicians: A social network analysis of a primary care practice. *Journal of General Internal Medicine, 22*(6), 794–798. doi:10.1007/s11606-007-0190-8 PMID:17404798

Kuziemsky, C. E., Laul, F., & Leung, R. C. (2005). A review on diffusion of personal digital assistants in healthcare. *Journal of Medical Systems, 29*(4), 335–342. doi:10.1007/s10916-005-5893-y PMID:16178332

Kuziemsky, C. E., Laul, F., & Leung, R. C. (2005). A review on diffusion of personal digital assistants in healthcare. *Journal of Medical Systems, 29*(4), 335–342. doi:10.1007/s10916-005-5893-y PMID:16178332

Lapointe, L., & Rivard, S. (2005). A multilevel model of resistance to information technology implementation. *Management Information Systems Quarterly, 29*(3), 461–491.

Laumer, S., & Eckhardt, A. (2012). Why do people reject technologies: A review of user resistance theories. In Y. K. Dwivedi, M. R. Wade, & S. L. Scheneberger (Eds.), *Information Systems Theory Explaining and Predicting Our Digital Society* (pp. 63–86). Springer. doi:10.1007/978-1-4419-6108-2_4

Lewin, K. (1947). Group decision and social change. *Readings in Social Psychology, 3*, 197–211.

Lottridge, D. M., Chignell, M., Danicic-Mizdrak, R., Pavlovic, N. J., Kushniruk, A., & Straus, S. E. (2007). Group differences in physician responses to handheld presentation of clinical evidence: A verbal protocol analysis. *BMC Medical Informatics and Decision Making, 7*(1), 22. doi:10.1186/1472-6947-7-22 PMID:17655759

Lu, Y.-C., Sears, A., & Jacko, J. (2005). A review and a framework of handheld computer adoption in healthcare. *International Journal of Medical Informatics, 74*(5), 409–422. doi:10.1016/j.ijmedinf.2005.03.001 PMID:15893264

Markus, M. L. (2001). Toward a theory of knowledge reuse: Types of knowledge reuse situations and factors in reuse success. *Journal of Management Information Systems, 18*(1), 57–93.

Martinko, M. J., Zmud, R. W., & Henry, J. W. (1996). An attributional explanation of individual resistance to the introduction of information technologies in the workplace. *Behaviour & Information Technology, 15*(5), 313–330. doi:10.1080/014492996120085a

McAfee, A. P. (2006). Enterprise 2.0: The dawn of emergent collaboration. *Engineering Management Review, IEEE, 34*(3), 38–38. doi:10.1109/EMR.2006.261380

McAlearney, A. S., Schweikhart, S. B., & Medow, M. A. (2004). Doctors' experience with handheld computers in clinical practice: Qualitative study. *BMJ (Clinical Research Ed.), 328*(7449), 1162. doi:10.1136/bmj.328.7449.1162 PMID:15142920

Medpac. (2004). *Report to the congress: New approaches in Medicare.* Washington, DC: Author.

Molm, L. D. (1997). *Coercive power in social exchange.* Cambridge Univ Pr. doi:10.1017/CBO9780511570919

Prgomet, M., Georgiou, A., & Westbrook, J. I. (2009). The impact of mobile handheld technology on hospital physicians' work practices and patient care: A systematic review. *Journal of the American Medical Informatics Association, 16*(6), 792–801. doi:10.1197/jamia.M3215 PMID:19717793

Rai, A., Lang, S. S., & Welker, R. B. (2002). Assessing the validity of IS success models: An empirical test and theoretical analysis. *Information Systems Research, 13*(1), 50–69. doi:10.1287/isre.13.1.50.96

Rindfleisch, T. C. (1997). Privacy, information technology, and health care. *Communications of the ACM, 40*(8), 93–100. doi:10.1145/257874.257896

Sackett, D. L., & Straus, S. E. et al. (1998). Finding and applying evidence during clinical rounds. *Journal of the American Medical Association, 280*(15), 1336. doi:10.1001/jama.280.15.1336 PMID:9794314

Saga, V. L., & Zmud, R. W. (1994). The nature and determinants of IT acceptance, routinization, and infusion. In L. Levine (Ed.), *Diffusion, Transfer and Implementation of Information Technology* (pp. 67–86). Amsterdam: North-Holland.

Scott, C., Seidel, J., Bowen, S., & Gall, N. (2009). Integrated health systems and integrated knowledge: creating space for putting knowledge into action. *Healthcare Quarterly (Toronto, Ont.), 13*, 30.

Shannon, T., Feied, C., Smith, M., Handler, J., & Gillam, M. (2006). Wireless handheld computers and voluntary utilization of computerized prescribing systems in the emergency department. *The Journal of Emergency Medicine, 31*(3), 309–315. doi:10.1016/j.jemermed.2005.09.020 PMID:16982373

Skowronski, J. J., & Carlston, D. E. (1987). Social judgment and social memory: The role of cue diagnosticity in negativity, positivity, and extremity biases. *Journal of Personality and Social Psychology, 52*(4), 689–699. doi:10.1037/0022-3514.52.4.689

Speier, C., Vessey, I., & Valacich, J. S. (2003). The effects of interruptions, task complexity, and information presentation on computer-supported decision-making performance. *Decision Sciences, 34*(4), 771–797. doi:10.1111/j.1540-5414.2003.02292.x

Teng, J. T., & Calhoun, K. J. (1996). Organizational Computing as a Facilitator of Operational and Managerial Decision Making: An Exploratory Study of Managers' Perceptions*. *Decision Sciences*, *27*(4), 673–710. doi:10.1111/j.1540-5915.1996.tb01831.x

Trimmer, K., Beachboard, J., Wiggins, C., & Woodhouse, W. (2008). Electronic medical records use - An examination of resident physician intentions. In *Proceeding of the 41 st Hawaii International Conference on System Sciences*, (pp. 249 - 261). IEEE. doi:10.1109/HICSS.2008.140

VanDen Kerkhof, E. G., Parlow, J. L., Goldstein, D. H., & Milne, B. (2004). In Canada, anesthesiologists are less likely to respond to an electronic, compared to a paper questionnaire. Canadian Journal of Anesthesia, 51(5), 449–454.

Vandenkerkhof, E., Hall, S., Wilson, R., Gay, A., & Duhn, L. (2009). Evaluation of an innovative communication technology in an acute care setting. *CIN Computers Informatics*, *27*(4), 254–262. doi:10.1097/NCN.0b013e3181a91bf6 PMID:19574751

Varshney, U. (2006). Using wireless technologies in healthcare. *International Journal of Mobile Communications*, *4*(3), 354–368.

Venkatesh, V., Morris, M. G., Davis, G. B., & Davis, F. D. (2003). User acceptance of information technology: Toward a unified view. *Management Information Systems Quarterly*, 425–478.

Wasko, M. M., & Faraj, S. (2005). Why should I share? Examining social capital and knowledge contribution in electronic networks of practice. *Management Information Systems Quarterly*, 35–57.

Westbrook, J. I., Gosling, A. S., & Coiera, E. (2004). Do clinicians use online evidence to support patient care? A study of 55,000 clinicians. *Journal of the American Medical Informatics Association*, *11*(2), 113–120. doi:10.1197/jamia.M1385 PMID:14662801

Wixom, B. H., & Todd, P. A. (2005). A theoretical integration of user satisfaction and technology acceptance. *Information Systems Research*, *16*(1), 85–102. doi:10.1287/isre.1050.0042

Yin, R. K. (2009). *Case study research: Design and methods* (Vol. 5). Sage Publications, Inc.

KEY TERMS AND DEFINITIONS

Dual-Factor Model: IT usage considerations among potential users is based on a simultaneous examination of enabling and inhibiting factors.

Healthcare Information Technologies (Health IT): Information and communication technologies used in the healthcare industry (e.g., electronic health records, clinical decision support systems) to improve the quality, safety, and efficiency of healthcare.

IT Acceptance: The individuals' willingness to use information technologies.

IT Resistance: Individuals' refusal to accept or comply with information technologies. Sometimes, individuals actively engage in actions to prevent the acceptance of the technology (e.g., hostility behaviours toward the change agent, a person or technology).

IT Privacy: Accidental disclosure and unauthorized intrusion of network systems.

Mobile Devices: The information technologies that are portable and use cellular communication and wireless networking (e.g., tablet computers, smartphones).

Social Exchange Theory: Proposes that social behavior is the result of an exchange process. An exchange indicates that one party provides something to another party. An implicit or explicit obligation is then created in the receiving party. The receiving party must provide some sort of benefit to the first in order to discharge this obligation. The returns may be either direct or indirect.

ENDNOTES

[1]   Evidence-based medicine (EBM) is defined as "the conscientious, explicit and judicious use of current best evidence in making decisions about the care of individual patients" (Sackett et al., 1996). Information technology is perceived as a key component of effective healthcare by creating the data framework for EBM. The EBM is expected to provide a systematic analysis of all available evidence in electronic format from an ever-changing, continually updated statistical dataset. These sets may include standard clinical trial models, publications on medical protocols and their efficacy, demographic and genetic data, and day-to-day in-field observations. This information would allow physicians to balance their experience and training with EBM data, which could provide real-time situational awareness and decision support (Rubel, 2008).

[2]   RAND stands for Research and Development. It is a nonprofit institution that conducts research on different topics such as education, labor and population and health. These statistics are sometimes challenged (Blumenthal, 2009).

[3]   A panel of experts in the healthcare industry examined the factors and rated a subset as being more applicable in this context. Details of this pilot study are found in the methodology section.

[4]   The hospital was in stage 3 out of 7. That is, the current capabilities of the EMR are nursing clinical documentation (flow sheets), CDSS (error checking), and picture archive and communication systems (PACS) available outside the Radiology department via organization's intranet. In stage 4, computer practitioner order entry (CPOE) are implemented and clinicians can then create orders and access to the second level of clinical decision support capabilities related to evidence based medicine protocols.

This research was previously published in Business Technologies in Contemporary Organizations edited by Abrar Haider, pages 210-235, copyright year 2015 by Business Science Reference (an imprint of IGI Global).

Chapter 77
Information Security Threats in Patient–Centred Healthcare

Shada Alsalamah
King Saud University, Saudi Arabia

Hessah Alsalamah
King Saud University, Saudi Arabia

Alex W. Gray
Cardiff University, UK

Jeremy Hilton
Cranfield University, UK

ABSTRACT

Healthcare is taking an evolutionary approach towards the adoption of Patient-Centred (PC) delivery approach, which requires the flow of information between different healthcare providers to support a patient's treatment plan, so the Care Team (CT) can seamlessly and securely access relevant information held in the different discrete Legacy Information Systems (LIS). Each of these LIS deploys an organisational-driven information security policy that meets its local information sharing context needs. Nevertheless, incorporating these LIS in collaborative PC care brings multiple inconsistent policies together, which raises a number of information security threats that can block the CT access to critical information across a patient's treatment journey. Using an empirical study, this chapter identifies information security threats that can cause the issue, and defines a common collaboration-driven information security design. Finally, it identifies requirements in LIS to address the inconsistent policies in modern PC collaborative environments that would help improve the quality of care.

INTRODUCTION

Population ageing is a demographic revolution affecting the entire world (United Nations Population Fund (UNFPA), 2014) due to medical advances, increased child survival, and improved health care. This is evidenced by figures published by the UNFPA (UNFPA, 2014); see Figure 1, which shows the increasing number of people aged 60 or over between the years 1950-2050 in the world's developed

DOI: 10.4018/978-1-5225-3926-1.ch077

Figure 1. Number of people aged 60 or over: World, developed and developing countries, 1950-2050 (UNFPA, 2014)

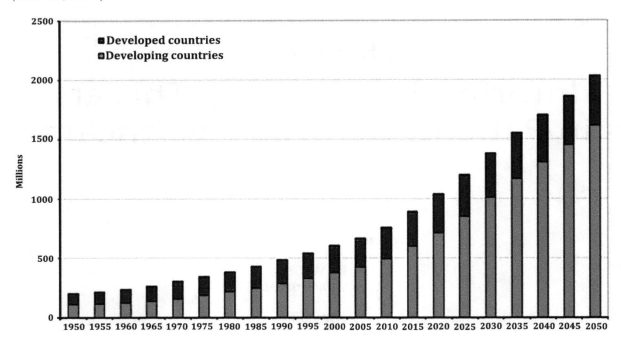

and developing countries (UNFPA, 2014). However, this does not mean that older persons should be a burden (UNFPA, 2014). Older people's health conditions require more holistic care as comorbidity is more prevalent in older patients than in younger ones (McGarrigle, H., Personal Communication, November 2013). Patients with comorbidity suffer from more than one condition at a time, and so they follow multiple treatment pathways. It is clear that healthcare delivery systems need to cope with this emerging need, and be ready for the ageing population, with modern integrated healthcare services that can cope holistically with a patient with more than one health condition.

Therefore, the delivery of healthcare in many countries has been shifting towards an integrated PC care using an evolutionary approach that incorporates Legacy Information Systems (LIS). PC healthcare is where care provision is tailored to meet an individual patient's needs holistically. It is the basis of modern healthcare collaborative environments today, and many countries are using an evolutionary approach to shift towards PC care by building integrated systems based on the sound foundations of the current LIS to support it. The movement towards PC using LIS creates a new information sharing context that is collaboration-driven and is different from local organisation-driven contexts of LIS. This new context, however, requires medical information to flow with the patient between different healthcare providers as they follow the patient's treatment plans and share information across healthcare organisations. This allows the CT to seamlessly access relevant information held in different discrete information systems so that a complete picture is available if required. Nevertheless, meeting this collaboration-driven information sharing context demands an information security context that can carefully balance between enabling seamless access to CT without invading the patient's privacy. This can be addressed using an information security design that ensures the confidentiality, integrity, and availability of patient information is preserved in this collaborative environment (Calder & Watkins, 2008; Mense et al., 2013;

Pfleeger and Pfleeger, 2003; Pipkin, 2000; Posthumus and von Solms, 2004; SANS Institute, 2001). Therefore, collaboration-driven information security should meet the overall care goal while retaining local information security for shared medical information among the CT. However, LIS were not designed to support a holistic view of a patient record needed in comorbidity, as they were developed to meet the needs of the disease centred approach at a time when information sharing was not common. LIS are unable to support seamless access to information because they are unable to comply with the information security of the shared information that is coming together in this collaborative environment supporting PC care, whether this information is related to a patient following one treatment pathway or one who has comorbidities. This is because the LIS incorporated in PC collaborative environments as part of the evolutionary approach are autonomous discrete information systems, where each of these systems protects its information using an information security context that is suitable for its local information sharing context. Consequently, a LIS may compromise on the availability of information by blocking a CT from accessing the information they need to care for the patient, and so interrupt care continuity. Thus, LIS require additional security features to cope with this emerging need if they are to participate in collaborative PC. This chapter aims to identify the range of information security threats that LIS present to PC care thus limiting its implementation, and derive a set of information security requirements in LIS to mitigate these threats, while being incorporated into collaborative PC care.

BACKGROUND

Modern integrated healthcare services are an essential part of e-health (Powell, 2009). They use ICT to enhance collaboration, communication and coordination in the health sector (Eysenbach, 2001; Powell, 2009). At the heart of this integration of care lies PC healthcare (Allam, 2006), defined as:

A collaborative effort consisting of patients, patients' families, friends, the doctors and other health professionals [...] where patients and the health care professionals collaborate as a team, share knowledge and work toward the common goals of optimum healing and recovery (International Alliance of Patient Organizations. (IAPO), 2004)

In the global adoption of PC care (Department of Health (DoH), 1997; Ellingsen & Røed, 2010; Skilton, 2011), patient treatment is shifting from a traditionally fragmented disease centred approach towards an integrated PC one (Al-Salamah et al., 2011; Allam, 2006; DoH, 1997; IAPO, 2004; Skilton, 2011). Disease-centred care is also known as traditional healthcare (Smith & Eloff, 1999), doctor-centred (IAPO, 2004), hospital-centred (IAPO, 2004), location-based, and clinic-centred healthcare (Beale, 2004). In a disease centred approach, healthcare professionals use a treatment approach reflecting the needs of the disease diagnosis. Care for the patient focuses on the needs of the professionals treating the patient (Dawson et al., 2009; Skilton, 2011). This leads to each professional using an information silo to store information about patients with the same disease, and this is held in their organisation and managed by an independent stand-alone system not integrated with any other disease silo (Dawson et al., 2009). Access to patient information is limited to the physical boundaries of the provider (Dawson et al., 2009). Any decision-making process is fragmented and based on limited available information, as each healthcare provider keeps patient information "hidden" from care providers in other areas (Skilton, 2011).

PC care has a more holistic view that considers the patient's condition as a whole in contrast to different healthcare professionals treating each diagnosed disease separately (Al-Salamah et al., 2011; American Cancer Society, 2008). The patient is kept at the heart of these healthcare services and care is integrated and tailored to the patient's needs and current state (Allam, 2006; Dawson et al., 2009; DoH, 1997, 2010b). It encourages healthcare professionals to adapt to these needs (DoH, 2010b) by collaborating as a CT (Al-Salamah et al., 2011) and using shared decision-making processes in regular Multi-Disciplinary Team (MDT) reviews (Skilton, 2011), mostly on a weekly basis. Also, each CT member collects and shares relevant information with other members. This collectively forms a complete patient record about the holistic condition of the patient, covering all the patient's multiple conditions in cases of comorbidity. This encourages using appropriate information-sharing mechanisms among CT members while still preserving information confidentiality. Thus, central to PC care is the appointment of a "Guardian" of person-based clinical information in each healthcare organisation to oversee the sharing arrangements and make decisions when it comes to the use and sharing of clinical information and patient identifiable information (DoH, 2010a). Therefore, each healthcare organisation with access to patient records is mandated to have a Caldicott Guardian (Health and Social Care Information Centre (HSCIS), 2013), who is:

The senior person is responsible for protecting the confidentiality of a patient and service-user information and enabling appropriate information-sharing. (HSCIS, 2013)

Each Caldicott Guardian plays a key role in ensuring the organisation satisfies the highest practical standards for handling patient identifiable information (DoH, 2010a; HSCIS, 2013). There is also an overarching lead Information Governance Caldicott Guardian whose role is to make sure all local Caldicott Guardians are consistent (Crosby 2012). Both traditional and PC approaches have different attributes: the key emphasis in disease-centred care is on record keeping (Dawson et al., 2009), while the PC approach, on the other hand, creates a "culture of open information" (DoH, 2010b) emphasising accessibility to patient information (Dawson et al., 2009), teamwork and collaboration (Al-Salamah et al., 2011), and shared decision-making (DoH, 2010b; Skilton, 2011). This led to PC treatment being referred to as "shared care" of a patient (Smith & Eloff, 1999).

TOWARDS PC CARE ADOPTION USING LIS

The movement towards PC healthcare is occurring in many countries. Most countries adopting PC care, including the UK, favour an evolutionary approach over a revolutionary one that involves using LIS, so that the LIS are gradually replaced with newer systems (Allam, 2006; Bisbal et al., 1999; DoH, 2000, 2010b; Morrey, 2013; Skilton, 2011). Bisbal et al. (1999) define an LIS as "any information system that significantly resist modification and evolution" (Bisbal et al., 1999). Although LIS are often brittle, slow, none extensible, expensive to maintain, and harder to integrate with other systems (Bisbal et al., 1999), they represent the backbone of the healthcare organisation's information, hence it must be used in this movement. Also, this evolutionary approach is less expensive and has a lower risk of failure than alternative approaches (Bisbal et al., 1999), where the LIS are totally discarded and replaced with newer ones, which can have a serious impact if the information becomes unavailable for a period or lost. Hence, it is important not to discard an LIS but evolve it (Bisbal et al., 1999; DoH, 1997; Morrey, 2013). Therefore, it is not a surprise that the transformation from LIS supporting a traditional approach to systems supporting PC care is a concrete challenge the UK National Health Service (NHS) is facing whilst modernising its health services (DoH, 2002; Skilton, 2011). Data in the old format is stored in stand-alone information silos and needs to be converted into the format required by the new integrated support systems (DoH, 2002). The evolutionary movement in the NHS is based on the principle of "keeping what works and discarding what has failed" (DoH, 1997) as it believes that what is working effectively should not be discarded. This means the new integrated systems are built on the foundations of the fragmented LIS (DoH, 1997). Thus, for the time being, the LIS will not be discarded (DoH, 1997, 2000; Skilton, 2011) but will be interfaced with the new support systems (DoH, 2002). Nevertheless, the NHS strategy towards integrated healthcare specifies that healthcare systems used by healthcare professionals working patient-centrally (whether totally new or combined with LIS) should have the five information principles in Table 1 (DoH & NHS Executive, 1998; Skilton, 2011).

These principles support integrated care in which the needs of patients, not the needs of support healthcare systems, are at the heart of the health services. However, meeting the above information principles in an integrated healthcare system requires a supporting collaborative environment (Shaller, 2007) that provides holistic records of a patient's health in which all CT members treating the patient can incorporate their contributions and the record is shared by the CT (Gaunt, 2009). This is to meet the needs of PC care information sharing and security contexts. This collaborative environment should operate effectively, ensuring accessibility and flexibility of healthcare services across the organisational boundaries of the NHS healthcare organisations providing the care, to ensure that individuals experience healthcare that is well integrated with smooth transitions between health services in different settings (Gaunt, 2009; Skilton, 2011). Nevertheless, such an environment raises key information security threats that are barriers to the implementation of integrated healthcare using LIS, and thus a more secure collaborative environment is required. This is caused by the LIS being designed to meet the needs of traditional treatment models (DoH, 1997), and not fully supporting the secure cross-organisational information sharing needed in collaborative environments generated by PC care. Therefore, LIS hinder the realisation of PC care in modern healthcare, and require enhancing to create a secure collaborative environment where CT members can seamlessly access all relevant information at the point of treatment of a patient without losing control over it.

Table 1. NHS Information Principles

NHS Principle Number	Description
NHS Principle #1	Information is person-based
NHS Principle #2	Systems are integrated
NHS Principle #3	Management information is derived from operational systems
NHS Principle #4	Information is secure and confidential
NHS Principle #5	Information is shared across the NHS

SOLUTIONS AND RECOMMENDATIONS

The study is carried out at different research stages using a mixture of different qualitative methods, including domain analysis, conceptual modelling, observations, and interviews.

1. **Domain Analysis:** Initially, a domain analysis (Fernandez et al., 2007) was conducted to understand the complexity of PC healthcare in a well-defined information sharing context, namely cancer care. This complexity is best investigated through a real-life treatment pathway. Therefore, to study the various complexities due to different treatment pathways, three different types of cancers were investigated: Hepatocellular (HC), Upper Gastrointestinal (UGI), and breast cancers. Their treatment pathways, also known as Integrated Care Pathways (ICP), were analysed. The pathways used are published in the Map of Medicine (MoM) (2013) clinical guidelines. HC cancer has a fairly simple one-page ICP, and UGI cancer has a more detailed two-page ICP while breast cancer is the most complex of these three cancers as it has a six-page ICP. Due to the complexity of breast cancer ICPs, it was studied in more detail using conceptual modelling to understand each treatment point.

2. **Conceptual Modelling:** Breast cancer is the most complex pathway of these cancers and could not be studied through its ICPs alone, and needed enrichment details, which required further investigation. A comprehensive conceptual model of the breast cancer ICPs is created, and part of this conceptual model was published in (Alsalamah et al., 2011). In the creation of this complex diagram, each treatment point was investigated to identify the healthcare professional's role, information collected and recorded at that point, and healthcare information system and health record used for storing this information. The development of this conceptual model provided a good understanding of how breast cancer treatment should be achieved in a PC manner.

3. **Observation of Current Practice and System Usage:** The investigations carried out on all three cancer ICPs highlighted that MDT reviews are essential elements in PC care and that some cancers have more than one MDT review. These reviews are the most intensive points for sharing information throughout the treatment pathways. According to a General Practitioner (GP) (Sheard 2011), the MDTs were introduced in the UK less than a decade ago as an essential step towards PC care. An MDT review consists of healthcare professionals from differing specialities who meet regularly (mostly on a weekly basis) to make shared decisions about patients' care plans (Sheard, 2011; Skilton, 2011). They are fundamental in most treatment pathways (Sheard 2011) and represent an important information sharing point as they create and monitor the care management plans. Therefore, to best understand PC care, a total of seven different MDT review sessions in the selected cancers' pathways were observed (see details in Table 2).

Table 2. Observed MDT Sessions

Cancer Type	MDT Review	Total no. of Hours	Total no. of Patients
Breast Cancer	4 Normal Breast Cancer MDT reviews	8 hours 30 minutes	Average of 35-40 patients per session reaching 50 sometimes (Patel, M., Personal Communication, November 2013)
	1 Metastatic Breast Cancer MDT review	1 hour	8 patients
UGI Cancer	1 UGI MDT review	1 hour	9 patients
HC Cancer	1 Hepatobiliary MDT review	1 hour 30 minutes	20 patients

MDTs helps understand the limitations of LIS in supporting decision-making processes at MDTs. Moreover, although LIS's support for MDTs is observed, further understanding of the architecture of these LIS is needed to understand how they are used to record and retrieve information outside MDTs in other points of treatment. Therefore, the use of three of the main information systems currently used in cancer treatments in the Welsh Cancer Centre were studied using observations inside and outside MDTs. These systems were:

- **CaNISC:** Short for Cancer Network Information System (Cymru), the stand-alone supporting system providing information to health professionals treating Welsh cancer patients across different NHS trusts in Wales (NHS Wales Informatics Service (NWIS), 2013). It is designated as the central repository of cancer data across Wales (Cancer National Specialist Advisory Group, 2012).
- **Centricity:** The radiology system at Velindre NHS Trust.
- **Clinical Portal:** The web-based support system is providing test results and letters to healthcare professionals at different NHS Trusts or hospitals. Each hospital has its separate implementation of the Clinical Portal to view local clinical information within the hospital's perimeter, and although they all have a similar idea, look, and feel, they are local implementations with some differences (Morrey 2013).

These observations and studies help gain a proper understanding of these LIS's structure, limitations and weaknesses, and their usage for information sharing to support PC cancer care. However, the outcomes do not fully cover the information security context outside the MDTs, and so, the information security context is investigated next and linked with the information sharing context using a different, more direct method of inquiry.

4. **Semi-Structured Interviews and Personal Communications:** Different interviews and various personal communications (including email and face-to-face communication methods) are conducted with healthcare professionals, information governance personnel, and senior employees in the NHS. They are chosen because of their knowledge of information governance and healthcare systems in the UK in general, and the treatment pathways used in cancer care. The interviewees cover the 18 different roles in Table 3. These interviews and personal communications cover how PC care was being supported by the current procedures linking to LIS from the interviewees' perspective and what would improve this support. The interactions are based on both the role of the interviewee and the problem being investigated.

Dr. Tom Crosby (2012), the Velindre Cancer Centre's Caldicott Guardian, is interviewed. His role as a Caldicott Guardian is itself part of the broader Information Governance at Velindre (DoH, 2010a). He is also Medical Director of the South Wales Cancer Network and plays a number of other leading roles, including: Clinical Director of the Velindre Cancer Centre, Chair of the Cancer Service Management Board, and Consultant Oncologist treating UGI cancer. The interview aims to identify the right balance of information security in information systems supporting cancer treatments pursuing a PC care, and the threats present in current information systems that would breach that balance. The synthesis from the Caldicott Guardian's interview is confirmed by a second interview with Dr. Crosby (2012), then assessed by the former head of the CIU (Morrey 2013), and an IT Lead at Velindre NHS Trust (Stockdale, 2013).

Table 3. Interviews and Personal Communications

Category	Role(s)
Senior roles in the healthcare organisation	Chair of the Cancer Service Management Board
	Clinical Director of the Velindre Cancer Centre
	Head of the Software Service Unit at Velindre Cancer Centre
	Head of Information Management & Technology (IM&T)
	IT Lead at Velindre Hospital
	Head of Clinical Information Unit (CIU) at Velindre NHS Trust
Information governance and support personnel	Cancer Centre Caldicott Guardian
	Information Governance and Security Specialist
	Information Governance Support Manager
Care team members	GP
	Breast Cancer Nurse Specialist
	Breast Cancer Consultant Clinical Oncologist
	UGI Cancer Consultant Clinical Oncologist
Care team support personnel	Normal Breast Cancer MDT Coordinator
	Metastatic Breast Cancer MDT Coordinator
	UGI cancer MDT Coordinator
	HC cancer MDT Coordinator

Also, breast cancer is selected to assess the results from the initial interview with the Caldicott Guardian. This is done by interviewing a Breast Cancer Oncologist (Borley 2013), Clinical Nurse Specialist in Breast Care (McGarrigle 2013), and the Normal Breast Cancer MDT Coordinator (Patel 2013). In the remainder of this chapter, a synthesis from all interviews regarding information security issues in LIS is presented.

The Right Balance of Information Security in Cancer Care

In very broad terms, according to Dr. Crosby (2012), information security implementation in healthcare must aim to carefully balance access to clinical information and patient identifiable information by those people who need to see it to support clinical decision-making, while protecting the clinical and patient identifiable information from those who do not treat the patient, and maintaining the accuracy of this information. He emphasised the need for this balance in information security to be on both levels - an individual case record basis, and also on a more population-wide group basis (Crosby 2012). Therefore, at one extreme, his role as clinical director of the cancer centre is to ensure when *clinicians and staff see patients they have the right amount of clinical information available,* and at the other extreme, as the Caldicott Guardian, he needs *to ensure that as much security is put in place that is reasonable and practical to ensure that is done safely* (Crosby 2012). This indicates that the balance of information security that Dr. Crosby is enforcing in the Cancer Centre is on a need-to-know basis, as highlighted in the NHS

Plan to modernise its healthcare system (DoH, 2003, 2010a), while complying with the Data Protection Act 1998 (DoH, 2003, 2010a) and a long list of other legislations (DoH, 2010a). This includes, but is not limited to, the Human Rights Act 1998, the Freedom of Information Act 2000, the NHS Code of Practice on Confidentiality 2003 and the inception of NHS Information Governance 2003 (DoH, 2010a). The Caldicott Guardian must ensure the implementation of this information access need by making sure the *use or flow of patient-identifiable information should be regularly justified and routinely tested against the principles developed in the Caldicott Report* (DoH, 2010a), see Table 4.

Information Security Issues Threatening the Balance

In fact, the "need-to-know" access rule has been the norm balance of information security in healthcare for decades, even in autonomous discrete information systems supporting traditional disease-centred care, each with its own information security rules deployed. A discrete LIS's local information security balance is already enforced within their physical perimeter on a "need-to-know" basis. However, each discrete information system has interpreted this high-level information access rule from the national guideline into their information security design and expressed it differently at the lower levels of the design to enforce it at the machine level. This situation of inconsistent interpretations of the information access rule is causing an information security issue that threatens the implementation of PC care using these systems. This was clearly highlighted by the Caldicott Guardian, when he said:

on a very high level I think because of varying interpretation of the guidance around information security, clinicians are often blocked from having the right information to treat a patient and I do not think enough weight is put on that (i.e. patients' rights of access to the best healthcare available because of variation in the interpretation of security rules). (Crosby 2012)

Therefore, moving towards PC care, where the medical treatment follows a treatment pathway with care at a number of locations, requires an overarching balance of information security that implements the "need-to-know" access rule at the collaboration level, without interfering with the inconsistent local implementations of this rule. This interpretation inconsistency is threatening the stability of the local balance once the information leaves the discrete LIS by compromising one or more of the security goals in many ways, along with other threats as described in the interview and discussed fully in the next section.

Table 4. Principles in the Caldicott Report

Caldicott Guardian Principle Number	Description
1	Justify the purpose(s) for using confidential information
2	Only use it when necessary
3	Use the minimum that is required
4	Access should be on a strict need-to-know basis
5	Everyone must understand his or her responsibilities
6	Understand and comply with the law

1. Threats to Information Integrity

LIS supporting cancer treatment are raising integrity issues as they fall short of preserving the accuracy of clinical information in that context. Among the causes of this situation are:

a.   **Human Error:** The integrity of patient information can be hard to preserve once the human error has occurred in the recording of the information for a patient being referred to different healthcare providers. If an oncologist at one organisation receives an incorrect code for the diagnosed cancer type (i.e. a code referring to a different cancer type), current systems do not allow him or her to change it. This is because the owner who recorded it works for a different healthcare provider, and edit access right is not granted to a consultant who works with a different organisation. Another major weakness in the current system is that it is not possible to track back to the owner of information at the point where the information was compiled. In addition, even if there is a need to write to the information originator (if known) to request an alteration, it cannot be changed remotely by the current system (Crosby 2012).

b.   **Inconsistent Results in Different Systems:** Regular MDT reviews are essential to cancer treatments as the most crucial information sharing point among CT members, as critical shared decision-making processes occur at the MDT. However, the use of different hospitals' discrete information systems in geographically distributed collaborative care affects the accuracy of the information. This was highlighted by an MDT coordinator (Patel 2013) who expressed extreme concern about information accuracy, which she finds difficult to preserve in the context of collaborative cancer care. She mentioned an incident in one of the MDT reviews when the pathologist did not have some patients' results, but the breast care nurse did. In such a case, the consultant who examined the patient is normally at the MDT review and she/he makes the decision as to whether the results from the nurse should be considered, or the patient's case should be rescheduled to the next review awaiting the pathologist's results. However, the consultant's absence, in this case, made it worse, and because patients cannot be left hanging, the MDT Coordinator had to make the decision, but she did not know what to do in this very confusing situation. Eventually, she put the patient on the following week's MDT list, and although this delayed the patient's treatment, if the diagnosis is reconfirmed, this decision has less risk for the patient than considering wrong results. Although such cases are very rare, they still happen, and it is critically important to deal with them professionally. However, the systems could help in these cases if information is organised in chronological order, to show the treatment points and compare the date when the nurse and the pathologist saw the patient with the date of the test results. This would help the coordinator make an informed decision.

LIS compromise on the integrity of PC information, and need the following requirements to restore the right level of information integrity to suit PC cancer care:

- Information organisation in chronological order to help track the information to the information owner and treatment points.
- Remote information update after dissemination to allow information owners to update the information in the case of a human error incident.

2. Threats to Information Availability

Information availability is critical in patient care management. According to the Caldicott Guardian, more harm is done to the patient through lack of access to relevant information than by misuse, due to the risk of information falling into the wrong hands, as it prevents informed clinical decisions using it (Crosby 2012). However, LIS supporting a PC care compromise on the availability of patient information for some reasons.

a. *Disconnected systems at major sharing points.* MDT reviews are one of the most sensitive sharing points in a treatment journey for most conditions and diseases, not only for cancer. However, in the context of cancer care, a patient's case is normally discussed at several MDT review points: the initial diagnosis of cancer, and at key treatment points such as chemotherapy and surgery. Normally, before an MDT review, consultants or nurses based on the patients care request the patient to be added to the MDT list with a note as to why the patient's case requires discussion and what information needs to be ready to enable the discussion. The MDT Coordinator prepares a list of all patients to be considered, and they will come from several organisations. The relevant Cancer Service Departments are then responsible for listing reports on CaNISC in the MDT Summary ready for the meeting, and the coordinator is responsible as overall coordinator for ensuring images and other information are available (Biscoe 2012). However, some MDT reviews are not very successful in achieving this goal because some systems are not connected. According to an oncologist (Borley 2013), this results in the MDT patient list that the MDT coordinator, surgeon, and pathologist have as being totally different. Therefore, the results of patients in the list the surgeon had expected and the results that the MDT coordinator and pathologist were expecting were not there, "so it was all a bit hopeless" (Borley, 2013). Moreover, in one of the observed MDT reviews, Twelve of the patients were not discussed because the information was not there at that point in time; although the patients had been referred, the information did not flow with them, and hence, was not available on time. In such a case, all the MDT members said was: 'we do not know why, so we are going to investigate why this is happening and come back next week.' However, a week's delay makes a huge difference to the patient's treatment as "the clock is ticking and the patients wouldn't understand that delay" (Morrey 2013).

b. *Inconsistent information security policies.* Many LIS in the UK were designed in 1948, when the NHS was established (DoH, 1997), to meet the requirements of a disease centred approach. All NHS Trusts and hospitals working under the NHS umbrella adopted the NHS national high-level policies and practice guidelines for the implementation of information access on a "need-to-know" basis, and each system adapted the policies and guidelines to achieve an organisation driven implementation of this access need locally (National Institute for Healthcare and Clinical Excellence (NICE), 2002) and implemented locally. This was achieved by interpreting high-level policies into lower-level ones, which can result in different inconsistent information security policies and rules at this level. Once information is shared, the different healthcare providers can have varying interpretations of the guidance around information security (Crosby 2012) (See Figure 2).

The Caldicott Guardian at Velindre explained this in an example:

Figure 2. Inconsistent interpretation of the "need-to-know" information access need among various hospitals working under the NHS umbrella

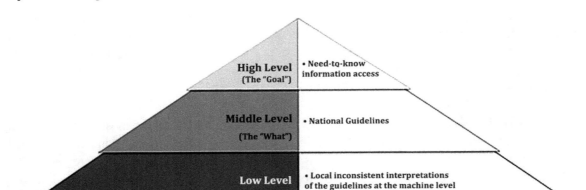

The South Wales service for hepatic surgery (liver surgery) is run here for patients with secondary cancers in their liver; the surgical service is based in Cardiff and the oncology is largely based here but we take patients from all over Wales. Patients are referred from West Wales to the surgeon who considers the case, using their films and x-rays sent electronically or by disk to Cardiff. They are discussed here by the MDT that you came to, or a similar one. However, Cardiff does not have direct access to those images because West Wales are only holding on to them as [...] the statutory owner of the information is the patient and the original healthcare organisation. Darren Lloyd, who is the Head of Information Governance, has said basically that it is a wrong interpretation of the rules; clinical information should be allowed to follow a patient. On a very high level I think because of varying interpretation of the guidance around information security, clinicians are often blocked from having the right information to treat a patient and I don't think enough weight is put on that (i.e. patient's rights of access to the best healthcare available because of variation in the interpretation of security rules). (Crosby 2012)

Also, current systems cannot override access permissions locally to allow access in such cases, so CT members must contact the originator to ask for relaxation of security rules (Crosby 2012). This interrupts treatment continuity, causes delays, and hinders effective communication of information.

- *Inflexible balance of information security in emergency cases.* The big challenge in information security solutions in healthcare systems is that life threatening emergency situations require resilience, most importantly when the patient is unconscious, and decisions can mean life or death. In such cases, there is a need to access any information stored about the patient at very short notice, in the hope that it will help save the patient's life. This may require trusted CT members to access information not normally required for their regular treatment role (Crosby 2012) and, therefore, there is a need to relax already assigned access rights to enable immediate access to information when every second counts, before restoring these levels of information security. A major weakness in current LIS is the inability to deal with such cases when the CT member's access is blocked, and writing to the original organisation requesting access (Crosby 2012) may delay or prevent the treatment happening in a timely fashion.

- *Inconsistent user-hostile information system design.* LIS supporting PC healthcare today have inconsistent information system design. Two widely used LIS in cancer care across Wales are: CaNISC and Clinical Portal. On the one hand, CaNISC is a disease-centred information system designed to hold cancer-related information for each patient to be used for all organisations and groups across Wales (Morrey 2013). Although CaNISC is an effective system for information sharing across systems, it is a disease-centred system that holds cancer-related information. Therefore, it was not designed to provide a holistic view of the patient's condition, especially if the patient has comorbidities. Also, the patient information is partitioned to each individual hospital (Morrey 2013). The Caldicott Guardian stated that: *the design of CaNISC is not intuitive; it's on a provider level and not a patient level. So you have to find your way around it* (Crosby 2013). He explained this in an example: *in Cardiff and Vale, if the surgeon puts in information, even if they put it into CaNISC, they'd put it under their provider episode. Moreover, you have to have a fairly good knowledge to navigate around the case note to find that if you were, say, a Velindre person* (Crosby 2013). This disease-centred design makes CaNISC a slow user-hostile system that requires intensive training to be properly used to locate relevant information (McGarrigle 2013). This was confirmed by a Clinical Nurse Specialist in Breast Care who said:

We are very simple people. You know, we are nurses and we are doctors, and none of us is stupid, but that is not our priority. This is supposed to be a tool for us. Need to be able to just help us do our job, not learn somebody else's job and we do not have much time to learn how to make it work. (McGarrigle 2013)

She summed CaNISC up as very difficult to find information, and hard work. She complained *CaNISC is not easy!* (McGarrigle 2013).

The Clinical Portal, on the other hand, is an organisation centred information system design providing test results and letters to healthcare professionals at different NHS Trusts or hospitals. Each hospital has its separate implementation of the Clinical Portal to view local clinical information within the hospital's perimeter, and although they all have a similar idea, look, and feel, they are local implementations (Morrey 2013). It has a similar but different structure to CaNISC (McGarrigle 2013). Users have to log into the system using the hospital number that gives access to all the test results conducted in the hospital for that patient (McGarrigle 2013). Thus, CT members may have to do several login attempts to different hospital portals to collect relevant information about a particular patient if the tests have been conducted in several hospitals. This is another issue for CT members, as explained by the Clinical Nurse Specialist: *the biggest problem [with] Clinical Portal is getting into it in the first place* (McGarrigle 2013). This is mainly *because if you do not have the hospital number, it does not like letting you in just with a name. It will sometimes, and you have to find out the right address* (McGarrigle 2013). Although the Clinical Portal is a more user-friendly system in comparison with CaNISC, according to the same Clinical Nurse Specialist, she said: *Portal is OK. Portal is quite quick* (McGarrigle 2013), however, its structure makes it an organisation-centred system that is unable to provide a PC view, like CaNISC.

- *Untraceable shared information.* To guarantee patient care continuity, systems supporting healthcare should reflect the patient's care management occurring in a number of healthcare organisations, and the flow of their information following the treatment pathway (Crosby 2012). This means these systems should not reflect the needs of an organisation the patient is treated in

(Clinical Portal is an organisation-centred system), nor a disease the patient is being treated for (CaNISC is a disease-centred system). Developing systems that reflect the patient's treatment pathway helps track patient treatment as a single business process. Currently, enhanced LIS supporting PC healthcare are designed to organise patient case note data in parallel on a healthcare-provider basis and not in sequence on a treatment-point basis (Crosby 2012; Patel 2013). Thus, information management is based on the healthcare provider and each patient's case notes are split into parallel partitions where each provider holds relevant information for a disease or part of the treatment in their partition (Crosby 2012). Each provider owns and controls their part of the information (Crosby 2012), and they give direct access to it by listing the CT member's names as having access (Crosby 2012). If a CT member happens not to be listed for access to the information (normally caused by the interpretation of security rules), he/she will have no access until the other provider grants permission (Crosby 2012). This not only makes it difficult to find relevant clinical information, but may also cause information duplication in the different partitions (Crosby 2012). For example, when each provider submits a stage of diagnosis with obvious differences, revealing a mistake, this can cause data inconsistency issues directly affecting the patient's clinical care, making it harder to locate and track relevant information at a point of care (Crosby 2012). Also, these problems can lead to losing track of patients and their information at some point in the treatment pathway. For example, it may be unclear which CT member is responsible for patient follow-up after treatment (Alsalamah et al., 2011; NICE, 2002) leading to the patient not receiving this necessary health service. Additionally, care management may be interrupted when information does not flow with the patient from one provider to another on the clinical pathway (for example, when patients are referred to Cardiff from Swansea, but their scan images do not follow; this can make critical information unavailable at a treatment point and cause incorrect treatment (Crosby 2012).

- *Manual management of referrals between healthcare providers.* According to a Breast Cancer Nurse Specialist (McGarrigle 2013), current systems do not automatically refer the patient to the CT member in charge, following a treatment plan. Early referrals in the treatment pathway come from the GP and are normally faxed to the hospital. Some GPs fill a pro forma with all the required information, including the last 10-15 visits to the GP, medical history, and medication they are on. The surgeon then looks at any of this information that is relevant to cancer, mostly medical history, and ignores what is not relevant. Although the faxed referral remains in paper-format, relevant information is added to the cancer record in the surgeon's local information system. Any referrals are happening after the initial GP referral are dictated letters that are transcribed by secretaries using a dictation system, for example from an MDT review to an oncologist. The Breast Cancer Nurse Specialist explained:

At the moment [...] the doctors see a patient, they dictate into a machine and say: 'I have just seen this lady...' and then the secretaries pick up the tape, and they put it into a machine and they play it back, and they type it in" (McGarrigle 2013). She complained that although the dictation systems are as accurate as typing, they are "causing the secretaries trouble when they dictate the letters and that is not the word they said at all. (McGarrigle 2013)

This ineffective referral approach may cause delays in information delivery, as well as exposing the information to human error, resulting in the information being inaccurate (McGarrigle 2013). It is clear that current systems are incapable of handling referrals and neither means today for referrals is practical. Therefore this aspect needs improvement. As such, an automated referral to a CT member's role that is picked up by the recipient with all information needed is also a key requirement in PC care.

LIS compromise on the availability of PC information and the requirements below will help restore the right level of information availability to suit PC cancer care.

- Common collaboration-driven information access needs to overarch the local organisation-driven policies.
- Consistent information organisation needs that provide a PC holistic view that gives easy access to a patient's clinical information.
- Automated referrals among different healthcare providers with the right information for the person.
- Gathering and filtering of relevant information to avoid overwhelming CT members with irrelevant information. This increases the chance of finding the right information at the right time.
- Resilience in emergency cases. This is a crucial requirement that speeds up access to information for decision making in a life or death situation.

3. Threats to Information Confidentiality

Current LIS compromise on the confidentiality of patient information.

- *Improper disclosure of medical information.* Information confidentiality is essential due to the movement towards a culture of open information, in which information access is a priority to healthcare professionals (DoH, 2010b; Skilton, 2011). A higher degree of information sharing is needed in PC care than in a traditional disease-centred approach (Crosby, 2012; Eysenbach, 2001; Skilton, 2011). Confidentiality can be breached in PC care if the information is improperly disclosed to unauthorised people (Crosby 2012). There are two factors increasing the risk of improper disclosure of information: the number of people having access to the information, and the value of this information (Anderson, 1996). PC care has a higher risk of medical information being disclosed to unauthorised people than in a traditional approach. This is due to the NHS planning to integrate separate systems run by 100 Health Authorities, around 3,500 GPs and over 400 NHS Trusts, in the modernisation of UK healthcare systems (DoH, 1997). Also, there is a direct correlation between valuable information and the risk of its disclosure (Anderson, 1996), mainly because if it is valuable to its owner, it will be valuable to someone else (Calder & Watkins, 2008). There are many reasons why systems are supporting healthcare store highly valuable information. First and foremost, clinical information has value as a basis for healthcare professionals' decision-making processes (Crosby 2012), and its corruption can lead to incorrect decisions that may harm or even kill a patient (Anderson, 1996). The systems hold extensive information about a patient, which may contain personal, embarrassing, and critical medical information (Alsalamah et al., 2011). This information has a longevity characteristic meaning it is highly sensitive and confidential at all times without decay, even after the patient is dead (Beale, 2004; DoH, 2003; Crosby, 2012; Smith & Eloff, 1999). Therefore, the nature of medical information means it should only be disclosed for permitted medical purposes (DoH, 2003). This puts PC information at great risk of improper disclosure (Anderson, 1996) and stresses the need to keep information protected from those not needing it, while ensuring availability of life-critical information about the patient's medical condition on a "need-to-know" basis at the time of care (DoH, 2003, 2010a).

- *Hospital-wide Access Control.* CaNISC has a security model that reflects its information system design. Dr. Morrey explains the security model developed in CaNISC:

The way that CaNISC operated it, was to say that once you got a referral into the organisation, then anybody in the organisation can actually see it, and the way we enforced that was there was a security log, so any time anybody reads anything or changes anything, it's recorded in the database. Moreover, everybody knows there is that full audit trail. (Morrey 2013)

This security model has a hospital-wide access control model that is causing some issues. Dr. Morrey highlighted these issues:

The problem we ran into was when you implement that then in terms of the security model, medical secretaries for an example, or sometimes maybe a nurse, would actually have wider access than the consultant [...] the reason is that the consultant belongs to his firm [i.e. hospital system], and he sees patients about his firm. The nurse or the medical secretary may need to cover for another medical secretary, who works in another consultant firm. So, you end up with a situation where the medical secretary or maybe the nurse in their role that spans consultant firms... have wider access than individual consultants. (Morrey 2013)

The following requirements paint the full picture of a PC collaboration-driven information security that restores the right level of information confidentiality.

- Common collaboration-driven information access needs. This requirement not only helps with information availability, but it also preserves its confidentiality as it defines the fine line between these two conflicting information security goals.
- Information security policies awareness in a culture of open information. This requirement raises the awareness of CT members as to how to look at another member's information within the collaboration to help preserve the confidentiality of shared information, especially in emergency cases.

The list of threats is summarised in Table 5.

4. Requirements in LIS for a Common Collaboration-Driven Information Security

The threats to PC information (shown in Table 5) highlight the fact that LIS fall short of meeting the information sharing and security contexts in PC care, due to the compromises they have to make in terms of information availability, integrity, and confidentiality. Although threats target all information security goals, there is more weight on the compromises to the availability of information in the PC information sharing context. Interviews showed that the current balance of information security in LIS used in cancer care is more concerned with information confidentiality and this may be working well locally, within its physical and logical perimeters, as this meets these systems' information sharing and security contexts. This is because information security implementation in discrete LIS focused mainly on information con-

Table 5. Information Security Threats in LIS

Threat Category	Threat Description
Information integrity threats	Human error
	Inconsistent results in different systems
Information availability threats	Disconnected systems at major sharing points
	Inconsistent information security policies
	Inflexible balance of information security in emergency cases
	Inconsistent user-hostile information system design
	Untraceable shared information
	Manual management of referrals between healthcare providers
Information confidentiality threats	Improper disclosure of medical information
	Hospital-wide access control

fidentiality and integrity as they were the information security issues at that time (Pfleeger & Pfleeger, 2003), whereas information availability was not. Pfleeger and Pfleeger recognise this phenomenon in LIS, and they add that it is not clear that a single point-of-control can enforce availability (Pfleeger & Pfleeger, 2003). Therefore, the key reason why LIS fall short of attaining a security balance in PC care is because information availability issues were only raised by the movement towards collaboration, when the need for information sharing started to emerge, making this information security goal a challenge in collaborative environments. Therefore, when this information leaves these autonomous LIS, there is a need for these systems to rebalance the information security to address the compromises it makes on the availability of information for the collaboration without interrupting the local balances of information security. To cope with this emerging need, LIS need additional requirements to define a collaboration-driven information security policy that can attain the new balance of information security that has more weight on information availability. The requirements are summarised in the following points:

1. Consistent information organisation needs that provide a PC holistic view that provides easy access to a patient's clinical information
2. Common collaboration-driven information access needs to overarch the local organisation-driven policies. This requirement helps with information availability, and, at the same time, preserves its confidentiality. This means it is the key requirements that define the fine line between these two conflicting information security goals.
3. Information organisation in chronological order to help track the information to the information owner and treatment points.
4. Gathering and filtering of relevant information, to avoid overwhelming CT members with irrelevant information. This increases the chance of finding the right information at the right time.
5. Automated referrals among different healthcare providers with the right information for the person.
6. Resilience in emergency cases. This is a crucial requirement that speeds up access to information for decision-making in a life or death situation.
7. Remote information update after dissemination to allow information owners to update the information in the case of a human error incident.

8. Information security policies awareness. This requirement raises the awareness of CT members in terms of how to look after another member's information within the collaboration to help preserve the confidentiality of shared information, especially in emergency cases.

These eight requirements aim to reduce the impact of the threats whilst attaining a common collaboration-driven balance of information security.

FUTURE RESEARCH DIRECTIONS

A proof of concept prototype has been implemented using workflow technology to proof the concept and show technically how the suggested requirements could be implemented. It tested information access needs and issues in healthcare collaborative environments through three cancer treatment pathways and included collaboration between different healthcare organisations when a patient is following a treatment pathway. This could be generalised to fit any possible treatment pathway for any health condition as long as the treatment points can be predicted. The scope of the implemented prototype excluded situations when information is related to more than one disease for patients following more than one treatment pathway, and this occurs when there is comorbidity. Comorbidity is part of the notion of PC care provision. Therefore, in the future it would be interesting to test how different information access needs are in such cases, when from a technical point of view, it comes to mapping the treatment processes together, but the decisions will be far complicated than in a single treatment process as no one knows at which point the interaction will happen.

This research drew boundaries around healthcare collaborative environments as it is believed to be one of the more complex environments if not the most. This is due to the fact that it involves a large number of users coming from geographically distributed environments where the fine line between information availability and confidentiality can easily get blurry. However, there are other applicable domains for these approaches with less complications, future research can study and test how general this solution is and whether it is applicable to other domains. The experiments conducted in this research suggests a number of characteristics that can predict the applicability of this research: large geographical area, large number of users with different roles, heterogeneous information systems with inconsistent information security contexts and AC models, and a common collaborative goal. Collaborative environments sharing these characteristics are more likely to suit this approach.

CONCLUSION

There is a global shift in healthcare delivery towards an integrated PC treatment approach to cope with the emerging needs of an ageing population worldwide. The adoption of PC care in many countries is achieved through an evolutionary approach using existing LIS, which were developed at a time when the sharing of information was not common. In collaboration with Velindre Cancer Centre, this research defines a common collaboration-driven balance of information security in PC care, identifies weaknesses in LIS used today in cancer care and uses them to achieve a secure collaborative environment. Results show that the threats they present compromise on information security goals. Initially, human error in shared information, and inconsistent results at different systems compromise the integrity of clinical information. In addition, inconsistent information security policies, the inflexible balance of information security in emergency cases, untraceable shared information, and inconsistent user-hostile information system design all contribute to compromising the availability of PC information among CT members. Finally, improper disclosure of medical information, and a hospital-wide access control compromise the confidentiality of patient information. Results also show that most of the information security issues are around the availability of clinical information. This means that information security implementation in discrete LIS focused on the confidentiality and integrity of medical information, as they were a key issue while availability was not. Thus, the key reason LIS falls short of attaining a security balance in PC care is because information availability only became an issue with collaboration. These threats led to the identification of eight requirements needed to assist LIS to reduce the impact of the threats and attain a common collaboration-driven information security to assist LIS safely implement PC care without being totally discarded. This is to improve the quality of care we all receive as patients for better health, a better nation, and a better tomorrow.

REFERENCES

Al-Salamah, H., Gray, A., & Morrey, D. (2011). Velindre Healthcare Integrated Care Pathway. In L. Fischer (Ed.), Taming the Unpredictable Real World Adaptive Case Management: Case Studies and Practical Guidance (pp. 183-195). Lighthouse Point: Future Strategies Inc.

Allam, O. (2006). *A Holistic Analysis Approach to Facilitating Communication between General Practitioners and Cancer Care Teams.* (Unpublished Doctoral Dissertation). Cardiff University, Cardiff, UK.

Alsalamah, S., Gray, A., & Hilton, J. (2011). Towards Persistent Control over Shared Information in a Collaborative Environment. In L. Armistead (Ed.), *Proceedings of the 6th International Conference on Information Warfare and Security (ICIW)* (pp. 278–287). Washington, DC: Academic Publishing International Limited.

Alsalamah, S., Gray, A., & Hilton, J. (2011). Sharing Patient Medical Information among Healthcare Team Members While Sustaining Information Security. In P. A. Bath, T. Mettler, D. Raptis, & B. A. Sen (Ed.), *Proceedings of the 15th International Symposium on Health Information Management Research (ISHIMR)* (pp. 553–554). Zurich, Switzerland: University of Zurich, University of St. Gallen and University of Sheffield.

American Cancer Society. (2008). *Holistic Medicine.* Retrieved February 20, 2013, from http://www.cancer.org/Treatment/TreatmentsandSideEffects/ComplementaryandAlternativeMedicine/MindBodyandSpirit/holistic-medicine

Anderson, R. J. (1996). *Security in Clinical Information Systems.* Cambridge, UK: British Medical Association.

Beale, T. (2004). The Health Record - Why Is It so Hard? In R. Haux & C. Kulikowski (Eds.), *IMIA Yearbook of Medical Informatics 2005: Ubiquitous Health Care Systems* (pp. 301–304). Stuttgart, Germany.

Bisbal, J., Lawless, D., & Grimson, J. (1999). Legacy Information Systems: Issues and Directions. *IEEE Software*, *16*(5), 103–111. doi:10.1109/52.795108

Calder, A., & Watkins, S. (2008). *IT Governance : A Manager's Guide to Data Security and ISO 27001/ ISO 27002* (4th ed.). London, UK: Kogan Page Limited.

Cancer National Specialist Advisory Group. (2012). *Welsh Breast Cancer Clinical Audit for Patients Diagnosed 2008*. Retrieved from http://www.wales.nhs.uk/sites3/Documents/322/Cancer_NSAG_WBC-CA_2008.pdf

Dawson, J., Tulu, B., & Horan, T. A. (2009). Towards Patient-Centered Care: The Role of E-Health in Enabling Patient Access to Health Information. In E. V. Wilson (Ed.), *Patient-Centered E-Health* (pp. 1–9). London, UK: IGI Global. doi:10.4018/978-1-60566-016-5.ch001

DoH. (1997). *The New NHS: Modern, Dependable*. London, UK: HMSO.

DoH. (2000). *The NHS Plan: A Summary*. London, UK: Stationary Office.

DoH. (2002). *Delivering 21 St Century IT Support for the NHS: National Strategic Programme*. London, UK: Stationary Office.

DoH. (2003). *Confidentiality: NHS Code of Practice*. London, UK: HMSO.

DoH. (2010a). *Caldicott Guardian Manual 2010*. London, UK: HMSO.

DoH. (2010b). *Equity and Excellence: Liberating the NHS*. London: HMSO.

DoH & NHS Executive. (1998). *Information for Health: An Information Strategy for the Modern NHS 1998-2005*. London, UK: Stationary Office.

Ellingsen, G., & Røed, K. (2010). The Role of Integration in Health-Based Information Infrastructures. [CSCW]. *Computer Supported Cooperative Work*, *19*(6), 557–584. doi:10.1007/s10606-010-9122-y

Eysenbach, G. (2001). What Is E-Health? *Journal of Medical Internet Research*, *3*(2), e20. doi:10.2196/jmir.3.2.e20 PMID:11720962

Fernandez, E. B., Yoshioka, N., Washizaki, H., & Jurjens, J. (2007). Using Security Patterns to 'build Secure Systems. In *proceeding of the 1st International Workshop on Software Patterns and Quality (SPAQu)* (pp.16-31). Nagoya, Japan: IGI Global.

Gaunt, N. (2009). Electronic Health Records for Patient-Centred Healthcare. In W. Currie & D. Finnegan (Eds.), *Integrating Healthcare with Information and Communications Technology* (pp. 113–133). Oxford, UK: Radcliffe Publishing Ltd.

International Alliance of Patient' Organizations (IAPO). (2004). *What Is Patient-Centred Healthcare? A Review of Definitions and Principles*. Retrieved from http://iapo.org.uk/patient-centred-healthcare

Kee, C. (2001). *Security Policy Roadmap - Process for Creating Security Policies*. Retrieved from http://www.sans.org/reading-room/whitepapers/policyissues/

Map of Medicine (MoM). (2013). *Map of Medicine*. Retrieved March 20, 2013 from http://mapofmedicine.com/

Mense, A., Hoheiser-pförtner, F., Schmid, M., & Wahl, H. (2013). Concepts for a Standard Based Cross-Organisational Information Security Management System in the Context of a Nationwide EHR. In C.U. Lehmann et al. (Ed.), *14th World Congress on Medical and Health Informatics (Medinfo)* (pp. 548–552). Copenhagen, Denmark: IMIA and IOS Press.

National Institute for Healthcare and Clinical Excellence (NICE). (2002). *Improving Outcomes in Breast Cancer - Manual Update*. Retrieved from https://www.nice.org.uk/guidance/csgbc/evidence/improving-outcomes-in-breast-cancer-manual-update-2

NHS Wales Informatics Service (NWIS). (2013). *Canisc*. Retrieved from http://www.wales.nhs.uk/nwis/page/52601

Pfleeger, C. P., & Pfleeger, S. L. (2003). *Security in Computing* (3rd ed.). Prentice Hall.

Pipkin, D. L. (2000). *Information Security Protecting the Global Enterprise*. Prentice Hall.

Posthumus, S., & Solms, R. V. (2004). A Framework for the Governance of Information Security. *Computers & Security*, *23*(8), 638–646. doi:10.1016/j.cose.2004.10.006

Powell, J. (2009). Integrating Healthcare with ICT. In W. Currie & D. Finnegan (Eds.), *Integrating Healthcare with Information and Communications Technology* (pp. 85–94). Oxford, UK: Radcliffe Publishing Ltd.

Shaller, D. (2007). *Patient-Centered Care: What Does It Take?* Retrieved from http://www.commonwealthfund.org/usr_doc/Shaller_patient-centeredcarewhatdoesittake_1067.pdf?section=4039

Skilton, A. (2011). *Using Team Structure to Understand and Support the Needs of Distributed Healthcare Teams*. (Unpublished Doctoral Dissertation). Cardiff University, Cardiff, UK.

Smith, E., & Eloff, J. H. (1999). Security in Health-Care Information Systems--Current Trends. *International Journal of Medical Informatics*, *54*(1), 39–54. doi:10.1016/S1386-5056(98)00168-3 PMID:10206428

United Nations Population Fund (UNFPA). (2014). *Population Ageing: A Celebration and a Challenge*. Retrieved from http://www.unfpa.org/pds/ageing.html

KEY TERMS AND DEFINITIONS

Caldicott Guardian: A senior person in the UK national healthcare system responsible for the confidentiality of patients' information.

Comorbidity: Simultaneous presence of more than one condition at the same time in a patient resulting in the patient following multiple treatment pathways in parallel.

Disease-Centred Healthcare Delivery Model: In this model specialists treat their patients in isolation according to their specialty, regardless of other illnesses and medications taken by their patients.

Information Security Threats: Indication or warning of possible security breach.

Information Governance: Action or manner of managing and controlling access to information.

Legacy Systems: Information systems that has been used in a place for some time and significantly resist modification and evolution.

Patient-Centred Healthcare Delivery Model: In this model specialist provide care tailored to meet an individual patient's needs holistically rather than manage separate diseases.

This research was previously published in M-Health Innovations for Patient-Centered Care edited by Anastasius Moumtzoglou, pages 298-318, copyright year 2016 by Medical Information Science Reference (an imprint of IGI Global).

Chapter 78
Monitoring Time Consumption in Complementary Diagnostic and Therapeutic Procedure Requests

Ana Alpuim
University of Minho, Portugal

Marisa Esteves
University of Minho, Portugal

Sónia Pereira
University of Minho, Portugal

Manuel Santos
University of Minho, Portugal

ABSTRACT

Over the years, information technologies and computer applications have been widespread amongst all fields, including healthcare. The main goal of these organizations is focused on providing quality health services to their patients, ensuring the provision of quality services. Therefore, decisions have to be made quickly and effectively. Thus, the increased use of information technologies in healthcare has been helping the decision-making process, improving the quality of their services. For an example, the insertion of Business Intelligence (BI) tools in healthcare environments has been recently used to improve healthcare delivery. It is based on the analysis of data in order to provide useful information. BI tools assist managers and health professionals through decision-making, since they allow the manipulation and analysis of data in order to extract knowledge. This work aims to study and analyze the time that physicians take to prescribe medical exams in Centro Hospitalar do Porto (CHP), though BI tools. The main concern is to identify the physicians who take more time than average to prescribe complementary means of diagnosis and treatment, making it possible to identify and understand the reason why it

DOI: 10.4018/978-1-5225-3926-1.ch078

occurs. To discover these outliners, a BI platform was developed using the Pentaho Community. This platform presents means to represent information through tables and graphs that facilitate the analysis of information and the knowledge extraction. This information will be useful to represent knowledge concerning not only the prescription system (auditing it) but also its users. The platform evaluates the time prescription, by specialty and physician, which can afterwards be applied in the decision-making process. This platform enables the identification of measures to unravel the time differences that some physicians exhibit, in order to, subsequently, improve the whole process of electronic medical prescription.

INTRODUCTION

The Electronic Health Record (EHR) is a Health Information System (HIS) that collects all the information of a patient from various information systems, including his medical history. The EHR covers several hospital departments and units, enabling an analysis of the clinical process. It should be noted that it is oriented to the patient and not the service unit or even the diseases to which they are subject, i.e., it stands with the firm intention of benefiting the patients (Duarte et al., 2011; Hasman, 1998).

The EHR is nothing more than a set of standardized documents used for the registration of medical procedures rendered to a given patient in a given hospital unit by health professionals. Essentially, it is a set of information compiled by health professionals, which corresponds to the full data record of a given patient, including all the existing information about him. Hereupon, it tracks the general state of the individual and allows the preparation of the same clinical history, chronologically, and it also enables remote and simultaneous access to any clinical process (Duarte et al., 2011; Hasman, 1998).

This HIS is seen as a set of registration annotations and use of clinical information for better delivery of healthcare services to the patient. This being the task of practically everyone who works in the hospital, they all contribute to a better delivery of services. The EHR integrates information from various sources, from other HIS or other applications based on Information and Communication Technologies (ICT) in all its aspects, in order to replace the part, improve and speed up the assistance to the patient to accelerate certain processes, prevent medical errors, and also ease the work of all health professionals (Duarte et al., 2011; Hasman, 1998).

Besides registration, consultation and research set of clinical information, resulting from the provision of healthcare to a given patient, the EHR system also allows the prescription of medicines and Complementary Diagnostic and Therapeutic Procedures (CDTP), called the Electronic Medical Prescription (EMP). The EMP is a procedure performed by the ICT through an application, the SAM – *Sistema de Apoio ao Médico* – (Support Medical System)[1].

The EMP reduces some existing problems by improving the legibility, which does not exist in handwritten requests – data security and confidentiality of data relating to patients – since access will be assuredly restricted. It also helps with revenue management and diagnostic tests (Ammenwerth et al., 2008).

The EHR integrates the data with other information systems via the internet: collects, processes and updates data; supports research and can return the information to patients in various ways. Finally, it also allows to obtain different types of reports with a variety of font types and sizes, and still images which simplifies and assists the perception of the diagnosis by health professionals (Duarte et al., 2011).

On the other hand, the change from a manual to an electronic record affects the established communication practices by changing the content and patterns of communication between departments. Communication via computers can increase the speed of communication between professionals but, in some cases, can also cause misunderstandings and consequently some flaws, by passing the manual records to digital format (Chiasson et al., 2007; Heeks, 2006).

SAM has a large potential for improvement and, despite some limitations, the use of electronic prescribing is clearly advantageous compared to manual prescription. This system has numerous potential, one of which being the registration times that health professionals spend for prescribing CDTP.

Every prescription is recorded at least once, at the time of the request, but may be recorded several times, regarding the tasks of each request. Each one of those tasks matches a required form, when prescribing a CDTP. The time of the request corresponds to a total time starting from the moment the professional registers the order of a CDTP, ending when the process is complete. In the meantime, when prescribing a CDTP, the physician is required to complete one or more forms, which vary depending on the test request. Particular examination may not even have an associated form. The task time refers to the period it takes the physician to answer all the questions of the form(s) and click OK. The request time is always higher, because it includes the times of the tasks.

Analyzing these times becomes an essential task for improving the EMP process. Thus, an evaluation and analysis of these times is necessary. By analyzing the times recorded in databases, it is possible to separate them, either by the prescribing physician of the CDTP as well as the various specialties. To solve this problem, a platform within CHP was developed. CHP is a large healthcare organization in northern Portugal, and their data are the source for the platform developed. This platform allows us to identify the professionals who take longer than the average time on CDTP prescription process, which is a time that is essential during the day-to-day queries. This platform was developed by using the Pentaho Community software, which is an open source BI tool.

BACKGROUND

Medical Record

The user's medical record (MR) is a rich source of data, often carried out by nurses for clinical research, acting as a repository of information of a user (Gregory & Radovinsky, 2012). It is often used as a primary source of data for epidemiological analysis purposes and it is also considered standard in any study to identify demographic, clinical data variables, specific aspects related to treatment and mortality schemes (Cassidy et al., 2002; Murray et al., 2003). Data collection through the MR involves the review of their specific sources. These include nursing, consultation notes, admission and high reports, laboratory tests, surgical reports, and other clinical and administrative documentation, which, however, is not easily done if the registration is manual. A good strategy before starting data collection is necessary (Eder et al., 2005; Gearing et al., 2006; Pan et al., 2005). The tool used in the EHR for data collection should be systematically organized and should be easy to use (Gregory & Radovinsky, 2012). The MR has always been recognized as a rich source of information for conducting clinical research, decision-making and identification of diagnosis. Nonetheless, researchers should include the development and testing of the tools used for the collection (Gregory & Radovinsky, 2012).

The data collected from the EHR is essential to establish a health history on users, in order to investigate the prediction of disease. It is estimated that every year numerous lives are lost due to poorly coordinated medical information (Chiasson et al., 2007). The advantages of using data obtained from the EHR through a retrospective analysis of the records include the ability to access large amounts of data at a relatively low cost (Gregory & Radovinsky, 2012).

Over the years, a variety of systems were developed and implemented in an attempt to improve the delivery of healthcare. These systems include EHR that replaces paper records storage and search of information. Every day that passes, healthcare is becoming increasingly complex (Waegemann, 2003). With the many advances in the ICT in the last 20 years, particularly in health, many ways have been discussed in EHR but, further, developed and implemented. Nowadays, many people involved in healthcare are expecting to move to a paperless environment. This is an important step but, at the moment, it has only been achieved with success in some institutions (Waegemann, 2003).

The ICT offer many advantages over manual records on paper for storage and searching of data of users. Although it has been possible, but not fully implemented, it is expected that in the future, all records will be stored and viewed on a computer and mobile devices (Tavakoli et al., 2011).

In the past few years, many organizations have underestimated the strategic importance of information and its associated technologies, which results in a lack of potential planning the ICT. In many cases, organizations have failed to realize the strategic benefits of the ICT because they have been considering them as a mere replacement of manual and administrative functions and not as a powerful strategic resource as it should be (Saleem et al., 2009).

The data collection can be done in a document or through an electronic register. Both types of data collection instruments have some advantages and limitations. Generally, in the department of medical records, a paper document is often more cost effective and easier to use to collect data (Allison et al., 2000). However, using a paper document requires that data has to be then introduced into an electronic database in order to analyze the knowledge through computers (Gregory & Radovinsky, 2012). For this purpose, the researchers usually send copies of MR on paper to the data center where data managers belong in the database. This routine paper has many drawbacks that results in the insertion of erroneous data in the database leading to a longer duration of the clinical trial, especially for a larger amount of data, since more data the longer it takes to insert them in an electronic register (Kawado et al., 2003; Paul et al., 2005). Even under the best circumstances, the data entry process is fraught with the possibility of error occurrence, and the analysis and the results of data studies will be influenced. Nonetheless, the collection of data directly from an electronic DB, reduces the possibility of errors in the input thereof, which may result in a more reliable collection and consequently a better analysis and decision-making is more reasoned (Worster & Haines, 2004). Furthermore, for large investigations, the collection from an electronic DB facilitates the centralization and access to them may be more profitable (Gearing et al., 2006).

When implemented correctly, the EHR has a great potential benefit to health systems and decision-making because they can improve the way the data of users are documented and organized. Consequently, the EHR provides better readability of the user data, simultaneous and remote access, and integration with other information sources (Powsner et al., 1998). Thereby, all of the points referred above contribute to improve the delivery of healthcare.

Fortunately, physicians and health professionals have been realizing the importance of the implementation of electronic records, verifying that they have benefits, such as accuracy, readability of data, complete information and reducing repetition of data entry (Munyisia et al., 2011).

Compared to the manual paper system, the electronic documentation resulted in improvements on users, i.e., greater usefulness of records to provide healthcare without compromising the results of users, which means that there are significant improvements in health (Rossi et al., 2014). Study results also show that the greatest benefit is the reduction in cost control and data management. Of course, the exact value depends on the estimation of parameters that affect the calculations (Pavlović et al., 2009).

Nevertheless, with both the manual records as the EHR, errors still occur. The failure of some EHR, already computerized, may be due to bad design information (Powsner et al., 1998). The existence of errors in medical documents is very common. The classification of these errors would help to understand their causes, their origin and, finally, develop support tools for understanding. The literature provides numerous examples of medical errors rating. These classifications are the basis for reporting errors and, therefore, to reflect the needs of specific areas of expertise. In addition to vary according to the area of specialization, error classification schemes differ in dimensions along which the classification is conducted (Tavakoli et al., 2011).

BUSINESS INTELLIGENCE

The implementation of Business Intelligence (BI) in healthcare organizations helps its managers and health professionals in their own decision-making processes through data analysis that provide relevant information about the processes and activities of those organizations. Thus, BI tools can improve the quality and safety in healthcare, and consequently the performance of the organizations (Bonney, 2013; Prevedello et al., 2010).

Many HIS as the EHR, contain large amounts of clinical information highly relevant for decision-making. Studies suggest that it is necessary to apply BI tools to ensure that the contents of the registers are efficiently used, since these tools allow the extraction of relevant information. Subsequently, the extracted data can be used by health professionals to support real-time decision, contributing to the improvement of healthcare (Bonney, 2013).

In most health organizations, data is stored in different systems and it is sometimes necessary to relate them. Typically, these systems are poorly integrated, making extraction a difficult operation. For this reason, there is interest in developing applications that make access and data extraction an easier process. BI tools are able to work efficiently with health data to generate information and knowledge in real time, this being the reason why these tools are used in the health sector. Over the years, the interest in the application of BI tools in the health sector has increased and different solutions have been created (Bonney, 2013).

Business Intelligence Systems

The term BI is assigned to an area of decision support systems that refers to the process of collection, compilation, integration, storage, analysis and presentation of data on the activities of a particular organization (Glaser & Stone, 2008; Prevedello et al., 2010). This type of representation of knowledge by the information submitted by BI systems can be relevant and strategic to support professionals in decision-making (Bonney, 2013). This technology provides the means to transform the data into relevant and strategic information, in order to constitute significant and important knowledge to support decisions of the organization's professionals. This allows the workers as executives, managers and analysts, to make better decisions quickly (Bonney, 2013; Loshin, 2013).

The main benefits of using BI systems are its flexibility and time reducing in data access and data analysis. Decision-making is supported by actual data, making it more likely that the assessment is correct and feasible (Bonney, 2013). The use of BI makes the quality of inputs increases. These systems have the ability to put the right information available to users at the right time, in order to help in the decision-making process (Mettler & Vimarlund, 2009). In this aspect, it becomes clear to identify the advantage in implementing these systems. BI systems must be able to integrate high amounts of data from various sources and, accordingly, providing analytical tools for data analysis, these being the two main tasks of the BI (Popovič et al., 2012).

BI systems provide tools relatively easy to use, which make this type of systems easily available to all its end users, revealing himself as an advantage for organizations that implement BI (Chaudhuri et al., 2011; Glaser & Stone, 2008; Prevedello et al., 2010).

Business Intelligence Steps

Throughout the recent years, it has been noticed a significant improvement in the development of BI tools. The speed of data collection has increased, as well as the sophistication and interactivity in handling the data and the report query in the tools used to present information. The BI technology includes various software features as Extraction, Transformation and Load (ETL), Data Warehouse, Online Analytical Process (OLAP), Data Mining (DM), reporting, query and virtualization of databases (Bonney, 2013). A BI system integrates data from heterogeneous sources, and converts them into a unified format to carry them to a DW. This process of extraction, transformation and loading of data, can be very complex and time consuming. After the implementation of the ETL process, the data stored in the DW can be used for analytical applications capable of aggregating them using OLAP (Prevedello et al., 2010).

ETL

Running the ETL process is one of the most difficult tasks for the settlement of a DW. It is complex, lengthy and consumes most of the time in the implementation of the DW. The process to populate a DW, running an ETL tool, consists of three steps. The first is extraction, where data are drawn from different sources. The second refers to transformation, which, as the name implies, consists in processing and cleaning the data. The third step commits the data to the load and DW is called by load. ETL tools are specialized in addressing issues of heterogeneity of information sources, and dealing with the cleaning and data transformation. The ETL is an essential step for loading large volumes of data and to ensure their quality and hence good results in the indicators presented by BI tools (Chaudhuri et al., 2011; El-Sappagh et al., 2011).

The ETL is a complex combination of processes and technologies that consume a significant amount of effort in the population of a DW. The ETL process is not a sporadic event. As the data sources vary, the DW will update itself periodically. That is, the DW will not change its structure, even if it is loaded with more information. For this, the ETL process will run again in order to maintain its value as a tool in aiding decision-making. Clearly, the ETL process must be designed to be easily modified (El-Sappagh et al., 2011).

As already mentioned, an ETL system consists of three consecutive steps, summarized in Figure 1:

- **Extraction:** It is the first step of the ETL process and it is responsible for extracting data from the different sources. Each data source has its specific features that have to be managed in order to effectively extract the data for the ETL process. The process should integrate the systems that may have different platforms, such as management systems with different databases, operating systems and communication protocols (El-Sappagh et al., 2011).
- **Transformation:** The second step of any ETL process includes cleansing, transforming and integrating data. This step cleans information, in order to obtain accurate data, i.e., correct, complete, consistent and unambiguous information. This process sets all the characteristics to which the data must obey (El-Sappagh et al., 2011).
- **Load:** Load data into the DW is the last of the three steps of the ETL process. It loads information into DW, which is a data structure prepared to receive the previously extracted and processed data (El-Sappagh et al., 2011).

Data Warehouse

The main component of a BI system is a DW; a repository of data from different sources that stores information about an organization activities (Loshin, 2013). The DW can store and consolidate data in a valid and consistent format for each organization. It also allows users to analyze and explore the data using other tools. The DW enables the integration of different data from heterogeneous sources. This allows an analysis of dimensions (properties). For the reasons above, the databases of DW are considered multi-dimensional and object-oriented to facilitate the use of information, the object being the set of information about a particular process in an organization. In addition to object-oriented, a DW has the ability to integrate data, which is one of its main features. Thus, the process of data entry enables the elimination of inconsistencies (Park & Kim, 2013).

The DW only performs two different operations, which are inserting and querying data. Because the data is loaded in a large DW volume, upgrading is not executed regularly. It can then be said that the DW is not volatile, i.e., the data are not deleted or updated. But the rate at which data is loaded, varies

Figure 1. ETL processes (El-Sappagh et al., 2011 adapted)

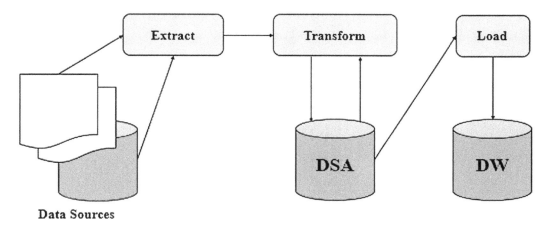

depending on the needs of each organization (Park & Kim, 2013). The storage of relevant data from different sources and formats can improve the speed and efficiency of knowledge discovery process, which makes the decision-making more correct and quickly due to the greater amount of information (El-Sappagh et al., 2011; Prevedello et al., 2010).

The data stored in DW is consistent and is available for analysis by BI tools in order to extract information and generate reports to apply in the decision-making process. The DW differs from those operational databases, because they are integrated, organized by theme and vary over time, which means that each entry in the DW corresponds to a specific point of time, allowing the temporal analysis of the data. In addition, the DW size is larger than the data marts and allows OLAP, being essentially used for decision support (El-Sappagh et al., 2011). Unlike operating systems, the DW was not designed for a quick and efficient transaction process, but rather for quick access to information for analysis and reporting purposes (Popovič et al., 2012).

The DW organizes its information depending on the dimensional model that the user defines. This model being the better and more efficient method to represent the data (Loshin, 2013). There are several different dimensional models, but the most common are as follow:

- **Star Schema:** In the star schema model, all tables are directly related to a central table, called by fact table, the others being referred as dimension tables. These links occur between the primary keys of dimension tables and foreign keys of fact table. The dimension tables contain the description of the measured facts, and these attributes are often used to identify headers in query results. This model is called Star Schema since the fact table is surrounded by the dimension tables, resembling a star. The fact table is the main element of the model and represents the events used to measure performance and outcomes of processes (Chaudhuri et al., 2011; Soler et al., 2008). The Star Schema model is shown in Figure 2 and can be constituted by more tables but they all have to be attached to the fact table.

Figure 2. Star Schema model of a DW

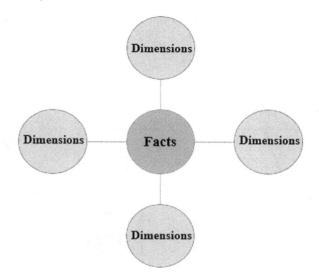

- **Snow Flake:** In this model, the dimension tables also relate to the fact table, but there are some dimensions that are not directly related to the fact table but related to other dimension tables, relating only between them. This purposes the normalization of dimension tables in order to reduce the space occupied by these tables. In the Snow Flake model, there are auxiliary dimension tables that standardize the main dimension tables. Building the database in this way, started to use more tables to represent the same dimensions, but occupying less disk space than the Star Schema model (Chaudhuri et al., 2011; Soler et al., 2008). In the Figure 3, the model demonstrated is the Snow Flake one given that the model may consist of more tables linked together.

The Snow Flake model reduces the space required for storage of data, but increases the number of tables to the model, making it more complex. As more tables are used, the access to data through queries will be hampered and it will take longer to be implemented, i.e., data access is slower than the previous model.

On the other hand, the Star Schema model presents simpler and easier navigation through the software, but wastes space and can repeat the same descriptions along the boards.

Therefore, it is more advantageous to use a Star Schema model, because it provides a faster and easier access to data, creating auxiliary tables for specific dimensions only when strictly necessary, i.e., namely when it is shown a benefit to justify the loss of query performance, which is not so great depending on how the tables are built. That being said, most DW use Star Schema model for representation of the data (Kimball & Ross, 2002; Loshin, 2013; Pardillo et al., 2010).

In Figure 4 the architecture of a DW can be observed.

Figure 3. Snow Flake model of a DW

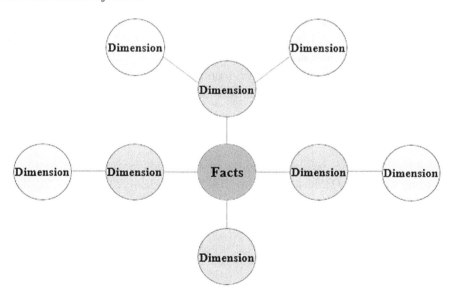

Figure 4. Architecture of a DW (Chaudhuri et al., 2011 Adapted)

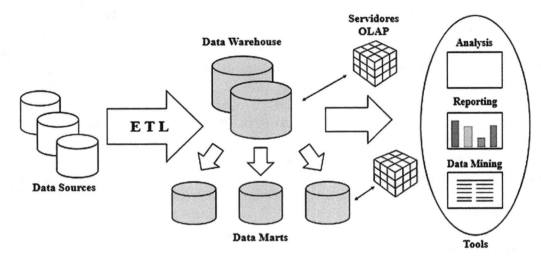

Data Mining

The DM in DB defines a process with a continuous set of activities that produce knowledge from DB. This set consists of five steps such as selection, pre-processing, processing, DM, and finally interpretation or evaluation (Heinrichs & Lim, 2003).

In the first step, there is a selection of key data to perform the DM. Secondly, comes pre-processing, including data cleaning and treating, in order to make them consistent and feasible for further processing. This cleaning process, also referred to as elimination of noise, noise reduction or elimination feature, can be made by ETL or other available techniques. According to the destination, the data is processed, this being the phase transformation. Finally, in the DM phase, the kind of result to be achieved and its purpose are defined. The interpretation or evaluation is the last step and consists in the interpretation and evaluation, as the name implies, of the patterns obtained. The validity of the results is checked by applying the standards found in new sets of data. In short, DM is the process of holding large amounts of data looking for consistent patterns as rules or time sequences, to detect relationships between information, thus finding new subsets of data (Heinrichs & Lim, 2003; Hema & Malik, 2011; PhridviRaj & GuruRao, 2014).

DM has evolved rapidly due to the introduction of new methods in various applications related to different fields including medicine (Heinrichs & Lim, 2003; PhridviRaj & GuruRao, 2014). As mentioned above, it is used to analyze the relationships between information and discover patterns from existing data. The main objective of DM is then to extract information from the data and make it understandable (Hema & Malik, 2011).

Pentaho Community

The software Pentaho Community was developed in 2004 by Pentaho Corporation and it consists in a BI tool that provides data integration, reporting, charts and dashboards based on data processing technologies. This software was created in the Java language and is the first with an open source version in the market of BI tools, this being the community edition version, but there is also another license, not free, which corresponds to the enterprise edition[2].

Most of the information presented by the Pentaho Community is shaped in dashboards that align the organization's strategy and the monitoring of their progress with the objectives of the different areas. The dashboards can have several uses ranging depending on the user. There are two types of dashboards: analytic and integral. The analytic allows obtaining reports and indicators from DM. This type of strategic dashboards are ways to analyze the areas surrounding unrelated environment, consisting in a query tool with the objective of presenting indicators (Sharma et al., 2012).

The BI tool, Pentaho Community, has different modules in the structure, among which, used in this work, CDE.

Pentaho CDE was created to simplify the processes of creating, editing and interpretation of dashboards. It is a powerful and complete tool that combines custom data sources and components with a visual interface to create a layout customized by the user, which can add several components from text boxes to graphics. These layouts of dashboards are simply created with a combination of rows and columns, *html* blocks, CSS, JavaScript and even images. Pentaho CDE has a graphical environment that allows access to information by users: essential information to understand and optimize the performance of an organization. Easy integration between Pentaho Reporting, Pentaho CDE and Pentaho Analysis modules is possible. The user can define the origins of the data represented by dashboards, that is, it is required to specify where the data comes from and how the user entails it to be shown[3].

The CDE plugin is divided into Layout, Components, Data Sources and Preview.

Layout

The layout section is defined by creating a framework for the user, formatting the dashboard structure through *html* code, allowing inserting functions in JavaScript or CSS. The CDE also has templates already defined that the user can choose to save time in creating the dashboard.

Components

It is in the components section that different components can be created and edited, to be inserted into the dashboard, and it is required in advance to assign a space for each component in the layout section. This section is divided into six categories, and it is through these that the user can choose the components that he wants to insert.

Data Sources

Each of these components, created in the previous section, will be associated with a DB in order to show its contents. This connection between the components and DB is made in this section, through which queries will only show the information that the user requires.

Preview

Finally, the preview section allows the users to preview the dashboard. However, for this to be possible, the user has to record the dashboard whenever making a change before the preview.

Advantages and Disadvantages of CDE

After the study of BI tools, it was possible to draw some conclusions regarding the module CDE of Pentaho Community such as:

- Flexible development options for the user;
- Allows connections to multiple data sources;
- The definition of the layout depends entirely on the user;
- Wide range of visual components, graphs, tables, text, selection, parameters, etc.;
- Interaction with the user in the solution itself;
- Share irreversibility;
- Do not need a DW, being chosen by the user to create one;
- Low technical documentation supporting the development.

CASE STUDY

This study applied data from CHP, a hospital in north of Portugal, covering thousands of people.

The Electronic Medical Prescription

The prescription of CDTP is a task of particular interest not only for screening of diseases but mainly in an attempt to find the cause of issues, presenting itself as a powerful task available to clinicians to the decision-making process and therefore the well-being of patients. The prescription of CDTP occupies a large percentage of consultation time, as well as a lot of the day-to-day of a healthcare professional. Thus, it is of major interest to minimize the time spent on prescription of CDTP, with a more rational and efficient use of all available resources to ensure the provision of healthcare with maximum efficiency and quality.

The generalization of the prescription process, in addition to promoting global dematerialization of the whole process of electronic prescribing and the adoption of electronic provision, also results in many benefits, for health professionals as well as users.

Among these benefits, there can be mentioned:

- Reduction in prescription errors;
- Orders placed in time;
- Streamlining and standardization of procedures;
- Reduced operating costs inherent in the process of prescribing CDTP.

Business Intelligence Platform

The business intelligence platform was developed in order to identify physicians who take longer in EMP processes. Nevertheless, to achieve this goal, the physicians' prescription time was not the only variable in study. It was also analyzed the number of requests among the numerous distinct specialties and sub-specialties, between 1st June 2013 and 31st March 2014. After the identification of these individuals, it was certainly essential to understand why such event occurs. One hypothesis is the unsuitable familiarization with the SAM platform that contains the application of CDTP prescription.

To obtain the final product of this study, the BI platform was carried out one series of steps, which are briefly described below.

Selection of Data

Understanding the data domain is the driver element to acquire knowledge in Database (DB), since existing knowledge can be complemented with the attained information in the discovery process. First of all, for this study, it was performed a selection and data collection at CHP, which required prior study to understand the outlook of this project so as to select the data you want to analyze, and finally collect them. The intent was to frame the dissertation project with the area of the organization, in this case the CHP, by defining the project goals, as well as acquiring fundamental concepts to perform it.

Before selecting the data, it is necessary to exploit it and understand it. However, access to tables does not imply that data is accessible to understanding the context of tables and the meaning of each attribute; hence, the need to understand all that is contained in the DB, since the designation of each table until the origin of the values of each attribute. After an understanding of the data, it will then be possible to select the relevant information to be used in the project.

Data Extraction

The data used in the study, corresponds to real data from CHP's DB, which was extracted after being selected. The application SAM aims to aid in medical activities allowing the integration of clinical applications, such as the EMP cited above. The SAM's DB contains various types of data spread across multiple tables.

Creating Tables

After the extraction of the CHP's data, the handling of DB was performed with Oracle SQL Developer, an integrated and free development environment. Several tables were created, with its primary keys and foreign keys. Subsequently, the data selected and extracted earlier, was loaded.

Creating Views

In order to create a Data Warehouse (DW), various views were built in aim to represent subsets of information existing in the created tables.

Data Warehouse

The finalization of DW was based essentially on SQL queries manipulation. After creating the views, they were loaded with the desired information. This step is carried out by crossing queries, shifting the data tables to views in order to obtain useful knowledge.

Platform Development

Initially, for the development of BI platform, it began by defining the structure in section layout of CDE (Community Dashboard Editor) from Pentaho Community, where is created a dashboard.

Then the best schemas were chosen to represent the information, which are bar graphs, point graphs and tables. Finally, so that these graphs contain information, it was necessary to establish a link between the data and the platform. That is, a connection between Oracle SQL Developer, to create queries, and module CDE of Pentaho Community.

Knowledge Extraction

During the study, it was performed the knowledge extraction (KE), in tables or graphs, from the platform built using the Pentaho Community software. This extraction was executed on the CDTP prescription orders, which allowed a better analysis and a broader view of the CHP's prescription service, in order to generate knowledge. This KE was carried out using the Oracle SQL Developer software. The aim is to analyze, through indicators, the average time registration for prescription of CDTP between the beginning of June 2013 and the end of March 2014. The indicators analyzed are:

- Number of requests by specialty;
- Number of requests by subspecialty;
- Number of requests by specialty per day;
- Average time tasks by subspecialty;
- Average time of each task by specialty and physician;
- Requests of CDTP by specialty;
- Requests of CDTP by physician.

Subspecialty relates to groups where each specialty is divided. It analyzed the average time applications in seconds and minutes, as well as the average time of tasks, knowing that a request may or may not have tasks. These analyzes are all made in seconds. Next, we analyzed the relationship between the time of application and the number of requests, time of the tasks and the number of applications. And, finally, it is possible to obtain the percentage of time that a physician uses in completing tasks on demand. This percentage value is obtained by the average ratio of the average of the tasks and applications. It should be noted that the analysis done by subspecialty is also made by physician. Ultimately, it allows identifying the physicians who spend more time in prescribing CDTP.

Comparison with Existing Studies

In the last years, a panoply of BI applications have been developed through BI tools, which are designed to store, retrieve, analyze, transform and present data for BI. In short, it corresponds to the analysis of data in order to provide useful information. The insertion of BI tools in healthcare environments assists managers and health professionals though decision-making, improving healthcare quality, safety, efficiency and delivery. These BI tools include spreadsheets, reporting and querying software, OLAP, digital dashboards, data mining, data warehousing and local information systems. In the market, there is a large set of application software that have been used to build BI applications including TACTIC, JasperReport, Zoho Reports, Palo, Tableau Software, BIRT and Pentaho, just to name a few.

The choice of the BI tool to use is an important decision which depends on what data is going to be analysed and how, so it can be provided with the right kinds of tools. Some of the basic needs that must be considered in the choice of a BI tool include speed, the kind of breadth expected out of the BI application and its usability, among others.

It is worth noting that the use of BI tools by industry widespread among all fields including engineering, mathematics, economics, computer science and, as already mentioned, healthcare. For instance, BI open-source tools were already applied in the field of Radiology to create a prototype model of a data warehouse for BI (Prevedello et al., 2010) and an HIV BI tool was used to provide a reporting system for population indicators, being an effective tool to monitor and further impact the epidemic (Snyder et al., 2014).

RESULTS

In this section, some of the results of the various case studies conducted through the platform are presented. They were obtained with the module CDE of Pentaho Community, which is a tool through which it is possible to treat and analyze data in order to provide useful information to extract knowledge and assist in decision-making. Several indicators were tested and they are displayed in the form of title's section of this chapter.

Number of Requests by Specialty

The chart in Figure 5 indicates to the platform users the amount of CDTP requests made in the period between 1st June 2013 and 31st March 2014, by specialty. Analyzing the graph, it shows that, during this period, applications of ten different specialties were made. If the study was carried out in a shorter time

Figure 5. Number of requests by specialty

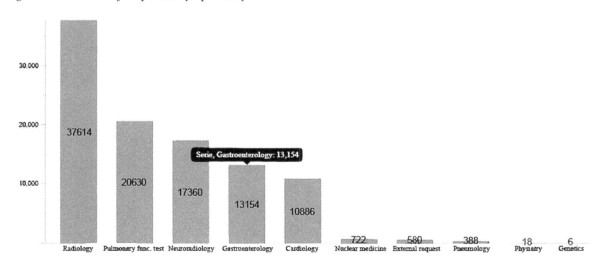

interval some of these specialty applications would not exist, and the number of graph bars would be lower. It can be verified that the radiology specialty, is, without any doubt, the one that has made most requests, with 37,614 requests. In contrast, the specialties of physiatry and genetics have only 18 and 6 requests, respectively.

Number of Requests for Subspecialty

In addition to the analysis of the number of requests by specialty, it was further done a more detailed analysis of the amount of orders. Therefore, it was used another indicator: the number of requests per subspecialty. This analysis was realized since a specialty may or may not be divided into others, as can be seen in the table of Figure 6, where the cardiology specialty is divided into six different subspecialties, being noninvasive arrhythmology, echocardiography, electrocardiography, hemodynamics, pacing and electrophysiology, and HJU. While the specialty of physiatry, for instance, has none. As can be seen, more than 60 CDTP requests have been registered per subspecialties.

Number of Requests by Specialty per Day

To study the amount of orders per day, it was created a picker, which allows the platform users to choose the day, between 1st June 2013 and 31st March 2014 to get the information. The number of bars also varies depending on the chosen days. In the example, the picker is on July 7, 2013, as shown in Figure 7. In this graph, only CDTP of three different specialties were prescribed: cardiology with two applications, neuroradiology, and finally radiology with eight applications. Moving the cursor over the bars, the platform identifies the number of applications for the specialty in question. In this case, on July 7, 2013, six applications of neuroradiology specialty were recorded.

Average Time Tasks by Subspecialty

Each request of CDTP may or may not require health professionals to fill forms at each prescription. This process, which involves filling out surveys or forms, is called task. An application may have no

Figure 6. Number of requests for subspecialty

SubSpecialty	NRequests
Cardiology - Noninvasive arrhythmology	732
Cardiology - Echocardiography	7146
Cardiology - Electrocardiography	1878
Cardiology - Hemodynamics	982
Cardiology - Pacing and electrophysiology	90
Cardiology - HJU	58
Genetics	6
Physiatry	18
Gastroenterology - Biofeedback	30
Gastroenterology - Liver biopsy	104

Show 10 entries   Search:

Showing 1 to 10 of 64 entries

Figure 7. Number of requests by specialty per day

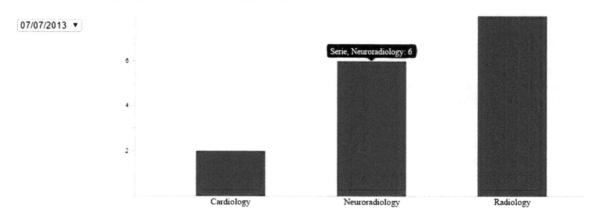

associated task, only one, or can have several tasks. Therefore, an indicator was created to analyze the average time of the tasks for each of the subspecialties. This information is presented on the dot plot in Figure 8 where each dot represents a subspecialty.

Due to the high amount of subspecialties analysis, the names of each subspecialty overlap in the x-axis, preventing the user to see them. In order to understand the information and extract useful knowledge, the user can explore the various points with the cursor, and the platform will show both the subspecialty as well as the average time of the tasks. As this procedure can be unpractical, the table shown on Figure 9 was built. That being said, the graph presented in Figure 8 shows that the tasks of echocardiography cardiology specialty takes an average of 56.3 seconds to be performed. All this information is represented in a readable way in the table of Figure 9, which identifies the subspecialty and the average time of the

Figure 8. Average time tasks by subspecialty

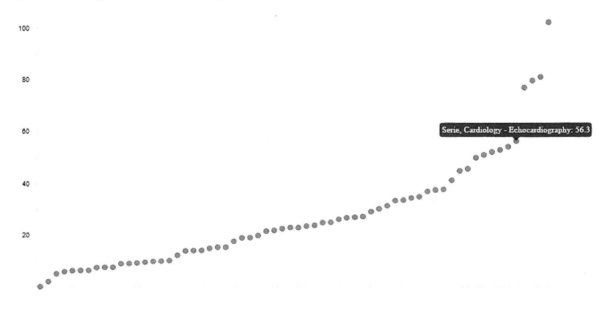

Figure 9. Average time tasks by subspecialty

SubSpecialty	AverageTime
Gastroenterology - HJU	125.6
Neuroradiology - Computed tomography	115.9
Cardiology - Hemodynamics	100.2
Gastroenterology - C.P.R.E.	95.5
Neuroradiology - Doppler ultrasound	94.9
Neuroradiology - Magnetic resonance imaging	92.7
Radiology - Computed tomography	91.9
Radiology/Neuroradiology - Magnetic resonance imaging	91.1
Gastroenterology - Liver biopsy	90.5
Gastroenterology - Upper endoscopy	90

Show 10 ▼ entries Search:

Showing 1 to 10 of 76 entries

tasks associated with it. This table is sorted descendingly by the time consumption that every subspecialty spends carrying out its tasks.

It can be seen that the request whose tasks take, on average, more time to perform, refers to the specialty of gastroenterology and request for HJU.

Average Time of Each Task by Subspecialty and Physician

The following study is certainly the most relevant for this project. Through indicator analysis, the average time of each task by specialty and physician shows which physicians devote more time in the prescription process, compared to their colleagues who prescribe the same requests. Thereafter, a few examples will be presented, but the platform has the ability to analyze more than 60 different requests for various specialties.

Again, the platform uses a picker, where the user has the option of subspecialty, as can be seen in Figure 10.

For example, in the chart represented in Figure 10, where physicians who prescribed one pacing and electrophysiology are analyzed, it can be seen that there are clearly two physicians who take longer than their colleagues to prescribe the same examination of cardiology specialty. These two individuals are identifiable through their ID's, but for confidentiality reasons, they cannot be revealed. However, it is easily noticeable that they are, from left to right, the first and the sixth individuals, respectively. As already mentioned, it is possible to move the cursor to a desired point of the graphic and get information. It appears that the selected physician spends an average of 45.3 seconds on the performance of the tasks of pacing and electrophysiology.

For examinations prescribed more often, the number of physicians who prescribe them is also higher. Thus, due to the large number of physicians who prescribe these tests, their ID's overlap in the x-axis, which makes it difficult to identify them, unless moving the cursor to the point where it is desired to get information. For this reason, once again, apart from the graph, a table that easily identifies the ID and the meantime was created, which is presented in Figure 11. This table is provided with a picker for the user to select the desired subspecialty. The average times are already ordered from highest to lowest, since the goal is to identify those that, on average, need more time in the prescription process.

Figure 10. Average time tasks by specialty and physician

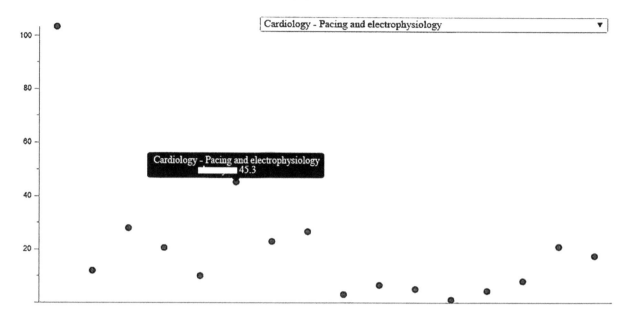

Figure 11. Average time tasks by physician

IDPhysician	AverageTime
	704.3
	573.5
	445
	377
	325
	298
	216.8
	186
	184
	179.5

Show 10 ▾ entries   Search:

Radiology - Computed tomography ▾

Showing 1 to 10 of 540 entries

Requests of CDTP by Specialty

In Figure 12, it is presented a detailed analysis of the average time in the log CDTP between 1st June 2013 and 31st March 2014. In this table the analysis is done by specialty, containing information on: the number of applications for each service; the total time spent in the prescription of all cases; the total time of the tasks of those requests; the average time in seconds of applications and tasks, respectively; the percentage of time that is spent on tasks during the prescription process; and finally, the total time applications in minutes, rounded to units.

Only to the top ten applications, it is possible to notice that electrocardiography is the request that occurs more often, with 9645 records. Despite being the examination with the greatest number of requests,

Figure 12. Average time on registration of CDTP by specialty

Show 10 ▾ entries   Search:

Specialty	SubSpecialty	NRequests	Time Requests (seg.)	Time Tasks (seg.)	AverageTime Request	AverageTime Task	% Tasks	Time Requests (min.)
Cardiology	Cardiology - Hemodynamics	793	116453	13250	146.85	16.71	11.378	1941
Cardiology	Cardiology - Pacing and electrophysiology	105	8160	328	77.71	3.12	4.02	136
Cardiology	Cardiology - HJU	248	4375	489	17.64	1.97	11.177	73
Cardiology	Cardiology - Electrocardiography	9645	103615	9858	10.74	1.02	9.514	1727
Cardiology	Cardiology - Noninvasive arrhythmology	2953	42035	2583	14.23	0.87	6.145	701
Cardiology	Cardiology - Echocardiography	5557	432083	36850	77.75	6.63	8.528	7201
Physiatry	Physiatry	1745	132	19	0.08	0.01	14.394	2
Gastroenterology	Gastroenterology - Liver biopsy	53	8712	1890	164.38	35.66	21.694	145
Gastroenterology	Gastroenterology - HJU	565	68139	5060	120.6	8.96	7.426	1136
Gastroenterology	Gastroenterology - Functional anorectal disorders	120	6145	727	51.21	6.06	11.831	102

Showing 1 to 10 of 64 entries

the echocardiography, with only 5557 applications, takes longer to be prescribed, as the total time of applications of echocardiography is superior to the electrocardiographs. For the tasks' execution time, once again, echocardiography presents the highest total time, although it is not the examination with the greatest number of applications. Thus, it can be concluded from this information that applications for echocardiography involve filling in more forms than requests for electrocardiographs.

On the other hand, the prescription of liver biopsy, the gastroenterology specialty, takes longer in the forms of prescription. For about 22% of the time the prescription is spent in performing the tasks.

Requests of CDTP by Physician

In Figure 13, a detailed analysis is presented, which corresponds to the average time of a CDTP registration by a physician, between 1st June 2013 and 31st March 2014. As shown in Figure 12, this is the same information about the number of requests, but this time for each physician.

As can be seen, in this period, requests were prescribed for more than 40,000 physicians, bearing in mind that a physician prescribes various applications, i.e., that does not mean that there are over 40,000 health professionals. Although, in the example shown, all physicians have prescribed noninvasive arrhythmologys (cardiology specialty), some have superior times.

For instance, the third doctor presented prescribed 16 noninvasive arrythmologys, all in a total of 201 seconds, which amounts to an average of 13 seconds per request. Compared to their colleagues, this physician is much less time consuming than, for example, the sixth physician in the table that takes 53 seconds on average per request. This is not to say that the fastest physician is more effective in the electronic prescription process. On the contrary, it is shown that the faster individual has a percentage value of task below 1%, while the term used for comparison in this example is about 8%. These values

Figure 13. Average time on registration of CDTP by physician

Show 10 ▼ entries

Search: _____

Physician ⇕	SubSpecialty ⇕	NRequests ⇕	Time Requests (seg.) ⇕	Time Tasks (seg.) ⇕	AverageTime Request ⇕	AverageTime Task ⇕	% Tasks ⇕	Time Requests (min.) ⇕
	Cardiology - Noninvasive arrhythmology	4	174	8	44	2	4.598	3
	Cardiology - Noninvasive arrhythmology	2	242	3	121	2	1.24	4
	Cardiology - Noninvasive arrhythmology	16	201	2	13	0	0.995	3
	Cardiology - Noninvasive arrhythmology	4	163	7	41	2	4.294	3
	Cardiology - Noninvasive arrhythmology	2	421	10	211	5	2.375	7
	Cardiology - Noninvasive arrhythmology	2	105	8	53	4	7.619	2
	Cardiology - Noninvasive arrhythmology	4	55	7	14	2	12.727	1
	Cardiology - Noninvasive arrhythmology	6	111	17	19	3	15.315	2
	Cardiology - Noninvasive arrhythmology	4	143	6	36	2	4.196	2
	Cardiology - Noninvasive arrhythmology	4	401	10	100	3	2.494	7

Showing 1 to 10 of 40,107 entries

may cast doubt on the third doctor of the list, because only approximately 1% of the prescription of time is devoted to tasks. The question that arises is: does this physician correctly fills all matters of forms?

DISCUSSION

With a review of the audit platform for their potential users, it is possible identifying physicians who spend more time in CDTP prescription process. With that being said, it is also achievable identifying the reasons which cause those physicians to perform, on average, a lower number of consultations within a period of time. This is of upmost importance since the prescription is an existing task in much of the consultations carried out in this country. With the extracted information through the platform, the organization's administrators can make decisions such as imposing the optimization of the prescription process. Reducing the prescription time, they will be able to reduce the time of the consultations, consequently. On the other hand, to decrease the time of a query, physicians will be able to give more consultations a day, which will bring benefits to consumers, as the waiting times decrease. In addition, consultations, in private health organizations, are most likely to reduce their costs, which is another considerable advantage for users.

Nonetheless, the platform SAM, which owns the EMP platform, is minimally evaluated since, in addition to the prescription platform, it has many other features. Nevertheless, this evaluation is done through an analysis with the aim to improve through the implementation of changes.

CONCLUSION AND FUTURE RESEARCH

Nowadays, it is essential on the part of all organizations the use of ICT in their services. These technologies are provided with automated mechanisms for data processing. The use of BI systems allows users to access the right information in the shortest time possible, making effective decisions, correcting processes and anticipating the needs of the institutions.

It is important to note that the use of EHR systems encompasses several groups of professionals in a hospital setting. Thus, such systems should be developed to meet their requirements, developing the interaction between all healthcare providers, and presenting itself as an improvement and benefit in the workplace.

The use of a BI system for the construction of a platform has proved to be useful in knowledge extraction process. In addition, the platform itself has several advantages, among which the decrease in the prescription process and consequently the reduction of appointment duration (after the decision-making by managers of health organizations). This means that it is possible to perform more queries per day, i.e., the productivity of physicians' increases and reduce waiting lists, which will probably lower the cost of these same queries.

After the development of the platform, it is clear that it will bring plenty of benefits such as the time decrease of the prescription process and, consequently, the reduction of appointment duration. Ultimately, this means that it is possible to perform more consultations a day, which probably will lower the consultations' cost, i.e., it follows that you can improve and make more efficient the entire process of EMP.

Future Work

As future work, it is suggested to analyze the forms associated with each request (i.e. to examine the issues of jobs and consequently analyze the responses of health professionals) as there may be physicians who, even in mandatory, do not answer questions in the most correct way, which may cause the times of the tasks and applications to decrease. Consequently, the below average physicians, identified as outliers by this platform, may even be those who respond to all questions of the form, and correctly.

It is suggested to even perform fieldwork, and measure the times of applications and tasks in the very act of limitation, in the query. Most likely because, while the doctor is making his request for the CDTP, he will not be completely focused on completing the tasks since he could, for instance, be talking to the patient. That is, the process of prescription requests and the tasks will not be continuous, which makes the results a less viable platform since the data is measured automatically. Hence, it is important to perform measurements on the ground, to get a sense of the times and the physicians that the platform points out as the most accurate.

On the other hand, it is also possible to study the self-limitation platform SAM, in order to predict potential improvements. Nonetheless, it may be needed to reformulate the questions of the various tasks, as there may be questions difficult to interpret, even by health professionals, as they may be interfering with time spent on the EMP process. After following these suggestions, it can be possible to ascertain with any certainty who the slowest physicians are in prescribing CDTP.

Moreover, it could be interesting to execute this same study but with other BI tools or explore more features of Pentaho Community.

Finally, it is believed that, using as a basis the work presented throughout this dissertation and considering the proposals submitted previously, it is possible to improve the efficiency of the entire EMP of CDTP process.

ACKNOWLEDGMENT

This work is funded by National Funds through the FCT - *Fundação para a Ciência e Tecnologia* (Portuguese Foundation for Science and Technology) - within project PEst-OE/EEI/UI0752/2014.

REFERENCES

Allison, J. J., Wall, T. C., Spettell, C. M., Calhoun, J., Fargason, C. A., Kobylinski, R. W., & Kiefe, C. et al. (2000). The art and science of chart review. *The Joint Commission Journal on Quality Improvement*, *26*, 115–136. PMID:10709146

Ammenwerth, E., Schnell-Inderst, P., Machan, C., & Siebert, U. (2008). The Effect of Electronic Prescribing on Medication Errors and Adverse Drug Events: A Systematic Review. *Journal of the American Medical Informatics Association : JAMIA*, *15*(5), 585–600. doi:10.1197/jamia.M2667 PMID:18579832

Bonney, W. (2013). Applicability of Business Intelligence in Electronic Health Record. *Procedia: Social and Behavioral Sciences*, *73*, 257–262. doi:10.1016/j.sbspro.2013.02.050

Cassidy, L. D., Marsh, G. M., Holleran, M. K., & Ruhl, L. S. (2002). Methodology to improve data quality from chart review in the managed care setting. *The American Journal of Managed Care*, *8*, 787–793. PMID:12234019

Chaudhuri, S., Dayal, U., & Narasayya, V. (2011). An overview of business intelligence technology. *Communications of the ACM*, *54*(8), 88. doi:10.1145/1978542.1978562

Chiasson, M., Reddy, M., Kaplan, B., & Davidson, E. (2007). Expanding multi-disciplinary approaches to healthcare information technologies: What does information systems offer medical informatics? *International Journal of Medical Informatics*, *76*, 89–97. doi:10.1016/j.ijmedinf.2006.05.010 PMID:16769245

Duarte, J., Portela, C. F., Abelha, A., Machado, J., & Santos, M. F. (2011). Electronic health record in dermatology service. In *Communications in Computer and Information Science* (Vol. 221, pp. 156–164). CCIS; doi:10.1007/978-3-642-24352-3_17

Eder, C., Fullerton, J., Benroth, R., & Lindsay, S. P. (2005). Pragmatic strategies that enhance the reliability of data abstracted from medical records. *Applied Nursing Research*, *18*(1), 50–54. doi:10.1016/j.apnr.2004.04.005 PMID:15812736

El-Sappagh, S. H. A., Hendawi, A. M. A., & El Bastawissy, A. H. (2011). A proposed model for data warehouse ETL processes. *Journal of King Saud University - Computer and Information Sciences*. doi:10.1016/j.jksuci.2011.05.005

Gearing, R. E., & Mian, I. a, Barber, J., & Ickowicz, A. (2006). A methodology for conducting retrospective chart review research in child and adolescent psychiatry. *Journal de l'Académie Canadienne de Psychiatrie de L'enfant et de L'adolescent* [Journal of the Canadian Academy of Child and Adolescent Psychiatry], *15*, 126–34. Retrieved from http://www.pubmedcentral.nih.gov/articlerender.fcgi?artid=2 277255&tool=pmcentrez&rendertype=abstract

Glaser, J., & Stone, J. (2008). Effective use of business intelligence. *Healthcare Financial Management : Journal of the Healthcare Financial Management Association, 62,* 68–72. PMID:18309596

Gregory, K. E., & Radovinsky, L. (2012). Research strategies that result in optimal data collection from the patient medical record. *Applied Nursing Research, 25*(2), 108–116. doi:10.1016/j.apnr.2010.02.004 PMID:20974093

Hasman, A. (1998). Education and health informatics. International Journal of Medical Informatics, 52(1-3), 209–216. doi:10.1016/S1386-5056(98)90133-3

Heeks, R. (2006). Health information systems: Failure, success and improvisation. *International Journal of Medical Informatics, 75*(2), 125–137. doi:10.1016/j.ijmedinf.2005.07.024 PMID:16112893

Heinrichs, J. H., & Lim, J. S. (2003). Integrating web-based data mining tools with business models for knowledge management. *Decision Support Systems, 35*(1), 103–112. doi:10.1016/S0167-9236(02)00098-2

Hema, R., & Malik, N. (2011). *Data Mining and Business Intelligence.* Bvicamacin.

Kawado, M., Hinotsu, S., Matsuyama, Y., Yamaguchi, T., Hashimoto, S., & Ohashi, Y. (2003). A comparison of error detection rates between the reading aloud method and the double data entry method. *Controlled Clinical Trials, 24*(5), 560–569. doi:10.1016/S0197-2456(03)00089-8 PMID:14500053

Kimball, R., & Ross, M. (2002). *The data warehouse toolkit: the complete guide to dimensional modelling.* New York: Wiley. doi:10.1145/945721.945741

Loshin, D. (2013). Business Intelligence: The Savvy Manager's Guide. Morgan Kaufmann. Retrieved from http://scholar.google.com/scholar?hl=en&btnG=Search&q=intitle:Business+Intelligence:+The +Savvy+Manager's+Guide#4

Mettler, T., & Vimarlund, V. (2009). Understanding business intelligence in the context of healthcare. *Health Informatics Journal, 15*(3), 254–264. doi:10.1177/1460458209337446 PMID:19713399

Munyisia, E. N., Yu, P., & Hailey, D. (2011). The changes in caregivers' perceptions about the quality of information and benefits of nursing documentation associated with the introduction of an electronic documentation system in a nursing home. *International Journal of Medical Informatics, 80*(2), 116–126. doi:10.1016/j.ijmedinf.2010.10.011 PMID:21242104

Murray, M. D., Smith, F. E., Fox, J., Teal, E. Y., Kesterson, J. G., Stiffler, T. A., & McDonald, C. J. et al. (2003). Structure, functions, and activities of a research support informatics section. *Journal of the American Medical Informatics Association, 10*(4), 389–398. doi:10.1197/jamia.M1252 PMID:12668695

Pan, L., Fergusson, D., Schweitzer, I., & Hebert, P. C. (2005). Ensuring high accuracy of data abstracted from patient charts: The use of a standardized medical record as a training tool. *Journal of Clinical Epidemiology*, *58*(9), 918–923. doi:10.1016/j.jclinepi.2005.02.004 PMID:16085195

Pardillo, J., Mazón, J. N., & Trujillo, J. (2010). Extending OCL for OLAP querying on conceptual multidimensional models of data warehouses. *Information Sciences*, *180*(5), 584–601. doi:10.1016/j.ins.2009.11.006

Park, T., & Kim, H. (2013). A data warehouse-based decision support system for sewer infrastructure management. *Automation in Construction*, *30*, 37–49. doi:10.1016/j.autcon.2012.11.017

Paul, J., Seib, R., & Prescott, T. (2005). The internet and clinical trials: Background, online resources, examples and issues. *Journal of Medical Internet Research*, *7*(1), e5. doi:10.2196/jmir.7.1.e5 PMID:15829477

Pavlović, I., Kern, T., & Miklavčič, D. (2009). Comparison of paper-based and electronic data collection process in clinical trials: Costs simulation study. *Contemporary Clinical Trials*, *30*(4), 300–316. doi:10.1016/j.cct.2009.03.008 PMID:19345286

PhridviRaj, M. S. B., & GuruRao, C. V. (2014). Data Mining – Past, Present and Future – A Typical Survey on Data Streams. *Procedia Technology*, *12*, 255–263. doi:10.1016/j.protcy.2013.12.483

Popovič, A., Hackney, R., Coelho, P. S., & Jaklič, J. (2012). Towards business intelligence systems success: Effects of maturity and culture on analytical decision making. *Decision Support Systems*, *54*(1), 729–739. doi:10.1016/j.dss.2012.08.017

Powsner, S. M., Wyatt, J. C., & Wright, P. (1998). Opportunities for and challenges of computerisation. *Lancet*, *352*(9140), 1617–1622. doi:10.1016/S0140-6736(98)08309-3 PMID:9843122

Prevedello, L. M., Andriole, K. P., Hanson, R., Kelly, P., & Khorasani, R. (2010). Business intelligence tools for radiology: Creating a prototype model using open-source tools. *Journal of Digital Imaging*, *23*(2), 133–141. doi:10.1007/s10278-008-9167-3 PMID:19011943

Rossi, M., Campbell, K. L., & Ferguson, M. (2014). Implementation of the nutrition care process and international dietetics and nutrition terminology in a single-center hemodialysis unit: Comparing paper vs electronic records. *Journal of the Academy of Nutrition and Dietetics*, *114*(1), 124–130. doi:10.1016/j.jand.2013.07.033 PMID:24161368

Saleem, J. J., Russ, A. L., Justice, C. F., Hagg, H., Ebright, P. R., Woodbridge, P. A., & Doebbeling, B. N. (2009). Exploring the persistence of paper with the electronic health record. *International Journal of Medical Informatics*, *78*(9), 618–628. doi:10.1016/j.ijmedinf.2009.04.001 PMID:19464231

Sharma, S., Osei-Bryson, K.-M., & Kasper, G. M. (2012). Evaluation of an integrated Knowledge Discovery and Data Mining process model. *Expert Systems with Applications*, *39*(13), 11335–11348. doi:10.1016/j.eswa.2012.02.044

Snyder, L., Mcewen Dean, L., Davidson, A., Thrun, M., Mccormick, E., & Mettenbrink, J. C. (2014). Integrating Data into Meaningful HIV Indicators Using Business Intelligence. *2014 Council of State and Territorial Epidemiologists Annual Conference.*

Soler, E., Trujillo, J., Fernández-Medina, E., & Piattini, M. (2008). Building a secure star schema in data warehouses by an extension of the relational package from CWM. *Computer Standards & Interfaces*, *30*(6), 341–350. doi:10.1016/j.csi.2008.03.002

Tavakoli, N., Jahanbakhsh, M., Mokhtari, H., & Tadayon, H. R. (2011). Opportunities of electronic health record implementation in Isfahan. Procedia Computer Science (Vol. 3, pp. 1195–1198). doi:10.1016/j.procs.2010.12.193

Waegemann, C. (2003). EHR vs. CPR vs. EMR. *Healthcare Informatics Online*.

Worster, A., & Haines, T. (2004). Advanced Statistics: Understanding Medical Record Review (MRR) Studies. *Academic Emergency Medicine*, *11*(2), 187–192. doi:10.1111/j.1553-2712.2004.tb01433.x PMID:14759964

ADDITIONAL READING

Coiera, E., Westbrook, J., & Wyatt, J. (2006). The safety and quality of decision support systems. *Yearbook of Medical Informatics*, 2006, 20–25. PMID:17051290

Fayyad, U., Piatetsky-shapiro, G., & Smyth, P. (1996). *Data Mining and Knowledge Discovery*, *17*(3), 37–54.

Ferreira, J., Miranda, M., Abelha, A., & Machado, J. (2010). O Processo ETL em Sistemas Data Warehouse. *INForum 2010 - II Simpósio de Informática* (pp. 757–765).

Inmon, W. H. (2002). *Building the Data Warehouse* (3rd ed.). New York, NY, USA: John Wiley & Sons, Inc.

Koh, H. C., & Tan, G. (2005). Data mining applications in healthcare. *Journal of Healthcare Information Management : JHIM*, *19*(2), 64–72. PMID:15869215

KEY TERMS AND DEFINITIONS

Business Intelligence (BI): Set of technologies capable of treating and analyzing data in order to present relevant and strategic information, helpful in the decision-making process of an organization.

Data Mining (DM): Process of discovering interesting and relevant patterns in large datasets.

Data Warehouse (DW): Component of a BI system that stores and consolidates data into a valid and consistent format and allows the analysis and exploration of that data using other tools.

Electronic Health Record (EHR): HIS that covers the different services and units of a healthcare institution and consists of a set of standardized documents for the registration of the medical procedures provided to a particular patient.

Extraction, Transformation and Load (ETL): Process that transforms and converts data coming from several sources to a unified format, fitted to the DW schema where these data will be stored.

ENDNOTES

[1]   http://www.min-saude.pt/portal
[2]   http://www.pentaho.com/product/product-overview; http://www.pentaho.com/solutions/healthcare
[3]   http://www.webdetails.pt/ctools/cde/

This research was previously published in Applying Business Intelligence to Clinical and Healthcare Organizations edited by José Machado and António Abelha, pages 208-240, copyright year 2016 by Medical Information Science Reference (an imprint of IGI Global).

Chapter 79
Smart Medication Management, Current Technologies, and Future Directions

Seyed Ali Rokni
Washington State University, USA

Hassan Ghasemzadeh
Washington State University, USA

Niloofar Hezarjaribi
Washington State University, USA

ABSTRACT

Medication non-adherence is a major healthcare challenge with irreversible consequences in terms of healthcare costs and quality of care. While recent years have seen some effort in developing sensor-based technologies to detect medication adherence and provide interventions, the community lacks a comprehensive study on the clinical utility, reliability, and effectiveness of such medication intake monitoring solutions. Furthermore, many opportunities inspired machine learning algorithms have largely remained unexplored. In an effort to highlight these knowledge gaps, in this paper, we take an interdisciplinary approach to (1) review and compare existing engineering products for medication intake monitoring; (2) discuss clinical applications where such technologies have demonstrated to be effective; (3) explore research gaps and shed light on unmet needs and future research opportunities in the area of medication management from both clinical and technology development points of view. The results of this paper may open several new avenues in the area of technology-based medication.

INTRODUCTION

Insufficient medication adherence is a big problem in medical field and contributes significantly to healthcare costs and poor quality of care, in particular in patients with chronic conditions. Studies show that medical prescriptions are never filled in almost 20% to 30% of the cases. Furthermore, 50% of medicines are not taken as prescribed for chronic patients (WHO, 2003), (Viswanathan et al., 2012).

DOI: 10.4018/978-1-5225-3926-1.ch079

Of all medication-related hospitalizations in the US, 33% to 69% are as a result of patient's insufficient adherence to prescribed medication (Lüscher & Vetter, 1990), which annually costs about $100 billion to $289 billion (Viswanathan et al., 2012). The consequences of medication non-adherence are enormous. In the United States, more than 10% of hospitalizations, approximately 125,000 deaths, and a substantial growth in morbidity and mortality are due to medication non-adherence. For example, studies show if the patients fill no discharge medications by 120 days after a post-acute myocardial infarction, the probability of death at 1 year will increase 80% (Jackevicius, Li, & Tu, 2008).

Improving medication adherence can potentially influence large patient populations and result in significant cost savings. Each American adult has at least one chronic illness and currently 75% of the total cost of healthcare accounts for patients with one or more chronic conditions (Chisholm-Burns & Spivey, 2012). Average adherence to medication in chronic illnesses is generally higher than that of acute diseases (Jackevicius, Mamdani, & Tu, 2002). As an example, half of the patients with acute coronary syndromes discontinue to take hydroxymethylglutaryl–coenzyme six months after they start therapy (Lüscher & Vetter, 1990). These observations show that novel clinical and technological approaches are needed to enhance medication adherence which will significantly decrease the costs associated with poor adherence in patients with chronic conditions.

According to 2003 report of World Health Organization (WHO) (WHO, 2003), interventions could be deployed to improve medication adherence in patients with chronic diseases, such as asthma, heart failure, diabetes. Technological advancement in intervention methods results in higher rate and improving assessing methods of adherence. Electronic intervention and monitoring approaches such as mobile and wireless technologies, electronic sensors, and web portals are developing very fast and aim to provide patients and healthcare providers with a potential rapid and organized form of gathering, manipulating, and analyzing adherence patterns with customized reports to enhance medication adherence behaviors. Taking advantages of technology in medication adherence is not only useful for patients' health, but also can be utilized by clinicians and researchers to improve their clinical decisions, development strategies, and methods of intervention.

With the recent advancements in electronics, sensor design, communications, and data analytics, we can potentially develop novel technological approaches to objectively monitor patients, assess their medication adherence, and provide effective and timely interventions. While recent years have seen some effort in developing sensor-based technologies such as wireless electronic pillboxes to detect medication adherence and provide interventions, the community lacks a comprehensive study on the clinical utility, reliability, and effectiveness of current such medication intake monitoring solutions. Furthermore, many opportunities inspired by computational models such as signal processing and machine learning algorithms have largely remained unexplored. In fact, the literature is lacking a comprehensive study of existing technology-related medication adherence solutions, an analysis of advantages and shortcomings of the state-of-the-art technologies, a study of promises that these systems provide, and future directions in this research area. In an effort to highlight these knowledge gaps, in this paper, we take an interdisciplinary approach to

1. Review and compare existing engineering products for medication intake monitoring;
2. Discuss clinical applications where such technologies have demonstrated to be effective;
3. Explore research gaps and shed light on unmet needs and future research opportunities in the area of medication management from both clinical and technology development points of view.

The results of this paper may open several new avenues in the area of technology-based medication management focusing on:

1. Establishment of new and robust clinical definitions for medication adherence; and
2. Development of more robust medication monitoring devices and services;
3. Development of signal processing, pervasive computing, machine learning, and wearable computing solutions that facilitate robust and accurate and effective medication monitoring and clinical interventions.

BACKGROUND

Medication Adherence: A Definition

Adherence to medication is commonly defined as patients take the amount of medicine prescribed by their health care provider; yet, the community lacks a concrete definition of medication adherence where number, duration, and frequency of medicine intake are all reflected in it. Furthermore, most current studies use a discrete metric to describe medication adherence where a patient is either adherent or not. Some of the concerns that the current definitions of medication adherence raise are the following. Sometimes the patients take all of monthly prescribed medicine in one day. It might be no constraint on using the medication at specific time A literature review reveals that definition and methods of assessing adherence to medication is different from one researcher to another (Jackevicius et al., 2008). Measuring adherence to medication is important to evaluate clinical and economic outcomes of low adherence. The rate of adherence often measured as percentage of amount of taken medication to prescribed amount of it. This measure could become more precise if combined with correctness-taking assigned pills for that specific day and promptness-taking medication at appropriate time (Chisholm-Burns & Spivey, 2012). Adequate adherence is different from one study to another or from one illness to another. For instance, several trails assume that an adherence rate of higher than 70% is admissible while other trails do not accept adherence lower than 95% (Jackevicius et al., 2008).

Methods to Assess Medication Adherence

There exist different methods for measuring patient's adherence but quantitative approaches can be divided into two different categories:

1. Direct methods;
2. Indirect methods (Lüscher & Vetter, 1990), (Fairman & Matheral, 2000).

Although direct methods such as a blood test are the most accurate measurement methods for short time, they are expensive, need cooperation of health care provider, and are sensitive to by the patient's abuse such as "white coat adherence" (Feinstein, n. d.). Indirect approaches such as questioning the patient or pill-count are objective; meanwhile, they can be sensitive to misrepresentation and tend to result in overestimation of patient's adherence by healthcare providers (Lüscher & Vetter, 1990). While there exists several methods for adherence assessment, none of them truly can be considered as a gold standard (Fairman & Matheral, 2000).

The selection of measurement methods depends on the type of disease and intervention, available resources and sometimes ethical and legal issues (Fairman & Matheral, 2000). Therefore, having a context-aware monitoring system is essential to improve medication adherence. For example, (Wagner & Arnfast, 2010), designing and testing a system to remind a patient to take his/her morning medication if the medication has not been taken within a fixed time interval after waking up. Although the study has been tested on 3 patients, the results show that weight sensor did not fully work as expected and also it is not really applicable and dependent to a gateway computer.

Commercially Available Electronic Pillboxes

Electronic pillboxes are perhaps the most common technology-based medication adherence monitoring solutions. In this section, we review existing electronic pillboxes briefly. In recent years, there have been many companies providing new pillboxes equipped with micro-electronic circuits, wireless connectivity, and several types of alarms to address the problem medication non-adherence. These commercially available pillboxes, can record information about date and time of cap opening. A summary of available products is shown in Table 1. These technologies, which are called "smart pillboxes", vary in different ways. Some, such as epill and iRemember, only provide reminders about the time of taking pills, while several others such as CleverCap and MedMinder provide mechanisms for reporting a history of medication adherence for each patient. Patients using AdhereTech have the option to receive customizable messaging and interventions, which is helpful in case of missing doses. In contrast with many other pillboxes, which only record data when the cap is opened, AdhereTech also records the number of pills or liquid remaining in the bottle.

Beside the clinical services they provide, different pillboxes appear to vary in their underlying technology for data communication and adherence detection. While MedSignal, doseCue and SIMPILL use a mobile phone as a gateway for data transmission, other products such as MEMS communicate with a reader connected to a computer. More recently, several products provide the ability to transmit adherence data directly by the use of cellular connectivity embedded into the pillbox, which eliminates the need for additional gateway. Such technologies intend to enhance robustness of data transmission by providing a continuous connection with the data server. Examples of such devices are GlowCap and SMRxT. Another technology difference is in the method used to detect whether the pill is taken or not. For example, eCAP and Quand Medication Compliance use RFID technology for detection while ePill cannot automatically detect that.

These electronic pillboxes provide different types of alarms. While talkingRx provides only audible alert message in addition to showing the clock, some others such as MedPro Pill Organizer provide light and audio alerts, calling, texting or sending emails in the condition of missing a pill as well as a web portal which reports a summary of the patient's adherence data.

Clearly, there is a tradeoff between the amount of service one receives and the cost associated with purchasing and maintaining the adherence monitoring technology. Packages such as Dose-Alert and didit are among inexpensive acting as a sticker on any available pillboxes. They, however, provide no more than a reminder service. On the other hand, AdhereTech or Med Pro, which are more expensive technologies, use more advanced technology and provide more extensive services and alerts such as reporting to family and caregivers.

Table 1. Available electronic pillboxes

Name	Transmission Technology	Additional Features
AdhereTech	Wireless transmission from bottle to server/ Real time analysis	
MedPro Pill Organizer/Automated Security Alert	Communicates through a cellular network and remote control using a web portal.	Reporting, History
iRemember	Bluetooth, Wi-Fi under development	
CleverCap	Connect to Wi-Fi, 2Net HUB	Linked to the cloud while in cellular range
eCAP/Med-ic	BT4, RFID, NFC/ Secure data report	
ePill	NA	Timer
GlowCap	AT&T Mobile Network	
Didit	NA	Manual Tracking Device
Adherence Solutions LLC/ Dose Alert	NA	Programmable Sticker on Bottle
MedMinder,Jon-Locked Pill Dispenser and Medical Alert	internal cellular modem	Weekly Report
doseCue	Bluetooth, mobile phone as gateway	Exception Report
SMRxT	Fits standard Rx vials/ Verizon telecommunication	
TalkingRx/Rex	NA	The pharmacist records up to 60 seconds of instructions when dispensing the medication
MedCenter	NA	Pill Organizer
Quand Medication Compliance	NFC and mobile phone	
Ubox	NA	
MedSignals	phone line	
MEMS 6 TrackCap/Aardex,..	Reader connected to computer	
SIMPill	Cell phone	

CLINICAL STUDIES WITH ELECTRONIC MEDICATION MONITORING

In spite of the rapid changes in technology and development of new products, there are still a few controlled studies that have actually been designed to demonstrate the using of technology, especially electronic devices, in improving adherence rates. Smaller number of studies shows that using electronic devices cannot result in meaningful improvements in adherence rates. In this section, we review exiting chronic conditions in which electronic approaches have been utilized for medication adherence. These clinical studies are summarized in Table 2.

Diabetes

Diabetes is a group of disorders which refers to high level blood glucose and needs precise monitoring of exercise, diet, and medication for achieving good glycemic control (Cramer, 2004). Complexity of diabetes treatment and duration of disease cause that healthcare systems often do not have sufficient

Table 2. Exiting chronic conditions using medical-adherence

Area	Source	Samples/Duration	Intervention	Results
Diabetes	(Morak et al., 2012)	59 samples/ 13 months	e-blister	Feasibility study
	(Cramer, 2004)	A literature search/ 38 years	MEMS; APREX	MEMS is useful in improving adherence
	(Franklin et al., 2008)	126 patient with type 1 diabetes / 1 year	Text message via SweetTalk software system	Sweet Talk may support intensive insulin therapy.
	(Brath et al., 2013)	53 patients (30 female)/ NA	Electronic blister	Feasibility of mHealth based adherence management.
	(Vervloet et al., 2012)	RCT on 104 type 2 diabetes patients/ 6 month	SMS reminder	Receiving text-message reminders led to significantly more doses taking and less miss doses comparing patients receiving no reminders.
HIV (antiretroviral therapy (ART))	(Horvath et al., 2012)	meta-analysis of Two RCTs from Kenya/ 48-52 weeks	Text Messaging	There is high-quality evidence that compared to standard care, text-messaging is efficacious in promoting adherence to ART.
	(Pop-Eleches et al., 2011)	431 adult patients Africa/ 48 weeks	SMS	During the 48 weeks, 53% of participants achieved adherence of at least 90%
	(Khonsari et al., 2014)	62 patients with ACS/ 8 weeks	SMS reminder	The risk of being low adherent among the control group was 4.09 times greater than the intervention group
Heart/ Hypertension	(Burnier et al., 2001)	41 Forty-one hypertensive patients/ 2 months	Electronic monitoring	During monitoring, in more than 30% of participants, blood pressure was normalized and in another 20% insufficient compliance was unmasked.
	(Patel et al., 2013)	48 patients/ 12 weeks	mobile-phone-based automated medication reminder	During the study, average blood pressure improved significantly from baseline.
	(Park et al., 2014)	90 patients with mean age more than 59.2 years/ 30 days	Text messaging	Using MEMS and text-message responses, adherence to antiplatelet therapy increased.
Asthma	(Spaulding et al., 2011)	5 children/ 6 months	MDILogII	The number of children who were correctly using their medications doubled
	(Burgess et al., 2011)	26 children aged between 6 and 14 years/ NA	MDILogI	Adherence in the intervention group was significantly higher (79% vs. 58%)
	(Bender et al., 2000)	27 children/2 months	metered dose inhaler (MDI) equipped with an electronic Doser	Monitoring adherence using electronic devices is more reliable than canister weight measures or self-report.
	(Ostojic et al., 2005)	16-week/ 16 patients	GSM-SMS	GSM-SMS is an appropriate tool for telemedicine can enhance asthma control when using with a written plan and standard follow-up.
Smoking	(Shi, Jiang, Yu, & Zhang, 2013)	92 participants/12weeks	mobile phone text-messaging	Higher rate of smoking reduction in the intervention group (66% vs. 35%) compared to the control group. Also, higher rate in moving to quitting stages (52% vs. 18%)
Schizophrenia	(Ben-Zeev et al., 2014)	33 individuals/1 months	Smart-phone App	Significant reductions in psychotic symptoms.

continued on following page

Table 2. Continued

Area	Source	Samples/Duration	Intervention	Results
General (Each day they took at least one medication twice)	(de Oliveira, Cherubini, & Oliver, 2010)	18 elders/ 6 weeks	SMS reminder	A significant correlation between self-report and SMS acknowledgements
VitaminC	(Cocosila, Archer, Brian Haynes, & Yuan, 2009)	102 subjects/ 1 month	Smart-phone App. A Social network	Improvement in promptness and compliance to take the medication
Several Chronic disease (e.g. arthritis, diabetes, hypertension, and COPD)	(M. L. Lee & Dey, 2014)	12 old adults/ 10 months	Real-time sensor-based feedback(pillbox + in-home visual feedback	With real-time feedback, promptness, correctness of individuals increases and variability of their medication taking decreased, compared to their own baseline and to a control group
Cancer	(Spaulding et al., 2011)	375 patients/ NA	Video game	Significant improvement in adherence to medication and indicators of cancer-related knowledge and self-efficacy
Kidney Transplantation	(Burgess et al., 2011)	20 stable adult kidney transplants /a mean of 9.2 weeks.	Ingestible Sensor System (ISS)	Ingestible event marker detection accuracy and adherence was near 100%

resources to provide support to individuals with diabetes. Electronic devices have potential ability to help patients and clinician to fight this chronic illness. According to (Cramer, 2004), which is a literature search from 1966 to 2003, there are several studies demonstrating that using Medication Event Monitoring Systems (MEMS) and APREX are useful in improving adherence rates. A feasibility study in (Morak, Schwarz, Hayn, Schreier, & Member, 2012) with 59 individuals shows that medication adherence monitoring based on mHealth and Near Field Communication (NFC) technology is feasible. During 13 months of the study, patients with diabetes were monitored using 1,760 electronic blisters. Those devices were able to record events and transmit data via mobile phones. Leveraging e-Blisters and mHealth in (Brath et al., 2013) shows promising results. The authors in (Brath et al., 2013) claim that using Electronic blisters is not only accepted by patients but also can help to increase adherence in patients. This improvement happened even in patients with high baseline adherence and, subsequently, resulted in improvement of other indicators such as cholesterol concentrations and blood pressure. Unlike studies that use e-blisters, (Franklin, Greene, Waller, Greene, & Pagliari, 2008) and (Vervloet et al., 2012) utilize text messaging, in (Franklin et al., 2008), a randomized controlled trial with 126 patients suffering from diabetes, clinic visits were supported by daily text-messages generated using the Sweet Talk software system. The results show Sweet Talk was associated with improved patient's adherence and self-efficiency. Beside all previously mentioned studies, results of (Vervloet et al., 2012) are very impressive. They investigated the consequences of these text message reminders on adherence to oral anti-diabetics by collecting data in a randomized controlled trial involving 104 patients suffering from diabetes with suboptimal adherence to oral anti-diabetics. According to this study, within selected time windows patients who received text-message reminders took significantly more doses than patients didn't received reminders.

HIV

More than ten millions of people are suffering from HIV infection. By development of antiretroviral therapy (ART) by combining at least three antiretroviral drugs, HIV is not still a fatal disease, but a chronically controllable illness. Although, ART can help HIV infected patients to live healthier and longer, it is difficult to keep patient's adherence to ART. Non-adherence to this therapy specially in people who, previously have started taking them is a cause of resistance development (Bangsberg, Kroetz, & Deeks, 2007). Therefore, taking advantage of technology has the potential to help reinforce adherence and increase the chance of therapy in these patients.

A meta-analysis in (Horvath, Azman, Kennedy, & Rutherford, 2012) has been performed to determine effectiveness of mobile phone text-messaging in promoting adherence to ART in HIV infected patients. In their literature review which two randomized controlled trial in Kenya have been done for 48 to 52 weeks, they found that mobile phone text messaging at weekly intervals enhance adherence to ART, compared to standard care. Also, (Pop-Eleches et al., 2011) provides other evidence of effectiveness of text-messaging to promote HIV medication adherence. They suggest that text-message reminders are potential tools to achieve better treatment response in resource-poor settings. They studied 431 adult patients who had started ART within 3 months, daily or weekly SMS reminders that were sent to the intervention groups. The results of this study show that during the 48 weeks, 53% of patients receiving weekly text-message reminders achieved at least 90% adherence.

Other studies conducted, conclude having detail understating of patients' adherence patterns is applicable using diary-corrected MEMS data. They compare various methods of adherence assessment including therapeutic drug monitoring, medication event monitoring system (MEMS) caps, data of pharmacy refills, pill count, questionnaires and diaries on 26 patients and found MEMS data is significantly correlated with patient's self-report and therapeutic monitoring results. Also, authors of (Miller & Himelhoch, 2013) surveyed 100 HIV-positive patients attending an urban HIV outpatient clinic and found that vast majority of patients in the survey use their own mobile phone to promote adherence interventions to HIV medication.

Cardiovascular

Non-adherence to medications has been documented to occur in more than 60% of cardiovascular patients (Khonsari et al., 2014). Effectiveness of using SMS as a mean of reminding patient with acute coronary syndrome (ACS) has been shown in (Khonsari et al., 2014). They studied 62 patients with ACS and found that risk of being low adherent among the control group was 4.09 times greater than the intervention group. In (Park, Howie-Esquivel, Chung, & Dracup, 2014) a study has been conducted on the same disease for 90 patients during 30 days and the results show that text messaging increase adherence to antiplatelet therapy.

Mobile phone reminder not only increases the medication adherence in patient with acute coronary but also in patients with hypertension. According to (Patel et al., 2013) study on 48 patients, using mobile phone reminders cause significant improvement in average blood pressure and level of control after initiation of the study. Also, in (Burnier, Schneider, Chioléro, Stubi, & Brunner, 2001) study has been shown that using electronic monitoring led to normalizing blood pressure in more than 30% of the patients and in another 20% insufficient compliance was unmasked.

Asthma

Adherence to asthma medication tends to be very poor, with the reported rates of non-adherence ranging from 30 to 70 percent. In two different studies MDILogI and MDILogII shown to be effective to increase asthma medication adherence among children. In (Spaulding, Devine, Duncan, Wilson, & Hogan, 2011), using MDILogII caused the number of children who were using their medications correctly within four weeks, changed from 28.6% to 54.1%. Similarly, taking advantage of MDILogI among 26 children aged between 6 and 14 years led to significantly higher adherence in the intervention group (79% versus 58%) (Burgess, Sly, & Devadason, 2011). According to (Bender et al., 2000), compare to self-report or canister weight measures, electronic adherence monitoring are significantly more accurate. In addition to previous studies, successful usage of audio-visual reminder and text messaging has been reported by (Charles et al., 2007) and (Ostojic et al., 2005).

Using mobile application or SMS increase adherence to medication among patients with different disease. For example, (Franklin et al., 2008) shows that using text messaging led to a significantly higher rate of smoking reduction among the intervention group (66% vs. 35%). Effectiveness of text messaging is not only in chronic disease but also in simple regimens such as taking daily Vitamin C (WHO, 2003). Also, After 1 month of using a specific smart phone application in patients with schizophrenia, results demonstrate significant reductions in psychotic symptoms (Khonsari et al., 2014). Some studies such as (Spaulding et al., 2011) and (Park et al., 2014) using a smart phone application, provide a type of competition and show significantly improved treatment adherence and the accuracy of the drug intake time.

CHALLENGES AND FUTURE DIRECTIONS

Challenges associated with current medication management technologies can be divided into these major categories:

1. Context-Aware Interventions;
2. Scalability;
3. Reliability.

Context-aware intervention refers to the need for providing interventions that incorporate various contextual needs to the patient and environment. For example, most current interventions are static in nature. Current approaches provide fixed-time reminders. Scalability refers to the lack of approaches to adapt new sensor or sensor modalities with minimal computational efforts such as retraining of a machine learning algorithm. Reliability refers to the lack of accurate approach to detect medication intake. In this section, after presenting the existing machine learning and reliability assessment techniques, we discuss a medication management monitoring framework that addresses shortcomings of the state of the art technologies.

Data Analytics in Medication Monitoring

The utility of data analytics in healthcare delivery and interventions is growing. According to a survey, only 7% of health plans use predictive analytics, but more than half of the surveyed insurers plan on incorporating predictive analytics into their intervention targeting (Jones, 2014). Data analytics approaches have potential to assist medication management programs in many ways. In particular, they can be used for predictive modeling, personalized interventions, and clinical decision support.

The purpose of predictive modeling is to provide early interventions based on predictions made through machine learning algorithms. Data analytics and machine learning techniques provide tools to medication management programs to detect patients who are more likely to be non-adherent to their medication and predict the most effective intervention for each individual patient. There are several studies that use machine learning to construct a machine learning model to predict patient's future. For example, authors in (Son, Kim, Kim, Choi, & Lee, 2010) attempt to identify predictors of medication adherence in heart failure patients using Support Vector Machine (SVM) algorithms. It has been also shown that SVM achieves acceptable result in predicting adherence to medication in elderly patients with chronic diseases (S. K. Lee, Kang, Kim, & Son, 2013).

Data analytics can be also used to develop personalized interventions. Patients' response to clinical interventions varies according to different contextual attributes such as medical history, age, race, income and education level and many other factors. These factors result in different source of non-adherence and need distinctive interventions. For example, authors of (Raparelli et al., n.d.) have shown that medication adherence is related to socio-economic status of individuals. Therefore, it is needed to design medication management programs that are tailored toward individual patient's behavior, and predict adherent versus non-adherent patients. Cleary, the subsequent interventions need to be personalized according to the adherence level and socio-economic attributes of the people. In the context of medication intake monitoring, providing effective prompts or reminders is an important intervention strategy to enhance adherence to medications. Authors in (Vurgun et al., 2007) designed a reasoning system to detect elders' context and send appropriate prompts to elders to take their medication. The result of this study reveals that context-aware interventions are more effective than static rule-based interventions.

Data analytics approaches can be utilized for clinical decision support purposes. Using machine learning techniques, we can potentially predict most effective interventions. According to findings in (Sboner & Aliferis, 2005), it is possible to predict physician judgments. This finding is useful for designing expert clinical systems that help fine tune intervention strategies based on patient's physiological and contextual attributes. It means that the outcomes of the interventions (e.g., successful versus unsuccessful medicine reminder) can be used to continuously improve the predictive model and provide better interventions for each patient.

Reliability of Medication Adherence Monitoring Systems

Sensor-based technologies that detect medication intake can be divided into these categories:

1. Sensors embedded in pillboxes;
2. Sensors deployed in environment;
3. On-body or wearable sensors;
4. In-body sensors. The majority of the products available in the market fall within the first category.

While sensor-based technologies such as smart blister, bottle packs or RFID-enabled computer chip technology, can help increase medication adherence rate, they suffer from several weaknesses. These technologies are most beneficial when patients are motivated on taking their medication but often forgets to take the medication. Besides their cost and their limitation which should be physically attached to the medications, they are unable to draw reliable conclusion regarding patient's compliance. These systems provide no solution for acknowledging that a patient is in fact ingesting or not. For example, a patient may open the bottle without taking the medication but it activates the technology and counts as taking medication.

Approaches such as (Bilodeau & Ammouri, 2011), (Huynh, Sequeira, Daniel, & Meunier, 2010) use captured videos of the subject to detect medication intake. These vision-based methods are limited to in-home or in-building settings due to their requirement of taking a medication within the field of view of a camera.

Wearable sensors have been also used to assess medication intake. There are other approaches which try to identify wrist movement in order to determine in order to detect pattern of opening the pillbox and taking medication. For example, in (Chen, Kehtarnavaz, Fellow, Jafari, & Member, 2014), authors designed a wearable sensor network for medication adherence to confirm pill intake by identify the two consecutive actions of "twist-cap" and "hand-to-mouth".

In order to precisely measure patient's adherence, it needs to record when a pill is actually taken, we can rely on the approach of ingestible event marker (Eisenberger et al., 2013), (Belknap et al., 2013). These methods unlike RFID chips, which transmit a signal through the air, rely on the conductive characteristics of tissues to send confirming signals to the receiver. The adhesive patch worn by the patient can collect data and detect when a particular pill was taken. The signal then passes to a gateway such nearby wireless phone to transmit data to central server.

Conceptual Framework

As we described above, medical adherence in recent works was only about having sensors on the pillboxes; however, the previous techniques have some drawbacks such as the pillbox might have been opened by someone else, and none or more than one pill might have been taken by the patient. Many uncertainties will arise when the sensors are only placed on the pillboxes; therefore, we envision that future medication adherence monitoring and intervention systems will include smart sensors integrated with the patient's body, living environment, and medicine containers; besides, advance machine learning algorithms will be involved which provide reinforcement mechanisms such as context-aware prompting, adaptive rewarding, and motivational feedback to enhance compliance to medicine.

1. **Accurate Context Inference:** In this block we try to detect the current context including the activity, location, and the context of the environment. The inferences for the activity is to discriminate taking pills with other activities such as opening a bottle of water and drinking it, opening a chocolate bar and eating it, and etc. Detecting the location is to recognize that this is the patient taking the pill or someone else opened the pillbox by calculating the distance of patient from the pillbox. In this block some context-specific reminders will be delivered in order to remind the patient about his/her state such as sending a reminder to take the pill, sending a message that the patient has taken the pill successfully, and etc. It uses the patient's history and the sequence of the context. The goal for this block is to develop a learning approach in order to accurately recognize patient' activity and infer his/her context.

2. **Plug-n-Learn:** As we explained above we want to develop a learning approach for recognizing the patient's activity. Now suppose we have a sensor trained with that approach and we want to add

a new sensor in order to improve the accuracy of the system. Obviously we don't want to do the entire learning process from the scratch; therefore, we will develop a transfer learning approach in order to adapt the other sensor to our algorithm. By doing this new sensor can be easily adapted to the system, instead of starting over for each sensor we can train our sensor using existing model, and adding new sensors will contribute to improve the overall performance of the system.

3. **Reliable Medication Intake Measurement:** In order to keep track of the patient taking the medicine it is required to monitor his/her activities. There are some available solutions which have their own pros and cons.

    a. **Video Camera:** Its accuracy is high; however, it will violate the patient's privacy and it is not applicable in all situations.

    b. **Movement's Pattern Detection:** We can integrate it with available sensors; yet, the sensors will be learned in the labs using limited amount of patterns and the patterns won't be comprehensive.

    c. **Ingestible Event Marker:** It is a device for prescription which saves the time-stamps. Although it is accurate, it is not popular based on patient's amenability.

CONCLUSION AND FUTURE WORKS

In this paper, we studied medication adherence and the challenges associated with non-adherence from both technology development and clinical point of view. We discussed the impact of medication non-adherence and advantages of technology-driven solutions in chronic diseases; also, we highlighted different approaches for maintaining medication adherence as a means for enhancing clinical outcomes. We reviewed the state-of-the-art solutions for medication intake monitoring, discussed clinical utility of such technologies, and proposed a conceptual framework to address shortcomings of the current technologies. Discussions in this article can help researchers better identify unmet needs in the area of technology-based medication management from a multi-disciplinary point of view. In particular, our discussions in this paper highlight research gaps and future directions in the important research area.

REFERENCES

Bangsberg, D. R., Kroetz, D. L., & Deeks, S. G. (2007). Adherence-resistance relationships to combination HIV antiretroviral therapy. *Current HIV/AIDS Reports*, *4*(2), 65–72. http://www.ncbi.nlm.nih.gov/pubmed/17547827 doi:10.1007/s11904-007-0010-0 PMID:17547827

Belknap, R., Weis, S., Brookens, A., Au-Yeung, K. Y., Moon, G., DiCarlo, L., & Reves, R. (2013). Feasibility of an ingestible sensor-based system for monitoring adherence to tuberculosis therapy. *PLoS ONE*, *8*(1), e53373. doi:10.1371/journal.pone.0053373 PMID:23308203

Ben-Zeev, D., Brenner, C. J., Begale, M., Duffecy, J., Mohr, D. C., & Mueser, K. T. (2014). Feasibility, Acceptability, and Preliminary Efficacy of a Smartphone Intervention for Schizophrenia. *Schizophrenia Bulletin*. http://doi.org/<ALIGNMENT.qj></ALIGNMENT>10.1093/schbul/sbu033

Bender, B., Wamboldt, F. S., O'Connor, S. L., Rand, C., Szefler, S., Milgrom, H., & Wamboldt, M. Z. (2000). Measurement of children's asthma medication adherence by self report, mother report, canister weight, and Doser CT. *Annals of Allergy, Asthma & Immunology: Official Publication of the American College of Allergy, Asthma, &. Immunology, 85*(5), 416–421. Retrieved from http://www.ncbi.nlm.nih.gov/pubmed/11101187

Bilodeau, G. A., & Ammouri, S. (2011). Monitoring of medication intake using a camera system. *Journal of Medical Systems, 35*(3), 377–389. doi:10.1007/s10916-009-9374-6 PMID:20703552

Brath, H., Morak, J., Kästenbauer, T., Modre-Osprian, R., Strohner-Kästenbauer, H., Schwarz, M., & Schreier, G. et al. (2013). Mobile health (mHealth) based medication adherence measurement - a pilot trial using electronic blisters in diabetes patients. *British Journal of Clinical Pharmacology, 76*(Suppl. 1), 47–55. doi:10.1111/bcp.12184 PMID:24007452

Burgess, S., Sly, P., & Devadason, S. (2011). Adherence with preventive medication in childhood asthma. *Pulmonary Medicine, 973849.* doi:10.1155/2011/973849 PMID:21660201

Burnier, M., Schneider, M. P., Chioléro, A., Stubi, C. L., & Brunner, H. R. (2001). Electronic compliance monitoring in resistant hypertension: The basis for rational therapeutic decisions. *Journal of Hypertension, 19*(2), 335–341. http://www.ncbi.nlm.nih.gov/pubmed/11212978 doi:10.1097/00004872-200102000-00022 PMID:11212978

Charles, T., Quinn, D., Weatherall, M., Aldington, S., Beasley, R., & Holt, S. (2007). An audiovisual reminder function improves adherence with inhaled corticosteroid therapy??in asthma. *The Journal of Allergy and Clinical Immunology, 119*(4), 811–816. doi:10.1016/j.jaci.2006.11.700 PMID:17320942

Chen, C., Kehtarnavaz, N., Fellow, I., Jafari, R., & Member, I. S. (2014). A Medication Adherence Monitoring System for Pill Bottles Based on a Wearable Inertial Sensor. *Proceedings of the International Conference of the IEEE Engineering in Medicine and Biology Society (EMBC)* (Vol. 1). doi:10.1109/EMBC.2014.6944743

Chisholm-Burns, M. A., & Spivey, C. A. (2012). The "cost" of medication nonadherence: Consequences we cannot afford to accept. *Journal of the American Pharmacists Association, 52*(6), 823–826. doi:10.1331/JAPhA.2012.11088 PMID:23229971

Cocosila, M., Archer, N., Brian Haynes, R., & Yuan, Y. (2009). Can wireless text messaging improve adherence to preventive activities? Results of a randomised controlled trial. *International Journal of Medical Informatics, 78*(4), 230–238. doi:10.1016/j.ijmedinf.2008.07.011 PMID:18778967

Cramer, J. A. (2004). A systematic review of adherence with medications for diabetes. *Diabetes Care, 27*(5), 1218–1224. http://www.ncbi.nlm.nih.gov/pubmed/15111553 doi:10.2337/diacare.27.5.1218 PMID:15111553

de Oliveira, R., Cherubini, M., & Oliver, N. (2010). MoviPill: improving medication compliance for elders using a mobile persuasive social game. *Proceedings of the 12th ACM international conference on Ubiquitous computing* (pp. 251–260). http://doi.org/ doi:10.1145/1864349.1864371

Eisenberger, U., Wüthrich, R. P., Bock, A., Ambühl, P., Steiger, J., Intondi, A., & De Geest, S. et al. (2013). Medication adherence assessment: High accuracy of the new Ingestible Sensor System in kidney transplants. *Transplantation*, *96*(3), 245–250. doi:10.1097/TP.0b013e31829b7571 PMID:23823651

Fairman, K., & Matheral, B. (2000). Evaluating Medication Adherence: Which Measure Is Right for Your Program? *Journal of Managed Care Pharmacy*, *6*(6), 499–506. doi:10.18553/jmcp.2000.6.6.499

Feinstein, A. R. (n.d.). On white-coat effects and the electronic monitoring of compliance. *Arch. Intern. Med., 150*, 1377–8.

Franklin, V. L., Greene, A., Waller, A., Greene, S. A., & Pagliari, C. (2008). Patients' engagement with "Sweet Talk" - a text messaging support system for young people with diabetes. *Journal of Medical Internet Research*, *10*(2), e20. doi:10.2196/jmir.962 PMID:18653444

Granger, B. B., & Bosworth, H. B. (2011). Medication adherence: Emerging use of technology. *Current Opinion in Cardiology*, *26*(4), 279–287. doi:10.1097/HCO.0b013e328347c150 PMID:21597368

Horvath, T., Azman, H., Kennedy, G. E., & Rutherford, G. W. (2012). Mobile phone text messaging for promoting adherence to antiretroviral therapy in patients with HIV infection. *Cochrane Database of Systematic Reviews (Online), 3*. doi:10.1002/14651858.CD009756 PMID:22419345

Huynh, H. H., Sequeira, J., Daniel, M., & Meunier, J. (2010). Enhancing the recognition of medication intake using a stereo camera. *Proceedings of the 3rd International Conference on Communications and Electronics* (pp. 175–179). http://doi.org/ doi:<ALIGNMENT.qj></ALIGNMENT>10.1109/ICCE.2010.5670705

Jackevicius, C. A., Li, P., & Tu, J. V. (2008). Prevalence, predictors, and outcomes of primary nonadherence after acute myocardial infarction. *Circulation*, *117*(8), 1028–1036. doi:10.1161/CIRCULATIONAHA.107.706820 PMID:18299512

Jackevicius, C. A., Mamdani, M., & Tu, J. V. (2002). Adherence with statin therapy in elderly patients with and without acute coronary syndromes. *Journal of the American Medical Association*, *288*(4), 462–467. doi:10.1001/jama.288.4.462 PMID:12132976

Jones, C. D. (2014). Medication adherence study looks at types of interventions. *Managed Care (Langhorne, Pa.)*, *23*, 38–41. PMID:25282863

Khonsari, S., Subramanian, P., Chinna, K., Latif, L. a, Ling, L. W., & Gholami, O. (2014). Effect of a reminder system using an automated short message service on medication adherence following acute coronary syndrome. *European Journal of Cardiovascular Nursing: Journal of the Working Group on Cardiovascular Nursing of the European Society of Cardiology*. http://doi.org/<ALIGNMENT.qj></ALIGNMENT>10.1177/1474515114521910

Lee, M. L., & Dey, A. K. (2014). Real-time feedback for improving medication taking. *Proceedings of the 32nd annual ACM conference on Human factors in computing systems CHI '14* (pp. 2259–2268). New York, New York, USA: ACM Press. http://doi.org/ doi:10.1145/2556288.2557210

Lee, S. K., Kang, B.-Y., Kim, H.-G., & Son, Y.-J. (2013). Predictors of medication adherence in elderly patients with chronic diseases using support vector machine models. *Healthcare Informatics Research*, *19*(1), 33–41. doi:10.4258/hir.2013.19.1.33 PMID:23626916

Lüscher, T. F., & Vetter, W. (1990). Adherence to medication. *Journal of Human Hypertension*, *4*(Suppl. 1), 43–46. doi:10.1056/NEJMra050100 PMID:2182868

Miller, C. W. T., & Himelhoch, S. (2013). Acceptability of Mobile Phone Technology for Medication Adherence Interventions among HIV-Positive Patients at an Urban Clinic. *AIDS Research and Treatment*, *670525*. doi:10.1155/2013/670525 PMID:23997948

Morak, J., Schwarz, M., Hayn, D., Schreier, G., & Member, S. (2012). Feasibility of mHealth and Near Field Communication technology based medication adherence monitoring. In *2012 Annual International Conference of the IEEE Engineering in Medicine and Biology Society* (Vol. 2012, pp. 272–275). IEEE. http://doi.org/ doi:10.1109/EMBC.2012.6345922

Ostojic, V., Cvoriscec, B., Ostojic, S. B., Reznikoff, D., Stipic-Markovic, A., & Tudjman, Z. (2005). Improving asthma control through telemedicine: A study of short-message service. *Telemedicine Journal and E-Health : The Official Journal of the American Telemedicine Association*, *11*(1), 28–35. doi:10.1089/tmj.2005.11.28 PMID:15785218

Park, L. G., Howie-Esquivel, J., Chung, M. L., & Dracup, K. (2014). A text messaging intervention to promote medication adherence for patients with coronary heart disease: A randomized controlled trial. *Patient Education and Counseling*, *94*(2), 261–268. doi:10.1016/j.pec.2013.10.027 PMID:24321403

Patel, S., Jacobus-Kantor, L., Marshall, L., Ritchie, C., Kaplinski, M., Khurana, P. S., & Katz, R. J. (2013). Mobilizing your medications: An automated medication reminder application for mobile phones and hypertension medication adherence in a high-risk urban population. *Journal of Diabetes Science and Technology*, *7*(3), 630–639. http://www.pubmedcentral.nih.gov/articlerender.fcgi?artid=3869130&tool=pmcentrez&rendertype=abstract doi:10.1177/193229681300700307 PMID:23759395

Pop-Eleches, C., Thirumurthy, H., Habyarimana, J. P., Zivin, J. G., Goldstein, M. P., de Walque, D., & Bangsberg, D. R. et al. (2011). Mobile phone technologies improve adherence to antiretroviral treatment in a resource-limited setting: A randomized controlled trial of text message reminders. *AIDS (London, England)*, *25*(6), 825–834. doi:10.1097/QAD.0b013e32834380c1 PMID:21252632

Raparelli, V., Proietti, M., Buttà, C., Di Giosia, P., Sirico, D., Gobbi, P., & Basili, S. et al. (n.d.). Medication prescription and adherence disparities in non valvular atrial fibrillation patients: An Italian portrait from the ARAPACIS study. *Internal and Emergency Medicine*.

Sboner, A., & Aliferis, C. F. (2005). Modeling clinical judgment and implicit guideline compliance in the diagnosis of melanomas using machine learning. *AMIA ... Annual Symposium Proceedings / AMIA Symposium. AMIA Symposium*, 664–8. Retrieved from http://www.pubmedcentral.nih.gov/articlerender.fcgi?artid=1560780&tool=pmcentrez&rendertype=abstract

Shi, H. J., Jiang, X. X., Yu, C. Y., & Zhang, Y. (2013). Use of mobile phone text messaging to deliver an individualized smoking behaviour intervention in Chinese adolescents. *Journal of Telemedicine and Telecare*, *19*(5), 282–287. doi:10.1177/1357633X13495489 PMID:24163238

Son, Y.-J., Kim, H.-G., Kim, E.-H., Choi, S., & Lee, S.-K. (2010). Application of support vector machine for prediction of medication adherence in heart failure patients. *Healthcare Informatics Research*, *16*(4), 253–259. doi:10.4258/hir.2010.16.4.253 PMID:21818444

Spaulding, S. A., Devine, K. A., Duncan, C. L., Wilson, N. W., & Hogan, M. B. (2011). Electronic monitoring and feedback to improve adherence in pediatric asthma. *Journal of Pediatric Psychology*, *37*(1), 64–74. doi:10.1093/jpepsy/jsr059 PMID:21852340

Vervloet, M., van Dijk, L., Santen-Reestman, J., van Vlijmen, B., van Wingerden, P., Bouvy, M. L., & de Bakker, D. H. (2012). SMS reminders improve adherence to oral medication in type 2 diabetes patients who are real time electronically monitored. *International Journal of Medical Informatics*, *81*(9), 594–604. doi:10.1016/j.ijmedinf.2012.05.005 PMID:22652012

Viswanathan, M., Golin, C. E., Jones, C. D., Ashok, M., Blalock, S. J., Wines, R. C. M., & Lohr, K. N. et al. (2012). Interventions to improve adherence to self-administered medications for chronic diseases in the United States: A systematic review. *Annals of Internal Medicine*, *157*(11), 785–795. doi:10.7326/0003-4819-157-11-201212040-00538 PMID:22964778

Vurgun, S., Vurgun, S., Philipose, M., Philipose, M., Pavel, M., & Pavel, M. (2007). A statistical reasoning system for medication prompting. *Lecture Notes in Computer Science*, *4717*, 1–18. doi:10.1007/978-3-540-74853-3_1

Wagner, S., & Arnfast, A. (2010). Context Aware Ubiquitous Medication Reminder System. *Hypertension*.

WHO. (2003). *Adherence to Long-Term Therapies, Evidence for action*. World Health Organization.

ADDITIONAL READING

Brown, M. T., & Bussell, J. K. (2011). Medication adherence: WHO cares? *Mayo Clinic Proceedings*, *86*(4), 304–314. doi:10.4065/mcp.2010.0575 PMID:21389250

Dayer, L., Heldenbrand, S., Anderson, P., Gubbins, P. O., & Martin, B. C. (2013). Smartphone medication adherence apps: Potential benefits to patients and providers. *Journal of the American Pharmacists Association: JAPhA*, *53*(2), 172–181. doi:10.1331/JAPhA.2013.12202 PMID:23571625

Granger, B. B., & Bosworth, H. B. (2011). Medication adherence: Emerging use of technology. *Current Opinion in Cardiology*, *26*(4), 279–287. doi:10.1097/HCO.0b013e328347c150 PMID:21597368

M., C. D., & Wendy, E. (2010). Thinking Outside the Pillbox — Medication Adherence as a Priority for Health Care Reform. *The New England Journal of Medicine*, *362*(17). doi:10.1056/NEJMp1002305

Orbæk, J., Gaard, M., Fabricius, P., Lefevre, R. S., & Møller, T. (2015). Patient safety and technology-driven medication - A qualitative study on how graduate nursing students navigate through complex medication administration. *Nurse Education in Practice*, *15*(3), 203–211. doi:10.1016/j.nepr.2014.11.015 PMID:25492454

Sabin, L. L., Bachman DeSilva, M., Gill, C. J., Zhong, L., Vian, T., & Xie, W. … Gifford, A. L. (2015). Improving Adherence to Antiretroviral Therapy With Triggered Real-time Text Message Reminders: The China Adherence Through Technology Study. *JAIDS Journal of Acquired Immune Deficiency Syndromes, 69*(5). Retrieved from http://journals.lww.com/jaids/Fulltext/2015/08150/Improving_Adherence_to_Antiretroviral_Therapy_With.6.aspx

Stirratt, M. J., Dunbar-Jacob, J., Crane, H. M., Simoni, J. M., Czajkowski, S., Hilliard, M. E., & Nilsen, W. J. et al. (2015). Self-report measures of medication adherence behavior: Recommendations on optimal use. *Translational Behavioral Medicine, 5*(4), 470–482. doi:10.1007/s13142-015-0315-2 PMID:26622919

Vollmer, W. M., Feldstein, A., Smith, D. H., Dubanoski, J. P., Waterbury, A., & Schneider, J. L. … Rand, C. (2011). Use of health information technology to improve medication adherence. *The American Journal of Managed Care, 17*(12), SP79–87. Retrieved from http://www.pubmedcentral.nih.gov/articlerender.fcgi?artid=3641901&tool=pmcentrez&rendertype=abstract

KEY TERMS AND DEFINITIONS

E-Health: An abbreviation of Electronic Health which is practicing medicine using electronic devices and communication.

Machine Learning: A field of computer science and artificial intelligence which enables computers to learn without being explicitly programmed.

Medication Adherence: The compliance of patients to the amount and process of medicine prescribed by their health care provider.

mHealth: An abbreviation of Mobile Health which is a subset of e-Health to practice medicine and patient health using mobile devices such as smart phone.

Remote Patient Monitoring: A technology which enable monitoring of patients outside of clinics.

RFID: An abbreviation of Radio-frequency Identification which enables identifying and tracking objects using electromagnetic fields.

Wearables: Sensors could be worn on body to acquire data of human context such as physical activity.

This research was previously published in the Handbook of Research on Healthcare Administration and Management edited by Nilmini Wickramasinghe, pages 188-204, copyright year 2017 by Medical Information Science Reference (an imprint of IGI Global).

Index

D

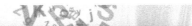
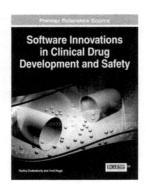
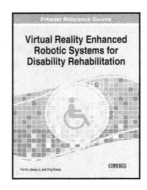
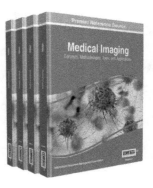
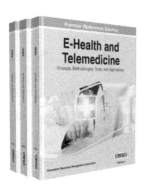
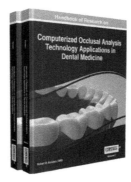
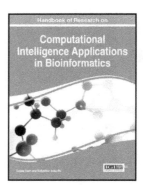
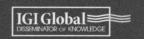

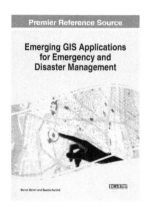 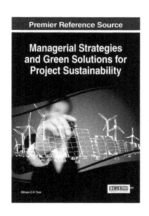 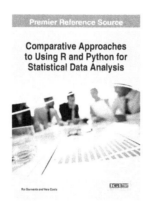 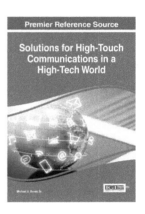

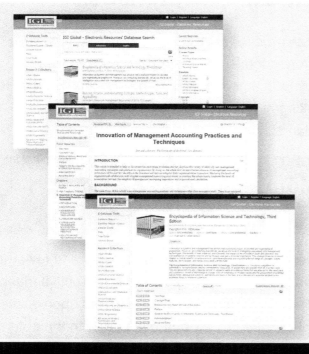
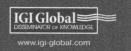

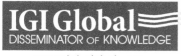
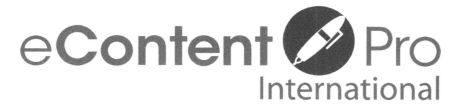

Printed in the USA
CPSIA information can be obtained
at www.ICGtesting.com
JSHW061356160923
48161JS00004B/337